Stuttering

Foundations and Clinical Applications

SECOND EDITION

Ehud Yairi

University of Illinois at Urbana-Champaign; Tel Aviv University

Carol H. Seery

University of Wisconsin–Milwaukee

PEARSON

Boston Columbus Indianapolis New York San Francisco Upper Saddle River
Amsterdam Cape Town Dubai London Madrid Milan Munich Paris Montreal Toronto
Delhi Mexico City São Paulo Sydney Hong Kong Seoul Singapore Taipei Tokyo

Vice President and Editorial Director: Jeffery W. Johnston

Acquistions Editor: Ann Davis

Executive Field Marketing Manager: Krista Clark

Senior Product Marketing Manager: Christopher Barry

Production Project Manager: Annette Joseph

Procurement Specialist: Linda Sager

Full-Service Project Management: Shylaja Gattupalli/Jouve India

Composition: Jouve India

Cover Designer: Suzanne Behnke

Cover Image: Anastasia B/Shutterstock

Credits and acknowledgments for material borrowed from other sources and reproduced, with permission, in this textbook appear on the appropriate page within the text.

Every effort has been made to provide accurate and current Internet information in this book. However, the Internet and information posted on it are constantly changing, so it is inevitable that some of the Internet addresses listed in this textbook will change.

Library of Congress Cataloging-in-Publication Data

Yairi, Ehud.
 Stuttering : foundations and clinical applications / Ehud Yairi, University of Illinois at Urbana-Champaign; Tel Aviv University, Carol H. Seery, University of Wisconsin-Milwaukee. — Second edition.
  pages cm
 Includes bibliographical references.
 ISBN-13: 978-0-13-335204-7
 ISBN-10: 0-13-335204-8
 1. Stuttering. I. Seery, Carol H. II. Title.
RC424.Y35 2014
616.85'54—dc23

2013044182

10 9 8 7 6 5 4 3 2

ISBN 10: 0-13-335204-8

ISBN 13: 978-013-335204-7

To my wife, Janie,

To our children, Micah, Dani, Keren, and to their families.

—E. Yairi

To my husband, Tom, and son, David.

To the memories of my father, David F. Hubbard, and my mother, Frances L. Hubbard.

—C. Seery

Preface

We wrote *Stuttering: Foundations and Clinical Applications* to serve both instructors and students in speech-language disorders and related fields as a single main text for a general course on stuttering. It is composed of three parts: the nature of stuttering, the explanations of stuttering, and the clinical management of stuttering. Many textbooks on stuttering are dedicated primarily to one or two of these subjects, but few address all three of them equally. We have undertaken to provide a balanced presentation across all three areas.

In addition, we offer a balanced perspective with regard to stuttering etiology, assessment, and treatment methods. We provide a comprehensive coverage of the options from the various viewpoints and relate them to specific age groups.

Finally, we sought a balance in using a written style that is easy to read yet deals with concepts and scientific material with appreciable depth. Whenever appropriate, we have shared examples from our own scholarly, clinical, and personal experiences to enrich the understanding of our readers.

We hope that reading this book enhances your knowledge, as it has ours in writing it.

New to This Edition

The entire text of the second edition of *Stuttering: Foundations and Clinical Applications* has been enhanced with editorial revisions for ease in readability.

Additionally, the new text highlights sections with the latest scientific knowledge of stuttering regarding:

- Incidence and prevalence
- Onset
- Natural recovery
- Genetics

Sections that have been completely revised include:

- Brain anatomy and physiology
- Motor aspects
- Cluttering

Other features modified for improved presentation:

- New case studies
- New tables and figures
- New outline format of treatment procedures
- Revised chapter order in the clinical management section

Instructional Materials

- New/modified slides and exam questions available to instructors

Acknowledgments

The authors are grateful for the generous personal input from Professors Luc De Nil, University of Toronto; Florence Myers, Adelphi University; Rosalee Shenker, McGill University; Anne Smith, Purdue University; and both Cecilia Lundstrom and Marie Garsten of Helsingborg Hospital in Sweden. Special thanks to Karly Klagos and Michelle Thiel for comments and to Marie Turner for comments and technical assistance with the references.

We gratefully acknowledge the project management of Annette Joseph, Lauren Carlson, and Shylaja Gattupalli. The publishers also obtained comments from the following reviewers: Paul Blanchet, SUNY Fredonia; Brent A. Gregg, University of Central Arkansas; Betty L. McMicken, California State University at Long Beach; and Jean Sawyer, Illinois State University. Their input is greatly appreciated.

Brief Contents

Contents

Chapter 1

What Is Stuttering?

LEARNER OBJECTIVES

Readers of this chapter will be able to:

- Discriminate definitions of stuttering as speech phenomena or as a complex disorder.
- Analyze concepts and issues related to defining stuttering.
- Evaluate the significance and influence of various stuttering definitions.
- Examine the context of stuttering identification with respect to normal speech and normal disfluency.
- Analyze the meaning of stuttering from different points of view, and identify sources of definitional diversity.

Defining Stuttering: Bases and Aims

At first glance, stuttering appears to be a phenomenon that would be rather easy to define. When most people think of stuttering, they typically recall speech that everyone would recognize, like the repetitive "I I I I um I um la-la-la-like um." Hence the common notion is that "everyone knows what stuttering is." Such, however, is not the case for scholars in the field. For them, the definition of stuttering is far from straightforward. The closer they have looked at stuttering, the more it has grown in complexity. But laypeople too may be confused. We had a case of a child brought to us by parents complaining about his stuttering. We concluded that the child exhibited cleft palate speech with no sign of stuttering. The parents concurred that what they called "stuttering" was the child's unusual articulation and voice quality. In another referral for a stuttering problem, we concluded that a fast speaking rate and mumbled articulation was the source of confusion, and diagnosed the child with a phonological disorder. Typically, however, identification of 'stuttering' needs a closer examination beyond these broad levels of discernment.

In this chapter, we discuss the diversity of the viewpoints about stuttering held by scholars. As professionals and researchers, we must clarify what we mean by the term *stuttering,* strive to agree on the scope of that term, and determine when it applies. Before attempting either to define stuttering or evaluate its definition, it is important to understand what definitions are for. The *New Oxford American Dictionary* (Jewell & Abate, 2001) emphasizes that a definition spells out the exact meaning of a word or the nature of something. Rather than relying on dictionaries however, we will offer examples of definitions that have been given by clinician-researchers over the years. The differences among the definitions will reveal how difficult it has been to specify an "exact" meaning of "stuttering."

Sometimes people use the term *stuttering* referring to the overt (surface) features: the speech events. But are those the only essence of stuttering? Another use of *stuttering* is referring to the covert (or hidden) features, particularly the speaker's experience of a loss of control and a host of negative emotional reactions. But must there be an underlying sense of helplessness every time a person stutters? Because stuttering encompasses both overt and covert features, there have been definitions intended to capture both aspects.

Although precision might seem the ideal outcome of our search, we hold that a definition should be a statement that expresses the *essential* rather than the *exact* nature or meaning of a matter, distinguishing it from other similar or related concepts. Thus, the aim of defining stuttering should be to state its fundamental properties and set forth the limits unique to this phenomenon. It is tempting to believe that a thorough definition of stuttering is the goal. But for professional purposes that usually involve measurement, the most useful definition may not be the one that is most thorough. Instead, the most useful definition of stuttering is one that remains free from opinion, explanation, or theory. This point is illustrated by analogy through various definitions of "water." If *water* is defined as "a tasteless liquid," we encounter the problem that "taste" is a matter of opinion. Or, if water is defined as "a liquid compound of hydrogen and oxygen," the application is limited because most "water" contains many other constituent elements. But if people agreed that "water" is the liquid form of what falls from the sky as precipitation, then the concept is ready for discussion, study, and description, including its numerous and ever-changing properties.

We must point out that a definition is not the same as a set of diagnostic criteria. Trying to define stuttering and undertaking to diagnose it are two different endeavors. Whereas a definition attempts to delineate the meaning of a term, the function of a diagnosis is to determine whether the presenting communication pattern constitutes a clinical problem or a risk for becoming one. Arriving at a clinical diagnosis often involves analysis of the frequency or intensity levels of the parameters found in the definition. For example, if the parameter that defined stuttering was syllable repetitions, the diagnostician would still have to determine whether the number of repetitions raised a need for concern. Specifications, such as the number of repetitions that cause concern, may vary with factors of age, time since onset, consistency, and so on. Researchers strive to study, identify, and enumerate these parameters with ever-increasing details.

Definitions of stuttering have varied for many reasons. Some have differed depending on the areas of expertise, interests, and needs of the definers. Others have been influenced by the many characteristics and dimensions of stuttering, typical age of onset, patterns of development, suspected etiology, and more. Over the years, many have boldly announced an answer, but to our knowledge no statement yet has attained the status of attracting unanimous or even a majority agreement. Still, we believe that the wide range of perspectives by the many who have tried to define it yield valuable information that may eventually help us solve the issue of what should be called "stuttering."

A useful definition of stuttering needs to be free of opinion or explanation so that it enables researchers to explore its various forms and features, and generate, confirm, or refute theories of its causes, all without changing the definition. Unfortunately, many of the definitions of stuttering have lacked these desired qualities, and therefore have not been sufficiently rigorous in support of research. In this chapter we review several definitions of stuttering and consider their content, application, benefits, and limitations, so that students of stuttering can appreciate and critically evaluate the issues involved.

Before we proceed, we offer a few words concerning terminology. To avoid frequent repetitions of the same term, the following abbreviations and referents for each group will be used interchangeably:

- People who stutter—PWS—stutterers
- Normally fluent speakers—NFS—nonstutterers
- Children who stutter—CWS
- Children who do not stutter—normally fluent children—NFC

Why is the Definition Important? Practical Implications

One study found that college students tend to pour beer and liquor in quantities that are larger than commonly used standards for single servings (White et al., 2005). One possible reason for the overpouring is students' lack of knowledge of the definition of standard serving sizes. This may pose unfortunate health risks and other hazardous consequences. From a scientific perspective, however, their weak knowledge about the actual serving size casts doubt on the accuracy of various studies of students' reports about their alcohol consumption. Critically, lacking a clear referent, students underestimate their drinking. This example highlights the potentially powerful influence of definitions.

Because definitions provide a reference and orientation to their conceptual topics, definitions of "what is stuttering" exert direct impact on theory, research, and clinical application. One method of specifying a phenomenon is to collect samples of cases people can agree on, and then determine features that the cases share in common. But if there has not been any clarity about which cases belong in the sample, then conclusions are apt to be misleading. Definitions impact (1) the population identified, (2) what is quantified about it, and (3) who receives treatment and how progress is evaluated. These three important functions of a definition are elaborated next.

Population Identification

This issue is encountered at the very early stage of stuttering research—identifying and counting the subpopulation of people who stutter. The specific definition, or the absence of one, can influence the findings concerning incidence and prevalence (to be discussed in Chapter 2), regardless of the data collection method. Consider, for example, the potential inconsistency in a survey that asks hundreds of schoolteachers around the country to report the number of stuttering children in their schools but that does not provide a definition of a child who stutters. Similarly, in the conduct of just about every study of stuttering, the investigator should follow some operational definition to determine who is qualified to be included as a participant who stutters. In comparative studies, it is also necessary to determine who does not stutter to be qualified as a control subject.

Unfortunately, many past studies failed to adhere to the basic definitional requirement. For example, participants were included because they were "regarded" as stutterers without further elaboration of what they had to exhibit to be viewed as "stuttering." When such studies have clinical implications, the use of a vaguely defined population makes it difficult to apply their results.

Quantification and Measurement

The implications of a definition extend beyond the selection of potential clients and research participants. Definition is important to those who look at changes in the phenomena. Investigators and clinicians interested in the amount or characteristics of stuttered speech under various conditions must define, in advance, what the "stuttering" is—that is, what will be the target measured. For example, Yairi and Ambrose (1999a) investigated changes in the frequency of stuttered speech events in preschool children. They defined stuttering as consisting of three observable speech elements: (1) repetitions of parts of words, (2) repetitions of single-syllable words, and (3) sound prolongations and blocks. They referred to these as "stuttering-like disfluencies." Their definition was based on a long history of investigations revealing a valid and reliable set of overt speech behaviors typical of children who were judged by their parents and clinicians to exhibit stuttering. By contrast, but no less valid, in a study of the effect of therapy on the speech of young children who stutter, J. Ingham and G. Riley (1998) defined stuttering in terms of what the experimenters *perceived* as stuttered syllables. No objective, observable characteristics were specified. Their definition was based on an extensive experiment revealing that well-trained examiners can perceptually identify instances of "stuttering" (no further definition) with valid and reliable judgments. Both sets of researchers have contributed significantly to the knowledge of stuttering, yet their scientific definitions were very different. Decisions about what stuttering is, and how it will be measured, affect which research can be consulted during clinical applications.

Evaluation of Clinical Progress

It should be clearer by now that definitions of stuttering have major implications in the clinical arena. Although the matter of diagnosis is separate from the issue of definition, critical decisions of whether a person is diagnosed as exhibiting stuttering and recommended for therapy on the one hand, and, on the other hand, whether he or she has stopped stuttering and should be discharged, hinge on its formal definition as well as evaluative criteria. Such decisions are more difficult when the person in question exhibits a mild stutter or presents a borderline case. Consumers of clinical services at all stages and levels need to be confident their concerns are not overlooked because of insufficient definitions and diagnoses of the disorder. Several definitions readers may encounter, such as "Stuttering is a transient disturbance in communicative, propositional, language usage," are not useful in practical situations. Clients and health-care agencies paying for treatment are entitled to insist on reasonable grounds for identification of the condition for which treatment is requested. Thus, in addition to theoretical, research, and clinical purposes, there is also a significant economic motive to establish a clear, acceptable definition of stuttering.

What to Define: Atypical (Abnormal) Speech or Complex Disorder?

When the term *stuttering* or a derivative (e.g., *a stutter*) is used, the referent may be to either atypical (abnormal) speech event(s) or to a complex disorder in which atypical speech is but one component. In the statement "Last night he was *stuttering*," the term refers exclusively to the occurrence of the surface (overt) phenomena: interruptions of the flow of speech that are perceived as atypical. By contrast, in the statement "She has had a *stuttering* problem for quite some time," it may have broader meaning. Here, stuttering may refer to a person who has habitually demonstrated atypical speech or it may refer to a disorder involving other important aspects, such as physiology, emotion, cognition, and social facets that have persisted, in addition to the occurrences of the atypical speech events. This is illustrated in Sheehan's (1958, p. 123) notion of the "stuttering iceberg": that what we perceive as stuttering events reveals only a small part of the disorder—that is, the tip of the iceberg.

Accordingly, "stuttering" has been defined by scholars as either of the two concepts stated above, although not always in a mutually exclusive manner. The stuttering literature, however, reveals far too many discussions that fail to establish what needs to be defined, overlooking the two conceptualizations of stuttering and leaving students of the subject bewildered. Thus we contrast two types of definitions of stuttering: (1) disordered speech phenomena and (2) a complex disorder. Taking this orientation, the definitional language referring to stuttering as a speech phenomenon generally describes what a person is *doing* when talking. The second, broader concept of stuttering necessitates an entirely different focus. Here, the definitional language usually contains statements about what a person *is* or *has*.[1] We develop these two concepts of stuttering further, in the next sections.

Stuttering as Atypical Speech

The event of stuttering only occurs in the context of attempting to speak. It is different from a hiccup that occurs whether a person is speaking or not. The most meaningful speech, like saying one's name, is more apt to be stuttered than a nonsense phrase made up of words in a mixed up order (Wingate, 1979). For many, the act of saying an isolated

---

[1]Johnson (1958) made comparisons between what a person is *doing* versus what a person *is or has*.

speech sound is far less apt to trigger stutter events than delivering a public address. For others, however, the mere attempt to make the sound of an isolated vowel will trigger stuttering. Stuttering is an involuntary disruption of the smooth execution of a speaker's intentional speech act. Because stuttering is so inextricably tied to the act of speaking, it will be beneficial to examine normal speech production and the concepts of speech fluency and disfluency, prior to defining stuttering.

Normally Fluent Speech Production

Normal fluency is recognized by the ease and ongoing flow of speech muscular movement and the resultant speech sounds. Speech produced fluently consists of suitable dimensions of (1) rate, the appropriate timing within and across words; (2) continuity, the smooth connections within and across words; and (3) tension effort, the appropriate regulation of exertion or force (Starkweather, 1987). Hence, various levels of the speech system must function properly and in close coordination.

Levels and Systems

Speech originates in the speaker's brain and involves complex processes, including formulation of an intended message, selection and ordering of words, sounds and syllables, and preparation of utterance rhythm, tempo, and vocal tone. The final spoken output depends on transmission of coordinated neurological commands from the brain to the peripheral motor and sensory mechanisms that regulate the desired speech signals and movements. The gross anatomical components of the peripheral speech system are the lungs, trachea, larynx, pharyngeal cavity, oral cavity, and nasal cavity. The pharyngeal and oral cavities are usually referred to as the *vocal tract,* beginning at the larynx and terminating at the lips. The nasal cavity begins at the velum (soft palate) and ends at the nostrils.

At the motor physiological level, normally fluent speech requires a series of precisely coordinated movements of respiratory, phonatory, and articulatory muscles. Prior to speaking, an optimal air volume within a certain range enters the lungs via inhalation. The air is then expelled into the larynx and the vocal tract. As air rushes from the lungs through the trachea, the vocal cords within the larynx approximate (i.e., are positioned near midline) and are set into gentle vibration, interrupting the airflow with quasi-periodic pulses that result in the sound that we call "voice." In the next stage, the relatively simple acoustic properties of the sound are modulated and filtered as they pass through the vocal tract, being shaped by the movement and positioning of the articulators, especially the tongue, lips, and jaw, creating recognized speech sounds, such as vowels. When the velum is lowered, the nasal cavities are acoustically coupled to the vocal tract to produce the nasal sounds of speech. Other sounds are generated by varying the shape and size at various locations in the vocal tract. For example, some consonants (i.e., fricatives) are formed by generating turbulent noise as the air is forced through various narrow constrictions shaped in the oral cavity, whereas others, such as plosives (or stops), are formed by quick releases of air pressure built up behind obstructions, such as closed lips. Sounds are filtered and modified still further as they blend

Figure 1.1   Motor Physiological Processes in Speech Production

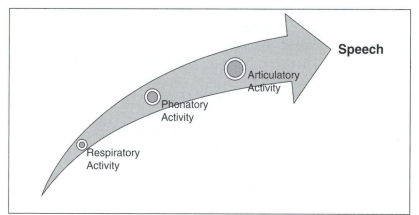

(e.g., for coarticulation) into syllables, words, and sentences. They are then further refined by changes in rate, pitch, intonation, and loudness, which combine alterations of the respiratory, phonatory, and articulatory systems as reflected in Figure 1.1. Thus speech output becomes acoustically complex in both the frequency and time dimensions, and as a function of the constantly varying length and cross-sectional area of the vocal tract, as well as the position of the articulators and durations of their movements. Finally, the speech output is also modulated by the speaker's own monitoring of proprioceptive, tactile, kinesthetic, and auditory feedback loops.

This account, which is probably familiar to many of you, is presented to make the point that stuttering, at least at the surface level, should be appraised against the larger normal complex structures and functions that are disrupted. It is the precise, delicate, coordinated, and timed array of movements and resultant normal flow of speech that may be disrupted at just about any or all levels of the speech motor system: respiration, phonation, and articulation. *It is for clinicians to appreciate that these are what speech therapy attempts to restore.* The disruptions frequently appear as various disfluencies described later or as complete cessations of speech, inability to initiate words, respiratory and phonatory irregularities (e.g., running out of air for speech, pitch raising, glottal fry, etc.), and others. Additionally, there is growing evidence to suspect that disruptions underlying disfluency also occur at higher levels of speech planning and control in the brain, as will be discussed in Chapter 7.

Normal Disfluency or Instances of Stuttering?

The various surface interruptions that occur in ongoing speech have been referred to as "disfluencies." For practical purposes, these events have been categorized using linguistic terminology or other descriptors applied to speech events. Among the most commonly referred to disfluency categories are word repetition, part-word or syllable repetition, sound repetition, phrase repetition, sound prolongation, blockage,[2] interjection, and revision. Some of these (e.g., phrase repetition) minimally interrupt speech continuity but they do slow down its progress.[3] A critical fact is that disfluencies occur not only in the speech of people who stutter but also in the speech of practically all speakers, especially young children (Johnson, 1961a; Yairi, 1981). It is important, therefore, to recognize from the outset that disfluency and stuttering, although related, are not synonymous. In most people and under most circumstances, disfluencies are not too frequent and are regarded as normal. But, when produced differently or under some circumstances, disfluent speech is regarded as abnormal or stuttering. Thus the terms *disfluency* and *disfluencies* refer to speech disruptions regardless of whether they happen to be normal or abnormal (stuttered) speech.

> Alternate spellings of some terms are found in the stuttering literature. Examples are "disfluencies" vs. "dysfluencies," or "disrhythmic phonations" vs. "dysrhythmic phonations." Although not all writers use the distinction, the prefix *dis* may be contrasted with *dys* on purpose. Wingate (2002) explains that the prefix *dis* is the Latin for "not"; *dys* refers to "disorder." Therefore when encountering *dys*, you should understand that the referent may be more closely tied to the disorder of stuttering. By contrast, the prefix *dis* commonly refers to all disruptions whether specifically stuttered or not.

The distinction between "normal disfluency" and "stuttering," sometimes blurred, stems from two sources, speech production and speech perception. From a production perspective there are abundant data showing that several disfluency types occur much more frequently in the speech of people who are regarded as exhibiting stuttering (Ambrose & Yairi, 1999; Johnson & Associates, 1959). Syllable repetition is a prime example. It is found in the speech of all speakers but its level is 10 times higher in the speech of children who stutter (CWS) than in the speech of normally fluent children (NFC). Single-syllable word repetition is five times higher. In many cases, disfluencies produced by people who stutter not only are more frequent but differ in other properties from those of the same type produced by normally fluent people. When a PWS repeats a syllable such as "an-an-and," or a single-syllable word, such as "but-but-but," the speed of the repetitions is three times faster than repetitions produced by NFS (Throneburg & Yairi, 1994, 2001), the number of repetitions per instance is greater (Ambrose & Yairi, 1995), and their distribution (clustering) within speech is different (Hubbard & Yairi, 1988; Sawyer & Yairi, 2010). From a perceptual perspective, the very same disfluency types also tend to be judged as "stuttering" by listeners (Young, 1984). Of course, the frequency of occurrence is very influential. One or two syllable repetitions per 100 words of running speech may be perceived as normal, but five syllable repetitions in the same amount of speech are likely to be perceived as stuttering (Sander, 1963). Still, listeners vary in how they perceive the same disfluencies as "normal" or "stuttering."

---

[2]The categories of sound prolongations and blocks are frequently merged in a single category, disrhythmic phonations.

[3]Disfluencies are described and discussed in more detail in Chapter 4.

Concerning disfluency types, all conventionally recognized and defined disfluencies found in people who stutter also occur in the speech of normally fluent children. But disfluency types that are most typical to stuttering have been dubbed as "core behaviors" (Van Riper, 1971). Yairi and Ambrose (1992a) refer to these types as stuttering-like disfluencies, or SLD ("stuttering-like" acknowledges that they are not exclusive to stuttering), and other disfluencies (OD), which are regarded as less stuttering-like and more typical to normally fluent speakers. These are listed in Table 1.1.

Table 1.1 Types of Disfluency

STUTTERING-LIKE DISFLUENCY	EXAMPLES
Part-Word Repetition	Bu-bu-but
Single-Syllable Word Repetition	And-and-and
Disrhythmic Phonation	Mo—mmy
OTHER DISFLUENCIES	EXAMPLES
Phrase Repetition	I like to—I like to . . .
Revision	It was, I mean . . .
Interjection	Uhm, well, er

From the speaker's perspective, the reason(s) underlying the behavior are also important. A normal speech disruption, common to those who do not stutter, is usually associated with reasons that the speaker recognizes, such as word-finding, a sentence-formulation decision, a reconsideration of message content, a distracting event nearby, and so on. When the speaker recognizes the reason for the speech disruption, he or she is apt to acknowledge it as a "normal disfluency." The experience of normal disfluency for reasons such as these is shared by the nonstutterer and stutterer alike. By contrast, when the word(s) to be said is fully decided and the speaker is intent to engage in speaking, but the production becomes "stuck" for what seems to be no apparent reason, it is then that the experience by the speaker is apt to fit the label of stuttering.

Perceptible differences may distinguish many moments of stuttering from normal disfluency, but some listeners may find it difficult to determine if a disfluency they have heard is normal or stuttered. Listeners seem to operate with different perceptual thresholds in regard to "how much is too much?" That is, how much disruption does it take to evoke a person's judgment that a repetition is "stuttering" rather than "normal disfluency" (Martin & Haroldson, 1981). Factors potentially affecting listener judgment include the type, duration, and intensity of the disfluency, as well as the context, past experience, and characteristics (e.g., gender) of the listener (Kawai, Healey, & Carrell, 2007). For example, a person who has relatives who stutter may be more sensitive to disfluencies and exhibit a lower threshold.

Defining Stuttering as Speech Events

The preceding discussion revealed a precedent for categorizing overt instances of speech disruption into *primary* (or "core") disfluency types commonly evident as signs of stuttering, and *secondary* (or "other") disfluency types, are evident when a speaker hesitates or reformulates for reasons that may or may not relate to stuttering. This two-class structure has been confirmed with empirical research (Lewis, 1991), and not surprisingly, a number of scientists have offered definitions of stuttering from the standpoint of criteria based on behavioral observations.

Examples of Definitions of Stuttered Speech

As early as 1931, Travis defined stuttering objectively as "a disturbance in the rhythm of speech; an intermittent blocking; a convulsive repetition of a sound." This definition, proposed at the beginning of the modern era of speech pathology, appears to have influenced Travis's students to coin the term *moment of stuttering*. Among them, Wendell Johnson was probably most responsible for the widespread adoption of the concept (Johnson, 1955a, p. 13). This terminology suggests that immediately before and immediately after the perceived stuttering, speech was normal, a questionable assumption. In our opinion the term *stuttering event* is preferable because it reflects the concept of *activity* rather than *time*.

Wingate offered one of the most well-known definitions of stuttering as speech events. At first, he provided a lengthy three-part definition in which the first part focused on core speech features: "The term stuttering means (a) disruption in the fluency of verbal expression, which is (b) characterized by involuntary, audible or silent, repetitions or prolongations in the utterance of short speech elements, namely, sounds, syllables and words of one syllable. These disruptions (c) usually occur frequently or are marked in character and (d) are not readily controllable" (Wingate, 1964, p. 488). Later, however, he argued that the essence of stuttering consisted of "silent or audible elemental repetitions and prolongations" (Wingate, 1988, p. 9). Although present also in the speech of normally fluent people, they are infrequently uttered, especially by adults, and also shorter. It is the frequent occurrence, and the length of these events in a person's speech that conveys the impression of stuttering. Hence, "a-ai" may be perceived as normal but the longer "a-a-a-a-a-ai" is more likely to be perceived as stuttering. Wingate's latter definition was helpfully succinct although still insufficiently definitive as to what is meant by "elemental," that is, sounds, syllables, and monosyllabic words creating some disagreement.

More recently, Guitar (2014) proposed that stuttering consists of "an abnormally high frequency and/or duration of stoppages in the forward flow of speech. These stoppages usually take the form of (a) repetitions of sounds, syllables or one-syllable words, (b) prolongations of sounds, or (c) 'blockages' or 'blocks' of airflow or voicing in speech" (p. 7). These statements offer additional characteristics not mentioned in Wingate's definition.

The American Speech-Language-Hearing Association (ASHA) has addressed the definition of stuttering as phenomena in a technical paper prepared for its Special Interest Division 4, Fluency and Fluency Disorders (1999). They discuss the issue of definition at greater length, but state that "stuttering refers to speech events that contain monosyllabic whole-word repetitions, part-word repetitions, audible sound prolongations, or silent fixations or blockages. These may or may not be accompanied by accessory (secondary) behaviors (i.e., behaviors used to escape and/or avoid these speech events)" (pp. 4-5). This definition also extends beyond pure speech characteristics to include secondary physical characteristics when applicable.

Yairi and Ambrose (2005, p. 20) considered the fact that normally fluent speakers also produce, at times, some disfluent speech. Therefore, they defined stuttering based on the statistical *probability* that certain speech patterns will be either produced by people who stutter or will be so perceived by listeners. In their words,

> we consider those speech characteristics that young children who stutter tend to produce, and those that are *likely* to be judged by listeners as stuttering. Thus, children considered to stutter are inclined to exhibit interruptions in the flow of speech in the form of repetition of parts of words (e.g., sounds and syllables) and monosyllabic words, as well as by disrhythmic phonations—prolongations of sounds and arrests of speech (blocks). We have referred to these overt speech phenomena as Stuttering-Like Disfluency (SLD). These are the most common disfluencies produced by children who stutter, as well as the speech events most *likely* to be perceived as stuttering.

Interestingly, a few scholars, such as Howell (2009) and Jiang et al. (2012), have raised reservations about the inclusion of monosyllabic words as stuttering. We disagree with them. For an expanded discussion of our view see Yairi (2013). Our own attempt at definition, which also treats stuttering primarily as atypical speech events, will be provided later in this chapter.

Fluent Speech of People Who Stutter

A substantial percentage, usually most, of the spoken message expressed by people who stutter is fluent. This fact is well-established. On average, only 10% of words in oral reading were found to be stuttered by adults (Bloodstein, 1944). Similarly, a mean of 11.84% stuttered words was found in conversation/storytelling or conversation/ reading contexts for children ages 5 through 12 (G. Riley & J. Riley, 1980). An inevitable question is whether a stutterer's fluent speech is also abnormal in other speech parameters. If yes, should this be considered in the definition? For several decades there has been growing evidence that the fluent portions of the speech of PWS differs from the fluency of NFS. For example, when all disfluent segments were removed from tape-recorded speech samples, listeners could still correctly identify the speech of stutterers from matched samples of nonstutterers (Wendahl & Cole, 1961). Research of the acoustic and physiologic properties of the fluent speech of stutterers has reported more convincing support. Vowel duration measures (Zimmermann, 1980a), second formant transitions (Robb & Blomgren, 1997), and vocal fold vibrations (Hall & Yairi, 1992) produced by stutterers in their fluent speech are different from those produced by normal speakers. These findings have been used in support of arguments against limiting stuttering definitions to disfluent speech characteristics. So far, however, the characteristics of fluent speech of PWS have not been incorporated into definitions of stuttering.

Overall, in spite of difficulties arising from a certain amount of overlap between normal disfluency and stuttering, speech-oriented definitions appear to be in reasonably close agreement on the essential elements (disfluency features) that should be included. Experimenters and clinicians are in a position of being able to apply some principles in formulating working definitions for their specific studies or clinical needs. Still, reflecting the incomplete state of knowledge, there are inconsistent applications, and definitions have failed to refer to fluent speech characteristics of PWS. Focusing on speech, they disregard other important aspects of stuttering and therefore may not cover certain cases, such as people with covert stuttering.

Regarding the role of speech-based definition, it was noted that "whatever else the clinical disorder of stuttering entails, there seems to be relatively little disagreement that the term 'stuttering' refers to the domain of motor speech production and its disruption by speech disfluencies. Physical, physiological, cognitive, and emotional components, regardless of how frequent or intense they might be, would not be labeled as 'stuttering' if they did not accompany a speaker's disfluent speech" (Yairi & Ambrose, 2005, p. 19).

Stuttering as a Complex Disorder

Multidimensional Characteristics of the Stuttering Disorder

The backdrop for defining stuttering as a complex disorder is its multidimensionality. It involves much more than the overt dimensions of disfluent speech. The multifaceted nature is apparent from the very first contact of a speech-language clinician with an adult who stutters who exhibits lip tremor during stuttering and reports strong anxiety prior to and during talking. For this particular client, the fear associated with stuttered speech is as much, if not more, of a problem than the speech aspects. Also children who stutter may exhibit physical body tension and secondary movements during stuttered speech, as well as avoidance behavior and social withdrawal. The reactions of parents must also be addressed. The clinician realizes that all these have to be described, and if possible quantified.

Six major dimensions of the complex stuttering disorder are distinguished:

1. **Overt speech characteristics:** Interruptions of the normal flow of speech that occur at the respiratory, phonatory, and articulatory levels but are evident

acoustically as repetitions of speech segments, prolongations, and/or cessation of sound, and so on.

2. **Physical concomitants:** Tense body movements, especially in the head and neck, but also in other parts of the body, often manifest in association with the overt speech events. These are known as "secondary characteristics." They are not necessary for stuttering to occur or be diagnosed, but may appear as the person struggles through a stuttering event.

3. **Physiological activity:** Stuttered speech is associated with changes in blood flow, skin reactions, pupil responses, brainwave activities, and other physiological changes. Many of these cannot be observed with the naked eye but have been well documented by means of sophisticated technology.

4. **Affective features:** Strong emotional reactions about talking, especially fears of speaking in many situations, are quite common. When these emotions become intense, leading to avoidance of speaking, the emotional dimension of the disorder could overshadow that of the atypical speech. Even children, particularly those with sensitive temperaments and slow adaptation to change, may react to their speech difficulties with fear of speaking, avoidance of speaking, sadness, and/or frustration.

5. **Cognitive processes:** Clinicians familiar with stuttering are likely to have heard parents, teachers, relatives, or other listeners comment that the person who stutters is "thinking faster than he can talk." A parent may comment, "He has so much to say and he just can't get it all out at once." These assumptions could be valid. The cognitive underpinnings of the selection, planning, preparation, and execution of speech may, in effect, present "overload" for the person who stutters, yielding stuttered speech. Second, the speaker's response to the experience of speech disruptions is influenced by his or her concepts about the nature of the disorder and the language used to characterize it. For example, a person may relate his or her perception of stuttering as "words getting stuck" in the throat, likening words to objects when actually, muscular activity and movement is interrupted.

6. **Social dynamics.** The function of speech is to communicate with others—listeners. Most speakers watch for the signs that their listeners hear, think, and respond to what was said to them. When stutter events are carried along with the message, both the speaker and the listener may change their communicative actions midstream. The speaker's communicative influence can be spoiled if listeners pay more attention to the stuttering than the message, or worse, if listeners make derisive or judgmental evaluations. These dynamics lead speakers who stutter to become more watchful of listeners, inspired by the fear of stuttering itself and the strong need to avert the undesired social impact of disrupted communication. In turn, the disorder of stuttering can have devastating effects on social interactions such as class participation, initiating conversations, answering the telephone, dating, adjustments to new environments, and making career choices.

Additionally, in complex ways, stuttering is also interwoven with the language and phonological development of some children. These aspects can have particularly important implications for clinical intervention during early childhood. Finally, all of the above are impacted by genetic factors, a topic we expand on in later chapters.

Diversity of Disorder-Oriented Definitions

Reviewing the plethora of definitions of the complex stuttering disorder, and the diversity encountered, one may raise the legitimate question of whether the experts who offered them were addressing the same condition. It also becomes evident that not all definitions have adhered to the expected purpose of clarifying the meaning, scope, and application of a term. Some digress to explain stuttering or merely offer a point of view regarding its etiology; others constitute descriptions of a few selected features. Even those that provide descriptions have not offered a characterization that sufficiently distinguishes the disorder of stuttering from other speech problems (e.g., apraxic speech, aphasic speech, cluttering, etc.). Before we proceed with examples of these definitions, we should understand the potential sources of the diversity among them.

Within the *complex disorder* conceptual framework, a further division of the definitions must be noted: Some are confined to a single domain, (e.g., neurologic factors), whereas others encompass interactions among multiple domains (e.g., motoric and psychologic). Until the 1940s, many professionals who expressed active interest in stuttering were psychiatrists, physicians representing other specialties, psychologists, and more. Understandably, these professionals operated from different knowledge bases, informational sources, general perspectives, entrenched conventions, and strong biases. Although they looked at many of the same facts, they arrived at different definitions that reflected their diverse backgrounds. They also were inclined to examine only one piece, or a few, of the stuttering puzzle, those that were more in tune with their particular area of expertise, eager for a clear-cut definition that also promoted their theoretical orientation. Having pointed this out, it is only fair to acknowledge that varying experiences and circumstances do indeed provide different types and amounts of information about any particular problem. For example, scholars and clinicians who work primarily with young children who stutter are likely to have a different perspective and understanding of the disorder than those who work exclusively with adults. If, however, people with different areas of knowledge and expertise work together to solve the multidimensional puzzle of stuttering, understanding of the disorder will continue to grow.

Examples of Definitions of Stuttering as a Complex Disorder

Different frames of reference, reflecting various theoretical positions that have influenced definitions of the stuttering disorder are organized here into six subcategories. Examples of organic, psychopathogenic, psychosocial, learning-based orientations, listener-based, and speaker-based perspectives (i.e., from the standpoint of the person who stutters) are presented next.

Organic Orientations

During much of the first half of the 20th century, the view that stuttering is organically based was popular as seen in West, Nelson, and Berry's (1939) reflection that stuttering, like left-handedness, twinning, or other atypical subpopulation characteristics, rests on some common heritable factor of structure or biochemistry. Years later, West (1958) was more specific in stating that stuttering is "primarily an epileptic disorder that manifests itself in dyssynergies of the neuromotor mechanism for oral language" (p. 197). In our view, this provides a good example of an attempted definition that, instead, ought to be classified as an explanation. In relation to the previous discussion, note that it does not treat stuttering as a surface phenomenon but as a disorder. Further, as such, it is focused on a single etiological variable, a faulty neurological system. It does not define stuttering as a complex disorder.

Also representing the organic orientation is Van Riper's (1971) definition that highlights the timing of muscle movement. He proposed that "stuttering is a disorder of timing . . . when a person stutters on a word, there is a temporal disruption of the simultaneous and successive programming of muscular movement required to produce one of the word's integrated sounds, or to emit one of its syllables appropriately" (p. 415). This definition treats stuttering as a disorder and focuses on a single variable. In the same source, however, Van Riper stated that "stuttering occurs when a forward flow of speech is interrupted by a motorically disrupted sound, syllable, or word or the speaker's reactions thereto" (p. 15). This definition has the advantage that it acknowledges the reality that stutter events can take many different behavioral forms (i.e., prolonged sounds, repetitions, etc.). Note, however, that it also encompasses the inner experience of a person who stutters. By combining these two elements of surface and covert features, it treats stuttering as a truly complex disorder.

Listener-Based Orientations

Most stuttering definitions are based on the listener's perspective. For that reason, many definitions focus on visible characteristics and take the form of this one found in *Churchill's Illustrated Medical Dictionary*: "A speech disorder affecting the fluency of production, often characterized by repetitions of certain sounds, syllables, words, or phrases, and by the prolongation of sounds and blocking of the articulation of words. Severer forms may be associated with facial grimacing, limb and postural gestures, involuntary grunts, or impaired control of airflow. The severity of symptoms may vary with the speaker's situation and audience." Reflecting its medical orientation, the dictionary goes on to state, "It is unusual to find evidence of neurological dysfunction in the confirmed adolescent or adult stutterer" (Koenisberger, 1989, pp. 1802–1803).

Psychopathogenic Orientations

Viewing stuttering as a psychopathological disorder was similarly popular during the first half of the 20th century. Although this theoretical orientation has lost much ground, a brief review illuminates the diversity of opinions. Coriat (1943a, p. 28) conceived stuttering to be "a psychoneurosis caused by the persistence into later life of early pre-genital[4] oral nursing, oral sadistic, and anal sadistic components." A quarter century later, Glauber (1958, p. 78) suggested that "stuttering is a neurotic disorder in which personality disturbance is in part reflected in speech. . . . Stuttering is a symptom of a psychopathological condition classified as pregenital conversion neurosis." Similarly, Murphy and Fitzsimons (1960, p. 17) stated, "First, stuttering behavior is primarily a psychogenically motivated symptom which manifests itself most discernibly in oral function." Again, all three definitions are primarily explanations, viewing stuttering as an underlying psychological disorder but limited in scope to a single essential factor.

Psychosocial Orientations

Another take on stuttering is seen in the attempts to define it as a psychosocial problem. As Fletcher (1928, p. 226) conceived it, stuttering is "a morbidity of social consciousness, a hyper-sensitivity of social attitude, a pathological social response." The main factors that operate here are fear, anxiety, inferiority feelings, and so on, in terms of social relationships, all of which have their genesis in specific experiences. The fears and anxiety are not general but in the anticipation of the necessity to speak under certain defined conditions that set off the pathological reactions. Another perspective of stuttering within the context of social interaction was offered by Eisenson (1958, p. 244), who proposed that "stuttering is a transient disturbance in communicative propositional language usage." This concept of stuttering emphasizes its social impact as a breakdown in conveying meaning when communicating with others. Again, the above are not definitions but descriptions and explanations.

Learning Orientations

In the 1950s, when psychological learning theories were popular, Johnson (1955a, pp. 23–24) offered his famous definition that the essence of stuttering was "an anticipatory apprehensive hypertonic avoidance reaction." Although the definition lacks specific reference to speech, Johnson's writings clearly point out speech as the cause of the anticipation. Accordingly, stuttering occurs when (based on past experience) a speaker anticipates stuttering and reacts by setting off an acquired (learned) array of cognitive, emotional, and tense physical responses that end up as struggled, stuttered speech. This experience is similar to the act of tight-rope walking. There is a circular, slightly troublesome, nature to this definition in that it necessitates another definition to characterize the stuttering events that prompted the initial reaction.

In this group of learning-oriented definitions we also cite Brutten and Shoemaker (1967, p. 61), who defined stuttering as "a form of fluency failure that results from conditioned negative emotions." This definition, as the previous one, would hardly aid anyone attempting to identify stuttering. It is merely a statement concerning the authors' belief about its cause: certain acquired (learned) emotions that trigger fluency failure.

---

[4]Pregenital refers to the organization of the child's sexual development during the early infantile period, before the genital zone became its focus.

The Speaker's Perspective

Stemming from a difference in basic conceptualization, another factor has impacted the diversity of stuttering definitions. Whereas most definitions assume a *listener-observer's* frame of reference, a few are based on the *speaker's,* that is, the person who stutters, point of view (e.g., Perkins, 1990a). Related to this matter, there are people who stutter severely yet never miss an opportunity to speak, and people who stutter very mildly but hesitate to speak at all, revealing a wide contrast in the *speaker's* perceptions of their stuttering problem. One can argue, therefore, that the personal point of view has implications for describing, diagnosing, and treating stuttering, and hence, also in defining it. This point of view was the subject of exchange between Brocklehurst (2013) as a proponent and Yairi (2013) presenting a skeptical position, particularly regarding research applications.

> One scholar recently suggested that the criterion for determining whether adults are identified as people who stutter is whether they identify themselves as such (Brocklehurst, 2013). Imagine the problems that this approach could create when conducting research. Suppose a team of investigators wishes to compare a group of people who stutter (PWS) with a control group of normally fluent speakers (NFS) on a particular parameter. In selecting participants for the experimental (stuttering) group all of the investigators perceive the speech of one volunteer as normal though the person insists that he stutters. Should they accept self-identification as a sufficient basis, and include him as a stutterer? Similarly, imagine that the investigators perceive stuttering in the speech of another volunteer who insists that she does not stutter. Should they accept her self-identification and include the volunteer as a nonstutterer? Our answer is negative in both cases.

One example of a succinct definition of stuttering that zeroes in on the speaker's perspective was offered by Perkins (1990a). He proposed that "loss of control of the ability to voluntarily continue a disrupted utterance is the essence of stuttering" (p. 376). Again from the perspective of the person who stutters, the speaker's feeling of loss of control of his or her speech is a key characteristic, but it is difficult to distinguish this problem from others such as an apraxia of speech or spastic dysphonia.

Another definition of stuttering from the speaker's point of view was adopted by the World Health Organization: "Disorders of rhythm of speech in which the individual knows precisely what he wishes to say, but at the time is unable to say it because of involuntary, repetitive prolongation or cessation of a sound" (World Health Organization, 1977). Here, considerable weight is given to the inner experiences of the person while it also includes the basic symptomatology. As is the case with the Perkins definition, however, it may be difficult to distinguish the defining characteristics from apraxia. The additional limitation of these definitions is that stuttering might constitute a variety of different experiences for different people who perceive themselves to stutter.

Figure 1.2   A Model of the Stuttering Disorder

Impairment	Disability	Handicap
•Stuttering events	•Unsatisfying communicative interactions	•Situational fears and avoidance of talking

Other Views

One approach to overcoming the challenge of individual differences among those who stutter was presented by Yaruss and Quesal (2006). They included components of body function and structure, personal and environmental factors, and activity/participation in their model of the stuttering disorder. They also describe three levels of the disorder: impairment, disability, and handicap. Figure 1.2 conveys the essence of these three levels. Based on the *International Classification of Functioning, Disability, and Health* (ICF; WHO, 2001) *impairment* is evidenced when body function and structure are impeded, *disability* is realized when speech performance does not conform to social expectations, and *handicap* is experienced when goals for social participation are not achieved. Their model, however, is mainly useful for considering what stuttering *involves,* rather than providing a definition of what it *is.*

Overall, the few definitions just cited that address stuttering as a complex disorder are sufficient to demonstrate a wide diversity in the ways the supposed essence of stuttering has been captured, conceiving of it as an organic/motor disorder, psychiatric disorder, psychosocial disorder, learned disorder, and a disorder affecting a speaker's intentional control. The definitions differ so greatly that one might almost wonder if all of them refer to the same disorder. From a practical point of view, although each definition depicts one or several relevant parameters of stuttering, none of them is sufficiently specific (precise) to be useful in the identification of people who exhibit the disorder.

Our Point of View

In the preceding discussion of how to define stuttering as a disorder, we highlighted its multidimensional characteristics. In view of its complexity and the vast individual and age variations across multiple dimensions, it is nearly impossible to formulate a definition to satisfy the desired criteria. With these reservations in mind, we nevertheless offer our own opinion.

An ideal definition of stuttering should endure even when diverse theories across time are proposed to explain it. We are inclined to define stuttering in as pure and as simple a form as possible, similar to how water has been defined, essentially as what falls as liquid precipitation. Such a definition should prove beneficial even if, just like water, stuttering is rarely encountered in a pure and simple form. Hence, stripped down to essentials, we define stuttering as *articulatory gestures in a holding pattern (repetition, prolongation, block) in an attempted delivery of syllables (including single-syllable words) or elements of syllables.*

> For research purposes, we define stuttering events when speech is characterized by periods of frequent and/or intense disruptions to the integration of syllable or elements of syllables as components of spoken utterances.[5] At its minimum, such disruptions consist of gestural holding patterns of repeated and/or elongated speech elements, including sound, syllable, or a single-syllable words. Examples of such disruptions include repetitions that are fast in tempo, especially those consisting of two or more extra iterations, prolongations that are longer than a half second, and complete articulatory blockages of speech sounds.

At its onset in young children, stuttering is a speech disorder (also known as "developmental stuttering" because of its childhood onset) in those who are prone to experience intermittent disruptions in the form of one or all of the speech events described above. These disruptions occur at levels sufficient to distract listeners and interfere with communication. The disorder is genetically based but highly responsive to environmental factors. When the disorder persists, it expands to acquire additional characteristics reflected in dynamic, multidimensional patterns of overt body tensions, motor-physiological adaptations, as well as emotional, cognitive, and social reactions. To the person who stutters, these additional aspects of the disorder may be more disturbing than the stuttered speech events.

Summary

The definition of stuttering has several very important research, theoretical, clinical, as well as financial implications. The term *stuttering* may refer to certain speech events or to the complex disorder. Defining stuttering, especially as a disorder, has proved to be a difficult task that has not yet been successfully accomplished. This is not surprising considering its multidimensionality. Several points were highlighted in this chapter:

- Disorder-based definitions have continued to reflect a wide diversity of perspectives from psychogenic to neurogenic to learning, and to that of the stutterer's subjective perception. Still, some progress has been made as reflected in the World Health Organization's view of the problem.

- Disagreement is considerably narrower regarding the definition of stuttering as a speech phenomenon.

- There was an early tendency that lasted for some time, to present a confusing picture of speech characteristics, overemphasizing overlap between normal disfluency and

---

[5]The concept of stuttering as a disruption to the integration of syllables was developed and supported most thoroughly by Wingate (1988).

stuttering. Considerable progress, however, has been made to clarify the differences between what is normal and what is not, and in zeroing on the essential features of disfluent events necessary for a definition.

- The diversity of opinion among scholars on (1) what stuttering is and (2) who is qualified as a "stutterer" has had a strong impact on how the disorder has been understood, investigated, and treated.
- The continuing conflicting views and the difficulties in arriving at a reasonable agreement could affect the overall progress in the field.
- Additional information about the fluent speech of people who stutter may strengthen future definitions of stuttering.
- The definition of stuttering may be improved in the future if speech scientists can find better ways to characterize and detect its overt and covert dimensions.

Study Questions and Discussion Topics

1. What is the purpose of a definition of a phenomenon?
2. Why is a definition of stuttering important? List and explain at least three reasons.
3. What are the two main categories of definitions of stuttering? Explain. Refer to two examples of each category.
4. What factors appear to have caused diversity in definitions of stuttering?
5. What are the similarities and differences between normal disfluency and stuttered speech?
6. Assume you will conduct a research project to study the effect of a new treatment on the frequency of stuttering. Which of the definitions cited in this chapter can be used for (a) selecting participants who stutter, and (b) measuring the frequency of stuttering?

Websites

Stuttering at the Web site for the National Institutes on Deafness and Other Communication Disorders. Accessed December 3, 2013, at http://www.nidcd.nih.gov/health/voice/pages/stutter.aspx

Stuttering at the Web site of the American Speech-Language-Hearing Association. Accessed December 3, 2013, at http://www.asha.org/public/speech/disorders/stuttering.htm

Suggested Readings

Brocklehurst, P. (2013). Stuttering prevalence, incidence and recovery rates depend on how we define it: Comment on Yairi & Ambrose' article Epidemiology of Stuttering: 21st century advances. *Journal of Fluency Disorders, 38,* 290–293.

Van Riper, C. (1982). Stuttering: Its definition. In *The nature of stuttering* (2nd ed., pp. 11–31). Englewood Cliffs, NJ: Prentice-Hall.

Yaruss, S., & Quesal, R. (2004). Stuttering and the International Classification of Functioning, Disability, and Health (ICF): An update. *Journal of Communication Disorders, 37*(1), 35–52.

Yairi, E. (2013). Defining stuttering for research purposes. *Journal of Disfluency Disorders,* 38, 294–298.

Young, M. (1984). Identification of stuttering and stutterers. In R. Curlee & W. Perkins (Eds.), *Nature and treatment of stuttering: New directions.* Boston, MA: College-Hill.

Who and How Many Stutter?

LEARNER OBJECTIVES

Readers of this chapter will:

- Understand the meanings of *incidence* and *prevalence* in general, and relate them to stuttering in particular.
- Understand population characteristics (e.g., age, gender) that influence the incidence and prevalence of stuttering.
- Understand the methodologies employed in incidence and prevalence studies of stuttering.
- Be familiar with incidence and prevalence findings and appreciate their implications as well as limitations.
- Evaluate implications of incidence and prevalence data toward an understanding of stuttering and its possible etiologies.

Incidence and Prevalence

The question of how many people experience the disorder of stuttering is one of the first raised by the professionals who study and/or treat it. The answer is not simple, because the question can be approached from different angles or contexts. Customarily, scientists distinguish between *incidence*—the probability that new cases of any disorder will develop over a period of time, and *prevalence*—the estimate of all the cases of the disorder at a given time. For example, many individuals in the population at large have had at least one ear infection at some point in life. The percentage of individuals who have *ever* developed an ear infection would be an estimate of incidence, and if by "ever" we mean at any time in life, then this would be the *lifetime incidence*. By contrast, a smaller percentage of people are apt to have ear infections at the particular time a population is examined. This would be the *prevalence* of ear infections when a survey is conducted (e.g., of 6-month-olds at a day-care facility). Naturally, the percentages will vary by age and season; for example, young children have more ear infections than older ones, especially during the winter months.

Interpretation of Incidence and Prevalence Data

For stuttering, examples of these measures are found in a study by Andrews and Harris (1964). In their longitudinal survey of 1,000 children who were followed for 16 years after the time of birth, the incidence of developmental stuttering, in this case *lifetime* incidence,[1] was approximately 4.5% because there were 45 cases of stuttering that

---

[1]The 16-year span is considered sufficient for "lifetime" incidence of developmental stuttering because it typically starts, and resolves for most, long before the 16th birthday.

Figure 2.1   An Example of Tracking the Incidence and Prevalence of Stuttering Cases

lasted any duration. By contrast, the *prevalence* of stuttering among the children surveyed at the end of the study was approximately 1%, reflecting the fact that only 10 were regarded as exhibiting stuttering at the time. The comparison just cited highlights the higher rates of stuttering incidence across the life span in contrast to the prevalence figures of those who stutter at a specific given time. Unfortunately, the stuttering literature has often confused the two terms, using *incidence* when the writer was actually referring to prevalence.

The change in incidence and prevalence for 30 children followed longitudinally over a 3-year period is illustrated in Figure 2.1. Data were collected from the same sample population on the same date, once a year. Each square in the grid represents one child. A minimum of 2 months of stuttering was required to count the case. In year 1, there were three cases of stuttering that began among the 30 children, for an incidence of 10% (3 of 30). In year 2, four new cases began, for an incidence of 13.3% (4 of 30). Because two children recovered naturally among the three previous cases, the prevalence of the disorder for that year is 16.7% (5 of 30). In year 3, there was a new incidence of 6.7% (2 of 30) but the prevalence drops to 13.3% (4 of 30) because three additional children recovered. The overall incidence of stuttering for the 3 years combined is 30% (9 of 30) with an average of 10% (3/30) per year. The prevalence also changed from year to year.

This example demonstrates that there are several ways of looking at incidence and prevalence data. It may be reported for specific, limited periods, for an overall period, or as an average across periods. Appropriate evaluation of the validity of incidence and prevalence estimates depends on a firm grasp of their definitions and the time frame involved for the target population. As with a number of other disorders (e.g., ear infections), cases of stuttering typically continue for a certain period of time and then subside. This additional dimension affects the estimates of incidence and prevalence and their interpretation. Recall that in the Andrews and Harris (1964) results, the lifetime incidence of stuttering was approximately 4.5%. This estimate was based on cases of stuttering that had lasted for *any* duration. By contrast, when the researchers examined only those cases that had lasted for *at least 6 months,* the incidence was only 3%. Thus incidence estimates may be influenced by an investigator's imposition of a minimal time that the disorder lingers in order to count a case. We hold that the true frequency of the phenomenon cannot be appreciated unless all cases that exhibit properly diagnosed stuttering, even for a short time, are counted.

Which is greater, the incidence of a disorder or its prevalence? It all depends on the time period used as a basis for comparison. When compared within a limited duration—for example, a 1-year span between the ages of 6 and 7—the incidence of only new stuttering cases that appear will be lower than the prevalence that includes all of the continuing cases. But when compared with the lifetime incidence, which is the number of people who have ever stuttered, the latter exceeds the prevalence, or number of people who currently stutter.

The Significance of Incidence and Prevalence

Information about the incidence and prevalence of stuttering in general, and with respect to specific factors such as age, gender, race, culture, and clinical subpopulations (e.g., those with hearing loss), has direct implications for understanding the magnitude of the problem, as well as its causes and dynamics. Beyond the theoretical significance, it also provides essential guidance in clinical decision making related to prognosis, counseling, and treatment recommendations. Because incidence estimates reflect the rate of new stuttering cases, they are especially important to studies concerned with the *prevention of* the disorder. Similarly, because prevalence estimates reflect the rate of currently existing cases, they are especially important to clinical processes of evaluation and *treatment* of the disorder. Incidence and prevalence data are vital in regard to research, professional training, clinical service delivery, public awareness, and funding of both clinical services and research.

Implications for Research and Theory

Incidence and prevalence data are crucial factors in designing research studies, evaluating their findings, and testing theoretical propositions. This is because the distribution of gender, age, skill domains (e.g., phonology), and natural recovery (without clinical intervention) among the sample of a study's participants ("subjects") can easily affect its outcome. For example, to be representative, sampled experimental groups need to include more males than females to reflect the gender ratio in the stuttering population. This gender disparity, however, changes with the ages of participants. Therefore, a representative sample of adults who stutter should include proportionately more males than a sample of preschool children. Consider another situation: a study of the language skills of young children who stutter. As explained, more boys than girls should be included in the samples. This, however, may yield inaccurate findings that children who stutter are below the norms because, as we know, boys may lag behind girls in typical speech and language development. It is essential in this situation to have a similarly gender-balanced control group.

Changes in the prevalence of stuttering with age and gender, and the influence of the rate and timing of natural recovery from stuttering, must be considered when interpreting results of clinical efficacy studies conducted with preschool children. If the natural recovery is overlooked, its effects may be confused and misinterpreted as being the outcome of treatment. If the different rates of recovery across genders are not considered in sample populations that have uneven proportions of males and females, there may similarly be misinterpretations of treatment outcomes.

Incidence and prevalence information are of immense importance to the theoretical foundations of stuttering. From an etiological perspective, gender distribution and percentage of natural recovery are essential for testing which of several genetic models best supports the notion that stuttering is hereditary. Furthermore, large deviations from the typical stuttering incidence found in certain subpopulations may provide relevant clues for making hypotheses about the nature of stuttering. For example, the low incidence of stuttering among deaf people draws attention to the role of auditory processes in stuttering. Similarly, a low or high incidence in certain cultures may suggest the influence of environmental factors, such as a high or low value placed on speaking skills affecting the level of pressure on children's speech. A high incidence in clinical subpopulations, such as people with Down syndrome, calls attention to a host of possible influences on stuttering, including chromosomal abnormality, low intelligence level, low muscle tone, and discrepancies in language skills during the critical stages of oral skill development.

Implications for Professional Training

Information about the occurrence of stuttering may influence both educational and clinical domains. For example, decisions concerning undergraduate and graduate academic curricula for students aspiring to become speech-language clinicians, as well as the amount of clinical practice required of them, are influenced by the incidence of the various disorders treated by these future professionals. Whereas many academic programs offer a course specifically devoted to language disorders in preschool children and a different course on language disorders in schoolchildren, such age-specific courses in stuttering may not be found. The relatively small size of the stuttering population was a reason the American Speech-Language-Hearing Association (ASHA) and many universities deemphasized academic and clinical training in fluency disorders required of students in speech-language pathology. For a period of several years, ASHA actually cancelled its traditional requirement for a minimum number of clinical practicum hours in the area of stuttering. It is encouraging that this professional-scientific organization resumed those requirements in the form of both knowledge and practical skill competencies so that future clinicians will be prepared to provide appropriate levels of service for individuals who stutter.

Incidence data impact the instructional content of courses taught on the topic of stuttering. The heightened occurrence of stuttering in early childhood, for example, would suggest the need to include parent counseling techniques in clinical curricula. Also, the focus of continuing education programs in stuttering mirrors the incidence of the disorder and its distribution. Not surprisingly, during the past two decades or so, there appear to be significantly more educational events focused on children than on adults who stutter.

Implications for Clinical Service Delivery

Information concerning the occurrence and distribution of stuttering, like that of many other disorders, is a major factor in both the planning of public and private clinical services and the availability of qualified personnel to treat the disorder. Considering the typical age of stuttering onset, which impacts the respective prevalence for that age range, health-care and educational systems should plan on providing more services for young children who stutter in early childhood centers and family community clinics than in clinical facilities where the majority of people served are adults. Additionally, clinicians need to be aware of the gender ratio to be sensitive to cultural aspects of communication for those they serve. For example, in counseling parents from cultures where boys are more highly desired in families, clinicians need to be prepared for the level of disappointment triggered by the parents learning that their son not only stutters but is at greater risk for persistence. This news may be received with more negative parental and societal reactions.

Incidence and prevalence data are also applicable in the interest of risk prediction. It is based on demographic factors such as age, gender, and familial distribution of the disorder. For example, if the lifetime incidence of stuttering is 5%, the risk for stuttering of a newborn infant is, on average, 5 in 100. But, adding our knowledge regarding the gender ratio of stuttering across the life span (about 4:1 in favor of males), and assuming an equal ratio of males and females in the population at large, a newborn boy has a risk of 8 in 100 and a newborn girl has a risk of 2 in 100 for stuttering at some time in life. Now, if the infant is born to a family with a history of stuttering, we know that the estimated risk is, on average, about 4 times higher (depending on the specifics of the history) as compared to a family without history of stuttering. A different prognostic application of incidence and prevalence data is seen in the question of whether a 5-year old boy who does not stutter is at a risk to begin stuttering. The answer: The chance is much smaller. Whereas Andrews (1984) concluded that 75% of the risk is over by age 6, Yairi and Ambrose (1999a) reported that over 90% of the risk for stuttering is over by age 4.

Other practical predictions can be made for children who have begun to stutter. Current data on incidence and prevalence, combined with other epidemiological information on the development of stuttering in early ages, allow us to provide a prognosis regarding a child's risk to develop chronic stuttering or to exhibit natural recovery.

We know, for example, that soon after onset, the chance for recovery is approximately 75%–80% or higher. After 2 years of stuttering, the recovery chance drops to 47%, and so on. Much more about all this will be offered in later chapters.

Implications for Public Awareness and Funding

Public concern about various health issues has influenced governmental agencies, as well as private foundations, in the distribution of money for research and treatment programs. For example, the sharp increase in the incidence of AIDS during the recent decades combined with increasing public awareness through the work of activists, philanthropic groups, and the media, have led to the consequent increase in financial resources dedicated to detecting and treating this disease. In many ways, inadequate information about stuttering and misconceptions about the size of the stuttering population, namely the prevailing notion that "only" 1%, or even less, of the population stutters, has diminished both public and professional attention to this communication disability. The 1% figure has produced an incorrect impression that stuttering is a "small" problem, although in children the percentage is considerably higher. It has been an important reason why stuttering was temporarily deemphasized by ASHA and affiliated academic training programs, as mentioned earlier.

Research Methodology for Incidence and Prevalence

Speech-language clinicians may serve as both the users and collectors of data related to the occurrence of stuttering cases. When evaluating incidence or prevalence figures related to stuttering, due attention must be given to the research methods employed. The fairly wide range of figures, 0.61% to 4.70% for prevalence, and 0.70% to 17.70% for incidence, reported across many studies (Bloodstein & Bernstein Ratner, 2008; Yairi & Ambrose, 2013) can most likely be attributed to the differences in the respective research methods used, including design, characteristics of the sample investigated, the definition of stuttering, or who identified stuttering and/or counted individuals who stutter.

Approaches to Prevalence Research

What methods are used to collect data about the occurrence of stuttering? By and large, prevalence research has been based on cross-sectional surveys of targeted groups, such as schoolchildren in different grade levels. Recall that in a cross-sectional study, data are collected from population samples at a single point in time. The most common procedure has relied on questionnaires returned by secondhand informers, such as schoolteachers, who are asked to list the children who stutter in their respective classes. Another method employs direct face-to-face evaluation by examiners who listen to participants' speech to identify stuttering. Although both the number of examiners and their professional experience with stuttering have varied, the face-to-face approach is expected to yield more valid and reliable information. A third approach is seen in several studies that applied multiple procedures, for example, using input from school personnel as well as individual screening by the investigators. It would be reasonable to assume that multiple inputs contribute to a higher degree of reliability. Ideally, all studies should be conducted in multiple sites to better reflect the broader population, settings, and geographic regions. Simultaneous sampling at the different sites and/or groups being surveyed ensures maximum uniformity in conditions. Still, variations abound. For example, Gillespie and Cooper (1973) obtained data on stuttering from just a single city.

The accuracy of statistics on stuttering is further complicated by the variation among studies in aspects such as their target sample populations. Preschool children, a single, narrow age group, were the focus of study by Proctor, Yairi, Duff et al. (2008). Others studied prevalence in a slightly wider age range of school-age children, such as grades 1 through 4 (Burdin, 1940), or among junior and senior high school students (Gillespie & Cooper, 1973). The most comprehensive studies include the widest age range, from kindergarten to 12th grade (e.g., Brady & Hall, 1976). Generally, these investigations used samples that were convenient to survey instead of randomly selected. An exception can be found in the 2002 Craig, Hancock, Tran et al. study that attempted a cross section of the entire population (all ages) of certain areas in Australia. The variations in target populations just described can be expected to result in a wide range of prevalence figures. In addition to age variability, several investigations have been conducted with specific subpopulations, such as African Americans (Proctor et al., 2008), individuals with cleft palate (Dalston, Martinkosky, & Hinton, 1987), and those with cognitive impairment (Preus, 1973), among others.

Cross-sectional prevalence surveys using questionnaires have made it possible to include large samples of participants. This is attractive because the sheer sample size may compensate for errors resulting from many possible uncontrolled variables. Examples of large-scale studies that used questionnaires and teacher input are Schindler (1955) sampling nearly 23,000 children, Wallin (1916) covering 89,000, and Glogowski (1976) with 875,000 children. Studies employing direct face-to-face observations, although potentially more valid and reliable, have been smaller in scope due to substantially increased costs for personnel, the time required for each interview, and difficulties in gaining entrance to schools and other institutions. Such studies include Gillespie and Cooper (1973), Mills and Streit (1942), and Proctor et al. (2008).

Approaches to Incidence Research

Data for stuttering incidence have been gathered by investigators who pursued one of two approaches: (1) longitudinal or (2) retrospective. With the first, the same group of individuals is followed for a period of time while being observed for newly emerging cases of stuttering. With the second, records are examined or informants surveyed are requested to obtain information about present as well as *past cases* (this is the retrospective aspect) of stuttering. Unquestionably, the first method holds the best potential for providing accurate information. It is, however, costly, difficult to execute, and bound to be limited in sample size and the number of years covered by the research. Also, although these investigations pertain to incidence, the researchers could not claim to have investigated the real *lifetime* incidence because, they included only portions of the life span.

The most famous longitudinal incidence study was carried out by Andrews and Harris (1964), who followed 1,000 children in the English city of Newcastle upon Tyne from birth to their 16th birthday. The children were visited at periodic intervals by health workers who noted when a child began stuttering and when the stuttering ceased. Those identified were also examined by speech therapists. The challenges and high costs involved in this type of study should be apparent. Although the first 16 years of life probably yield most of the information about stuttering incidence, any possible late onsets are missed. Another investigation that is unique was reported by Månsson (2000). His team assessed the incidence of stuttering by screening the *entire* population of 1,040 children who were born on the Danish island of Bornholm during 2 consecutive years. The children, however, were followed for only 5 years. The team repeated the study several years later (Månsson, 2005).

The retrospective approach to incidence research is illustrated in the 1971 Dickson study in which parents of almost 4,000 children in kindergarten through grade 9 were asked whether their children were stuttering at the time or if they had a history of *previous* stuttering. In the Craig et al. (2002) investigation, nearly 4,689 families comprising over 12,000 individuals participated in telephone interviews. Whereas it was possible to assess current stuttering (prevalence) via the telephone, identification of past stuttering cases (a major portion of the incidence) depended solely on the recollection of family members or individuals who used to stutter.

Overall, both longitudinal and retrospective studies suffer from flaws related primarily to vague descriptions of procedures, content of questionnaires, referrals, details of the personal examination of participants, and other factors. Surveys that are confined to school-age children can be expected to report a lower stuttering incidence than surveys that are confined to the preschool ages when stuttering typically begins. If human races differ in respect to stuttering, a study conducted in schools where races are not proportionally represented will yield misleading overall figures. In very young ages when the stuttering is often intermittent, some children may be missed in direct examination if they happened to experience a fluent period at the time of the study. Large up-and-down fluctuations in stuttering are common in the early stage of stuttering. Considering all these influences, direct comparisons among many of the studies are difficult. Although their cumulative data are useful in providing a reasonable idea of the range of the magnitude and distribution of the disorder of stuttering, ideally more carefully designed, executed, and reported research will be carried out in the future.

Defining Stuttering

As alluded to in Chapter 1, varying definitions of stuttering employed in incidence and prevalence research studies may have had some, or substantial, impact on their outcome and thus on the knowledge base of the profession. Consider the analogy of the challenges that arise when defining the common cold. There are colds with runny noses and sore throats, and there are colds with congestion and coughs. In turn, there may be differences in the prevalence or incidence of various colds reflected in the differences among cold symptoms. Similarly, not all stuttering is characterized by the same symptoms, and across research studies stuttering was not uniformly defined. Furthermore, in the survey conducted by Louttit and Halls (1936), no guiding definition was provided. It was left open to the individual opinions of the many people who carried out the survey. Louttit and Halls recognized the problem in their honest statement that "the teacher's judgment is the basis of the raw figures, so our whole analysis must rest on this somewhat insecure foundation" (p. 74).

Gillespie and Cooper (1973) improved on this method by conducting questionnaire surveys supplemented with a face-to-face meeting with each of 5,054 junior and senior high school students. Judgment of a student's stuttering was based on conversational speech and reading. Other studies defined stuttering more carefully and restricted their counts to cases that met behavioral criteria. Brady and Hall (1976) provided teachers participating in a questionnaire survey with the following definition: "Stuttering is a communication disorder characterized by excessive involuntary disruptions or blocking in the flow of speech, particularly when such disruptions consist of repetitions or prolongations of a sound or syllable and when they are accompanied by avoidance struggle behavior" (p. 76). In yet another study, Dickson (1971) defined stuttering as "repetitions of sounds and words and getting stuck on or between words" (p. 100). The questionnaires he used requested parents to provide specific information about disfluency as well as secondary stuttering characteristics. In the 2002 Craig et al. study, mentioned earlier, stuttering was defined as "repetitions of syllables, part or whole words or phrases; prolongations of speech; or blocking of sounds" (p. 1100). They also included information about secondary physical characteristics and the emotional components, such as embarrassment and anxiety.

Selecting Informants

Informants are people who gather the raw data. They determine who stutters based on their own observations or indirect data provided by other sources, such as a family's oral history. These have been teachers, health professionals, parents, and/or other family members. The accumulated data about stuttering prevalence or incidence have been gathered by people of different backgrounds and experience. Over the 70-year span between the studies of Louttit and Halls (1936), and Van Borsel, Moeyaert, Rosseel et al., (2006), many investigations relied on schoolteachers, sometimes hundreds and thousands of them (e.g., White House Conference, 1931). Those teachers had no professional training in speech pathology or in identifying stuttering, or even a brief preparatory training for the survey. The combined effect of so many people applying an individual perception of what constitutes stuttering without the benefit of a guiding definition raises doubts about the findings.

In other studies, information was gathered from parents of children (e.g., Reilly et al., 2013) or from other members of the families surveyed (Craig et al., 2002). In this respect, it is interesting to note that parents' diagnosis of stuttering and rating of its severity was found to align closely with that of experienced speech-language clinicians (McLeod & McKinnon, 2007; Yairi & Ambrose, 2005). One advantage of using parents as informants is that they are in a position to report an eruption of stuttering that lasted for a relatively short period. Such cases, occasionally quite severe, are typically missed by other methods, leading to *underestimates* of incidence or prevalence.

Another class of informants includes professionals who conduct direct observations of those being surveyed. There are, however, appreciable differences in the qualifications and number of these informants. As early as 1942, Mills and Streit employed 10 examiners to conduct individual testing of children in their school survey. All examiners had at least a year of training in speech pathology, and at least two were present at the testing of each child. The disadvantage: This team managed to screen only 25% of the pupils. In the Andrews and Harris (1964) study, only one of several health-care workers visited each child's home. Furthermore, in a good number of cases the examiners did not meet with the children but had to rely only on a parent's report instead of face-to-face evaluation. Proctor et al. (2008) used multiple sources to identify each child, including day-care staff, parental reports, and direct speech screening by a speech-language clinician. Stuttering was confirmed by the judgment of two clinicians. Obviously, corroboration by many informants strengthens the confidence in data validity.

Prevalence: Findings

Having reviewed a range of research methodology issues, the question is what has been found? To provide historical perspective, the findings of a good number of studies have been arranged in four groups according to general chronological order. These are presented in Table 2.1.

Early Investigations

Pioneer Reports

Considering the many experimental hazards we have discussed, it is intriguing to learn that early investigations of the school-age population yielded findings that are similar to better-designed modern studies. More than 100 years ago, four large studies with a total of nearly 660,000 participants, conducted in a variety of geographic regions around the world, revealed remarkably comparable results. In Europe, Lindberg (1900) surveyed 212,000 Danish schoolchildren, finding a stuttering prevalence of 0.90%, whereas von Sarbo (1901) studied 231,468 Hungarian children, reporting a prevalence of 1.02%. In the United States, Hartwell (1895) surveyed 129,060 schoolchildren in the Boston area, reporting a prevalence of 0.77% while Conradi (1904) surveyed approximately 87,440 schoolchildren in six cities, yielding a prevalence of 0.87%. We have calculated the mean prevalence of the four findings to be 0.89% (see Table 2.1).

Table 2.1 Reports on Stuttering Prevalence*

Study	Sample**	Prevalence
INITIAL REPORTS		
Lindberg (1900)	212,000	0.90%
Von Sarbo (1901)	231,000	1.02%
Hartwell (1985)	129,000	0.77%
Conradi (1904)	87,000	0.77%
Subgroup Mean		**0.89%**
EARLY 20TH CENTURY		
Blanton (1916)	5,000	0.72%
Wallin (1916)	89,000	0.70%
Watzl (1924)	136,000	0.60%
White House (1931)	3,500,000	0.70%
Louttit & Halls (1936)	200,000	0.77%
Subgroup Mean		**0.70%**
LATE 20TH CENTURY		
Gillespie & Cooper (1973)	5,000	2.12%
Leavitt (1974)	10,000	0.84%
Brady & Hall (1976)	187,000	0.35%
Hall, Mielke, Willeford et al. (1976)	39,000	0.80%
Glogowski (1976)	875,000	1.82%
Subgroup Mean		**1.18%**
21ST CENTURY		
Preschool		
Okalidou & Kampanaros (2001)	1,100	2.20%
McLeod & Harrison (2009)	5,000	5.60%
Proctor, Yairi, Duff et al. (2008)	3,200	2.60%
Subgroup Mean		**3.46%**
School		
Van Borsel, Moeyaert, Rosseel et al. (2006)	21,000	0.58%
McKinnon et al. (2007)	10,000	0.33%
Boyle, Boulet, Schieve et al. (2011)	119,000	1.60%

(continued)

Table 2.1   (Continued)

Study	Sample**	Prevalence
Subgroup Mean		**0.83%**
Lifetime		
Craig, Hancock, Tran et al. (2002)	12,000	**0.72%**

* The first three subgroups of studies were conducted with various ranges of school to high school grades.

** Rounded figures.

Early 20th-Century Reports

Information continued to come in during the first third of the 20th century. As can be seen in Table 2.1, five studies conducted between 1916 and 1936 yielded a mean prevalence of 0.70%. This group includes the largest of them all, a part of the White House Conference on Child Health and Protection (1931) where data were obtained for various speech disorders in a whopping sample of 3.5 million children from grade 1 to grade 12. Although many teachers served as informants, the finding of 0.70% prevalence was confirmed through a face-to-face reliability control study of 10,000 pupils.

Current Research

Late 20th-Century Reports

Studies conducted during the last third of the 20th century yielded a wider range of prevalence estimates, extending from a low of 0.35% to a high of 2.12%. The mean of the five studies listed for this period is 1.18%. Not counted in the calculation is an Australian study by Still, Harasty, and Reed (1994) that surveyed only 437 pupils.

21st-Century Reports

A comprehensive review of the literature (Yairi &Ambrose, 2013) has revealed seven prevalence studies published so far during the current century, all but one were relatively small in size compared to many previous investigations. As seen in Table 2.1, these are broken up according to age groups. The first three studies focused on preschoolers with a total of over 9,000 participants and yielded a mean prevalence 3.46% whereas the next three studies that covered over 150,000 school and high school pupils yielded a mean prevalence of 0.84%. The last study listed in the table (Craig et al., 2002) was carried out in Australia via telephone interviews with one person from each of 4,689 families, totalling 12,131 members ranging in age from under 1 year to 99 years. It is the only one that covered the entire age range. As could be expected, the highest prevalence was among the younger children, about 1.4% decreasing to 0.37% for ages 51+. The lifetime prevalence was of 0.72%. Overall, comparisons of the findings of the three subcategories within this subgroup also confirm the decline of prevalence with age.

Incidence: Findings

Estimates of the incidence of stuttering are likely to be less accurate than estimates of prevalence. The reason is that valid longitudinal or retrospective data are more diffi-cult to obtain than cross-sectional data used in prevalence research. Ideal incidence estimates require prospective longitudinal studies that track large samples of children representative of the population at large, starting from *prior* to the low end of the age when stuttering onsets occur, approximately 18 months, so as to capture all cases before natural recovery occurs.

To date, ideal longitudinal incidence data encompassing the entire age range, do not exist. Nevertheless, a handful of prospective investigations have provided gen-eral estimates. Already mentioned is the Andrews and Harris (1964) study with an initial sample of 1,142 babies, born and resided in a British city, who were tracked from birth to their 16th birthday (end of age 15). Tracking was conducted by health workers and speech clinicians through periodic home visits. No speech samples were recorded, and the evaluators had only brief contact with the child at each visit. As noted earlier, quite often parental reports substituted for the direct contact. Over the 16-year span, 43 children were identified as exhibiting stuttering, amounting to 4.9%[2] of the participants. It appears that more than any other finding, this one has influenced the generally accepted notion (e.g., NIH, 2010) that the lifetime incidence is approximately 5%.

The British study received strong support from another European investigation under the leadership of Hans Månsson (2000). Having a unique access to the birth records of *all* children born on the Danish island of Bornholm with its 45,000 low-mobility popu-lation, the Månsson team conducted direct speech, language, and hearing screenings of nearly the entire population of 1,040 children born during two years: 1991 and 1992. This was done within a month or two following their third birthday. Månsson found that 4.9% of the children exhibited stuttering, a figure identical to that of Andrews and Harris (1964) in a sample of a similar size. By age 8, after two follow-ups, it rose to 5.09%. Månsson (2005) repeated his survey among 928 newly the born population dur-ing the years 1995 and 1996. Extremely careful procedures were employed, including identical diagnosis by parents and two speech-language clinicians of current cases, and detailed parent reports of past stuttering that could not have been more than 18 months prior to the survey. This time the resultant incidence was a high of 17.7%. Although doubts may be raised, their methods were considerably more direct and verifiable than

---

[2]The 4.9% was calculated for the average size of the group, 875, to account for attrition.

those employed, for example, in the Craig et al.'s 2002 telephone survey to be discussed later. Support for higher than the conventional 5% incidence was recently provided by an ongoing longitudinal investigation of more than 1,600 Australian children, starting at 8 months of age. By age 4, incidence had already reached 11.2%. Here, parents' diagnosis was confirmed by speech clinicians (Reilly, Onslow, Packman et al., 2013).

An appreciable amount of the available incidence data, however, comes from questionnaires or interview studies using indirect retrospective methods, that is, informants reporting whether members of their family currently stutter or *have ever* stuttered, or by means of direct retrospective accounts, when informants are asked to report own history. The accuracy of these data may have been compromised by their secondhand nature, informants' use of different criteria, lost information about the familial history, and lapses in memory. Therefore, the resultant risk estimates tend to suffer from *underreporting*. We have selected four studies to present.

Glasner and Rosenthal (1957) interviewed parents of 996 children entering the first grade. The critical question was whether their child had *ever* stuttered. Of the sample, 153 (15.3%) were so reported. Nearly half had already stopped stuttering and could not have been objectively verified, but more than half (7.9%) of the sample was actively stuttering. A very different outcome was reported by Sheehan and Martyn (1970) whose team of clinicians interviewed 5,000 university students, observing speech and taking history of past speech disorders. Approximately 2.9% either exhibited present or reported past stuttering. Without parental input, however, it is rather likely that a number of these adults were not aware that they stuttered during early childhood.

Indication of incidence higher than 5% was provided by Felsenfeld, Kirk, Zhu et al. (2000), who investigated people listed with the Australian Twin Registry. As many of 3,768 young adults who stuttered (about 60% female and 40% males) responded to mailed questionnaires with the critical question if they had ever stuttered, revealing 8.8% incidence. More recently, a large longitudinal twin study in the United Kingdom used follow-up questionnaires from parents when their children were 2, 3, 4, and 7 years of age. Parents of 12,892 children identified at least 8.4% as having "ever stuttered" (Dworzynski, Remington, Rijsdijk et al., 2007).

Finally, the most inclusive investigation of lifetime incidence of stuttering was carried out by Craig et al. (2002). In a telephone interview with one member from each of 4,689 Australian families, their data totalled 12,131 persons younger than 1 year to 99 years of age. Interviewees were given a description of stuttering and asked if anyone residing in their home stuttered. Stuttering was identified from a recorded speech sample and an affirmative answer to at least one of several questions. To obtain lifetime incidence, interviewees were asked whether anyone in the household had *ever* stuttered. Adding the number of people who stuttered at the time to the number of those reporting past stuttering yielded an incidence of 2.21%. Table 2.2 summarizes the recent incident studies.

Although estimates of the lifetime incidence of stuttering in the United States, Western Europe, and Australia vary greatly, the 5% figure appears to be holding in

Table 2.2   Recent Stuttering Incidence Studies

Study	N	Target	Incidence
Felsenfeld et al. (2000)	3,768	Twins	8.80%
Månsson (2000)	1,040	Newly born	5.10%
Craig et al. (2002)	12,131	Life time	3.20%
Månsson (2005)	928	Newly born	17.70%
Dworzynski et al. (2007)	12,892	Young twins	8.40%
Reilly et al. (2013)	1,619	Preschool	11.20%

popularity. Reviewing studies published during the current century, Yairi and Ambrose (2013) observed "that four of the six recent incidence studies indicate a trend to up its estimate from the 5% level, with a central figure of 8% or higher. What is important to re-emphasize is that data obtained in early childhood are certainly more valid than data obtained at any other age because of the proximity of observers, both laypersons and professionals, to newly identified cases. Such data constitute minimum estimates because later onsets only add to the reported statistics for early life data" (p. 72). Bloodstein and Bernstein Ratner (2008, p.91) share this view, concluding that the lifetime incidence is *at least* 10%. If valid, the higher incidence for early ages contrasted with a lower incidence for older ages adds credence to high levels of natural recovery as will be discussed in Chapter 3.

Biological Factors in Stuttering Prevalence and Incidence

Familiality

Stuttering tends to occur more frequently than average in families whose members stutter or used to do so. A person who stutters is likely to have one, several, or many relatives with a history of stuttering. This pattern has been reported in many studies. In their review, Yairi, Ambrose, and Cox (1996) concluded that the majority of 28 studies reported between 30% to 60% of people who stutter had a familial incidence of the disorder compared with fewer than 10% of normally fluent people. It appears that the risk for a family member of a person who stutters to also stutter is 3 to 4 times higher than the risk for a family member of a person who does not stutter. Although these studies did not account for differences in family size, and contain other methodological problems, the general picture is clear. Note again the implications of these statistics for clinical risk prognosis. Interestingly, male relatives of a person who stutters are more likely to stutter than female relatives. Kay (1964) found that 39% of male relatives stuttered as compared to 15% of the female relatives. Similar findings were reported by later investigators.

In the past, the familiality of stuttering received psychosocial explanations that supported learning theories of stuttering. For example, Johnson (1955b) suggested that families with stuttering histories may have developed concerns about stuttering that affect their reactions to their children's normal disfluency, reactions that in turn trigger stuttering. Currently, however, ample evidence indicates a strong genetic component to stuttering (see review by Kraft & Yairi, 2012), a topic to be discussed in Chapter 7. The above is a clear example of how incidence data can be, and have been, used to enhance theories of stuttering.

Age

Age is among the strongest risk factors for stuttering mainly because in a very large proportion of cases the disorder erupts during the preschool period. The age factor is also seen in the decline of stuttering incidence and prevalence throughout the life span. Therefore, overall prevalence figures, such as the commonly held 1%, or our own estimate of 0.70% or 0.75%, mask important information. This is illustrated by the following examples. Whereas the Craig et al. (2002) investigation estimated the average prevalence across the life span at 0.72%, the data according to age groups indicated a substantial decline from 1.4% in young children to 0.53% in young adults to only 0.37% in older adults. A more recent study in Belgium, confined to the elementary school through high school population, also found prevalence to decline from 0.78% in the 6- to 10-year olds, to 0.53% in the 11- to 15-year olds, to 0.27% in the 16- to 20-year age group (Van Borsel et al., 2006). An even sharper contrast is seen when we compare the average prevalence of 0.75% with the 2.6% prevalence among 2- to 5-year-old children of either African American or European American heritage (Proctor et al., 2008). An obvious implication of these statistics is a call for greater emphasis on preparing clinicians for working with early childhood stuttering (Craig & Tran, 2005).

The decline in stuttering prevalence with age is directly related to two factors on which we further elaborate in Chapter 3. The first is the sharp reduction in new stuttering incidence after age 4. The second is natural recovery that may occur within weeks after onset but for most children within 3–4 years. Therefore, it is not surprising that the prevalence figures are highest among preschool- and school-aged children, decline during adolescence, and are lowest among adults. A point of interest: The high incidence between ages 2 and 4 has caused various speculations about some relationship between rapid speech and language development and stuttering onset.

Gender

It has been widely recognized that the prevalence of stuttering differs substantially between the genders, being more prevalent in males than in females. In one of the earliest studies, Conradi (1904) found a male-to-female ratio of 3:1. Thirty years later, Louttit and Halls (1936) reported a 3.1:1 ratio, and, after an additional 40 years,

Brady and Hall's (1976) survey yielded, according to our calculations, a ratio of 3.63:1.[3] Interestingly, all three studies covered children from kindergarten to grade 12. In their review, Bloodstein and Bernstein Ratner (2008) conclude that the overall gender ratio is approximately 3:1, which seems reasonable to us. Craig et al. (2002) reported a lower overall estimate of 2.3 males to every female who stutters. However, the most recent relevant study (Van Borsel et al., 2006) yielded a male-to-female ratio of 4.6:1 for a school population of up to age 20.

Why does the gender ratio increase with the advance of age? This may be attributed to a tendency for boys to begin stuttering later than girls, an unsupported speculation, as well as the greater occurrence of natural recovery among girls than boys documented by Yairi and Ambrose (2005). There have been, however, a few exceptional reports. Craig et al. (2002) found a gender ratio decline post adolescence. Also Van Borsel and colleagues (2006) found smaller male-to-female ratios in older groups within the age limits of their study.

> There is an interesting interaction between gender and age. Some of the variations among findings can probably be attributed to the fact that the gender ratio varies with age. For this reason, the ages targeted in incidence and prevalence studies influence their outcome. Most reports have shown a strong trend for the male-to-female ratio to increase appreciably with age. Gender ratio estimates range from approximately 2:1 in preschool-age children (Yairi & Ambrose, 1992b, 2005) to as high as 5.5:1 in 11th and 12th graders (Bloodstein & Bernstein Ratner, 2008 p. 92). Craig et al. (2002) upheld this trend, reporting a range from 2.3:1 in children under age 5 years to 4:1 in youth/young adults.

The gender ratio is particularly interesting because it strongly suggests a genetic contribution to stuttering (Kidd, Kidd, & Records, 1978). A study by the Illinois Stuttering Program (Suresh, Ambrose, Roe et al., 2006) demonstrated that males and females who stutter had different chromosomes on which the strongest signs for the possible presence of genes underlying stuttering were found. There is also increasing evidence for both functional and structural gender brain differences in the general population. For example, substantial differences in gray matter volume and concentration were reported in a large study by Good, Johnsrude, Ashburner et al. (2001). Indeed, research has shown functional brain regions that differ between males and females who stutter (Ingham, Fox, & Ingham, 2004).

It is worth noting that more males than females have been identified in various disabilities, and, generally, also in communication disorders (e.g., Broomfield & Dodd, 2004; Law, Boyle, & Harris, 2000). Other potential factors contributing to gender

---

[3]They mistakenly reported a ratio of 3.9:1

differences could be culturally based, such as different performance expectations for boys and girls, with higher standards and more pressure placed on boys (Schuell, 1946). Also, could there be a tendency for males to be identified and referred to experts at higher rates than females? None of these has received serious attention by research.

Geography, Race, and Culture

Readers should understand that the factors of geography, race, and culture tend to be intermingled. Although race per se is biologically determined, most of the black population lives in sub-Saharan Africa, most whites reside in Europe and America, whereas most Mongoloids populate East Asia. Keep in mind, however, that all the races share 99.99+% of their genetic materials. Also cultural differences are associated with geography, race, and ethnicity. Hence, our attempt to present each of these factors separately should be viewed with these reservations in mind.

Geography

Stuttering is found worldwide. Whereas previous sections in this chapter have focused on data from North America, Europe, and Australia, the professional literature testifies to the presence of the disorder in many geographic locations, including Asia, Africa, and South America. The October 18, 2005, issue of the *ASHA Leader* featured articles written by clinicians and investigators in India, Taiwan, Japan, Cameroon, Brazil, and other countries, describing the local status of the disorder and its treatment. Similarly, research-based data obtained in these and other countries provide additional evidence of the universality of stuttering. Research on incidence and prevalence in Asia, Africa, and South America, however, has been sparse. From what has been done, the results approximate those found in the Western world. For example, a sample of 140,000 Japanese schoolchildren revealed a 0.82% prevalence (Toyoda, 1959); in a much smaller Japanese study it was 0.98% (Ozawa, 1960). In Egypt, prevalence was reported at 0.93% (Okasha, Bishrey, Kamel et al., 1974). In South Africa, 6,581 pupils ages 5–21 yielded prevalence of 1.26% (Aron, 1962). The single study (to our knowledge) reported for the whole of Latin America was carried out in Colombia. Questionnaires were distributed to nearly 1,900 college students, of whom 2% reported stuttering (Ardila, Bateman, & Niño, 1994). The results should be viewed with skepticism due to the many possibilities of errors, including the likelihood that a good number of disinterested normally fluent students did not respond. The equal gender ratio found, quite unlike virtually all past studies on adults, reinforces our concern.

Because of the strong evidence for genetic factors in stuttering, noticeable incidence differences among subpopulations, if found, are not surprising. In particular, small and close groups with high levels of intermarriage, may exhibit a higher percentage of stuttering if the disorder was present in the original founders. The Hutterites, an isolated religious group that left Europe in the late 1800s and settled in the northern Midwest United States is an example (Wittke-Thompson, Ambrose, Yairi et al., 2007).

Alternatively, theoretical perspectives oriented toward learning and environmental explanations of stuttering would also lead to the expectations of marked differences among various cultural and social groups. In addition to the possibility that cultural factors actually influence the occurrence of stuttering, they may contribute artificially to variations in incidence/prevalence data if there is a tendency for community beliefs and values to influence the extent to which people admit that they or others stutter.

Race

Only a few published studies have specifically investigated stuttering in African American children (e.g., Carson & Kanter, 1945; Gillespie & Cooper, 1973). Additionally, few master's and doctoral theses have explored the disorder's prevalence among African American children (Madding, 1995; Neely, 1960). All of these studies surveyed elementary school children, except for Gillespie and Cooper (1973), who focused on adolescents. Overall, the findings tended to support the belief that stuttering occurs more frequently in African American than in European American children (Cooper & Cooper, 1998). Of course, all weaknesses we have attributed to prevalence research in stuttering in general also apply to research concerned with race: The studies are dated, contain many potential measurement errors, and the range of methodological variability creates difficulties in comparing results. Additionally studies conducted prior to 1967 took place in racially segregated school systems, and it is highly probable that the children spoke African American English (AAE). In this dialect, several types of disfluencies, such as revisions, repetitions, and prolongations, represent distinct semantic functions that could have been mistakenly regarded as stuttering (Proctor et al., 2008). A similar concern has been raised for studying Spanish-speaking preschool children, because these nonstuttering children exhibit higher frequencies of all types of disfluencies than monolingual English-speaking children (Watson & Anderson, 2001).

Recent years have seen a renewed interest in this area with a study by Proctor et al. (2008), the only study that zeroed in on preschool children, the age when most stuttering cases have their onset. Using a three-pronged approach that included clinician screening of children, teacher identification, and parent identification, data were collected on 3,164 children ages 2 to 5, 2,223 African Americans and 941 European Americans. The prevalence of stuttering was 2.6% for the African American, and 2.44% for the European American children. The difference was not significant. A few years later, however, scientists at the USA Center for Disease Control and Prevention (Boyle, Boulet, Schieve et al., 2011) surveyed parents and guardians of 119,367 children, age 3–17 years, asking if their child had any of several childhood disabilities, including stuttering (during the past 12 months only). For the white group, prevalence was 1.27%; for the black group prevalence was more than double at 2.63%; and for the Hispanic groups it was 1.96%. The difference between the white and black groups was statistically significant. Keep in mind, however, that the main source was parent reports with no firsthand verification. It would appear, therefore, that at the present the race factor in stuttering, limited here to African American, remains open, requiring more carefully planned investigations. A difficult question is the definition of races in the United States in view of the many individuals presenting various degrees of mixed races. To better examine the contribution of race in stuttering, large, careful incidence and prevalence studies in black Africa would be very helpful (Yairi & Ambrose, 2013).

Culture

For several decades, especially from the 1940s to the 1960s, beliefs that cultural values can significantly influence the incidence of stuttering were popular among speech pathologists and anthropologists. They argued that competitiveness, social pressure, and especially attention to speech skills, increase the incidence and vice versa. These ideas were in line with the influential *diagnosogenic theory* that assigned the cause of stuttering to parents' attitudes toward a child's speech (Johnson & Associates, 1959). Indeed, early reports claimed that certain Native American tribes did not stutter and did not even have a word for stuttering (Snidecor, 1947), whereas other tribes displayed a high incidence of stuttering (Lemert, 1953). Based on his impressions, Lemert (1962) also provided examples of cultural effects on either higher (Japan) or lower (Polynesian islands) occurrence of stuttering. More recently, Ujihira (2011) revisited that line of thinking, suggesting that the incidence/prevalence of stuttering in Japan is low. Unfortunately, his account was not based on hard incidence data.

Evidence eventually emerged for the presence of stuttering, as well as for a word for it, in Native American tribes previously regarded as stuttering-free (Zimmermann, Liljebald, Frank et al., 1983). Furthermore, as mentioned in the previous section, more scientific surveys in several countries did not show markedly different prevalence from American and European studies. These were conducted in countries such as Egypt, Japan, and South Africa, characterized by cultures different from Western cultures.

In the 1940s, Wendell Johnson and John Snidecor claimed they had found a society in which there was no stuttering. Interviews with the Bannock-Shoshone American Indians led them to conclude that the Indians had no word for stuttering and had never seen anything like it (when modeled). Later, in the 1960s, anthropologist Art Frank found conclusive evidence that the tribes had words for stuttering and that there had been people who stuttered present among them. What was the source of the discrepancy? The people in the tribe needed to feel sufficiently safe and trusting of the outsiders before they would admit their knowledge and experience with stuttering. Thus the validity of data collected from cross-cultural interviews depends on investigator rapport with informants.

The cultural domain may also be expanded to include stutterers' socioeconomic status, a factor that attracted some attention several decades ago. At the time, Morgenstern (1956) reported that among 29,500 Scottish schoolchildren, there was a statistically significant tendency for those coming from lower socioeconomic status groups, especially families of semiskilled workers, to be affected by a higher prevalence of stuttering than children from the middle or upper classes. A favorite explanation, fitting well within the then-prevailing diagnosogenic theory, was that upward mobility pressure exerted in these social layers, that is, parents pressuring their children to do better than they have done, causes more children to stutter than in higher classes. These findings and interpretations, however, have failed to gather much, if any, support.

Bilingualism

The ability to speak colloquially in two languages is another cultural aspect that has received some attention in relation to stuttering. Does the introduction of a second language pose a risk factor for stuttering? The available data are scant and suffer from weaknesses identified earlier. Most of the past findings suggested that stuttering is more prevalent among bilingual than among monolingual speakers. Travis, Johnson, and Shover (1937) reported a prevalence of 2.8% and 1.8%, respectively, in 4,827 schoolchildren. In South Africa, stuttering prevalence among bilingual schoolchildren was 2.16% as compared to 1.66% among monolinguals (Stern, 1948). More recent studies that corroborate this trend are lacking. An Internet survey by Au-Yeung, Howell, Davis et al. (2000) of nearly 800 individuals from 40 countries did not support past reports. The percentage of speakers reporting either current or past stuttering was almost identical among monolingual and bilingual speakers, 21.74% and 21.65%, respectively. The validity of this study is questionable for several reasons, including the fact that the majority of the respondents were females, a very atypical sample of people who stutter. A recent study by Howell, Davis, and Williams (2009) sampled children who stutter, ages 8–12+ years, in southeast England. They reported that among 38 bilingual children who stuttered, 36 (95%) stuttered in both languages, and that among 23 children with bilingual development since birth, recovery was lower compared to the monolingual and bilingual children who did not start to acquire the second language until they entered kindergarten. These results should be viewed with caution due to methodological and reporting deficiencies.

Prevalence in Clinical Subpopulations

We turn now to very different subpopulations than the ones discussed in the previous section. Each of these is characterized by a certain abnormality. Knowing the incidence and prevalence of stuttering within these subpopulations might contribute relevant information to our understanding of stuttering. In a well-known review of the stuttering literature, Andrews et al. (1983) noted that various disorders, especially obvious neurological conditions such as cerebral palsy, are associated with a higher than expected prevalence of stuttering. Consequently, they entertained the idea that more subtle central nervous system (CNS) dysfunctions may be causative factors of disfluent speech. Taking a different angle, several researchers investigated how many people who stutter also exhibit other disorders. Indeed, they found that stuttering tends to be associated with a host of other disorders (Arndt & Healy, 2001; Blood, Ridenour, Qualls et al., 2003). This raises the prospect that stuttering may be either a causative agent or a co-occurring disorder that shares a common cause. Regardless, we have emphasized the value of understanding incidence and prevalence differences in various groups. Either unusually high or unusually low figures could provide clues concerning the causes, precipitating factors, and treatment of stuttering. Several such groups are discussed next.

Hearing Impairment

One of the most interesting phenomena within our topic of incidence and prevalence is that people who suffer substantial loss of their hearing sense exhibit little or no stuttering. This could be a form of indirect evidence regarding the nature and cause of stuttering. In other words, if sufficient auditory acuity is needed to stutter, one may infer that processes involving auditory self-monitoring of speech play a role in the disorder.

Two early teacher surveys of schools for the deaf (as these were called), with a total student population of 28,000, yielded only 14 cases, a prevalence of only 0.05%, or a 20th of 1% (Backus, 1938; Harms & Malone, 1939). It is important to point out that only oral communication was considered. Since then, Montgomery and Fitch (1988) carried out the last prevalence study in this population; they also sought information for stuttering in manual communication. Responses to a questionnaire survey from 77 schools for the hearing impaired with a total of 9,930 students revealed only 12 children who stuttered: 3 in the oral mode, 6 in the manual mode, and 3 in both modes. Stuttering in the manual mode occurs as repetitive or prolonged movements of the hands or arms while signing language. The prevalence of 0.12%, is still considerably lower than that in the population at large. Of interest is the finding that the perceived manual disfluency was more prevalent than the oral disfluency. Silverman and Silverman (1971) too reported on the presence of "manual stuttering" among deaf people. According to the experience of one of us (Seery), however, clinicians should not be surprised to encounter people with moderate hearing loss who stutter.

Anecdotal observations by professionals who had extensive contact with this group have supported the conclusion pertaining to the rarity of stuttering in deaf people. Gutzmann (1912) commented that this was a well-known fact, and Bluemel (1913) noted that Gallaudet, a famous educator of the deaf, had stated that in 50 years of experience he could not recall ever encountering a deaf person who stuttered. Thus a connection between stuttering and audition is strongly suspected.

The hypothesis of a stuttering–audition link has been reinforced because high-level masking noise, which in effect reduces hearing, often results in a temporary reduction, or complete suppression, of stuttering, a phenomenon that has been applied in therapy. The theoretical views and recent research of the relation between stuttering and audition and related brain structure and function are discussed in Chapter 7.

Cleft Palate

Another clinical group with an apparently low occurrence of stuttering is that of individuals born with cleft palate and hypernasal speech. Here again, if this finding is upheld, it may have implications for the underlying causal factors of stuttering. The relevant literature, however, is limited. Bloodstein (1981) observed that stuttering in individuals with cleft palate is uncommon but did not provide substantiating data. Schwartz (1976) discussed a single case of a child with cleft palate who stuttered when wearing a corrective appliance. Blood and Seider (1981) reported that in a sample of 1,060 stutterers identified in the caseload of 358 speech-language clinicians, only 1% was composed of cleft palate patients. This finding, however, pertains to the occurrence of cleft palate among people who stutter, not the occurrence of stuttering in people with cleft palate.

The only direct study on this population was conducted by Dalston et al. (1987), employing retrospective examinations of the records of 534 patients, ages 3–66 years, all with structural anomalies that affected the velopharyngeal closure. Only one person in the sample, less than 0.2% of the total, was identified by speech-language clinicians as manifesting stuttering. Such a low occurrence of stuttering in individuals likely to experience considerable parental intrusive behavior and concern about their speech (Long & Dalston, 1983) raises questions about theoretical positions that claim negative environmental reactions to speech cause stuttering (e.g., Johnson & Associates, 1959). The phenomenon, however, gives rise to physiological considerations, for example, the possible relation between the duration of intraoral pressure drop and speaking rate. It is known that the overall speaking rate of people with cleft palate is slower than normal. Slowing down the speaking rate also increases fluency in people who stutter.

Cognitive Impairment

Whereas those with cleft palate and those who with hearing impairments present a lower incidence of stuttering than the general population, on the other end of the spectrum is the population of people with low mental abilities (called "mentally retarded" in past terminology) as classified by intelligence tests and other assessments. Several studies have reported considerably higher than normal incidence in this population. In the general group of cognitive impaired, early studies indicated 14% to 17%[4] prevalence (Gottsleben, 1955; Schlanger & Gottsleben, 1957), whereas later findings suggested lower figures of 2.5% to 7.0% (Chapman & Cooper, 1973; Schaeffer & Shearer, 1968). Apparently the prevalence of stuttering increases with the severity of the impairment. According to Boberg, Ewart, Mason et al. (1978), stuttering was twice as frequent among the trainable mentally retarded (TMR; IQs of 25 to 50) compared to the educable mentally retarded (EMR; IQs of 50 to 70). Similar results were reported by Brady and Hall (1976). They found 1.60% stuttering cases among those with relatively higher IQs; it was twice as high, 3.08%, for students with lower IQs.

---

[4]In a small study of only 74 children, Schlanger (1953) reported that more than 20% exhibited stuttering.

Most interesting are data pertaining to the Down syndrome subgroup, for whom surveys yielded prevalence estimates ranging from 15% (Schubert, 1966) to an extreme of 53.20% (Preus, 1973). Although some have argued that the high prevalence figures may have resulted from possibly confusing cluttering, hesitation, and expressive language difficulties for stuttering, others have maintained that stuttering characteristics exhibited by this subpopulation are similar to those observed in the population at large. Those with cognitive impairment who stutter, however, show low emotional reactivity to their stuttering (Preus, 1973, 1990). Otto and Yairi (1976) reported that children with Down syndrome, even if they are not regarded as exhibiting stuttering, produce very disfluent speech, including repetitions of syllables and words.

The high prevalence of stuttering in people with Down syndrome calls attention to a host of possible influences on stuttering, for example, chromosomal abnormality and/or motor deficiencies caused by low muscle tone during the critical stages of oral skills development. A genotyping study by Suresh et al. (2006) found the strongest indications for possible genes underlying stuttering was for females who stutter, and that sign was located on chromosome 21, the one that has also been implicated in Down syndrome. At the present, however, whether these two facts are related remains unknown. Additionally, the frequent occurrence of stronger vocabulary skills than expressive language abilities among children with Down syndrome provides clues that differences in the level of skills seen in certain areas of language proficiency may be an important factor in stuttering.

Although much of the data concerning stuttering among the cognitively impaired were collected more than 30 years ago, there has been recent support in a study conducted in Belgium. Among the 1,272 pupils attending special schools, including the so-called mentally handicapped, 2.28% were reported to stutter, 4 times more than in the regular schools surveyed. This group, however, also included children with emotional and physical problems (Van Borsel et al., 2006).

Other Groups

Scattered information has been published about other clinical groups showing either higher or lower prevalence than in the population at large. Higher prevalence was found for people with epilepsy (Gens, 1951), brain damage (Bohme, 1977), and psychosis (Freund, 1955). Lower prevalence was found for people with diabetes (Boldon, 1955). Generally, however, all pertinent surveys are outdated, small, not well documented, and sometimes contradictory.

Summary

We learn about how many and who stutter by studying aspects related to the incidence and prevalence of stuttering. Prevalence and incidence data are very useful for understanding the nature and possible cause(s) of stuttering, guiding the preparation of clinicians to specific needs of subpopulations, overall planning of clinical services at the national and local levels, and for obtaining financial resources for both research and clinical purposes. Thus they are important to the development of both theory and treatment for stuttering. Key points made in this chapter include:

- *Incidence* is the estimate of the chance of occurrence of any disorder. *Prevalence* is the estimate of how many people exhibit the disorder at a specific time period. Data on these two parameters are essential for designing studies of people who stutter, constructing genetic models of stuttering, and understanding its developmental trends.

- Appropriate interpretations of incidence and prevalence estimates require an appreciation of the varying methods that may have influenced the available data. Target populations have varied widely, and different approaches have been used, including cross-sectional, longitudinal, and retrospective studies.

- Methodological dissimilarities across studies have been related to the definition of stuttering, the specific technique of data collection (e.g., mailed questionnaires; direct examination), and the people providing the information about who stutters.

- Although 5% has been commonly cited as the lifetime incidence of stuttering, more recent findings indicate the possibility that it is as high as 8% or even higher. More research is needed to verify this new estimate.

- The overall prevalence of stuttering appears to be lower than the traditionally accepted 1% level and is probably closer to 0.70%.

- Children who stutter often are born into families that have other members who stutter. The strong familiality of stuttering has given rise to several interpretations of the disorder, among which genetics has prevailed.

- Incidence and prevalence data reveal clear evidence for an age factor in stuttering. With possible slight variations, both incidence and prevalence decline across the life span.

- The age-related diminution in the number of people who stutter reflects the combined factors of (a) declining new incidences in older ages, and (b) the growing number of natural recovery cases.

- Among preschoolers, prevalence may be larger than 2%, nearly three times higher than the average prevalence across the life span. Therefore, it would seem justified to alter the common perception that stuttering is a "small" problem. From a practical point of view, more resources should be directed to the study of stuttering in young children and for the preparation of clinicians to treat them and provide parent counseling.

- Both the incidence and prevalence of stuttering are gender-influenced with males running twice the risk of females to exhibit the disorder initially; the risk for them to sustain stuttering over years or even for life is much greater.

- The male-to-female gender ratio is smallest in very young children, generally increasing with age (small ratio fluctuations between specific age brackets are possible). Overall, older age brackets include fewer stutterers, mostly males.

- The combined effect of the age and gender factors is to shrink the stuttering population as it matures and to greatly increase its male predominance. Such extensive changes in the composition of people who stutter should be kept in mind prior to reaching conclusions about the "nature of stuttering" when based on observations of a narrow, adult population segment.

- Several clinical groups reveal large deviations, up or down, from the prevalence of stuttering in the population at large. Better understanding of such departures may provide relevant clues about the causes and nature of the disorder.

- Although there have been some indications for differences in the occurrence of stuttering in diverse cultural and racial populations spread over diverse geographic regions, much of the available information or reported impressions have not been adequately substantiated. Furthermore, it is not clear that, even if large differences exist, they are indeed due to cultural factors. Although culture may be a factor, genetic factors underlie incidence in specific groups is a serious alternative.

Study Questions and Discussion Topics

1. Test your knowledge of incidence/prevalence by answering questions about hypothetical data, presented in the table here, from a combined longitudinal and cross-sectional study of children 3 to 5 years of age.
   a. You will notice that one group of children was sampled longitudinally for all 3 years of the study (no attrition). How many children were in that group?
   b. Does this table offer information about incidence or prevalence? Why?
   c. What would you need to know in order to estimate the other kind of information (from Question C)?
   d. How do the estimates change most, according to year or according to age?

Hypothetical Cases of Stuttering in 3,400 Children Ages 3 to 5 Years in Each Year, 2102 to 2104

	Age 3 Years			Age 4 Years			Age 5 Years		
Year	Stuttering Cases	Pop. Sample	%	Stuttering Cases	Pop. Sample	%	Stuttering Cases	Pop. Sample	%
2102	20	400	5.0	15	600	2.5	15	900	1.67
2103	28	700	4.0	12	400	3.0	8	600	1.33
2104	32	800	4.0	14	700	2.0	6	400	1.50
Total	80	1,900	4.21	41	1,700	2.41	29	1,900	1.52

2. What are the advantages and disadvantages of surveying reports of schoolteachers to study the prevalence of stuttering?

3. What is a retrospective study? What are the limitations of retrospective studies in gathering incidence data?

4. Does stuttering vary across populations with the following characteristics? If so, how?
   a. Geographic region
   b. Gender
   c. Age
   d. Hearing impairment
   e. Cleft palate
   f. Cognitive impairment
5. Which figure is apt to be larger, prevalence or lifetime incidence of stuttering?
6. What are the research and clinical implications of incidence and prevalence data for stuttering?
7. What are plausible explanations for the variations in the sex ratio that occur with age in the stuttering population?
8. What factors may account for differences in the incidence of stuttering among cultures and races if, indeed, such differences are confirmed?

Websites

Incidence and Prevalence of Speech, Voice, and Language Disorders in Adults in the United States: 2008 Edition at the American Speech-Language-Hearing Association Web site. Accessed December 3, 2013, from http://www.asha.org/Research/reports/speech_voice_language/

Research on Incidence and Prevalence of Stuttering at the Stuttering Foundation of America Web site. Accessed December 3, 2013, from http://www.stutteringhelp.org/research-incidence-and-prevalence-stuttering

Suggested Readings

Craig A., Hancock, K., Tran, Y., Craig, M., & Peters, K. (2002). Epidemiology of stuttering in the community across the entire life span. *Journal of Speech-Language-Hearing Research, 45,* 1097–1105.

Lubker, B. B. (1997). Epidemiology: An essential science for speech-language pathology and audiology. *Journal of Communication Disorders, 30*(4), 251–267.

Månsson, H. (2000). Childhood stuttering: Incidence and development. *Journal of Fluency Disorders, 25,* 47–57.

Van Borsel, J., Moeyaert J., Rosseel, R., van Loo E., & van Renterghem T. (2006). Prevalence of stuttering in regular and special school populations in Belgium based on teacher perceptions. *Folia Phoniatrica et Logopaedica, 58,* 289–302.

Proctor, A., Yairi, E., Duff, M, & Zhang, J. (2008). Prevalence of stuttering in African American preschool children. *Journal of Speech, Language, and Hearing Research, 50,* 1465–1474.

Yairi, E., & Ambrose, N. (2013). Epidemiology of stuttering: 21st century advancements. *Journal of Fluency Disorders. 38,* 66–87.

Chapter 3

When and How Does Stuttering Begin? How Does It Develop?

LEARNER OBJECTIVES

Readers of this chapter will be able to:

- Describe features of stuttering onset with respect to age, type of onset, gender, and other factors.
- Explain the theoretical and clinical significance of information concerning stuttering onset.
- Characterize stuttering at onset in terms of disfluent speech, physical concomitants, emotional and physical health, and concomitant disorders.
- Identify potential developmental progressions and paths of stuttering.
- Differentiate phenomena of natural recovery from and persistence in stuttering.
- Evaluate research methods employed in the study of onset.

Theoretical and Clinical Significance

Among the most challenging issues regarding stuttering has been its beginning, or "onset." The desire to know and understand the details of when, how, and what begins is natural for speech-language clinicians and researchers alike. The potential theoretical significance of the onset event is seen in its relationship to the age factor. If stuttering typically began after age 25, then parental behavior and attitudes would receive minimal consideration as potential causative agents. However, because it typically begins in early years of life, when (1) children are under the heavy influence of their immediate environment, (b) anatomical structures for speech are growing quickly, and (c) speech and language skills are expanding sharply, then the possibilities of a parental role and/or vulnerabilities in the speech fluency system due to developmental processes, should be considered. It is understandable, therefore, why a theory depicting the young child's home environment as the cause of stuttering attracted much attention (Johnson & Associates, 1959) or, as explained by others, stuttering arises when various demands, both internal and external to children, exceed their motor, linguistic, cognitive, and other capacities to sustain fluent speech (Adams, 1990; Starkweather & Gottwald, 1990). More about these theoretical notions is explained in Chapter 6. In a similar vein, we may look at what we call the *manner* of onset. Whereas sudden onsets may give rise to suspicions of organic or psychogenic agents being involved, gradual onset favors learning explanations of stuttering (e.g., Wischner, 1950) because habit-forming processes take time. Another possibility is that a sudden or gradual onset of stuttering represents a sudden or gradual shift into adopting a new speech motor strategy or new language structure. Other examples could be cited to illustrate why good scientific information on onset is pertinent for theories about the disorder of stuttering.

Similarly, professionals' strong interests are directed to what happens after stuttering has begun: the early features (symptomatology) of stuttering, how they change with time, and the duration of the disorder. Here too, several examples will illustrate how stuttering features at onset and early developmental paths have theoretical and practical significance. If very early symptomatology does not reveal psychological problems or emotional reactions (e.g., anxiety) specifically when the child stutters, then theories that propose emotional maladjustment or anxiety as the etiology of stuttering lose ground. This same evidence is also relevant for the kind of treatment selected, such as play-based psychotherapy versus speech therapy. Also, if some children's symptoms run only a short course and then recede and vanish, whereas others' persist for a long time, it will be extremely helpful to identify these subgroups and distinguish them early on to facilitate clinical decision making. Furthermore, if stuttering persists, does it follow one or several courses? Is it possible that different patterns of onset and/or development indicate the presence of several stuttering subtypes? Information pertaining to these questions will have important theoretical and clinical implications.

In spite of the importance of issues involving the onset and development of stuttering and its symptoms, for many years they attracted limited scientific research. One reason is that both topics have proved to be difficult to investigate due to a variety of factors discussed later. Still, encouraging progress has been made, especially in the past 25 years.

Yairi and Ambrose (1992a, 2005) explain that unlike disordered language and phonology resulting from a child's failure to adequately develop those skills, and therefore having no identifiable onset, stuttering usually appears *after* a child has already demonstrated the skill of normal speech fluency. With stuttering, major changes *have* occurred. The child has suffered a loss: his or her fluency. The loss of an important function is easily observable and has dramatic effects. Parental alarm and panic reactions to the pronounced negative changes are common, adding a major emotional element to the problem. Also the child may be reacting, although unable to communicate this effectively. In contrast, children with disordered phonology did not possess good phonology that they then lost.

Onset

General Issues and Research Methods

As stated in Chapter 1, the vast majority of developmental stuttering cases begin in early childhood. In this respect, it is one of several communication disorders affecting young children. There is, however, an important distinction in that many cases of stuttering have an identifiable onset observed by parents or others. The fact that there is a general recognition of an event called the "onset of stuttering," has justified scientific effort to investigate it.

Scientific studies of stuttering onset are difficult because (a) there are no warning signs that onset is about to occur, and therefore (b) investigators cannot predict the right place and time to objectively document the very earliest stuttering or secure data even shortly thereafter. Yes, there have been a few individual case study reports (e.g., Mowrer, 1998) in which the investigator had access to a child close to the time of onset. The quality of these studies, however, varies in terms of the detail of the recorded observations and provision of quantified speech data. Although such reports provide insight, the small number of cases and limited information make results insufficient for generalization. To improve the chances for closer observations, Dutch scientists investigated onset in children from families in which one or both parents had stuttered themselves. This was done because, due to genetics, their chance of having children who stutter is much higher than for the population at large (Kloth, Janssen, Kraaimaat et al. 1995). One weakness of this method is that those families represent a biased sample of the stuttering population. Typically, fewer than 40% of those who stutter have a parent with a history of stuttering. In the Kloth et al. study, 100% of the children had at least one parent who stuttered.

An alternative research method would attempt to create stuttering onset intentionally in normally speaking individuals. This approach, however, would be unethical. An accusation was made that a master's thesis study conducted by Tudor (1939) under the mentorship of the late Wendell Johnson, a notable scientist in the field, attempted and succeeded at doing just this (Silverman, 1988). Johnson hypothesized that when parents

---

Many years later, the unpublished Tudor study was brought to light and heavily criticized for its harmful effects. Several U.S. newspapers repeated the accusation that the experiment caused stuttering (e.g., the *San Jose Mercury News* in its June 10 and 11, 2001, editions). Subsequently, two independent scientists (Ambrose & Yairi, 2002) carefully scrutinized the text and data in Tudor's master's thesis at the University of Iowa. They concluded that contrary to the accusations, the objectives of the study were not intended to turn normally speaking children into stutterers but to observe whether disfluency frequencies changed from their preexperimental levels (some of which were already rather high). Furthermore, the levels of stuttering-like disfluency (SLD), the most pertinent to stuttering, were not significantly altered from pre- to postexperimental analyses. Perceptual ratings of the level of disfluency by a group of judges also did not change. Hence no evidence was found that stuttering was the specific outcome of the study. All in all, the scrutiny of the study objectives, procedures, and results failed to support the accusations that the experiment actually caused stuttering (Ambrose & Yairi, 2002). Unfortunately, Silverman (2004) continued to sway newspapers and laypersons' opinions to the opposite opinion, while completely ignoring the work of other scientists in this regard.

or other adult listeners respond negatively to a child's normal speech hesitations and repetitions, the child reacts with tension in his or her speech that eventually develops into real stuttering. In the Tudor study, orphanage staff members were instructed to create such conditions by conveying overt concern, even correcting certain children when they hesitated or repeated words. Tudor collected speech samples and severity ratings at the beginning and at the end of one school semester so that comparisons could be made. Although a discerning examination of the data should have raised stronger doubts about the effects of the staff's reactions, the discussion of results in Tudor's thesis was slanted in favor of Johnson's hypothesis.

Other studies by Johnson relied on the most common approach to childhood stuttering onset: retrospective reports by caregivers of past observations. Typically, information is elicited through often lengthy, face-to-face interviews with parents of children who stutter. Questions such as the following usually are included: (1) When did your child first begin stuttering? (2) Who was the first to notice it? (3) What were the speech characteristics of the first stuttering? (Parents are also asked to mimic the early stuttering.) (4) How severe was the stuttering? (5) Was the first stuttering associated with physical illness or emotional stress? (6) Was the early stuttering associated with body tension? This approach runs several risks, too. The first potential problem is cases that are missed when only children who have stuttered for a set minimum period of time (e.g., 6 months) are identified and recruited for the study. Because many children who begin stuttering will stop within a short time after onset, participant selection criteria should not eliminate these cases, some of which can be quite severe. Typically, this appreciable subpopulation was not tapped in most past onset studies.

A second problem is that often data were obtained from parents a long time after the onset. A British study by Andrews and Harris (1964) used 80 children between 9 and 11 years of age. Because stuttering typically begins between ages 2 and 4, parents had to remember details of events that occurred years in the past. In the United States, Milisen and Johnson (1936) interviewed parents nearly 20 years after their children began stuttering. Apparently many parents prefer to adopt a wait-and-see strategy before seeking the services of a speech-language clinician. Perhaps they listen to a pediatrician's advice that the stuttering will go away (Yairi & Carrico, 1992). The end result is that genuine early stuttering is rarely observed in research. This raises the risk of obtaining low-accuracy data based on parents' vague, if not faulty, memory of significant details. For example, whether the first stuttering was composed of syllable repetitions or also of sound prolongations, how many times did the child repeat a syllable or a word (two? four?), and whether secondary characteristics, such as eye closing, were noticed. Few may appreciate the fact that the difference between repeating a syllable twice or four times is indeed a large one in this context and has a very significant impact. At the time of onset, parents are not particularly tuned in to such fine details; hence they may not offer the most accurate information later on.

Studies Concerning Onset

Systematic research of stuttering onset probably began with a little known study by Taylor (1937) at the University of Iowa in which parents of 47 stuttering children, ages 3 to 7 years, were interviewed concerning the circumstances of the onset and the early characteristics of the stuttering. A series of three studies then followed, all conducted at the same university. In 1942, Johnson reported findings also based on retrospective interviews of parents of 46 stuttering children; so did Darley (1955) for parents of 50 stuttering and 50 nonstuttering children. The largest investigation was carried out by Johnson and his colleagues (1959) using an extensive 840-item questionnaire to interview both parents of 150 children who stuttered, ages 2 to 9, and their nonstuttering peers. The standard interviews in all three studies probed into the onset of stuttering, child development, health history and status, child-rearing practices, home environment, and more. Their drawbacks were the wide age range of the children (2 to 9 years of age) and the long time gaps between the onset and the time when interviews were conducted (e.g., 50 months in the 1955 Darley study; 18 months in the 1959 Johnson & Associates study). Another significant study was conducted in Britain with 80 children ages 9 to 11 (Andrews & Harris, 1964). Limited information was also provided by Glasner and Rosenthal (1957), who interviewed parents of 153 young CWS. They, however, asked only four questions.

Several decades later, parent interview studies of stuttering onset were carried out at the University of Illinois at Urbana-Champaign. The first one by Yairi (1983) included only 23 stuttering children. Results for a larger sample of 87 children exhibiting early stuttering onset were reported by Yairi and Ambrose (1992b). Finally, in 2005 these two investigators presented data for 156 children. The Illinois investigations mark significant procedural improvements in that they were conducted directly with children (in addition to the parents) within a narrow age range (ages 2 to 5), and within 5 months, on the average, from the time of onset; some within days and weeks. The 5-month post-onset period was less than one third of the interval in the Johnson studies. Therefore, parents' reports were less colored by the passage of time. Also, recorded speech samples provided hard evidence about the stuttering, supplemented by data related to language and phonological skills.

The renewed interest in onset is also seen in European countries: Britain (Buck, Lees, & Cook, 2002), the Netherlands (Kloth et al., 1995), and Denmark (Månsson, 2000, 2005). Each of the two Månsson studies surveyed nearly all newborn children on Bornholm, a Danish island, and included approximately 1,000 children born during 2 consecutive years (1990–1991 and 1995–1996). Soon after their third birthday, the children were examined and their parents interviewed concerning stuttering. The Danish studies, too, represent important improvements in procedures because entire populations, not just samples, participated, and direct observations, as well as parent interviews, were conducted close to the time of onset. The most recent, and still ongoing, investigation has been carried out in Melbourne, Australia (Reilly et al. 2009; 2013). Here, 1,613 families in the community have agreed to participate in a longitudinal study of the language and speech development of their children, beginning at 8 months of age. Parents who suspected that their child began stuttering had to contact the investigators for verification. Minimal data about onset were secured in other studies (e.g., Howell, Davis, & Williams, 2008).

When Does Stuttering Begin?

In assessing research concerned with when stuttering begins, the age of the sample must be considered. Samples of children 2 to 6 years old will miss a few later onsets and are likely to yield a lower mean age at onset than samples of 6- to10-year-olds, even if both span a 4-year period. The younger sample will detect the many cases of very early onsets who recover naturally before they reach age 6. This is illustrated in the following studies: Yairi (1983) studied children under age 4 and found the mean age at onset was 28 months; Johnson and associates (1959) studied children under age 9 and found a mean onset age of 42 months; and Andrews and Harris (1964) studied children 11 to 13 years and the mean age at onset climbed to 60 months. We hold that the younger sample yields the most valid data because it captures cases that would have been otherwise lost to investigators due to large natural recovery, a phenomenon discussed later.

With the qualifications just listed in mind, data from various onset studies report a wide age range when stuttering begins, from as young as 18 months (Milisen & Johnson, 1936; Yairi, 1983) to the older teenage period (Preus, 1981). After age 9, however, the frequency of onsets is low. Stuttering onsets in adults are rare and typically linked to clear origins, either emotional traumas (Mahr & Leith, 1992) or brain damage (De Nil, Jokel, & Rochon 2007). They have been distinguished from developmental stuttering in children because of the likelihood they have a different etiology.

The available research and clinical evidence indicates that most stuttering onsets occur prior to age 5. In one study of 179 stuttering children, only 5 had onset later than age 4 (Månsson, 2000). Differences in sample sizes and procedures make it difficult to arrive at an overall mean age at onset. Recent studies conducted with considerably greater rigor than past ones indicate that the mean onset falls prior to the age of 3 years. Gender does not seem to exert influence on the age at onset.

Table 3.1 presents data for mean age of onset for five studies that used younger children and three studies that used older children. The mean age at onset for the first group is 32.4 months. The mean age for the second group is 52.6 months. This difference emphasizes our point concerning the influence of participants' age on the

Table 3.1 Mean or Median (*) Age in Months at Stuttering Onset

Study	Sample Size	M/F Ratio	Age	Age at Onset		
				Total	**Boys**	**Girls**
Månsson (2000)	53	1.65	by age 8	33.0	34.0	31.0
Buck, Lees, & Cook (2002)	61	2.2	by age 7	36.3	35.1	39.1
Månsson (2005)	179	1.34	by age 4	30	30.5	32.9
Yairi & Ambrose (2005)	163	2.1	by age 5	33	33.6	32.9
Reilly et al. (2009)	137	1.58	by age 3[1*]	29.9	29.3	29.7[2]
SUBGROUP MEAN				32.4		
Johnson & Associates (1959)	150		by age 9	42	42.4	41.2
Andrews & Harris (1964)	80		ages 11–13	60		
Howell, Davis, & Williams (2008)	76	5.33	ages 8–12	54.8	54.0	58.5
SUBGROUP MEAN				52.7		

[1*] All but two children began stuttering by 3 years of age.

[2] The gender breakdown was provided by Reilly in a personal communication (2012).

resultant mean age at onset. In our judgment, the mean of 32 months is much more reflective of the great majority of onsets. This is also apparent as we study the age distribution for onset. Some studies reported that nearly 60% of onsets take place between 24 and 36 months of age, the 3rd year of life, increasing to 85% by 42 months of age, and to 95% by age 48 months, the 4th birthday (Yairi & Ambrose, 2005). These data are relevant to other issues because in many cases the onset of stuttering parallels a critical period of fast growth of the child's speech mechanism as well as his or her speech and language skills. Indeed, links between stuttering and these factors have been suggested (Bernstein Ratner, 1997a).

How Does Stuttering Begin?

The view that stuttering always begins gradually, almost inconspicuously, with easy repetitions, no tension, and with the child being unaware of it, has been entrenched for over 100 years (Bluemel, 1913). Froeschels (1943) even stated that only in rare cases did stuttering onset deviate from this pattern, and Johnson and associates (1959) further promoted the concept. Contradictory observations were ignored, perhaps under the influence of learning theories that savor reinforcement dynamics whereby the initial easy disfluency gradually turns into full-fledged stuttering.

The traditional view, however, was somewhat contested when sudden onset was reported by Van Riper (1971) for 10% of 114 cases and by Preus (1981) for 17% of 100 cases. More recent data have further and drastically altered the picture. In a careful study of 87 children and parents soon after onset, Yairi and Ambrose (1992b) reported that for 44% of the children onset was judged by parents as sudden, with 31% describing it as an abrupt change over a single day. Later, these authors reported that nearly 30% of 163 children exhibited abrupt onset that took hold in a single day. Adding onsets that occurred over 2 to 3 days, the total sudden onsets exceeded 40%. Intermediate onsets (1 to 2 weeks) comprised 33% of the cases, with only 28% reporting gradual onset longer than 2 weeks. Males and females were distributed similarly also in respect to onset type (Yairi & Ambrose, 2005). Finally, in the Reilly et al. (2009) study of 169 children, 50% had sudden onset: 37.2% within one day and 12.4% within 2 to 3 days. In short, during the past 20-plus years, conventional concepts of the onset of stuttering have been altered with gradual onsets found to be the *least,* not the most, frequently reported.

I am desperately trying to find help for my preschooler. Denise will be 4 years old in approximately two months and has always excelled at speaking. She is the oldest of three children, one of them is only one year younger. She suddenly developed severe stuttering a week ago. She never stuttered at all before this, nor was she slow in speech development in any way. It was as if someone had flipped a light switch, and her speech dramatically changed. She is very, very smart. I know that all parents think that their child is intelligent, but mine really is (Ha Ha). Honestly though, I would get comments all of the time from complete strangers about how well she was talking and communicating. She stutters so severely now (and it has only been 7 days) that at times she will just quit trying to say the word she is stuck on and become silent. I will then say, "It's OK, baby, what were you saying?" And she will reply, "I can't." When she is stuck on a word, she will look at me with terrified eyes, and it is almost as though she CAN'T stop trying to say the word.

I have tried with great patience to follow all of the advice I can find from Web sites. They tell me not to acknowledge the stuttering, slow my speech, not finish her sentences, remain calm, etc. Nothing has helped in any way and it is dramatically worse even in these short 7 days. She asked me today, "Mommy, why can't I talk right?" (This question was a struggle that literally took at least a minute and a half to get through.) Her stuttering is so severe that it is literally robbing her of the ability to communicate with me. Although she diligently tries for a VERY long time to finish her thoughts, she is starting to quit talking and remain quiet.

I am desperate. I have an appointment today with her pediatrician and am thinking of enrolling her in speech therapy. However, with all of the conflicting reports out there, I don't know if I should ignore the stuttering and act as though it is not happening (I don't want to exacerbate the condition even more), or if I should proactively insist on speech therapy. The studies are totally conflicting. Although I do not show her my anxiety, I must tell you that I am completely overwhelmed and saddened. If you have any advice, I would be grateful to receive it. Please let me know what you have found to be helpful for a child in her situation. I cannot understand how this could literally start overnight and yet be so devastating.

Thank you so much for your time. Also, please let me know of any reference material that is beneficial.

In addition to more variation in the manner of onset, large-scale research also contradicted the traditional view that early stuttering is characterized by mild, if not normal, repetitions. Far from this, the Illinois studies reported that most parents said the early stuttering was moderate to severe, associated with some degree of force, even severe tension, and more than 20% thought their child was aware of the problem (Yairi & Ambrose, 1992b, 2005). The following letter received from a mother (personal details altered) vividly illustrates the above findings concerning abruptness of onset, severity of stuttering at onset, and early awareness of the stuttering. Also note the expressed parental anguish.

Features of Early Stuttering

Having briefly discussed when and how stuttering begins, the next question is what are its early speech characteristics and other features. What can the speech-language clinician expect? These are presented next.

Types and Frequency of Disfluencies

From the early research of stuttering onset and beyond, there has been considerable agreement about its most common features. Already in 1937 Taylor found that 85% of parents reported repetitions, especially of whole words, as the initial symptom of concern. A few years later, Johnson (1942) reported that 90% of parents described early stuttering as repetitions of parts of words, whole words, or phrases, typically at the beginning of speech attempts. Darley made a similar report in 1955. Johnson and associates (1959) stated that the most frequent features of early stuttering recounted were syllable repetitions (60% of parents) and word repetitions (50% of parents). In the Yairi (1983) study, parents of 95% of the children recalled syllable repetitions at onset and 40% also recalled word repetitions. Nevertheless, the symptomatology at onset is not confined to repetitions as writers have emphasized for a long time (e.g., from Froeschels in 1943 to Packman, Code, & Onslow in 2007). Just about all investigators reported other stuttering-like disfluencies observed by parents. Between 8% and 16% of the children exhibited what were described as sound stoppages, complete blocks, prolongation, and articulatory fixations (Darley 1955; Johnson & Associates, 1959; Taylor, 1937). Yairi and Ambrose (1992b) found that 36% of the children had sound prolongations at the time of onset, 23% had conspicuous silent periods, and 14% had blocks.

Recall that the preceding descriptions are based on retrospective reports. Quantified objective information became available only in the past 30 years when Yairi and Lewis (1984) insisted on (1) identifying children within 2 months of onset, (2) using children representing a narrow age range (25 to 39 months of age), and (3) recording speech for direct observation and analysis.[1] They found large differences in the disfluencies produced by children who stuttered and normally fluent peers, providing strong evidence

---

[1]Johnson and Associates (1959) also provided valuable information based on analyses of recorded speech of 89 children but these were taken up to 3 years post-onset.

that speech at onset is far from being normal as claimed by adherents to Johnson and associates' (1959) theory of stuttering. Their findings were confirmed by other investigators (e.g., Schwartz, Zebrowski, & Conture, 1990), as well as in larger studies at the University of Illinois (e.g., Ambrose & Yairi, 1999). Overlap between the two groups in the stuttering-like disfluencies was small.

Data on the disfluency frequency and types typical of children near stuttering onset as compared with normally speaking peers are shown in Table 3.2. As you can see, the gap between the two groups on the three disfluency types called *stuttering-like disfluency* is large. The two groups, however, are very similar with respect to *other disfluencies* i.e., interjections, revisions, phrase repetitions.

Length/Extent of Disfluencies

The numbers (frequency) and types of disfluency are not the only parameters of interest. The length of disfluent events is also important, often critical. Take two children, each of whom repeats the word *and* on five different words within 100 words. One child repeats the word only one extra time (and-and) on each occasion, whereas the second child repeats four extra times (and-and-and-and-and) on each occasion (each extra iteration is called a "repetition unit"). Although the count of disfluent words, 5, is the same, their disfluent speech is vastly different in quantity, and listeners will perceive it so. The first, a normally fluent child, would have uttered the word *and* a total of 10 times (5 × 2) as compared to 25 times (5 × 5) for the second child who exhibits stuttering. Hence information on the frequency of disfluency alone may be insufficient. Both Johnson (1942) and Darley (1955), two well-known researchers of stuttering onset, commented that parents described the early stuttering as two to four iterations of syllables, words, or phrases. The investigators referred to such

---

Table 3.2   Mean per 100 Syllables for Stuttering-Like Disfluencies (SLD) and Other Disfluencies for Stuttering and Normally Fluent Children

Disfluency Type	Stuttering Children, Mean (*N* = 103)	Normally Fluent Children, Mean (*N* = 52)
Part-word repetition	5.64	0.55
Single-syllable word repetition	3.24	0.79
Disrhythmic phonation	2.42	0.08
Total SLD	11.30	1.41
Other disfluencies	5.79	4.48

Source: Adapted from *Early Childhood Stuttering* (p. 320) by E. Yairi and N. G. Ambrose (2005), Austin, TX: PRO-ED. Copyright 2005 by PRO-ED, Inc. Adapted with permission.

disfluencies as "brief" and basically normal. They were badly mistaken because two to four iterations are far above normal. In short, they overlooked the fundamental significance of the length factor.

Years later, objective data obtained by other investigators from careful analyses of tape-recorded speech samples revealed extremely important information in this regard. The mean number of iterations for children who stutter is less than two, that is, less than "you-you-you." The mean for normally fluent children is just a fraction above one rep-etition unit, translated as slightly more than "you-you" (Ambrose & Yairi, 1995). This is a big difference. Furthermore, when the number of extra repetitions is two or more, the gap between children who stutter and normally fluent peers grows much wider. Whereas members of the first group do occasionally repeat three to five times, such instances are not common for the normally fluent children. In fact, it was concluded that the length, or extent, is often a more powerful discriminant between normal and abnormal disfluency than the number of disfluent events (Yairi & Lewis, 1984).

Physical Concomitants

The nonspeech body movements that accompany stuttering events have been referred to as concomitant (co-occurring) behaviors or, more often, "secondary" character-istics. For a long time, researchers believed that these emerge years after onset, as the older child tries ways to cope with, or avoid stuttering events. Examination of the past onset studies, however, makes us question this assumption. The percent-age of children with secondary characteristics at onset, particularly head, face, and neck movements reported by parents, varies from 11% (Taylor, 1937) to 53% (Yairi & Ambrose, 2005). The latter investigators wrote that "most parents of the 146 chil-dren we saw within one year of onset reported that their children exhibited at least one specific physical component at stuttering onset" (p. 69). Such parental reports were corroborated by frame-by-frame analyses of videotaped speech samples that identified and classified the different secondary characteristics (Schwartz et al., 1990; Yairi, Ambrose, Paden et al., 1996). Because a few secondary characteristics are often present from early on, even among children who later recover, it is not unreasonable to entertain the thought that they may be an integral aspect of stuttering, not neces-sarily "secondary." This possibility has not been specifically addressed in research studies.

Emotional and Physical Health

The notion that stuttering onset is associated with specific emotional stresses and health problems has been around for a long time and has risen and fallen in terms of scientific support. According to an early estimate, 28% of a 1,000-child caseload suf-fered emotional antecedents, such as shock or fright, prior to onset (Makuen, 1914). Another investigator reported emotional shocks prior to onset in 27% of her caseload of 200 children (Katsovaskaia, 1962). Similarly, physical illness prior to onset in 20% of the children was reported by West et al. (1939), and in 35% of the children by Katsovaskaia

(1962). A very different picture is seen in the Iowa studies, which concluded that in only a few of the 246 stuttering children were there associations of onset with either physical illness or emotional upheaval, and that the health histories revealed no more childhood diseases than those of normally fluent control children (Johnson & Associates, 1959). British investigators were in agreement, reporting no significant difference in the incidence of diseases between 80 stuttering children and their control peers (Andrews & Harris, 1964). Although some parents have reported to us that their children revealed strong emotional reactions associated with moments of stuttering soon after onset, such emotions appeared after the disorder has erupted.

The past 25 years have witnessed yet another turn concerning physical and emotional health issues associated with onset. For example, Poulos and Webster (1991) found that 37% of people who stutter *without* a family history of stuttering reported childhood incidences of anoxia, head injuries, and so on, that could have resulted in early brain damage. In contrast, such incidences occurred in only 2.6% of stutterers *with* family stuttering. Also, the most recent pertinent investigation found that 14% of the children were reported to experience health problems, such as respiratory problems, surgery, or illness that required medical treatment just prior to onset. Over 40% experienced emotionally upsetting events such as parents' divorce, death of a beloved pet, difficult day-care situations, and others. The authors opined that "if a child possesses predisposing (i.e., genetic) factors to stutter, aggravating physical or emotional stresses might very well trigger the onset" (Yairi & Ambrose, 2005, p. 63). So far, little, if any, in-depth research of health problems associated with the onset of stuttering has been done. Such information could enhance understanding biological and environmental forces in the emergence of stuttering.

Child temperament is another factor to consider. Johnson and associates (1959) reported that the stuttering children were rated by their parents less favorably than the control children on 35 of the 36 items depicting social development and temperament. More recently, investigators have reported several statistically significant differences in temperament traits between 31 young CWS and age-/gender-matched NFC (Anderson, Pellowski, Conture et al., 2003). Compared to controls, children who stutter were hypervigilant (i.e., less distractible), less adaptable to change, and had irregular biological functions. A larger study that followed 1,619 Australian children during their first 4 years of life yielded no significant differences between the 158 who began stuttering and those who did not on a temperament questionnaire administered to parents within 6 months prior to onset (Reilly et al., 2009; 2013). A recent study by a European team (Eggers, De Nil, & Van den Bergh, 2010) compared temperament scale scores for children who stutter and their normally fluent peers. Because participants were 3 to 8 years old, however, the study cannot be considered as exclusively pertaining to onset. Regardless, keep in mind that data for these studies were obtained from parents' responses to questionnaires, not directly from the children; hence validity may be limited. In view of the contradictory findings, the role of temperament at onset remains uncertain. More on this topic is in Chapter 6.

Phonology and Language

The scientific literature makes many references to a wide range of disorders that are present concomitantly with stuttering; those involving articulation/phonology and language skills are the most frequent. Much of the better incidence data in this regard have been reported for school-age children. A large survey of pupils who stutter revealed that 46% had articulation/ phonology disorders and 26% had language disorders (Blood et al., 2003). Surveys of the status of language and phonology in the school population (see Chapter 4), however, have limited bearing on stuttering onset that typically occurs years earlier. The following discussion is limited to preschool children, especially near stuttering onset, if possible.

> The overlap between the most common period for the onset of stuttering and the period during which there is an explosion in speech and language development, ages 2 to 4, raises the proposition of stuttering-language-phonology links. These potential links are of theoretical interest and are discussed in Chapter 6. If present, other speech-language difficulties during early stuttering are also relevant to clinicians' choice of a treatment regimen. For further study of the potential stuttering-language-phonology links, see Bernstein Ratner (1997a); Byrd, Wolk, and Lockett Davis (2007); Hall, Wagovitch, and Bernstein Ratner (2007); Paden (2005); and Watkins, 2005.

Disordered Phonology and Articulation

Are disorders of articulation or phonology[2] present at the time of stuttering onset or shortly thereafter? This is a justifiable question in light of the obvious overlap between the most common period of stuttering onset, 18 to 42 months of age, with the period when a child's development is rapidly advancing physically and in almost every capacity, including phonological and language skills. It tempts one to suggest co-influences, that is, that any interference in one domain could have multiple effects. Specifically, difficulties with fluency could co-occur with phonological deviations because the presence of one facilitates the manifestation of the other or because the two share common etiologies.

A general clinical observation of frequent speech articulation difficulties during the early stage of stuttering was made by Van Riper (1971), especially in one subgroup designated as Track II. Yet, our own experience with hundreds of children has not revealed parents commonly mentioning phonological issues when describing stuttering onset or problems that preceded it. So what has been the pertinent research evidence? You may be surprised to learn that in spite of strong interest in stuttering-phonology relationships, not a single study of a sizeable sample has investigated the basic question of whether the

---

[2]For many years, the term *articulation disorder* was applied to inabilities to produce, or correctly produce, speech sounds. As of the 1980s, it is now reserved for disorders in which there is a clear motor involvement. The term *phonological disorder* or *phonological delay* is applied to the majority of difficulties in sound production during childhood where motor interference is not apparent. These difficulties are presumed to reflect delay in the child's subliminal awareness of the different classes of sounds and problems in central planning of speech (Paden, 2005).

incidence of phonological deficiencies in children *near the onset* of stuttering (e.g., within 6 to 12 months) is different from that of a random control group of normally fluent peers or from available normative data. A study by Yaruss, LaSalle, and Conture (1998), for example, had 85 boys and 15 girls tested on the average 18.5 months post-onset, but no control group was employed. The few small studies have not supported such differences.

Throneburg, Yairi, and Paden (1994) observed that among 75 children who stuttered, ages 29 to 59 months, seen close to onset, none had profound phonological deficits and only 7% had severe phonological disorders. Similarly among the 50 normally fluent controls none exhibited profound phonological deficits and only 6% had severe phonological disorders. The authors asserted that "if there is a strong relation between stuttering and disordered phonology it would be expected that a larger proportion of stutterers than non-stutterers would have severe and profound phonologic disorders" (p. 508). Nonsupportive findings were also reported by Bernstein Ratner and Silverman (2000), who assembled children with a mean age under 36 months, all seen very close to the onset. They were matched with normally fluent children by age, gender, and socioeconomic status. The articulation abilities of 15 such child pairs were evaluated with the Goldman and Fristoe (1986) test, on which the CWS scored in the 56th percentile and the NFC in the 63rd percentile. The difference was not statistically significant. Such negative findings have been reinforced by studies that have failed to show relationships between the level of stuttering severity and the level of phonological skills close to onset (Gregg & Yairi, 2007, 2012).

Several investigators looked at the specific characteristics of phonology and stuttering. Louko, Edwards, and Conture (1990) reported that children who stuttered exhibited more phonological processes than normally fluent children (especially more consonant cluster reduction) than control children. Still, the mean number of processes per child in the two groups was similar. Wolk, Edwards, and Conture (1993) found that children who exhibited stuttering and disordered phonology had more similar than different phonology to that of normally fluent controls with disordered phonology. But, the atypical velarization and glottal replacement processes were more common for the children who stuttered. Comparing children who stutter with and without phonological deficits Yaruss and Conture (1996) found no differences in the frequency, duration, or severity of disfluencies during conversational speech.

Although a stuttering-phonology deficiency link at the time of onset or during the early stage of the disorder remains unclear, a subgroup of children who stutter appears more vulnerable. Indeed, two studies conducted at the University of Illinois, one with 36 children who stutter (Paden & Yairi, 1996) and one with 84 of them (Paden, Yairi, & Ambrose, 1999), tested within a year after onset, showed that the mean phonological performance of the small subgroup of children who later developed persistent stuttering lagged behind that of children who later recovered naturally, as well as behind normally fluent controls. The differences, however, were a matter of slower acquisition, not of abnormal developmental pattern and subsided within two years (Paden, Ambrose, & Yairi, 2002). Studies that dealt with phonology in young children who stutter are summarized in Table 3.3.

Table 3.3 Studies of phonological abilities in young children who stutter

Study	Sample Size	Age	Males/ Females	Controls	Findings
Louko, Edwards, & Conture (1990)	60	2.4–7.4 years	30/30	30	18 processes present, 12 of the 30 CWS exhibited disordered phonology.
Wolk, Edwards, & Conture (1993)	21	4 to 5 years	21/0	3 groups (a) stuttering & normal phonology abilities (S+NP), (b) stuttering & disordered phonology (S+DP), and (c) normal phonology & disordered phonology (NF+DP)	S+DP group produced significantly more sound prolongations than the S+NP group. Differences were noted between the S+DP and NF+DP groups in phonological behavior.
Throneburg, Yairi, & Paden (1994)	24	29 to 59 months	15/9	50 "normally speaking"	Only 7% demonstrated profound/severe phonological disorders.
Paden & Yairi (1996)	36	27 to 65 months	24/12	12 who recovered early, 12 who recovered late	Poor phonological ability in early stages, but wide individual variations in scores suggest additional factors are necessary for reliable prediction.
Yaruss & Conture (1996)	18	3 to 6 years	18/0	9 CWS with normal phonology	CRH predictions that utterances with faster articulatory rates or shorter response time latencies are more likely to contain speech errors/disfluencies
Paden, Yairi, & Ambrose (1999)	84	49 to 83 months	58/26	62 recovered children without clinical intervention	Persistent group moved more slowly in phonological progression and was more delayed in phonological development.

(continued)

Table 3.3 (Continued)

Study	Sample Size	Age	Males/ Females	Controls	Findings
Bernstein Ratner & Silverman (2000)	15	27 to 47 months	12/3	15 normally fluent	Showed a slight, but non-significant difference in favor of normally fluent children.
Wolk, Blomgren, & Smith (2000)	7	4 to 5 years	7/0	None	Disfluency on clusters with phonological errors was more common than on clusters without errors.
Ryan (2001a)	22	2; 4 to 5; 10 years	14/8	None	No significant difference in articulation test scores between recovered and persistent groups.
Paden, Ambrose & Yairi (2002)	84	49 to 83 months	58/26	62 recovered children without clinical intervention	Persistent stuttering group improved more than recovered group. At two-year visit, mean percentage of phonological errors for the two groups was identical.
Anderson, Wagovich, & Hall (2006)	24	3; 0 to 5; 2 years	18/6	12 CWNS	Nonword repetition skills differed for CWS compared with CWNS, and findings cannot be attributed to (a) weak language performance on the part of CWS, or (b) the occurrence of stuttering in the course of nonword production
Gregg & Yairi (2006)	28	25 to 38 months	20/8	None	No statistically significant differences were found for either of the two factors (minimal deviations-moderate deviations in phonological skills).
Byrd, Conture & Ohde (2007)	52	3 and 5 years	Gender matched between CWS & CSNS groups	26 CWNS	CWS are delayed in making the developmental shift in phonological encoding from holistic to incremental processing, a delay that may contribute to their difficulties establishing fluent speech.
Gregg & Yairi (2012)	29	29 to 49 months	20/9	None	No statistically significant differences in the stuttering characteristics of the two groups near onset.

A different picture is seen for school-age children who stutter. Some data indicate increased phonological difficulties among this population. Perhaps as the children who develop chronic stuttering grow older, they reveal other speech vulnerabilities. Such a scenario is seen in a British study of speech sound accuracy, comparing 37 children who stutter and 113 normally fluent controls over several years (Morley, 1957). Close to stuttering onset, fewer CWS had errors than NFC. The trend was reversed , however, at the more advanced age:

- At 3:9, errors were present in 50% of the CWS and 58% of the NFC.
- At 4:9, errors were present in 25% of the CWS and 36% of the NFC.
- At 6:6, errors were present in 14% of the CWS and 5% of the NFC.

These data add support to the view that children who persist in stuttering are at greater risk for phonological and articulation disorders. More on phonological disorders in school-age children who stutter is presented in Chapters 4 and 6.

Disordered Language

The idea of links between stuttering and language in young children is intuitive due to the fact that stuttering onset coincides with a time of rapid expansion in expressive and receptive language ability in young children. Bloodstein (2002) opined that children may reveal their tenuous grip on language by stuttering. Does this link mean that stuttering is associated with language disorders? The perspective that children who stutter are likely to have language skills that are inferior to those of their normally fluent peers has a long history in the field. One literature review generalized that "stutterers performed more poorly than nonstutterers on some tests of language development" (Andrews et al. 1983, p. 230). Recall, however, that most large-scale surveys were conducted with school-age populations, with the most recent one reporting 26% of those who stutter also exhibited language disorders (Blood et al., 2003). Although a recent analysis of 22 studies concluded that CWS scored lower than NFC on normative measures of both receptive and expressive language (Ntourou, Conture, & Lipsey, 2011), many of these studies included children who were up to 8 years of age, several years beyond the most typical age at onset of stuttering.

Only a few investigations have narrowed their focus to the presence of language problems in preschoolers near the time of stuttering onset. Although some statistically significant differences were detected, they did not reveal language problems for children who stutter. Their language skills are found to be within average range. For example, in one study, 20 preschool children who stuttered scored lower than normally fluent controls on several language measures but they were still within norms for receptive language and just slightly below norms for expressive skills (Ryan, 1992). Another small study similarly found that CWS scored lower than NFC and had a greater expressive-receptive language score discrepancy (Anderson & Conture, 2000). Nonetheless, they performed within the average range of language abilities. This team had similar results with another group of 16 CWS who scored lower than controls but within normal limits

(Anderson & Conture, 2004). Bernstein Ratner and Silverman (2000) reported language test data for 15 three-year-old CWS, all within less than 4 months post-onset, whose scores were within normal limits although somewhat lower than those of control peers. Similar findings in a larger study of 45 CWS and matched controls were reported by Anderson, Pellowski, and Conture (2005).

Relevant information from a different perspective was reported by the Illinois studies. In a large investigation of 84 children, ages 2 to 5, tested near stuttering onset, data derived from spontaneous language samples and standardized tests yielded mean scores at or well above norms. Children who continued to stutter, however, showed greater variability and atypical patterns of language production compared to those who later exhibited natural recovery. It was intriguing that on the standardized Preschool Language Scale (Zimmerman, Steiner, & Pond, 1979), scores near onset were higher than normative values on both comprehension and expression components (Watkins, Yairi, & Ambrose, 1999). A team of scholars in Germany similarly found that preschoolers who stuttered tended to have language skills at or above age expectations (Hage, 2001; Rommel, Hage, Kalehne, & Johannsen, 1999). In discussing the Illinois longitudinal studies of language development in CWS, Watkins (2005) concluded that "there is virtually no evidence that language development is vulnerable in any significant number of young children who stutter" (p. 246). Furthermore, she offered that advanced expressive language skills may be a risk factor for the onset of stuttering in some children, perhaps by placing excessive demands for language production on an immature speech motor system.

Overall, as was the case with phonology, current data do not seem to indicate gross, or widespread, language deficiency associated with the onset of stuttering. Inasmuch as conflicting notions are found in the literature, it may be traced, in our opinion, to mixing data for older school-age children with data for children close to onset. Also, Watkins and Johnson (2004) suggested that much of the controversy may have been fueled by methodological issues, such as inadequate control groups or lack of comparison with normative data, which yielded some differences. In a review of the literature, Nippold (2012a) concluded the existence of a stuttering-language connection was not supported. She posited an alternative perspective that CWS have a compromised motor control system making it difficult to move forward in speech. Hence, the tie to language lies not in a deficient linguistic system but in difficulty expressing the intended meaning via a fully functional speech system.

Nevertheless, we suggest it is important to recognize that the global nature of the various measures of language skills employed yield only superficial information about participants' language abilities, particularly in handling the online demands of language use in context. Perhaps closer examination of individual patterns of performance and finer language tasks may be important in clarifying the developmental relation between language and stuttering. Indeed, it has been demonstrated that the speech motor instability of individuals who stutter, including preschoolers, compared with normally fluent peers, is disproportionately increased by heightened syntactic and phonological complexity (MacPherson & Smith, 2013; Smith, Sadagopan, Walsh et al., 2010).

We conclude this section on the onset of stuttering with a rare, day-by-day, parental account of the event. It was recorded at the time by one of the authors (Yairi) as it was unfolding many years ago and involved the author's own son.

Micah (age 3 years, 6 months) began to show unusual disfluencies on December 20. December 21: Disfluencies continued, were quite frequent, and consisted of 6–7 repetitions of short words or just the initial syllable of a word. We noticed this with some concern.

December 22: Disfluent speech greatly increased. It is stuttering, at times severe. Short words, particularly /if/, /on/, /and/, and /in/ are often repeated 5–6 times, even up to 10–12 times. Also repetitions of initial syllables beginning with /l/ and /k/. There is a struggle behavior in that at times he closes his eyes. Most outstanding are Micah's reactions to the difficulties he had in talking. He would stop after a number of repetitions of a word and say "I cannot remember" and then just drop it. We are quite alarmed. The disfluencies do not always occur and there are sentences, and longer speech stretches, of only fluent speech. When disfluencies occur, they tend to be in groups. We decided to minimize his talking when severe disfluencies occurred (not asking questions, etc.) and be lax with demands and discipline. We also paid him more attention than usual. Except for the fact of my own, and my family's, history of stuttering, there was no apparent change in our life, or another reason of which we were aware, for the sudden stuttering onset.

December 23: There was considerable improvement. Spent much of the day in the nursery school. The babysitter who came in early evening reported later that his speech was rather fluent and that several instances of disfluency were quite mild. The nights of the 23rd and the 24th he wet the bed. This was the first time in several weeks. During the entire week he woke up at least once during each night, got out of bed, but went back to sleep.

December 24 and 25: We stayed at home. Disfluent speech was back. Up, but not as bad as on the 22nd. When disfluencies occurred, at times they gave a clear impression of stuttering because of the number of repetitions, 7–8, although no overt tension could be observed, nor closing of the eyes. Most of the speech was fluent and he talked slowly. The comment he made earlier, "I cannot remember," was not repeated after December 22. We continue to make special efforts to reduce all pressure. Often talked to him slowly. I tried rhythmic speech, which he liked. Although it was Christmas week, we do not celebrate this holiday, so there was no unusual tension at home.

December 26: In the morning, speech was fluent except for a few instances of easy repetitions that contained 3–4 iterations. He spent 7 hours in the nursery school. Back at home, speech continued to be good during the early evening. Later, when we went out for dinner, he had severe stuttering in the car as well as in the restaurant. We felt that people were noticing him. When we returned home, speech was good again.

December 27: A good day in terms of speech with only occasional repetitions of a word or sounds, 3–4 iterations.

December 28: Speech was relatively good with several instances of repetitions of 3–5 iterations. More stuttering in the car was noticed again. On one occasion, however, he repeated 15 times. No apparent reaction on his part.

December 29: Micah had several instances of severe repetitions in the morning and early afternoon, with 10–15 units at times. These occurred consistently on groups of 3–4 words. He seemed to be reacting to a TV program where the animals were drowning in the water. Each attempt to say the word "animal" was very difficult. He kept talking about it for quite a while. I took him to the park for 2 hours. Speech was fine for the rest of the afternoon and evening. We are concerned and upset by there-occurring of the stuttering even though most of the speech is normal.

December 30: Speech during the morning was normal. The nursery school teacher did not observe anything unusual except that he exhibited some jealousy of his younger brother (17 months younger). In the evening, though, and on December 31, there were random incidences of disfluent speech, primarily repetitions of 3–5 iterations but also 2–3 instances of over 10 units. At times he partially closed his eyes. Because most of the time his speech is fluent, we are not sure if he has a "stuttering problem."

January 1: We noticed Micah talking to himself (very slowly) for several minutes while playing in his room. This occurred several times. When talking to us, instances of stuttering, involving shutting of the eyes, were frequent. We were very concerned and tense about it. We began to do with him some rhythmic speech activities. Also, we began talking slowly to him and continued to avoid demands, relax discipline, and show more patience. On January 2, speech was very good all day. I took him out during early evening and let him do whatever he wanted to. Told him a story at bedtime. He was very affectionate and we were relieved. Speech was normal for 2 weeks or so.

January 18: Stuttering appeared again suddenly. Frequent excessive disfluencies. At times Micah stuttered on almost all words. This took the form of syllable (often beginning with consonants) repetitions, upward pitch shifts, closing eyes, and turning the head downward. He often stuttered on the same words: "marbles," "cookies," "Savta," and others. Struggle behaviors were very obvious; also his awareness of the speaking difficulties. He would stop without finishing the word, avoided words, and even substituted words. For example, he would try saying "marbles," repeating "ma-ma-ma-ma-ma-ma- ma- ma-" stops and say "the game." There were variations in the stuttering from situation to situation. Stuttering remained pretty consistent for the week with some day-to-day variations. The staff at the nursery school, as well as other people, also commented on the stuttering. We found out that one of the teachers reacted and told him to "stop mumbling," etc. She was advised to avoid all reactions, corrections, or suggestions."

Micah continued to stutter for approximately 10 weeks, during which he exhibited a wide range of stuttering severity. Stuttering stopped as quickly as it began and never occurred again. For the record, Micah's speech was relatively late to develop although his fine motor skills were excellent if not outstanding. According to notes taken at the time by his mother, a speech/language clinician, at 23 months of age expressive vocabulary was still mainly jargon with just a few words. Between 24 and 26 months of age, however, there was an apparent change. The notes indicate a sudden jump in expression, with many more single words. He finally began combining 2–3 word sentences. His language, however, was very advanced, and described as "wonderful." Indeed, receptive language test scores placed him at the 94th percentile. These observations are of interest in view of the controversy regarding possible links between stuttering onset and speech/language development.

Development

Once stuttering has emerged, what follows? This is an important question not only in regard to understanding the basic nature of disorder but also for practical clinical purposes. A clinician examining a 3-year-old child who began stuttering a few weeks earlier should be able to provide educated answers to parents' typical questions like these: "What is going to happen with this stuttering? Will it stop before he goes to kindergarten? If he goes on stuttering, for how long? Will it improve or get worse?" The clinician should also be able to respond to these questions when examining a child who has already stuttered for 2 or more years. His or her answers, however, are likely to be different because, as we will soon see, stuttering may change extensively with time. Aside for parent counseling purposes, information about the development of stuttering may be critical for making intervention decisions, such as whether to initiate or postpone therapy, or what kind of program fits the particular status of the disorder at any given time.

Some information pertaining to the questions just posed and clinical needs has been provided through a variety of sources including clinical observations, cross-sectional retrospective research, and direct longitudinal studies. But first let's consider several traditional concepts of the course of stuttering.

Traditional Models of Developmental Progression

Similar to the traditional portrayal of the onset of stuttering, the development of the disorder has also been pictured stereotypically. For a long time, the developmental outlines presented a unidirectional path that begins mildly and then, in a stepwise succession, increases in abnormality. Froeschels (1921) offers a very detailed account that emphasizes the escalating tempo of the repetitions as stuttering persists. A classic depiction of this view is expressed in Robinson's (1964) statement that "stuttering seldom remains static. It grows. And as it grows, it tends to change form and severity. Early patterns are replaced, obscured, or supplemented by more pronounced and abnormal behavior. Repetitions or prolongations become troublesome blocks" (p. 47).

The notion that stuttering progresses through prescribed stages has been particularly popular. Unfortunately, it emerged from unsystematic observations and subjective impressions by several influential clinicians, such as Bluemel (1932). His developmental system included two phases: *primary stuttering*, which is a pure speech disorder characterized exclusively by easy repetitions, and *secondary stuttering*, marked by considerable physical tension in speech and the child's awareness of the stuttering that leads to fear and avoidance of speaking. Although the transition time from primary to secondary stuttering varies among individuals, all follow a similar developmental pattern. In 1954,

Van Riper modified the Bluemel system by adding two intermediate stages. Essentially, he appears to have endorsed the concepts of primary and secondary stuttering. As indicated earlier in this chapter, however, recent data pertaining to onset negate the position that all early stuttering is "simple" repetitions, devoid of tension and emotional reactions. In our view, Bluemel's sharp stage dichotomy is not a valid depiction of the disorder.

A well-known four-phase developmental sequence was presented by Bloodstein (1960b) based on changes in five parameters: type of disfluency, loci of disfluency, physical tension, cognitive awareness, and emotional reactions. He used information from diagnostic reports for 16 subgroups, each of 30 children, representing 6-month age intervals between ages 2 and 16. Among the essential features of phase I (preschool ages), for example, are (1) repetitions of syllables and words occurring on functional short words at initial phrase positions, (2) up-and-down cycles in the stuttering with possible complete amelioration for days or weeks followed by resumption of stuttering, and (3) little evidence of awareness and concern. During phases II and III (school ages), (1) stuttering becomes chronic, (2) children identify themselves as stutterers, (3) stuttered speech increases in complexity and severity to include sound prolongations and blocks, (4) stuttering occurs throughout the sentences and on other types of words (nouns, verbs, adjectives, adverbs), and (5) fears and anticipation of stuttering emerge. By phase IV (adolescence and adulthood), strong emotional reactions take over as individuals exhibit avoidance of speaking prior to stuttering and shame and embarrassment afterward.

In spite of Bloodstein's recognition of individual differences in the age and timing of the disorder's progression, its overall uniformity and linear directionality is cardinal to his model. That is, only one sequence is recognized in which the disorder is worsening. In our opinion, this system, which is based on cross-sectional data, is seriously flawed because the methodology employed is grounded in an erroneous premise that successively older subgroups all represent members of the youngest subgroup (the 2-year-olds) as they grow and their stuttering continues. Such a premise is acceptable in research of the development of height or weight for children in the general population. It does not, however, apply to cross-sectional studies of the development of stuttering due to the high rate (75%+) of natural recovery. Because most young children stop stuttering within 2 to 4 years, they never progress to Bloodstein's phase II and beyond. This means that the older age groups in the Bloodstein study represented a very different subpopulation than the group at Phase I, when stuttering begins. These older groups were populated with a highly biased sample consisting of those who persisted in stuttering. We conclude that the four phases may, at best, describe the development of the small minority of children who continue to stutter for many years. Furthermore, among them are some whose stuttering remains steady or decreases. This is illustrated in Figure 3.1. Table 3.4 summarizes the main features of several stuttering development systems.

Figure 3.1   Schematic Showing That Children Who Stutter Tested at Later Times Do Not Represent the Same Group Tested Earlier

Testing: 1st Time	Testing: 6 Months Later	Type of Subject	Key
		Original child who stutters	
		New child who stutters	
		Control child who does not stutter	

Testing: 1 Year Later	Testing: 2 Years Later		

Note: Previous children who stuttered and recovered had to be replaced by new ones from persistent stutterers. With time this group represents mostly those who persist, a small fraction of the stuttering population. Control children who do not stutter remained the same.

Differential Developmental Models

The developmental systems reviewed earlier share the concept of uniformity in upward progression of stuttering. Not only have these systems made little provision for alternative developmental sequences, they have also reinforced the notion that stuttering is a homogeneous disorder, a concept that has had far-reaching research and clinical implications. This thinking is puzzling considering the ample contrarian evidence (e.g., children whose stuttering took the opposite path leading to complete recovery, or children whose stuttering changed little over time, or those whose initial stuttering was severe, or those who indicated awareness from early on). Perhaps the traditional developmental ideas were so strongly influenced by learning theories that contradictory evidence was simply ignored. If one believes that stuttering is a learned behavior, then it should be expected to be continuously reinforced and to grow. An important clinical implication of such models would be to recommend intervention as soon as possible to lessen the expected negative changes in the stuttering.

Table 3.4   Developmental Models of Stuttering That Described Sequential Stages

Source	Phase 1	Phase 2	Phase 3	Phase 4
Froeschels (1921)	Slow easy, even tempo "clonic" repetitions	Tense, fast tempo, irregular repetitions	Tense, forced, "tonic" postures, halted repetitions	Inhibited symptoms due to social pressures
Bluemel (1932)	"Primary" stuttering: easy repetitions of initial syllables	"Secondary" stuttering: tension, effort, awareness, fear	N/A	N/A
Van Riper (1954)	Slow easy, even repetitions and some prolongations	Faster, irregular repetitions; some prolongations; brief awareness	Tense, effortful stuttering; full awareness, fear, avoidance	N/A
Bloodstein (1960b)	Episodic; mostly repetitions of initial syllables; increases with excitement; little awareness or concern	Chronic; a variety of symptoms with more tension; still increases with excitement; aware but little concern	Chronic; complex symptoms; varies by sound, word, and situation; negative emotion but not fear; does not avoid talking	Chronic; complex symptoms; avoids sounds, words, and situations of talking; fear and shame; personal and social impact

N/A = not applicable.

A significant departure from the traditional model took place in 1971 with Van Riper's developmental system. It recognized diversity according to four alternative tracks. His new system drew from clinical notes recorded over time in the files of 44 children, not by means of controlled research procedures. Table 3.5 summarizes the main features of the four tracks. Note that the system seems to be based on four variables or risk factors: (1) age at onset: early-late, (2) type of onset: gradual-sudden, (3) pattern of stuttering: repetitions-blocks-tension, and (4) concomitant speech-language problems. For example a combination of early and gradual onsets with repetitions as the dominant symptom (Track I) had better chances for recovery than the combination of sudden onsets, blocks, prolongations, and physical tension (Track III). Children with delayed speech (Track II) were also slower to improve than those with "otherwise normal speech." An important advantage of models that recognize developmental diversity according to risk factors is in allowing for differentiation in clinical decisions concerning intervention and counseling. Treatment is considered a priority for those in Track IV.

Table 3.5 The Main Features of Van Riper's (1971) Developmental Tracks

	Features
Subtype Track I	High incidence: 48% (21/44)
	Early onset (2.5–4 years)
	Gradual, episodic, previously fluent
	Starts with easy repetitions
	Normal speech rate, good articulation
	Lack of awareness of speech disruption
	High recovery
	Persistent cases progress to fast, irregular repetitions, prolongations, and tension; awareness, fear, and avoidance later on
Subtype Track II	Medium incidence : 25% (11/44)
	Later onset than track I, as phrases and sentences emerge
	Gradual, chronic, not ever very fluent
	Part and whole-word repetitions, pauses, revisions
	Rapid rate (spurts), poor articulation, mumbled speech
	Lack of awareness of speech disruption
	Hesitations, revision, and false starts are added to hurried, irregular repetitions
Subtype Track III	Low incidence: 11% (5/44)
	Onset later like track II
	Sudden onset, chronic, previously fluent
	Blocks (laryngeal fixations, silent prolonged postures)
	Slow, careful rate, normal articulation
	Highly aware; many progress to complex and intense fears and avoidance patterns
Subtype Track IV	Lowest incidence: 9% (4/44)
	Later onset (usually after 4 years of age)
	Sudden, episodic, previously fluent
	Unique patterns of speech disruption
	Many iterations of initial whole words and phrases
	Normal rate, normal articulation
	Even if frequency increases, symptoms remain consistent
	Highly aware, but no avoidance
	No remissions

Note: Three of 44 cases did not fit any of the tracks.

Natural Recovery

A most remarkable aspect of stuttering is its disappearance in a large percentage of affected young children. The label *spontaneous recovery* has been the most commonly applied to this phenomenon, implying that the recovery occurs without treatment. The term *natural recovery*, however, might be more suitable. Whereas spontaneous recovery implies biological healing processes, natural recovery considers the possibility of environmental factors being responsible, at least in part, for the phenomenon, with parental correction of the child's stuttering being one such possibility (Ingham & Cordes, 1998). Among the first calling attention to natural recovery was Johnson (1934), whose clinical observations led him to estimate natural recovery of 30% to 40% among children who begin to stutter by age 8. Similarly, a 40% natural recovery by age 8 was estimated by Bryngelson (1938) on inspection of 1,492 case files. These figures, as well as data reported in a number of surveys, were often based on a single person's impression and without specifying any criteria.[3]

Of course, there is the all-important question as to who should be considered "recovered." Recent investigators of this phenomenon listed a number of criteria, both objective and subjective, all indicating no stuttering for *at least a year,* and that no formal treatment should have been received by the child (Yairi & Ambrose, 1999a, 2005):

Criteria for Natural Recovery

- No stuttering present for a minimum of 12 months as judged both by parent and clinician
- Parental rating of stuttering severity as less than 1 on an 8-point scale (0 = normal; 1 = borderline; 8 = severe)
- Clinician rating of stuttering severity as less than 1
- SLD observed and reported as fewer than 3 per 100 syllables
- Maintained no stuttering for 4 years to demonstrate stability of "recovered" status

Information about the high percentage of natural recovery rests on four types of evidence: (1) statistical inferences, (2) retrospective reports, (3) indirect longitudinal observations, and (4) direct longitudinal observations.

The Statistical Evidence

The statistical inference relies on the difference between the conventional 5% stuttering incidence and the 1% prevalence figure (see Chapter 2). The meaning of this comparison is that only 1 of 5 children who begin stuttering continues to do so. Put differently: About 4 of 5 children who begin stuttering (80%) recover, presumably naturally. Recall, however, that Chapter 2 highlighted recent data suggesting the incidence could be higher,

---

[3] An interesting review of recovery can be found in Wingate, 1976. A summary table of reports is provided in Bloodstein & Bernstein Ratner, 2008, p. 86.

perhaps 8%, while the prevalence is lower, about 0.70%. If true, the recovery level rises to 91% (7.3 out of 8). Although some participants in incidence/prevalence studies received therapy, most likely their numbers were small within the large-scale surveys conducted in the past, when clinical services for stuttering were sparse. Certainly, the number of those receiving therapy worldwide is still quite small. The careful longitudinal studies described below, serve to confirm the high recovery as deduced from data on the population at large.

Retrospective Evidence

Early systematic data on natural recovery were reported by investigators who employed retrospective methods. For example, information solicited about themselves from high school students and adults who stuttered in the past yielded nearly 79% recoveries (Sheehan & Martyn, 1966). In other studies, parents were asked about their children's stuttering history but no further objective forms of evidence, such as speech samples, were gathered, no criteria for stuttering or recovery were employed, and there was no verification of either the initial stuttering diagnosis or of remission. For example, in the Glasner and Rosenthal (1957) study, parents' retrospective reports indicated that only 31% continued to stutter habitually when they were about 6 years old, young enough to expect additional recovery cases. Dickson (1971) found 54% recovery as reported by parents of children in kindergarten through junior high school. More recently an incidence survey of approximately 4,700 families with 12,000 members spanning the entire age range also asked about past cases of stuttering. The finding indicated 70% recovery over lifetime (Craig et al., 2002).

Indirect Longitudinal Evidence

Longitudinal investigations that follow children for several years provide considerably more valid recovery evidence than retrospective studies, but some employed indirect data based only on parent reports. Johnson (1955b) followed 46 preschool-aged children who stuttered for up to 5 years (mean = 30 months). Most had stuttered for less than a year at the first parental visit. Information about the children's stuttering was obtained through several follow-up contacts, but was derived solely from parents' reports, not from direct observations by the investigators or from tape-recorded speech samples. In this study, 72% experienced complete recovery and 13% decreased their stuttering. None received speech therapy during the course of the study. A few years later, Johnson and Associates (1959) used a similar methodology with 118 stuttering children ages 2 to 7 at the time of the first interview, with a follow-up conducted 30 months later. Improvement was reported for 88% of the children, with 36% exhibiting complete recovery. In only 4% of the children did the stuttering severity increase, negating the traditional view that stuttering *typically* grows in complexity and severity. We believe that the more advanced age of the children (age 7) when entering this second study yielded lower full recovery rates because a good number of them had already stuttered for a long period and were persistent when they entered the study.

The largest and most recent investigation concerning recovery and persistency has been carried out in the United Kingdom by Dworzynski et al. (2007). Parents of

12,892 pairs of twins responded to a questionnaire regarding child health and development at each of four ages: 2, 3, 4, and 7. Some items pertained to stuttering. Children for whom stuttering was positively indicated in an earlier age and who were still stuttering at age 7 were considered persistent stutterers. By age 7, 1,085 of the 12,892 children were marked for stuttering with 950 (87.55%) recovered and 135 (11.39%) persisting.

Finally two longitudinal studies that were also conducted in the United Kingdom are problematic in that the starting point was age 8, after much recovery typically has occurred. Not surprisingly, one study with 76 CWS reported 50% recovery after a single follow-up 4 years later (Howell et al., 2008), while a repeat study with 206 CWS found 52% after 6 years (Howell & Davis, 2011). In spite of weaknesses, these studies show that recovery continues during the school-age years.

Direct Longitudinal Evidence

Much more valid and reliable evidence has been generated by longitudinal studies that employed direct monitoring of children's stuttering from near onset for a period of several years. These, too, have varied in methodological strength, such as how closely and how directly were children monitored, and how stuttering and recovery were determined.

A critical parameter is the starting point of the longitudinal observations in relation to the time of stuttering onset. The longer the time gap, the more misleading the findings are likely to be. Children who recover early are not accounted for among the participants because (1) they do not stutter and investigators are not aware of them, and (2) if the investigators are informed about these already recovered children (e.g., by parents who already have a child who stutters in the study), there is no way of going back in time to capture the necessary direct data. Hence the reported percentage of natural recovery is in danger of being much smaller than it is in reality. Illustrating this point is a study of 91 school children conducted in Sweden that found 47% recovery over 10 years (Fritzell, 1976). Other weaknesses aside, it is hopelessly faulty because many were first observed between ages 7 and 9, some even older. As we know, most recovery occurs before this age. It does, however, show that additional recovery occurs at later ages.

A well-known investigation conducted in England followed approximately 1,000 children from birth to their 16th birthday (Andrews & Harris, 1964). During this period, 43 children were identified to exhibit stuttering. Health professionals (e.g., nurses, social workers) who visited the children's homes evaluated their speech periodically. Often, however, the examiners had to rely on parents' reports. Furthermore, the children's speech was never recorded for objective evaluation. Regardless, 79% of the children who stuttered recovered without treatment.

Four European studies were published more recently. In the Netherlands, investigators found 70% natural recovery among 23 children who stuttered and whose families were at high risk for stuttering, having at least one parent who stuttered (Kloth et al., 1995). Because, as we explain later, children of parents who exhibit persistent stuttering would also have a higher chance to persist in stuttering, the 70% recovery is a likely biased underestimate for the greater population of children who stutter. In Germany, 65 children were tracked for several years, beginning at age 5. After 3 years, 71% of the group had recovered (Rommel et al., 1999). A year and a half later, recovery climbed to 77% (Johannsen, 2001). It is quite likely that the 77% recovery is an underestimate due to the late first evaluation that took place at age 5. Finally, in Denmark, a longitudinal study of 53 preschool children yielded 71.6% recovery after 2 years. By the 5-year follow-up, recovery had climbed to 85% (Månsson, 2000). In a second study of 179 CWS, the same investigator reported 94% recovery (Månsson, 2005). High levels of natural recovery found in Europe were echoed in two small American longitudinal studies: 80% after 5-year follow-ups (Panelli, McFarlane, & Shipley, 1978) and 68% after only 2-year follow-ups (Ryan, 2001a). In these studies the children did not receive therapy.

The Illinois Studies

Perhaps the most intensive long-term longitudinal investigation of the development of childhood stuttering was conducted at the University of Illinois at Urbana-Champaign. It obtained objective firsthand data in the form of audio- and video-recorded speech samples, as well as language, phonology, and many other data collected directly from the children and their parents. Another important advantage was that children were identified and initially recorded close to the stuttering onset. Therefore, it was possible to document cases of early natural recovery. The first study tracked 27 preschool children from approximately 6 months after onset, at 6-month intervals over 2 years. At that time, 67% exhibited complete recovery. Three years later, recovery reached 89% (Yairi & Ambrose, 1992a). A second study included only 16 children but they were very young, 2 to 3 years of age; all exhibited moderate to severe stuttering, and they were first recorded within just 12 weeks after stuttering onset (mean = 8 weeks). For this group, the investigators focused only on the first 6 months following the initial testing. Within this very brief period, three children (19%) exhibited recovery according to the most stringent criteria. If just one less of the multiple criteria were considered, 38% had exhibited recovery (Yairi, Ambrose, & Niermann, 1993). Of course, maintaining these achievements for a longer time was required to ascertain stable recovery. The importance of this study lies in demonstrating a strong trend for a quick, sharp decline in stuttering even within a few months following onset.

The largest Illinois study included 89 preschool children who stuttered, 23 to 65 months old (mean = 38 months) at the first visit, all seen close to onset (Yairi & Ambrose, 1999a, 2005). As with the earlier studies, speech samples and other measures of stuttering were secured at 6-month intervals for the first 2 years. Next, data were secured at a yearly interval for years 3 and 4, and at the final visit several years later. Recovery was determined using multiple criteria, including frequency of stuttering-like disfluencies in the recorded speech, clinician and parents' ratings of stuttering, and agreement among all. To avoid false classification of recovery, a failure to meet a single criterion, or if there was any doubt whatsoever, was sufficient for classifying a child as persistent. The overall natural recovery rate at the end of the study was 79%, identical to the English findings (Andrews & Harris, 1964) and just under the Danish data (Månsson, 2000).

Significantly, although reduction in stuttering may have begun within a few months or even weeks after onset, the time period needed to reach complete natural recovery varies. Only 9% of the children fully recovered during the first year, an additional 22% during the second year, and so on. At the 4-year point, natural recovery occurred for 74% of the sample, and it reached 79% by the 5th year. None of the recovered children received any formal speech therapy; children who persisted did receive therapy. Yairi and Ambrose (2005) concluded that "given a child who has just begun stuttering, we can thus say that he/she has about a 65–80% chance of natural recovery by three to five years after onset, or a 20% chance of persistence" (p. 168). It is important to note that the 70% to 80% recovery rate applies to children seen early in the course of their stuttering. It is lower for those evaluated later. Finally, natural recovery continues to occur throughout the years into adulthood although at much smaller percentages (Sheehan & Martyn, 1966; Wingate, 1976). It appears that few people of senior ages stutter habitually. Table 3.6 summarizes longitudinal studies concerned with recovery.

Table 3.6   Recovery Data for Longitudinal Studies

Study	Country	N	% Recovery
PRESCHOOL CHILDREN			
Johnson (1955b)	United States	46	72%
Andrews & Harris (1964)	United Kingdom	43	79%
Panelli, McFarlane, & Shipley (1978)	United States	15	80%
Yairi & Ambrose (1992)	United States	27	89%
Kloth, Janssen, Kraaimaat et al. (1995)	The Netherlands	23	70%
Månsson (2000)	Denmark	53	85%
Ryan (2001a)	United States	22	68%
Johannsen (2001)	Germany	65	77%
Yairi & Ambrose (2005)	United States	89	79%
Månsson (2005)	Denmark	179	94%
Dworzynski, Remington, Rijsdijk et al. (2007)	United Kingdom	1,085	87%
OLDER CHILDREN			
Johnson & Associates (1959)	United States	118	36%
Howell, Davis, & Williams (2008)	United Kingdom	76	50%
Howell & Davis (2011)	United Kingdom	206	52%

A testimony for natural recovery is presented here from the same mother who described the onset of stuttering in her daughter, Denise (not a participant in our study). Her initial letter was cited earlier in the chapter. This follow-up account was written 2 years after onset.

I would like to let you know that Denise is doing fine now. Better than fine, actually. She is in kindergarten and is reading at a 3rd- to 4th-grade level. She *never* stutters, and that nightmare has now, thankfully, become a thing of the past. When I reread the letter that I sent to you 2 years ago, it brought tears to my eyes. I was absolutely devastated at that time. It was heart wrenching. Denise was talking at an early age, and she has always been highly intelligent. To see her reduced to silence and tears overnight was more than I thought I could bear. Thank you so very much for your help and compassion. You will never know the comfort that you brought to me and my family during that time. I wrote to you out of sheer desperation. I honestly did not expect a response. (You did not know me or Denise, and you are probably very busy, etc.). Your letter back to me was my lifeline. I want to personally thank you again for your help.

I am so thankful that there are those of you in the field who are genuinely making inroads into this disability.

I do feel stuttering is a genuine disability. My baby was forced to stop communicating with us. I genuinely feel that stuttering is traumatic. The suddenness and the severity of it was staggering. Denise was 100% fine, and then WHAM! She was not experiencing any new routines (no new school, new friends, different home environment, etc.). Looking back, I can honestly say that I can see nothing that precipitated it in any way. I do not know what brought her out of it. We did our best to follow your suggestions. It was like her speech and her brain were at an impasse or something, and the signals were getting hopelessly stuck and circulated again and again along the same pathway. I am not sure what caused this, but I would be interested to hear your thoughts. I am still in awe of how severe it was. It was not an occasional word, but rather, OCCASIONALLY she would be able to speak a word WITHOUT stuttering. I am a registered cardiac nurse, and it reminds me of a certain cardiac condition where the impulse conduction for the heart gets "trapped" in a sense, and is constantly in a reentry or circular loop. I don't know if that makes sense or not; in my mind it does (ha ha). But, that is what it reminded me of. She would literally look at me with these crazy wide eyes, like she were unable to stop speaking a particular word at times (not just stop the stuttering, but like she actually wanted to just stop speaking that particular word and her mouth just wouldn't stop). It frightened her. Usually, she would just stop talking, but there were times when I swear she couldn't stop speaking a particular word. Of course, she was so young, it would have been impossible for me to ask her this question and have her understand what I was asking (I also was afraid to draw attention to it). However, as a mother, I am confident that this was the case.

Denise is, in fact, a great communicator now. Her reading level is astounding, even to us. She finishes her grandfather's word-find puzzle books, and we never see any signs of stuttering. In answer to your question, Denise did NOT receive speech therapy. We followed your recommendations and made sure that everyone else from her grandparents to her preschool teachers knew exactly what your recommendations were as well, so that we were all aboard the same train. She seemed to overcome the severe stuttering within a few months. She did, however, still stutter at times, especially when tired or not feeling well. Then, thankfully, one day it disappeared and never returned. It was such a bizarre thing.

I did not realize that your son also had an affliction of stuttering. I now know that you completely understand, not just from a clinical perspective, but from the perspective of a parent. I am so glad that your son recovered. As I mentioned before, she is doing well now. She excels in reading, spelling, and even math. At our first kindergarten conference a few weeks ago, her teacher told us that she was "very advanced." She also commented to us that Denise was doing so well, that she was, "far above all of her peers," and that "none of her peers are even close to being her intellectual equal." I don't say this to brag (although I am very proud of her), but rather to let you know, in case this somehow plays a factor.

Denise was also a very abstract thinker, which my father and others noticed at a very young age. For example, one day when she was maybe 15 or 16 months old, my husband and she were at the park. It was fall, and the sky was filled with birds flying south for the winter. My husband and her looked up at the sky, and Denise said, "Look Daddy . . . a 'V.'" She did not say, "Look Daddy! Birdies!" She said strange stuff like that all of the time. One day they were walking around the railroad ties that encircle the playground. She was 18 months old. She kept saying, "See Daddy! Octagon!" My husband was looking all around the playground trying to see where this supposed octagon was. After a short while, she became frustrated with him, because he kept saying, "Where baby? Where is the Octagon?" Finally, she pointed to the railroad ties and said, "See Daddy! Octagon!" As it turns out, the railroad ties that encircle the entire playground just happen to be in the shape of an octagon. However, the space is so large, that unless you could look down ON them from the sky, you'd never know it. But, she knew it just by walking on them while holding her Daddy's hand. These examples may mean nothing in relation to stuttering. If not, please forgive me for the rambling. However, in the off chance that they could, I thought that I would mention them.

Thank you again for all of your compassion, and your dedication to the field. My hope is that, one day, stuttering will be able to be treated so efficiently that no child has to suffer with it. I wish you the best of luck in your pursuits, and those of your students and colleagues. If, in your research, you find a link, please let me know, as I have heard that stuttering can be familial in nature. (Just in case stuttering rears its ugly head in our family again with another child, niece or nephew.)

Warm Regards.

Here we present parental testimonies illustrating how stuttering can substantially improve over a course shorter than one year, The first letter was received from a father shortly after onset, the second about 10 months later.

Letter 1: Roy is now 3 years and 4 months old. Suddenly he began stuttering earlier in this month (November). It started over the course of a couple days, and within that time period he very quickly developed severe problems. He would get hung up on a word, repeating it several times. At first, he would repeat a word a few times. Then, it grew to several times, and eventually became a matter of repeating the word 10–15 times before he would either get through it or give up completely. This was a daily occurrence, over and over many times throughout the day. At the time he stuttered more than he spoke without stuttering. He clearly struggled with it, closing his eyes, tensing his body. As it became worse, he would just stop himself and say, "Oh,

I just can't talk anymore." For a 3-year-old, we thought that was a remarkable statement, that he was so very aware and conscious of the onset of his stutter, and aware that it didn't always used to be that way. I would rate his stutter at that time as moderate, based on my limited experience with this. Aside from my own mild stuttering issues as an adolescent, I know a good friend of my sister's who has a very severe stutter which completely prevents him from carrying on any sort of fluid conversation without constant interruptions. To me, that seems very severe, but there may be worse?

Stuttering continued to worsen from November through to the present (January). Within our nuclear family, we have grown accustomed to it and are very conscious not to add to any stress he might have been experiencing, in particular with regard to his own awareness of the stuttering. For example, we have not called attention to the stuttering, we let him work through it and wait patiently for him to complete his sentences without interruption. We spoke privately with our two daughters, ages 9 and 7, to remind them not to make fun of Roy and to be patient while he speaks without interrupting him. They are very concerned about him, too, knowing that his stuttering was unusual and came on suddenly.

Letter 2: Little Roy turned 4 years old approximately 2 months ago. Since writing to you, his stuttering has changed fairly dramatically. He still gets hung up on words, but doesn't repeat them 10–20 times and no longer completely shuts down in frustration (which was so sad to see him tearfully exclaiming things like "Oh, I give up, I just can't talk anymore," etc.). I would say that currently he has a mild stutter repeating a sentence 2–3 times until he gets it out. This happens often in conversation with him a couple dozen times daily. He doesn't seem to get hung up on individual words, rather he seems to get hung up on a concept or the subject matter in general to which he can often substitute words or phrases thus changing his tactic or approach to delivering his sentence. He has long pauses mid-sentence, as if to collect his thoughts, during which it seems he changes direction and alters what he was saying. He obviously has developed many compensatory mechanisms for it. Not being an expert in any way, I'm sure that I don't pick up on all the ways he has dealt with it, but here are a few examples: When he starts to get hung up, he substitutes another word, or immediately changes direction and attacks the concept from another angle. He often will still start a sentence over when he senses that he has made a speech mistake, and when that happens it is common for him to repeat the beginning of a sentence 2–4 times before he gets the concept out, if he doesn't take a new approach completely. He has also "adopted" or mimics a vocal throat tic from his older sister (8 years), which is sometimes interjected as a mild pause in his speech, which seems to be commensurate with moments when he is struggling to get through a word. He repeats phrases often, almost as if practicing them. Also, he hums and sings much of the day. I would say, however, that today most people, adults and kids alike, do not notice a significant deviation from whatever "normal" speech is when they hear Roy talk, but that if pointed out, they could see clearly that he is making conscious adjustments to his speech. We did not seek other professional help, other than my note to you, but it may have been very helpful if we had.

When his stuttering was at its worst, he was 3 years, 4 months old, and I talked to him about it and explained what it was. He seemed reassured. He seemed glad that somebody was talking to him about it. I was concerned that talking about it with him might make things worse if he was to feel ashamed, or, I wondered if I could increase the high level of anxiety it was already clearly causing him. He's a smart little kid, and I explained that I stuttered as an adolescent but it seemed to have gone away on its own. I also said that a lot of kids go through this when they're young and their brains are growing and learning so much. I said it would go away, knowing that it might not. He then went through a couple of months where it became clear he was really trying to work through it, perhaps merely coincidentally with our discussion of the issue, and sure enough, much of it went away or has since been masked by his compensatory responses.

At age 4, he still has a hard time forming certain sounds with his mouth, but I don't think that's particularly unusual for his age group and certainly not unusual compared to the speech progression of his two older sisters. For example, he has a hard time saying the "kr," "L," "th" sounds as in *Christmas* ("kisst-mus"), *lightning* ("white-ning"), and *then* ("when") respectively. However, we have certainly noticed that Roy has a very good vocabulary for his age, and a remarkable ability to express even complex thoughts very clearly. He is, considering all things, a gifted little speaker. We also try to reduce his anxiety by not calling attention to his stuttering and let him work through it on his own without interrupting him, and I have never called attention to any of his compensatory strategies. He is not yet in school, but like our two other children, we will be looking to see if the classroom environment causes things to re-present, start up again, or get worse. We know that the classroom has typically been a very stressful place for the girls (now ages 8 and 10) and many of their tics and behaviors only appear in that environment. Interestingly, and sadly, the teacher(s) tend to handle them as disciplinary issues regardless of consultations in tic disorders.

Implications of Developmental Findings

Current information concerning the development of stuttering, natural recovery, and persistency has significant implications for theory, research, and clinical intervention. In the theoretical domain, it suggests the possibility that differences in etiological factors create at least two stuttering subtypes: those who persist and those who recover naturally. As we discuss in Chapter 7, recent research has provided supportive evidence of differences in the genetic makeup of these two subtypes. In the research domain, it would seem advisable that studies with young children be designed so as to distinguish between potentially recovering children and those destined to persist. For example, these subgroups should be differentiated in studies of the early language skills of children who stutter, or, in studying various characteristics of their parents. Taking natural recovery into consideration is especially important in studies that focus on the evaluation of therapies. Was a positive therapeutic outcome due to the treatment or, at least partially, to the strong likelihood for recovery? One way to answer this question would be to follow a nontreated control group. Also, parent counseling and decisions concerning priority and timing for initiating treatment should be significantly influenced by the findings on natural recovery. For example, knowing that many children who begin stuttering recover on their own, should all parents be advised to seek therapy for their child? Should clinicians be more selective when recommending who should receive therapy immediately and who may wait a while before rushing into unnecessary treatment? In other words, is it possible to predict the future development of early stuttering and use such information for clinical decisions and management?

Predictive Factors

Several attempts have been made to offer prediction criteria for future recovery or persistency. Pioneers in this area were Stromsta (1965), relying primarily on speech acoustic characteristics; Glyndon Riley, in his 1981 Stuttering Prediction Instrument for Young Children; and Cooper and Cooper (1985) in their list of prediction indicators covering a wide range of variables. These and other formal and informal means of predicting persistency and recovery are covered in Chapter 9, which focuses on the clinical evaluation of early stuttering.

An extensive effort in this direction has been made at the Illinois Stuttering Research Program based on longitudinal studies described earlier and summarized in Yairi and Ambrose (2005). The investigators showed that several biological factors provide various degrees of predictability. One of these is age. Children who persisted in stuttering tended to have somewhat later onsets than those who recovered, a trend supported by Buck et al. (2002). Gender is a stronger predictor. The 2:1 male-to-female ratio at the time of stuttering onset grew to 3.75:1 among children who a few years later persisted in stuttering. By comparison, the ratio among children who recovered was considerably smaller: 2.30:1. This means the rate of natural recovery for females is higher than for males. Furthermore, girls also recovered sooner than boys. On average, boys stuttered for 29.5 months prior to recovery as compared to only 24 months for girls. Perhaps the strongest predictor reported by the Illinois studies was the specific type of the child's family history of stuttering. Children who had a familial history of recovered stuttering had a 65% chance of following this pattern themselves. By contrast, children who had a familial history of persistent stuttering also had about a 65% chance of following their familial pattern. Adding this to even more direct evidence (Ambrose, Cox, & Yairi, 1997), it was concluded that recovery and persistency are influenced by genetics. Later hints of chromosomal differences between persistent and recovered stuttering have reinforced this conclusion (Suresh et al., 2006).

Another group of predictors was derived from speech factors. A strong one is the difference in the change in stuttering-like disfluencies (SLD) between children who recover naturally and those who persist. As you can see in Figure 3.2, at the earliest stage of the disorder, there is no distinction in the amount of SLD exhibited by children in the two groups. By 7 to 12 months following onset, however, there are signs of divergence. From this point on, differences are clear and significant. Generally, the level of SLD decreases in those who recover, eventually reaching normalcy. For children whose stuttering persists, the mean SLD remains constant for a while but later also declines somewhat, although several of them do increase their level. Hence the overall direction of SLD somewhere between 7 to 12 months post-onset is important for predicting the future course of stuttering.

Also of interest are the findings that the levels of Other Disfluencies (more typical to normal fluency) were not different among persistent, recovered, and normally fluent children during the first 2 years after onset. This class is not an important component in the clinical evaluation, development, and prediction of stuttering, at least in

Figure 3.2 Stuttering Frequency: Persistent, Recovered, and Control Groups

Ctl = control; Per = persistent; Rec = recovered; SLD = stuttering-like disfluency; Wt = weighted. *Source: Early Childhood Stuttering* (p. 78) by E. Yairi and N. G. Ambrose (2005), Austin, TX: PRO-ED. Copyright by authors, 2013.

young children. What counts are the up-and-down dynamics of SLD. Several additional speech disfluency features, such as type, length, and clustering, as well as secondary characteristics, are other potential predictors but appear to be weaker in power. The process of recovery seems to be associated not only with declining frequency of SLD but also with declining SLD length, fewer secondary characteristics (Throneburg & Yairi, 2001), and shorter disfluency clusters (Sawyer & Yairi, 2010).

In regard to linguistic factors, it appears that, on average, near the onset of stuttering, these children's language skills are at or above age norms. The Illinois studies revealed the interesting finding that within 3 years post-onset, the language performance of children who recovered naturally did not remain above average, whereas the language of children who persisted in stuttering tended to stay above average (Watkins, 2005; Watkins et al., 2000). If true, it means that advanced language may be a risk factor for persistency. At present, however, the predictive power of a child's language skills is not clear. The predictive power of phonological skills is also limited. During the very early phase of stuttering, phonological skills distinguish between those who will eventually recover and persist, but by the second year of stuttering, the difference between groups is greatly diminished and no longer statistically significant (Paden, 2005; Paden et al., 2002).

Summary

Onset

Improved scientific methods employed during the past 30 years have shed new light on the onset of stuttering. It appears that more than 60% of the children who stutter begin doing so prior to age 3, a figure that climbs to 85% by 4 years of age. These are earlier ages and within a narrower range than has been previously assumed. The findings reinforce the notion that, by and large, stuttering is a disorder that begins in early childhood. The overlap of many stuttering onsets with the period of fast development of the speech mechanism, rapid acquisition of complex articulatory movement, and expansion of syntactic and other language faculties raises the specter of stuttering-articulation-phonology-language links. These, however, have not been clearly established. Onset of stuttering after age 4 may involve a different interaction of etiological factors.

Recent data on the symptomatology of very early stuttering dispel traditional views of the event of onset. Clinicians should be prepared for:

- Heterogeneity in the characteristics observed and the manner in which it begins.
- Children whose onset is quite sudden; this is not parental imagination.
- Early stuttering that is rather advanced in the wealth of its characteristics and, in some cases, is quite severe.
- Whereas repetitions of initial syllables and short words are almost universal, stuttering may begin with or without sound prolongations, blocks, accessory physical tensions, and with or without awareness and emotional reactions.
- The early characteristics of stuttering negate the diagnosogenic theory (to be discussed in Chapter 6) that suggests stuttering begins as normal disfluencies that turn into stuttering due to the reactions of overanxious parents.
- Because the onset of stuttering marks a definite change in the child's normally fluent speech, parents may be quite apprehensive about its development.

Development

As we have seen, great variability is also the hallmark of the development of stuttering after it has begun. Whereas some children present more severe and complex overt stuttering with the passage of time, accompanied with various emerging, often strong, emotional components, others continue stuttering at a low level or stop stuttering altogether. Most importantly, the current solid evidence contradicts the traditional depiction of the disorder as always increasing in complexity and severity. Data clearly indicate the following:

- The most typical developmental trend of early stuttering is downward, decreasing in severity.
- The majority of children who stutter recover completely without clinical intervention. Thus early childhood is not only the period when most stuttering begins; it is also the time when the disorder stops due to natural remission.
- Emerging information regarding predictive factors for recovery and persistency in stuttering is important to the understanding of stuttering in general and has major practical implications for research purposes, parent counseling, and treatment decisions.

Study Questions and Discussion Topics

1. What is the theoretical significance and what are practical implications of information concerning the onset of stuttering?

2. What major changes in information (e.g., in terms of age, gender, suddenness, severity, concomitant behaviors) about the onset of stuttering have resulted from recent pertinent studies?

3. What is meant by sequential developmental models of stuttering? What is the major premise of the various developmental schemes that have been offered? Which more recent research findings make that premise questionable?

4. What are the main findings concerning natural recovery in terms of timing, percentage, and other factors (e.g., age, gender, etc.)?

5. What are the implications of information concerning natural recovery for clinical decisions? For the identification of sample populations in research?

Suggested Readings

Ambrose, N. G., & Yairi, E. (1999). Normative disfluency data for early childhood stuttering. *Journal of Speech, Language, and Hearing Research, 42,* 895–909.

Ambrose, N. G., & Yairi, E. (2002). The Tudor study: Data and ethics. *American Journal of Speech-Language Pathology, 11*(2), 190–203.

Månsson, H. (2000). Childhood stuttering: Incidence and development. *Journal of Fluency Disorders, 25,* 47–57.

Yairi, E., & Ambrose, N. (2005). *Early childhood stuttering* (Chapters 3, 4, and 5). Austin, TX: Pro Ed.

Chapter 4

Where Does Stuttering End? What Are Its Advanced Characteristics?

LEARNER OBJECTIVES

Readers of this chapter will be able to:

- Identify speech and physical behaviors associated with advanced stuttering.
- Understand research regarding the characteristics of people who stutter.
- Recognize the dynamics of stuttered speech as reflected in various phenomena and rules of stuttering.
- Develop appreciation of the emotional and cognitive aspects of advanced stuttering.

Advanced Stuttering

In Chapter 3, the characteristics of early childhood stuttering were described with just a few references to late occurring changes as depicted in Bloodstein's (1960b) developmental system. Although we commented that a good number of features seen in older individuals can also be observed in some young children, there are still marked disorder differences between children and adults who stutter. These include the proportions of certain disfluency types, the loci of stuttering, cognition, affective reactions, and others. Age and experience impact the stuttering disorder. For example, whereas 3-year-old children who stutter rarely experience negative reactions from others their age, many older children, as well as adults who stutter, do experience such reactions. Also, young children's limited cognitive abilities and brief history of the disorder may limit their anticipation of stuttering events as compared with adults. As stuttering lingers on and becomes chronic, additional and more consistent features appear and/or old ones crystallize to present a more complicated disorder. Furthermore, strong interactions among multiple systems can become firmly rooted beneath the surface of stuttering. Although Bluemel (1932) opined that incipient stuttering is a "pure" speech disturbance (and our definition agrees with him), we have alluded to stuttering as a complex disorder with multiple dimensions, especially when it persists. This chapter presents the broad range of symptoms and dynamics that are encountered in advanced stuttering. Acknowledging its essence, however, stuttering is typically classified as a speech disorder (ASHA, 2008b). Therefore, in accounting for its advanced characteristics, we begin with the obvious attributes of stuttering: speech features. These are rich in quantity and quality, and they include speech disfluency as well as other disruptions to suprasegmental properties.

Speech Disfluency

The interruption in the flow of speech, often referred to as speech disfluency, is the cardinal feature of stuttering. There is no stuttering without it. All the other characteristics frequently associated with the stuttering disorder, combined, would not be sufficient to amount to something that would merit the label "stuttering." As we explained in Chapter 1, however, the terms *disfluency* and *stuttering* should not be equated. Disfluency has a wider meaning in that it covers all speech interruptions. Some of these are regarded as typically normal, whereas others are regarded as typically abnormal, mostly stuttering. The distinction is complicated in that not all disfluent events in the speech of people who stutter are necessarily stuttering; some are normal. Types of disfluencies usually regarded as stuttering, however, are sometimes present in the speech of normally fluent speakers.

A bit of history. The term *nonfluency*, later referred to as *disfluency*, was first used by Wendell Johnson in the mid-20th century. Because he was convinced that stuttering moments evolved from normal disfluencies, he used the term *nonfluencies* in his published works, for example, throughout *The Onset of Stuttering* (Johnson & Associates, 1959). Prior to that time, stutter events mainly had been called *spasms* (Johnson & Leutenegger, 1955; Van Riper, 1992). Johnson later adopted the term *disfluency* after Van Riper argued with him that it did not make sense to identify or count "non-somethings" (Van Riper, 1992, p. 83). In the 1960s, the term *disfluency* began to appear in publications by Johnson and his colleagues, as in the title of the Iowa Speech Disfluency Test (Sander, 1961).

An important issue related to use of the term *disfluency* arises because research has shown that judgments of "stuttering" or "normal" are influenced by a host of factors. The label "stuttering moments" implies a value judgment by the listener. Various factors affect a listener's identification of a speech interruption as either normal or stuttering. Some are rooted in the objective properties of the speech segment in question, such as the specific type of disfluency. Sound prolongation, for example, is more apt to be perceived as stuttering than interjection (Young, 1984). Another property is the extent or duration of the segment. If the syllable *pa* in the word *patient* is repeated five times, it is much more likely to be judged as stuttering than if it is repeated only once or twice.

Other factors are rooted in more subjective influences, such as the listeners' background, life experience, and their cognitive set at a particular time. The same disfluent speech event may be judged differently by another listener or even by the same listener at different times or circumstances. In a well-known study, listeners were asked to mark down all stuttered interruptions in a speech sample. Other listeners were asked to mark down all normal speech interruptions. The investigators found that a majority of events were counted either as normal or stuttered, depending on the instructions. When asked to listen for stuttering, more events were so marked. When asked to listen for normal disfluency, more events were so marked (Williams & Kent, 1958). Similarly, a person who has family members who stutter may be more sensitive and inclined to judge speech interruptions as stuttering (Sander, 1968). Therefore, clinicians, older clients, and family members need to be aware that perceptions can be swayed by what the listener expects to hear. According to one theory, if the normal-abnormal distinction of speech interruptions is blurred, and an overly concerned parent perceives a young child's speech interruptions as abnormal and erroneously labels them as "stuttering," the distressed reactions could give rise to real stuttering (Johnson & Associates, 1959).

In contrast to value-laden judgments, identification of speech disruptions according to descriptive disfluency types does not involve labeling them as "stuttering," "normal," "desirable," or "undesirable." Typical disfluency classes simply describe the speech behaviors (e.g., *syllable repetition* or *sound prolongation*). The listener is focused on objective dimensions. It then becomes possible to address questions about which disfluent speech classes are more typical in the speech of people who stutter and which are more typical of normally fluent speakers. The answer is therefore a matter of statistical probability, not subjective judgment (Bloodstein, 1970; Yairi & Ambrose, 2005).

Types of Disfluency

Clinicians and researchers have not yet agreed on a particular taxonomy of disfluency classification. This fact was illustrated when Kully and Boberg (1988) sent a set of 10 speech samples (8 from stutterers, 2 from nonstutterers) to clinics in the United States, Canada, Australia, and Great Britain. Across the nine respondents who returned their analyses, there were pronounced discrepancies in the stuttering, disfluency, and syllable counts. Although we challenge their conclusions that ignore these authors' own data,[1] the study highlights potential problems regarding communication among professionals who employ a wide variety of procedural systems.

Disfluency classification systems began to appear in the literature in the late 1930s when several students of Wendell Johnson (e.g., Branscom, 1942; Davis, 1939) investigated speech interruptions in normally fluent preschool-age children. Due to the technical limitations of audio recording in that period, their archaic repertoire included only three types: syllable, word, and phrase repetition. Since then, a number of classifications have been offered, but they mostly represent variations of the eight disfluency types employed by Johnson and associates (1959). To cover speech interruptions found in

---

[1]Kully and Boberg (1988) emphasized the disagreement among clinics in identifying stuttering and disfluencies. The data in their Table 2 reveal that the average agreement between the two clinics that counted "percent disfluency" was 81.7%, a respectable level that was considerably better than agreement among clinics that counted "percent stuttering."

advanced stuttering, as well as in normally fluent speakers, we list and briefly describe types of disfluency.

Types of Speech Disfluency

I. **Part-word repetitions.** Repetitions of sounds or syllables. No distinction is made between these two. For example, "a-ai," "f-five," "ba-baby," "mo-mo-mommy." Various speech sounds may be repeated including vowels and consonants of different types.

II. **Single-syllable whole-word repetitions.** For example, "but-but," "and-and." Here, and in all other repetitions of speech segments, it is important to distinguish disfluency from what is not. Some repetitions are not disfluencies when they are words intended for emphasis such as: "It's so good, good, good!" (enthusiastically).

III. **Multiple-syllable word repetitions.** Repetition of longer words, such as "Because–because." Similar exceptions for emphasis apply. For example, in "She is very, very nice," the word *very* is not counted as a disfluency.

IV. **Phrase repetitions.** Repetition of any segment longer than one word, "I was–I was going," and even a word plus a sound or syllable of the next word as in "Once up–once upon" are examples of this type of disfluency.

V. **Prolonged sounds.** These are audible elongations of vowels as in "a>>>>>ai like to go," or elongations of consonants, such as in "M>>>>>>y name is." Or "S>>>>ometimes." Prolongations may be voiced or voiceless.

VI. **Blocks and broken words.** The articulators (tongue, lips) or the vocal cords are held in fixed positions, either at the beginning of a word, such as in "C———cake," or in the middle of a word as in "The ta———able is set." Typically, the blocks are silent or accompanied with minimally audible sound. They are *within-word* phenomena.

VII. **Tense pause.** These are unusual breaks that occur *between* words, associated with tense sounds, such as escaping air (e.g., I like to————go home").

VIII. **Interjections.** Those are extraneous sounds such as "um," "uh," "er," and "hmmm." Interjection, too, may be repeated such as in "um-um." Words and phrases such as *like, well,* or *you know,* are not considered disfluencies but become of interest if they are so frequent as to be distracting.

IX. **Revisions and incomplete utterance.** A revision is when an utterance is modified but the general content remains the same (e.g., "I like—I want this ball"). An incomplete (abandoned) utterance occurs when there is an apparent change of thought in the middle of the utterance (e.g., "The baby is—let's do that").

The physiological correlates of disfluencies vary. Obviously, repetitions involve articulatory gestures that are integral to the production of the specific sound except that they are unnecessarily repeated. Examples include approximation of the lips ("Mo-Mo-Mommy"), elevation of the back of the tongue ("ka-ka-kite"), movement of the whole tongue and jaw ("I-I-I") and tip of the tongue ("Da-Da-Daddy"), and others.

Often, however, these movements involve observable and/or audible tension. When the repeated sounds are voiced, more tension in the larynx may be associated.

Some disfluencies may involve abnormal articulatory positioning. Those labeled as tense pauses, for example, are associated with *blockages* or *blocks* of the vocal tract to the point that no air can pass through and no sound, or only barely audible sound, is emitted. Such silent blocks may occur at one of several levels: larynx, tongue, or lips, or sometimes at multiple levels. In "K——kite," the initial movement of the back of the tongue against the hard palate is legitimate, but it stays in tight contact too long. This is also referred to as *articulatory fixation*. When the vocal folds are tightly fixed, they are either in the abducted or adducted position—a *laryngeal fixation*. The specific disfluency examples given in the category of sound prolongations also involve *articulatory fixation*. The initial approximation of the articulators may be basically right, but they stay fixed in place for too long. In a prolongation, however, the fixation does not completely block the airflow, allowing for voiced prolongation such as "M>>>>an" or "Z>>>>>ebra," or for a voiceless prolongation such as "S>>>>nake." Van Riper (1982) stated, "These blocking and closures are some of the most important phenomena in the multifaceted disorder of advanced stuttering. The stutterer senses such closure very vividly. For a moment he feels impotent, out of control" (p. 122).

Over the years, the various disfluency types have been combined, renamed, or removed altogether. In 1968, Williams, Silverman, and Kools combined sound prolongations, blocks, and broken words into a single category labeled *disrhythmic phonation*. Also *revision* and *incomplete phrase* were merged. In 1981, Yairi separated word repetition into two different types: *monosyllabic word repetition* and *multisyllabic word repetition*. Campbell and Hill (1987) divided part-word repetition into *sound and syllable repetition* and added *hesitation,* and Ambrose and Yairi (1999) combined *multisyllabic word repetition* with *phrase repetition* into a single type and eliminated *tense pause,* which had low identification reliability.

Major Disfluency Classes

Scholars in the field have realized that disfluencies differ in the degree to which they are prevalent in the speech of people who stutter and normally fluent speakers, as well as in the extent to which they are perceived as stuttering or normal. Consequently, several attempts for grouping the various disfluency types to reflect such differences have been made. For example, Conture (2001) distinguished between *within-word disfluency* (including sound repetition, syllable repetition, and prolongation), which are more likely to be "stuttering," and *between-word disfluency* (all other types), which are more likely to be "normal disfluency." Campbell and Hill (1987) distinguish between *more typical* and *less typical* disfluency. They describe their classification as a continuum of disfluent speech behaviors. On one end of the continuum are the typical disfluencies of hesitations, interjections, revisions, and phrase repetitions; on the opposite end are the atypical disfluencies of sound repetitions, prolongations, blocks, and other signs of increased tension. In the middle are the "crossover" behaviors that could be either typical or atypical, depending on such features as numbers of repetitions per instance, or tension level. These disfluencies include part-word and one-syllable word repetitions. We find this classification problematic because the terminology employed uses "normal" (*typical*) as the reference within a framework of a continuum. It may imply that stuttering is merely a change in degree of what normal speakers do, not something unique to the disorder. In our opinion, although there is some similarity in format (e.g., repetitions), the nature of the production of stuttering is different (Throneburg & Yairi, 2001).

The classification proposed by the Illinois Stuttering Research Program (Ambrose & Yairi, 1999) also consists of two disfluency classes, *stuttering-like disfluency* (SLD) and *other disfluency* (OD), and each includes three types. These are listed next.

The Illinois Disfluency Classification System	
Stuttering-Like Disfluency	**Other Disfluency**
Part-Word Repetition	Interjection
Single-Syllable Word Repetition	Multisyllable-Word and Phrase Repetition
Disrhythmic Phonation	Revision/Abandoned Utterance

By using the terms *stuttering-like* and *other,* the authors underscore that certain disfluencies are neither exclusively stuttering nor exclusively normal. The distinction between the two classes is accomplished by implying the greater statistical probability of (a) their occurrence in the speech of the respective group of speakers, and (b) being perceived by listeners as different, the first type as stuttering and the second one as normal. Indeed, speech of children and adults who stutter contains a high proportion of disfluency types referred to as SLD. Also, it appears that the proportion of disrhythmic phonation (sound prolongations, blocks, and broken words) within the SLD is increased from early to advanced stuttering (Bloodstein, 1960b). Good-to-high interjudge (between different judges) reliability for SLD, reflecting agreement on the specific type and location of each disfluent event, has been reported in several studies as 0.86 and 0.89 or even higher (e.g., Ambrose & Yairi, 1999; Gregg & Yairi, 2007). It is recognized, however, that errors may occur when counting/classifying disfluencies. A small percentage of SLD may not represent stuttering whereas more normal disfluencies, such as interjections and short phrase repetitions, may be perceived as stuttering under certain circumstances.

In all, the three disfluency classifications (Conture, 2001; Gregory & Hill, 1999; Yairi & Ambrose, 2005) are in close agreement about the central characteristics of stuttering in terms of core speech features. They also recognize that a distinction between what is stuttering and what is normal can sometimes be difficult. Hence a small percentage of errors can be expected (Conture, 2001). Also, identification of a particular type of disfluency is sometimes challenging. For example, differentiating a repeated interjected "uh, uh" from a repeated article "a, a," or making a judgment of how to categorize a sound that is prolonged as it is being pulsed in a repetitive manner. Is it a prolongation or repetition? Strangely, a few scholars (e.g., Brocklehurst, 2013) have asserted that whereas syllable repetition, such as "bu-bu-bu-but," is stuttering, monosyllabic word repetition, such as "but-but-but-but" is not. We disagree. For opposing arguments, see Yairi (2013).

Dimensions of Disfluency

Frequency

The frequency of occurrence of each of the disfluency types and their total count has been its most commonly examined and reported dimension and is typically reported in terms of either the (1) *number* of disfluencies per 100 syllables or 100 words, or the (2) *percent* syllables or words that contain disfluency. (Methods for quantifying disfluency and stuttering are discussed in detail in Chapter 8.) Keep in mind, however, that even in advanced stages of the disorder, most of the speech of people who stutter is fluent. Bloodstein (1944) reported that, on average, only 10% of the words emitted by adults who stutter contain disfluencies regarded as stuttering.

It is equally important to realize that figures for the average, or mean, frequency of occurrence are likely to be misleading due to large daily and situational fluctuations often observed within each individual who stutters. Perhaps the most remarkable variations are seen in several conditions recognized to have an almost universal effect of temporarily reducing, or eliminating, the occurrence of stuttering. These include speaking alone, speaking to animals or babies, speaking in the presence of high-level noise, singing, talking in rhythm (as paced by a metronome), talking in unison, and whispering, Some of these, especially noise, have been richly investigated and are discussed later in the chapter. Other factors, however, seem to have the influence of increasing stuttering, for example, time pressure (Guitar, Schaefer, Donahue et al., 1992), the level of meaningful information in a message (Wingate, 1975), language complexity (Jayaram, 1984), and the size of audience (Young, 1985). Many other conditions are highly individualized. Some people increase the frequency of stuttering when speaking to specific persons, the opposite sex, or people in authority, or in specific physical environments, and so on. One of us had experienced more stuttering when lecturing in a particular classroom. Bloodstein and Bernstein Ratner (2008, p. 262) concluded that "what we know about the way stuttering varies in frequency can be generalized by saying that it is affected by communicative pressures."

Duration

One measure of length is the *duration* from the beginning to the end of a disfluent event. It can be applied to all disfluency types (e.g., sound prolongation or syllable repetition, or across both of them). Experienced clinicians are likely to have observed disfluencies lasting 30 seconds or longer. These certainly impact listeners. Such long disfluencies, however, are not too common.

Studies found that most disfluent events in the speech of adults who stutter are short with an overall mean of 1 second (Bloodstein & Bernstein Ratner, 2008). In one study, the mean length for individual participants ranged up to 3.7 seconds with a group median of 0.9 second. Only 25% of the 30 participants exhibited means longer than 1.4 seconds (Bloodstein, 1944). This is not much longer than the mean duration of all disfluency types for preschool children, about 1.1 seconds, reported by Yairi and Ambrose (2005). Not much change seems to have occurred over time in this respect. Beyond the mean, there is interest in looking at the extreme ends of the range. Johnson and Colley (1945) reported that the mean of the 10 shortest blocks was 0.41 seconds, whereas the mean of the 10 longest was 4.1 seconds. It seems like a rather narrow range unless one considers that people produce as many as a dozen words in 4 seconds.

Interestingly, listeners' perceptions of the length of disfluencies complement the speech production measures. Studies have found that sound prolongations lasting 1 second or longer are most apt to be perceived as stuttering (Lingwall & Bergstrand, 1979). Some prolongations are judged as stuttering after only a half second (Kawai, Healey, & Carrell, 2007). This should not be surprising because normally a single syllable in connected speech is uttered in less than one fifth of a second.

Examination of the age effect on the duration of sound prolongations shows only modest changes as stuttering advances. Mean durations near stuttering onset were approximately 632 milliseconds whereas 36 months later, nearing school age and stuttering persistence, the mean was elevated to 824 milliseconds. Although both means were less than 1 second, their relative values indicate that as stuttering continues, prolongations increase in duration (Throneburg & Yairi, 2001). With further advancement in age, the mean length of prolongations in school-age children and adults is about 1 second for either age group (Zebrowski, 1994). The high mean for individual adults, however, could reach 3 or 4 seconds as indicated above. This, however, is not clear because the investigators lumped together several disfluency types, not just prolongations.

Although repetitive disfluencies (e.g., syllable or word repetition) could also be measured for their duration in time, usually their length is determined by counting the number of extra iterations of the syllable or word. This measure is referred to as *repetition*

> The length of repetition type disfluencies is measured by the number of extra iterations of a speech segment. The concept underlying the measurement of repeated units, however, is not what people expect. The repeated units are not the segments said after its first utterance. Instead, the extra repetition units are the ones uttered *before* the sound or syllable is finally blended with the intended word. Hence, the sound or syllable eventually spoken as the fluent word is not counted (e.g., "but" in "b-b-b-but"), whereas the extra sounds or syllables uttered before the fluent word are the ones that are being counted (e.g., "b-b-b-" in "b-b-b-but"). This concept helps prevent an error in counting. Examination of the extra sounds or syllables at the start makes it easier to find the three units in the example.

units (Ambrose & Yairi, 1995). For example, "a-and" has one extra production of the vowel segment, which is counted as one repetition unit. If a speaker utters "a-a-and," it is counted as two repetition units. The number of repetition units also has an impact on the perception of stuttering as well as its severity (Sander, 1963). Obviously, a person saying "but-but-but-but-but-but-but-but-but" is bound to attract more attention and have his or her stuttering regarded as more severe than a person who says only "but-but-but."

Unfortunately, many studies of disfluency in people who stutter have focused only on the frequency of disfluent events, neglecting information about length. For example, several investigations by Onslow and associates (e.g., Onslow, Andrews, & Lincoln, 1994) reported the percentage of syllables stuttered but not the length or number of repetition units. If only the number of disfluent instances is considered, then the sentence "I-I am go-going ho-ho-me now" and the sentence "I-I-I-I-I am go-go-go-go-going ho-ho-ho-ho-home now" yield the same count: three instances of repetition. But were these of the same stuttering severity? Obviously not. Unfortunately, important information is lost in research studies, clinical evaluations, and progress reports.

Although our clinical experience has included samples of disfluencies containing more than 20 repetition units for a word or a syllable, these are the exceptions. The mean repetition units for preschool stuttering children was between 1.53 and 1.70. For normally fluent peers, 80% to 87% of their repetitions had only one extra unit ("a-and"), with a mean of about 1.16 (Ambrose & Yairi, 1995; Yairi & Lewis, 1984). These investigators concluded that the number of repetition units was the measure that best differentiated the young children who stutter from their normally fluent peers. School-age children who stutter had a mean of 2.45 units per instance (Zebrowski, 1994). Unfortunately, no data have been reported for adults.

Clusters

Another feature of stuttered speech, discussed in Chapter 3, is the tendency of disfluent events to occur in clusters of two or more on the same word or adjacent words. As mentioned, young children who stutter produce more disfluency clusters than normally fluent children (Hubbard & Yairi, 1988; LaSalle & Conture, 1995; Sawyer & Yairi, 2010). Limited information has been made available for advanced stuttering. Two investigations supported a tendency for clustering in adults (Fein, 1970; Still & Griggs, 1979), but a study of school-age children did not (Taylor & Taylor, 1967). The latter study, however, applied different definitions and analysis methods. Robb, Sargent, and O'Beirne (2009) observed clusters in adults who stutter but did not evaluate cluster frequencies with a model of what could be expected by chance. They found that clusters significantly increased with frequency of disfluency and with length of utterance. Mixed clusters (i.e., SLD-OD) were significantly more frequent than within class clusters (i.e., SLD-SLD or OD-OD). The significance of clustering is that it may contribute to the perceptual impression of "stuttering" or suggest greater severity. Further research is needed to explore clustering and its significance in advanced stuttering.

Physical Concomitants

We made reference to the physical concomitants of stuttering in Chapters 1 and 3. *Secondary* or *accessory characteristics* are other common terms referring to such concomitants. These are various body movements and postures that accompany stuttering events. Physical concomitants are many and appear in numerous variations among and within individuals who stutter. Tense body movements, especially in the head and neck, are often involved, but other body parts are involved too. Some are easily observed; others are covert. One individual reported that listeners have no idea that his toes are curling inside his shoes during moments of stuttering. Undoubtedly, physical concomitants contribute to the effect of tense, struggled speech, the perception of stuttering severity, and the overall degree of abnormality. A list of the most common observable characteristics is provided next.

Physical Concomitants (Secondary or Accessory Characteristics)	
Head jerks	Head turns (side; down)
Forehead tension	Nostrils flaring/constricted
Eyes closed; squinting	Eyes widely open
Facial contortions	Lips pressured
Jaw closed tightly	Teeth grinding
Jaw wide open	Rotational or sideways jaw movement
Tongue protrusion	Throat tightened
Body swaying	Hand and/or arm movements
Stepping sideways or backward	Clenching hands
Raising shoulder	
Irregular exhalation (blowing) during speech	
Irregular inhalations (gasping) in the midst of speaking	

The occurrence of most of these secondary characteristics during stuttering events in the speech of individuals ages 14 to 23 was investigated and confirmed by means of a motion picture camera, followed with a fine frame-by-frame analysis of the films (Prins & Lohr, 1972). The study, however, was confined to the head and neck. One finding was that the number of areas within the head and neck region involved in stutter events had a significant weight on the severity factor. It is important to understand that movement and/or postures regarded as concomitants are not necessary for the production of the intended speech. For example, engaging in a laryngeal block, the mouth may be widely open and some jaw movement observed. These gestures would have nothing to do with the production of the intended /i/ vowel. Closing the eyes or jerking the head sideways has nothing to do with the production of any speech sound.

Another physiological component sometimes observed in advanced stuttering is *tremor*. We have seen tremor in several clients, especially in the lips or jaw. Tremor is typically defined as a rhythmic, involuntary, oscillating movement of a body part. Physiological tremor is a normal phenomenon that affects all people when they engage in a sustained effort of muscle contraction. The typical oscillation rate of tremor is from 8 to 10 Hertz (Hz). In some situations (e.g., being anxious or very tired), tremors can become exaggerated. In a person who stutters, tremors appear to occur in the speech musculature when tension increases in antagonistic muscles. Research of tremor has shown evidence of oscillations in electromyography (EMG) activity ranging from 5 to 15 Hz in the upper lip, lower lip, or jaw structures of children and adults who stutter (Kelly, Smith, & Goffman, 1995; Smith, 1989). These findings could reflect instabilities in their speech motor systems. Chapter 7 has more information on this topic.

Why are physical concomitants viewed as *accessory* and *secondary*? According to Van Riper (1971), they are accessory because they are not "basic"; that is, they are not part of the central stuttering core of sound/syllable repetitions and prolongations. And, they are secondary because they occur late in the disorder's development. Reflected in much of the literature is a strong assumption that those accessories are acquired "behaviors" that are reinforced via instrumental learning (e.g., Brutten & Shoemaker, 1967). We take a skeptical view toward interpretation of physical concomitants as reinforced secondary reactions. As we discussed in Chapter 3, these supposedly "secondary" characteristics have been observed in young children from early stages of their stuttering. The possibility that these movements constitute an integral part of the neuromuscular disturbance in stuttering has not been ruled out.

Originally, so the thinking goes, secondary behaviors were used by the person who stutters to help cope with, or "get out of," stuttering blocks. At a critical moment, the behavior happened to coincide with relief from a speech block and was immediately reinforced. Over time the behavior was deeply integrated with the complex stuttering block, making it more severe. The stutterer's false feeling that the behavior provides relief from the block overrides any recognition that it actually does the opposite. Some clinicians have included secondary characteristics as targets for treatment (e.g., directly attempting to eliminate them). Other clinicians, however, have argued that this is not necessary; reducing the stuttered speech will automatically result in lessening these secondaries (Webster, 1980a).

Other Speech Characteristics

Voice

As stuttering persists, the speaker displays difficulty regulating dimensions of voice and speaking rate in addition to disfluency. Various vocal phenomena, such as monotone, sudden sharp shifts in the vocal pitch, occasional vocal fry,[2] and strained voice,

---

[2]Vocal fry, also known as glottal fry, refers to the low-pitched, creaky sound of air weakly bubbling up through the vocal folds. It has a pulsating sound like the effect of running a finger along the teeth of a comb.

are common in advanced stuttering. We have also observed cessations of phonation and changes in resonance quality, for example, the voice becoming quite denasal during stuttering. Some of these, such as vocal fry, are not abnormal but occur more frequently than in typically normal speech. Such characteristics are usually related to problems with regulating tension. Tense muscles are stiff, and stiffness offers resistance to movement. Excess tension could account for the speaker's sensation that the voice or speech mechanism is "stuck." Pitch inflection, an uncontrolled sudden rise in pitch on a voiced speech sound, is a possible acoustic outcome of excess tension in the voice.

Monotonous vocal pitch and a number of other changes in vocal quality may be used as avoidance to guard against stuttering. Vocal fry and monotonous pitch further add to the decline in overall quality of communication by the person who stutters. It is more difficult for listeners to focus on what the person is saying when, in addition to stuttering, the voice is flat and rough. Clinicians should be attentive to these dimensions in their overall therapeutic approach.

Acoustic and physiological research has supported laryngeal involvement in stuttering. In the 1970s and 1980s, there were many studies of both vocal reaction time (VRT), the interval between presenting a stimulus to the subject and the beginning of a vocal response, as well as of voice onset time (VOT), the gap between the release of a consonant and the beginning of vocal fold vibration on the following voiced sound (e.g., Adams, 1987). Although findings were inconsistent, Ward (2006) concluded that, overall, adults who stutter (1) tend to exhibit longer VRT and VOT, and (2) evidence less control (greater variability) in this respect than normally fluent speakers. Studies that investigated electrical activity in the larynx of people who stutter using EMG techniques, found a higher level of muscle tonus and simultaneous contraction of antagonistic opening and closing muscles during fluent speech (Freeman & Ushijima, 1978; Shapiro, 1980). Other investigators, however, reported that people who stutter reduced EMG activity during fluent speech (Smith, Denny, Shaffer et al. 1996). Conture, McCall, and Brewer (1977) used motion pictures to observe the larynx and also reported abnormal positioning during stuttering. The importance of such research is reflected in the fact that laryngeal control has long been recognized in therapy. For example, easy voice onset is an important target in several current prominent therapeutic programs. These are discussed in Chapter 12.

Speaking Rate

One traditional measure of verbal output is referred to as *overall speaking rate*. It is a global indicator of the amount of speech (number of words or syllables), including pauses and disfluencies, that a person utters in a given time. The overall speaking rate is lower (slower) for people who stutter than for normally fluent speakers. This is understandable because repeating the word *and* five times instead of just saying it once, and having additional interruptions, takes a longer time. Research has confirmed this common impression. Moderate to moderately high negative correlations of −0.72 and −0.88 between frequency of stuttering and overall speaking rate were reported by investigators a long time ago (e.g., Aron, 1967). Therefore, overall speaking rate can be clinically useful in evaluating stuttering as well as in monitoring therapeutic progress.

> Early on, Bloodstein (1944) reported the mean overall speaking rate during reading for adults who stutter was 122.7 words per minute (wpm), substantially slower than the mean of 170 wpm for normally fluent speakers (Walker, 1988). The difference in the two means is an excellent reflection of the growing communication problem as stuttering persists. Of course, diversity of rate is found in both groups. For people who stutter, the range is particularly wide, extending from 42 to 191 wpm. A satisfactory range for oral reading usually extends from 150 to 180 wpm (Fairbanks, 1960). It can be logically inferred that the slower the rate, the more stuttering.

The slower than normal overall speaking rate of people who stutter has raised the question of whether their speech movement during fluent speech also differs from normal. To this end, another indicator, *articulatory rate,* is used to measure the speed of speech after pauses and disfluent segments are disregarded. Some data along this line have been provided for adults but usually in the context of another topic of research (e.g., Logan, Roberts, Pretto et al., 2002; Prins & Hubbard, 1990). School-age data comparing CWS and NFC were reported by Logan, Byrd, Mazzocchi et al. 2011). Articulatory rates have been reported in terms of either syllables per second or phones per second. A reduction in the variability of articulatory rate has been suggested as an indicator of posttreatment improvement (Onslow, van Doorn, & Newman, 1992). Logan et al. (2011) found that articulatory rates of school-age CWS and NFS were not significantly different. Instructions for measurement of articulatory and speaking rates are presented in Chapter 8.

Durations of articulatory movements, measured kinematically, tend to be slower in adolescents and adults who stutter than in normally fluent speakers (e.g., Archibald & De Nil, 1999; Zimmerman & Hanley, 1983). This slowness, also seen in acoustic measures, appears to be present across all transitions between consonant and vowel segments (Prins & Hubbard, 1990). The clinical implication of slower fluent speech is counterintuitive. If the speech of people who stutter is already slower, why is it therapeutic to slow their speech further? Some ideas are presented in Chapters 6 and 7 that deal with theories of stuttering. This paradox, however, is not unique to stuttering remediation. Treatment of dysarthria, which is also slower than normal speech, is achieved with further slowing by the speaker.

Emotional Characteristics and Cognition

Emotional Reactions

One of the most commonly recognized characteristics of advanced stuttering is the complex emotionality that evolves over time (Bloodstein, 1960b; Bloodstein & Bernstein Ratner, 2008). These emotions may include fear, dread, anxiety, being trapped, panic, embarrassment, shame, humiliation, anger, resentment, and other unpleasant feelings. The type of emotions varies in time relative to the stuttering event:

Prior to stuttering—fear, dread, anxiety, panic.
During Stuttering—blankness, being trapped, panic, frustration.
After stuttering—shame, humiliation, anger, resentment.

Whereas many laypeople might believe that people stutter because they are emotional, it would appear to be just the opposite: People become emotional because they stutter. Research has confirmed that heightened emotional reactions are common in people who stutter. Both *state* and *trait* anxiety are greater among those who stutter than in the general population (Craig, Hancock, Tran et al., 2003). State anxiety is an emotional tension triggered by specific situations; trait anxiety is a relatively stable tendency to be emotionally tense in situations.

At what stage of the disorder does stuttering evoke these feelings? As indicated in Chapter 3, typically young children do not react to stuttering with the wide range of emotions and intensity that older children and adults do. As emotional reactions build up, three factors are apt to influence the level and timing of a child's reactions: (1) the child's sensitivity to stuttering, (2) other's reactions to stuttering, and (3) the child's reactions to others. Thus emotions emerge after the speaker becomes aware that stuttering is unpleasant to him or her. The fear escalates when a simple attempt to communicate deteriorates by means of a stutter into a terrifying feeling of being trapped, after attracting an upsurge of unwanted listener reactions, be they real or imagined. Loathing of stuttering develops after the stuttering beast has made mountains out of molehills.

Awareness is a complicated construct, and more knowledge is needed regarding its development. The mind is primed at an early age to detect novel stimuli. Seven-month-old infants tend to stare longer at novel stimuli than habituated stimuli (Fagan, 1984). At 14 months, infants who are shown actions with no opportunity to imitate them display recall of those modeled actions 4 months later (Meltzoff, 1995). At 2½ years of age, children can provide verbal descriptions of unique events they experienced 6 or more months in the past (Fivush, Gray, & Fromhoff, 1987). Children must be older, however, before biographical memories endure. Older children and adults find that autobiographical memories prior to age 3 or 4 are forgotten (West & Bauer, 1999). One's biographical memories become reliable at about 7 years of age (Rubin, Wetzler, & Nebes, 1986). Research has shown that a child's awareness of stuttering markedly increases between the ages of 4 and 5 years (Ambrose & Yairi, 1994; Ezrati-Vinacour, Platzky, & Yairi, 2001). Hence it would appear that sometime between the ages of 5 and 7 years, specific experiences of stuttering begin to have a lasting impression in a person's biographical memory. A study of awareness in 1,122 Belgium children ages 2 to 7 years found a gradual increase in awareness with age (Boey, Van de Heyning, Wuyts et al., 2009).

It is no wonder that as a person who stutters repeatedly experiences the many emotions prior to, during, and after stuttering, he or she often wants to avoid speaking situations, hold back from talking, mask stuttering with other behaviors, avoid looking at listeners, fear and think the worst of listeners, use unusual voice characteristics, or say things in circuitous ways. Individuals vary in their emotional responses to stuttering, as all people do toward their negative experiences. Individuals develop fears to specific situations, people, words, and even speech sounds. Answering the telephone, for example, creates a specific situational fear experienced by many people who stutter. An example of specific word fear is saying one's own name when introducing oneself. One of our clients, an economics major, had a specific fear of the sound /m/. Hence he stuttered on many words beginning with /m/, especially on *millions*. Another client scheduled to make a brief presentation in front of a class could not sleep the whole night before and was unable to eat breakfast until after the presentation was over. Nonetheless, people who stutter share remarkable empathy with each other concerning the emotional impact of stuttering. Feelings of anxiety about speaking, guilt over not having better speech control, and self-doubts about the ability to handle communication situations are common themes in group therapy or self-help group meetings. Many eventually choose their profession and particular job driven by the avoidance of speaking demands.

Avoidance behavior is one of the most predominant characteristics of advanced stuttering. One example is holding back from responding to questions in class, even when a student knows an answer quite well, for fear of the humiliation of stuttering. Or if there is an expectation of being called on, that student is apt to make an excuse to leave the room for the same reason. One young woman explained that she drove across a large city to ask one quick question just to avoid stuttering on the phone. She later explained that it was that incident that led her to realize just how much she was letting stuttering control her life, and that she never wanted to let it push her that far again. In a study of 200 adults who stutter, 20% reported turning down a job or promotions because of their fear of stuttering (Klein & Hood, 2004). The excellent movie *The King's Speech* provides a vivid example of how George VI was afraid of becoming king of England because of his stuttering.

Research evidence suggests that stuttering increases anxiety (Ezrati-Vinacour & Levin, 2004). The extent of negative reaction varies widely among people who stutter, ranging from little to no anxiety to the opposite extreme of social phobia. Studies of adolescents and adults who stutter found they report greater anxiety than the general population but less anxiety than people with social phobia or psychiatric disorders

(Kraaimaat, Vanryckeghem, & Van Dam-Baggen, 2002; Mahr & Torosian, 1999). More severe stuttering tends to be associated with a greater state anxiety than mild stuttering (Ezrati-Vinacour & Levin, 2004). The emotional reactions associated with advanced stuttering may grow in some individuals to such an extent that they become more of a handicap than the overt stuttered speech. In such cases, perhaps the strongest characteristic of advanced stuttering is avoidance behavior that may seriously affect day-to-day life and may lead to some social withdrawal. We believe that the emotional reactions should be considered when therapy is planned.

Cognition

The cognitive impact of stuttering has received limited attention in research but recent years have seen some growing interest. Not surprisingly, the results have been mixed. In 1963, Froeschels and Rieber reported reduced visual and auditory perception during stuttering events but Perkins (1969) failed to confirm this. Kamhi and McOsker (1982) found reduced comprehension of the material read when the person stutters. People who stutter were found to have poorer time estimation of verbal tasks in which they were engaged (Ezrati-Vinacour & Levin, 2001). In another study, accuracy of time estimate declined as the level of disfluency increased (Barasch, Guitar, McCauley et al., 2000). Increased disfluency during competing tasks, such as repeating syllables and doing mental addition tasks, led Bosshardt (1999, 2002) to conclude that stutterers are more sensitive to interference in attention than nonstutterers. Contradictory findings were indicated, however, by reduced stuttering during a competing task of playing computer games (Vasic & Wijnen, 2005). Similarly, some problems in the ability to focus were detected by the Posner Test of Covert Attention Shifts in a study by Heitmann, Asbornsen, and Helland (2004) but a trait study by Subramanian and Yairi (2006) did not find supportive evidence.

Although lower self-esteem and social anxiety might be expected among those who stutter, some studies have surprisingly demonstrated opposite results that showed self-esteem among stutterers was similar or more positive than among age- and gender-matched controls (Hearne, Packman, Onslow et al., 2008). Alternatively, one study found that adults who stutter rate themselves significantly lower on self-efficacy (Bray, Kehle, Lawless et al., 2003). The negative attitudes of people who stutter toward speech and communication have been surveyed through a variety of attitude scales. De Nil and Brutten (1991) found that 70 CWS, 7 to 14 years of age, had significantly more negative attitudes about communication than NFC. They tended to believe, often based on their life experiences, that others do not like the way they talk and will be unkind or make fun of them for stuttering.

The nonscientific literature on stuttering attributes a number of attitudes as common to people with advanced stuttering. One example is the tendency to think of one's self as a *giant in chains*. That is, the person tends to believe, "If only I didn't stutter, I would have been successful at that endeavor." Stuttering skews one's perspective on how much of life's struggles would still be present without stuttering. The stuttering attracts the blame for social or vocational setbacks. Another common belief is the tendency to expect and fear that stuttering will occur. The phenomenon of *expectancy* is described later in this chapter. In therapy, managing one's cognitive responses can be as critically important to remediation as addressing strategies for speaking (Menzies, O'Brian, Onslow et al., 2008).

Concomitant Disorders

As we discussed in Chapter 3, there has been a debate about whether young children who stutter also tend to exhibit other disorders, especially phonology and language, with greater frequency than is found in the population at large. Whereas the pool of data for school-age children is much larger than that for preschool-age children, there has been little interest in this domain as far as advanced stuttering in adolescents and adults is concerned. Among the larger sources, a survey of 358 speech clinicians who treated 1,060 school-age children who stutter found that 44% had one concomitant disorder, and an additional 24% had two or more concomitant disorders, adding up to 68% of the group (Blood & Seider, 1981). The percentage of children who exhibited only one of each concomitant disorder, as compared to population expectancy data according to ASHA, is shown in Table 4.1.

These data were supported by another survey of 241 clinicians from 10 U.S. states who treated 467 CWS (Arndt & Healey, 2001). They reported that 44% had one or more verified speech/language problem(s) to accompany stuttering. Three disorder subgroups—phonology only, language only, and phonology and language disorders—each constituted nearly 15% among the total group. The clients, however, ranged in age from 3 to 20 years, making it difficult to draw inferences specifically to advanced stuttering. In a more recent and considerably larger survey, 1,184 school speech-language pathologists in 46 U.S. states identified 2,628 children who stutter in kindergarten

Table 4.1	**Comparisons of the Prevalence of Various Disorders in People Who Stutter and in the Population at Large**	
Disorder	**PWS (%)**	**General Population (%)**
Phonology	16	6
Language	10	7
Learning disabilities	7	7
Reading disabilities	6	6
Other disabilities	5	N/A

N/A = not applicable; PWS = people who stutter.

through 12th grade. Nearly 65% had at least one concomitant disorder. The distribution according to disorders was as follows: articulation, 33.5%; phonology, 12.7%; language (expressive), 13.5%; and language (receptive), 12.1%. Among other disorders were learning disabilities, 11.4%; literacy disorders, 8.2%; attention deficits, 5.9%; auditory processing, 3.8%; neuropsychological, 2.9%; behavioral, 2.4%; and sensory, 2.1% (Blood et al., 2003). Males displayed the greater proportions of nearly all types of disorders.

> What does it mean that older children who stutter tend to have multiple disorders more often than the prevalence in the general population? Perhaps other speech-language problems make a speaker more vulnerable to fluency breakdown and stuttering. In contrast, stuttering itself may create the risk for developing additional speech-language problems. Finally, both stuttering and other speech-language problems may be related to yet another common underlying etiology. Research has not yet determined which of these possible implications are correct. Answers are also needed regarding whether certain aspects of treatment for other speech-language disorders put a child at risk for stuttering.

Such research has been criticized for its potential inflation of estimates because children with multiple needs are more apt to be referred and identified for services. Reviewing the literature concerning the co-occurrence of stuttering and language disorders Nippold (2004, 2012a) listed other limitations, such as failure to match the groups on gender and socioeconomic status, excluding control children if they showed signs of a language disorder yet including CWS regardless of language status. Although no direct links between stuttering and these disorders have been demonstrated, and they may well be completely independent of stuttering, clinicians who provide therapy for stuttering should probe for the presence of concomitant disorders to ascertain whether there are complicating conditions and to determine the therapeutic approach.

One reason why little research has been pursued related to concomitant language disorders in adults is because there has been no apparent reason to suspect that they exhibit poor language skills. Nevertheless, the past few years have seen growing interests in the language processing of this age group. For example, Scott, Trautman, and Cairns (2003) found that under time pressure, adults who stutter may have poorer language organization. Kleinow and Smith (2000) found that the speech motor stability of adults who stutter decreased when the speaking materials were more complex. They concluded that "language formulation processes may affect speech production processes and that the speech motor systems of adults who stutter may be especially susceptible to the linguistic demands required to produce a more complex utterance" (p. 548). Weber-Fox and Hampton (2008) concluded that whereas linguistic abilities are normal in adults who stutter, underlying brain activity mediating some aspects of language processing may function differently.

The Dynamics of Advanced Stuttering

Patterns of Occurrence

Among the established phenomena of advanced stuttering are the patterns of stuttering occurrence relative to previous stutter events. Three patterns demonstrate its predictability, revealing certain rules which show that stuttering is not as random as it often appears to listeners. Knowledge of the rules of stuttering is sometimes clinically useful. Better understanding should contribute more to its future clinical management.

Adaptation

Johnson and Knott (1937) were the first to publish the observation that when a passage is read aloud several consecutive times, stuttering declines with each rereading. This phenomenon is known as *adaptation* and its characteristics are fairly consistent. The greatest reduction of stuttering is evident on the second reading, followed by a more gradual decline that levels off after five readings. The typical result is a 50% reduction in stuttering from the first to the fifth reading. All types of disfluency decline, not just the stuttering-like disruptions (Silverman & Williams, 1971), and stuttering severity (e.g., intensity and duration of the prolongations) usually decreases along with frequency (Trotter, 1955).

Like most conditions that reduce stuttering, the decline is only temporary. After a sufficient period, the original level of stuttering returns. Some adaptation occurs even if a speaker keeps on talking without saying the same words. Speaking words that are always changing, however, yields much less, about a 10% to 20% reduction (e.g., Gray, 1965a). Finally, adaptation can take place whether successive readings are separated by 20 minutes, 1 hour, or even 24 hours (Leutenegger, 1957). This fact means that clinicians and researchers must be careful about evaluating progress with the same reading passage pre- and posttreatment. Rather than improving, the client may merely be adapting.

How has adaptation been explained? From a learning theory perspective, the adaptation curve seen in stuttering is similar to the extinction curve seen in experiments with animals where an acquired behavior is made to disappear when reinforcement is removed (Wischner, 1950). From a psychological-emotional perspective, it was suggested that once stuttering occurs, the fear of exposing stuttering is reduced, resulting in less stuttering in the following readings (Sheehan, 1958). Another explanation proposes that some form of motor-sensory rehearsal is responsible: An articulatory-vocal "set" becomes established as a speaker repeats spoken material (Max & Caruso, 1998). A recent explanation of the adaptation effect depicts it as involving basal ganglia processes (Alm, 2004b).

How is the adaptation effect useful? Some believe that the phenomenon might serve as a predictor of progress in therapy. Others have suggested that it could represent a basis for stuttering subtypes (Newman, 1963; Prins & Lohr, 1972). In certain circumstances it might be employed for clinical purposes. One such situation is when the client needs to present a paper to a class or a project to a company's executives. Rehearsing the materials several times out loud in conditions similar to the actual situation, immediately before the upcoming event, might help to reduce stuttering. Anecdotal reports suggest that mental rehearsal is less effective than rehearsing aloud. Adaptation appears to be aided by the sensory experience of speaking.

Not all people who stutter display the adaptation effect however, and among those who do, the amount varies (Kroll & Hood, 1976; Moore, Flowers, & Cunko, 1981). Perhaps for those who do not adapt, stuttering on the first reading is more threatening than they anticipated, and so their reactive responses are heightened for the next readings. Surprisingly, milder stutterers tend to show greater adaptation than more severe stutterers (Gray, 1965a). Perhaps adaptation reduces the reactive components that people who stutter mildly are already managing more successfully.

Which speech motor-sensory feedback systems (i.e., articulation, phonation, audition) might be essential to the adaptation effect? It appears that phonation could be the most important because oral rehearsal results in greater adaptation than either lipped or whispered rehearsal (e.g., Bruce & Adams, 1978). If the speaker needed to rehearse the articulatory pattern alone, then lipped or whispered rehearsal should be just as effective as voiced rehearsal. Other evidence supports the conclusion that suprasegmental (vocal) rather than segmental (phonemic) elements are crucial. For example, although the same words are repeated, adaptation can be prevented if commas are relocated to alter the rhythm and phrasing of the passage (Wingate, 1972).

Consistency

Another pattern of the stuttering dynamics during repeated oral readings is the tendency for words stuttered on the final readings to be those that had been stuttered initially. It is known as the *consistency effect.* This phenomenon has been reported in a number of studies over many years (e.g., Johnson & Knott, 1937; Wingate, 1986). Although stuttering frequency and severity decline, the words still stuttered in the last reading tend to be among those stuttered during the first one. The *consistency index* is calculated by dividing the number of words stuttered in the first reading that were also stuttered in the subsequent reading, by the number of words stuttered in the first reading. Johnson and Leutenegger (1955, p. 211) reported a mean consistency index for adults who stutter of 69.3%. Again, the effect shows that stuttering does not occur randomly but follows certain rules. Like adaptation, it has been interpreted in terms of learning theory, in that once a word has been associated with stuttering, it acquires the role of a stimulus to trigger stuttering on subsequent occasions (Johnson & Knott, 1937).

Adjacency

Stuttering is never eliminated completely by adaptation, and the remaining stuttering events appear to be strongly tied to the word locations. The mystifying power of these locations became the occasion for yet another phenomenon observed by Johnson and Millsapps (1937), the *adjacency effect*. It means that stuttering tends to occur at the same locations as before, even when previously stuttered words are removed from the reading passage being rehearsed. That is, stuttering tended to occur on the words adjacent to locations where stuttering had occurred before.

Expectancy

The previous three effects dealt with the patterns of stuttering events relative to their own occurrence. The phenomenon of *expectancy* is different in that it implies some impact of the person's cognition on the actual occurrence of stuttering. Specifically, expectancy refers to the ability of the person who stutters to scan ahead and predict with a good measure of accuracy, although not perfectly, what words or parts of words will be stuttered. This phenomenon was revealed when subjects were instructed to mark a passage according to places where they thought they would stutter. When an unmarked passage was later presented for them to read, a majority of locations had been predicted accurately.

Expectancy is very commonly experienced by many people who stutter: They know when, sometimes how, they will stutter. Like other phenomena described earlier, expectancy suggests that anticipatory anxiety is important to stuttering. It produces danger signals that lead to apprehension that lead to physical tension in preparing to cope with the upcoming stuttering. As Johnson (1948) opined, it is this tension that actually causes the stuttering. Therefore, reducing the emotional threat of stuttering would appear to be a worthwhile therapy goal. But because client predictions of stuttering are incorrect on a fair proportion of instances, they may also benefit in therapy by gaining more realistic expectations of when stuttering is apt to occur. As we discuss in Chapter 11, the ability to anticipate stuttering has been used in therapy, training clients to begin changing expected stuttering behavior before it actually occurs.

Loci of Stuttering

Adaptation, consistency, and adjacency phenomena demonstrate that there are forces that influence the occurrence of stuttering in the stream of speech, some under certain conditions, some more generally. The elements of spoken language also offer a certain degree of power to predict when stuttering events occur in general communication situations. Early investigators examined the linguistic variables associated with the specific locations (loci) of stuttering events, hoping that, to the extent stuttering could be predicted, its governing rules might be better understood and the disorder better treated.

In 1945, Spencer Brown reported that the occurrence of the stuttering of adolescents and adults was not random but commonly associated with specific language structures. Analyzing speech samples, he observed that stuttering tended to occur on (1) content words (versus function words), including nouns, verbs, adjectives, adverbs; (2) long words (versus short words); (3) consonant-initial words (versus vowel-initial word locations); and (4) sentence-initial (versus final locations). The more factors congregate in a single word, the higher its chance to be stuttered. These locations became known as "Brown's four factors" because they supposedly accounted for most stuttering instances.

Unfortunately, this type of research is confounded by the proportions of occurrence of the factors and the extent to which they overlap. For example, most content words are longer words, and most content words are consonant-initial. Later researchers concluded that the effects of these factors were not independent of each other (Quarrington, 1965; Soderberg, 1967). Initial sentence position was primarily responsible for the locations (Brown, 1945; Wingate, 1988). Other types of locations have been shown to attract stuttering, including words conveying "prominent" or important information (Lanyon & Duprez, 1970), unfamiliar words (Hubbard & Prins, 1994), and stressed or accented syllables and words (Prins, Hubbard, & Krause, 1991; Wingate, 1984).

Stuttering loci observed in adults are not the same as those in children. Prior to age 8, they are not as predictable and almost run in an opposite fashion. Children often stutter on function words, short words (most of their words are short), vowel-initial words, and familiar words (Bloodstein & Grossman, 1981; Natke, Sandrieser, van Ark et al., 2004). Consider the child who says, "I I I I I want to go." The first word *I* fits all four of these categories. Research suggests that the shift in stuttering locations to the advanced pattern may begin as early as age 5, be mostly complete by age 12, but continue to progress into adulthood (Au-Yeung, Gomez, & Howell, 2003). Table 4.2 provides a list of typical

Table 4.2   Examples of Typical Loci of Stuttering (Shown in Bold and Italics) for Adults and/or Children

Stuttering Location	Utterance Example	Typical Age Group
On the first three words of the utterance	"***The Galapagos Islands*** offer a ***warm*** respite from the vicissitudes of life."	Both adults and children
On initial sounds or syllables of the words	***The Ga***lapagos ***I***slands ***o***ffer a ***w***arm respite ***f***rom ***the*** ***vi***cissitudes ***of*** ***li***fe."	Both adults and children
On the content words (nouns/verbs/adjectives/adverbs)	The ***Galapagos Islands offer*** a ***warm respite*** from the ***vicissitudes*** of ***life***."	Adults, not children
On longer words (more sounds/letters)	The ***Galapagos Islands*** offer a warm ***respite*** from the ***vicissitudes*** of life."	Adults, not children
On consonant-initial words	***The Galapagos*** Islands offer a ***warm respite from*** the ***vicissitudes*** of ***life***."	Adults, not children
On unfamiliar words	The ***Galapagos*** Islands offer a warm respite from the ***vicissitudes*** of life."	Adults, not children
On the stressed syllables (after the first three words[3])	The Galapagos Islands ***of***fer a warm ***re***spite from the ***vi***cissitudes of life."	Adults

[3]See Hubbard (1998).

stuttering loci and whether they are common only in adults or in both children and adults. Examples of each of the loci are also given.

In sum, the locations of advanced stuttering can be divided into word-based factors and utterance-based factors. Word-based factors include initial position, sound class (consonant), length (in phones, letters, or syllables), syllabic stress, word familiarity, propositionality, and phonological complexity. Utterance-based factors include initial position (first three words), grammatical class, length (in syllables, words), propositionality, clause type (verb phrase), clause boundaries, and initiation of phonologic words. The vulnerability of early word and utterance position as a common location of fluency breakdown has led some researchers to notice its uniqueness as the time when the highest demands are placed on speech planning systems, both linguistically and motorically. The loci phenomenon is discussed further in Chapter 6 in regard to theories of stuttering.

The loci suggest a strong link between stuttering and language, although many of the locations are also typical of normal disfluencies (Silverman & Williams, 1967). Some researchers propose that stuttering locations reveal more about the nature of speech-language production itself than stuttering because other so-called speech errors (not disfluencies) also tend to occur at these same locations. Hence these loci may merely inform us where the pieces of speech-language structure can be fit together or taken apart. There remains much more to understand about why speech breaks apart, *when* it does, and *the way* it does (i.e., as SLD or other).

Conditions That Diminish Stuttering

One of the most mystifying but fascinating characteristics of the disorder of stuttering is its amelioration, that is, its improvement, in an extensive array of diverse conditions. It has been supposed that finding the common link among the various ameliorating conditions would unlock the nature of stuttering. Furthermore, such a discovery would provide important information concerning therapeutic methods. Unfortunately, researchers have not yet found that link. It is also unfortunate that the reduction in stuttering is usually only experienced while the condition is present; when removed, the stuttering resumes its previous level. This aspect, however, has barely been investigated.

For more than half a century, scholars have been aware that many conditions may induce fluency. Bloodstein (1950) surveyed 204 PWS, ages 16 to 44 years, regarding the conditions in which they experienced diminished stuttering. The participants reported experiencing reduction of stuttering in a total of 115 conditions. The following list (Table 4.3) presents some of these conditions and the percent of people who reported that they experienced absent or hardly any stuttering.

Table 4.3 Percent of People Reporting Conditions That Ameliorate Stuttering

More Than 90%	75%–90%	50%–75%	25%–30%
Singing	Swearing	Whispering	Reciting from memory
Reading in unison	Speaking alone	Monotone speech	Speaking at a higher/lower pitch
Speaking to animals	Reading alone	Suddenly frightened	Talking with an object in mouth
Speaking to infants	Inconsequential remarks	Imitating a dialect	Talking to persons regarded inferior
Rhythmic speech		Feeling calm/relaxed	Speaking on the telephone

Another question addresses the magnitude, or the size of the effect these conditions have on the frequency of stuttering: How much stuttering is eliminated? Some data were reported by Andrews, Howie, Dozsa et al. (1982) for three adult men. Examples of the average reduction levels experienced by these men are as follows (Table 4.4). As can be seen from the combined results, two conditions, singing and speaking in rhythm were selected by the highest percentage of participants and also experimentally resulted in the largest reduction in stuttering.

Table 4.4 Percentage of Reduction in Stuttering Under Certain Conditions*

More Than 90%	50%–80%	Less Than 50%
Singing	Arm swinging	Speaking when relaxed
Unison reading	Speaking alone	Speaking with topic cards
Shadowing	Speaking in a dialect	Speaking while writing
Slowing	Masking noise	
Response-contingent conditions	Talking to an animal	
Prolonged/delayed auditory feedback (DAF)		
Syllable-timed (rhythmic)		

* Based on information from Stuttering: Speech pattern characteristics under fluency-inducing conditions by G. Andrews, P. Howie, M. Dozsa, and B. Guitar. *Journal of Speech and Hearing Research, 25,* 208–216. Copyright 1982 by American Speech-Language-Hearing Association. All rights reserved.

Table 4.5	Ameliorating Conditions of Stuttering Used for Therapeutic Intervention Purposes		
Altered Sensory Information	**Altered Mental Reactions**	**Altered Speaking Pattern**
Delayed auditory feedback	Hypnotic suggestion	Metronome-timed speech
Masking noise	Emotionally distracting/intense stimuli	Reduced speaking rate
EMG biofeedback	Same words repeated over and over	Monotone speech
Response contingent stimuli	Voluntary stuttering, especially if repeated to gain control	Singsong speech

Relevant to clinicians in particular, several of the ameliorating conditions have indeed been employed for purposes of treatment of stuttering. Those conditions, some of which we describe in later chapters concerned with stuttering therapy, are listed in categories of altered sensory information, mental reactions, and speaking pattern (Table 4.5). Note that a good number of them are created by instrument-generated stimuli.

Two examples from scientific literature illustrate how research of this phenomenon can aid our understanding of stuttering. First, Stager, Jeffries, and Braun (2003) compared the brain activity patterns using PET (positron emission tomography) in adults who stutter with adults who do not stutter under two fluency-inducing conditions, singing and pacing speech. Results showed that, during the fluency-inducing conditions, auditory association brain areas that process speech and voice, and motor regions related to control of the larynx and oral articulators, were more active. This was true for both participant groups. The activation, however, was more robust in the left hemisphere of those who stutter prompting the authors to suggest that that under the fluency-inducing conditions, speakers are self-monitoring speech production more closely (a primarily left hemisphere function). Because both groups showed similar patterns, it was proposed that the sensory-motor and cognitive demands of self-monitoring for the tasks, not the task itself (i.e., singing) were responsible for fluency.

A second example of research that applied knowledge of ameliorating conditions was conducted by Sparks, Grant, Millay et al. (2002). The fluency of four adolescent speakers, two with mild and two with severe stuttering, was studied under slow and fast speaking rates with DAF or without DAF as a control condition. Fluency for the speakers with mild stuttering was the same for the two conditions; for speakers with severe stuttering it decreased by 90% for the two DAF speaking conditions as compared with no DAF. It appears that the severity of stuttering could be an important indicator of whether a speaker will respond to a fluency-inducing condition. Those with more severe stuttering may be more likely to benefit. The findings raise the possibility that the fluency-inducing effect of DAF is not necessarily its tendency to slow speech down.

Conditions That Increase Stuttering

Situations of communicative pressure tend to trigger more frequent or worse episodes of stuttering (Bloodstein & Bernstein Ratner, 2008). Such situations include having to say one's name, telephone calls, repairing miscommunications, responding to "What did you say?", addressing large audiences or groups and authority figures, prolonged anticipation time prior to a talking turn, and words or sounds believed to be difficult. Each speaker, however, may perceive communicative pressure in different ways. Some have difficulty speaking with the opposite sex and others with the same sex. Many have difficulty speaking to large groups and do much better one on one, but others have trouble with face-to-face individual encounters and do much better in front of large groups. Detailed information on how an individual person who stutters responds could enhance the planning and execution of therapy, for example, in planning desensitization programs (see Chapter 10).

Summary

As stuttering progresses into later childhood and beyond, the fully developed characteristics of advanced stuttering become more evident. This can be seen across the various domains of the disorder. Phenomena associated with the advanced disorder indicate that stuttering is governed by certain rules still waiting to be understood. Among the main points reviewed:

- A variety of disfluency types was detailed. The elements of frequency of occurrence, event durations, and clustering were highlighted.
- A wide array of physical behaviors associated with the stuttered speech becomes more visible, adding to the complexity and apparent abnormality of the disorder.
- Suprasegmental characteristics of voice quality, prosody, and speaking rate are also influenced by stuttering.
- A critical aspect of advanced stuttering is the tremendous growth in the emotional reactions that people who stutter develop, primarily negative emotions that lead to avoidance of speech and possible social withdrawal.
- Recent evidence hints that cognitive functions, such as reduced attention, may also occur during stuttering.
- Several predictable phenomena can be observed, such as adaptation, consistency, and adjacency. These may have some clinical implications.
- Unlike early stuttering, the stuttering loci in more advanced stages tend to be associated with language characteristics of longer, less familiar content words.
- The role of language in the occurrence of advanced stuttering is not well understood. Investigating the potential stuttering to language link may shed much light on the disorder.

- Stuttering can be greatly decreased, albeit temporarily, under various unique conditions, a number of which can be incorporated in treatment.

Study Questions and Discussion Topics

1. What are the main changes that occur in the speech characteristics of advanced as compared to early stuttering?
2. What are the main developments in the emotional and social domains?
3. What considerations should enter into the selection and application of a disfluency classification system and why?
4. Does anxiety cause some stuttering and/or does stuttering cause some anxiety, and what evidence exists to support either? What is the difference between state and trait anxiety?
5. What are possible reasons why the loci of stuttering shift from their typical patterns in early childhood to their different pattern in older childhood and after?
6. Do you think that the various ameliorating conditions of stuttering are apt to share one common underlying cause, or are they more likely to produce their effects for a variety of different reasons? Why?

Suggested Readings

Andrews, G., Howie, P., Dozsa, M., & Guitar, B. (1982). Stuttering: Speech pattern characteristics under fluency-inducing conditions. *Journal of Speech and Hearing Research, 25,* 208–216.

Blood, G., Blood, I., Maloney, K., Meyer, C., & Qualls, C. (2007). Anxiety levels in adolescents who stutter. *Journal of Communication Disorders, 40,* 452–469.

Bloodstein, O., & Bernstein Ratner, N. B. (2008). *A handbook on stuttering.* Clifton Park, NY: Delmar. See Chapters 10 and 11, which discuss stuttering as a response.

Wingate, M. E. (1976). *Stuttering: Theory and treatment.* New York, NY: Irvington. Chapter 8.

Chapter 5

Why Do People Stutter? Evaluating Theories and Models

LEARNER OBJECTIVES

Readers of this chapter will understand:

- The nature of scientific theory.
- Why stuttering theories have been numerous and diverse.
- Criteria that may be applied to evaluate the credibility of theories and models of stuttering.
- The potential role of subtyping in the characterization of stuttering.
- Factors to consider when evaluating why a particular individual stutters.

Theories and Models

In Part I of this book we presented some answers to the general questions of what stuttering is and who stutters, but now we turn our attention to the question of what causes stuttering and what controls its dynamics. To address this topic, we start by examining the scientific methods that help us arrive at reasonable theories and models. We address the more elementary question of what makes a good theory in general and then address the specific considerations of what makes a good theory of stuttering. Subsequent chapters then provide an overview of specific theories and models of stuttering.

Applying the scientific method is important to speech-language clinicians because it not only serves to reveal the nature of speech disorders in general, it also sheds light on associated factors specific to individuals who are served. Central to the scientific method is the process of skilled observation. By engaging in carefully controlled conditions of repeated observation, our theories of the factors underlying speech disorders can be tested and our understanding of those disorders enhanced.

Much of our knowledge of phenomena is dealt with on two levels: theoretical and practical. Musical knowledge illustrates this point. Music theory, among other things, describes the elements, such as notes and keys, and the relationships among them, such as scales, intervals, or chords. On the practical side, the elements and relationships permit musical compositions to be created, played, or sung. The aim of our theoretical knowledge of stuttering is to describe the relevant elements and the interrelationships of those elements. Theoretical knowledge, in turn, will facilitate our practical management of stuttering: its prevention, assessment, and treatment.

Before a scientist or practitioner engages in study of a phenomenon, it is customary to formulate a theory about what will be observed. Once observational evidence has been collected and analyzed, the theory can either be accepted or rejected. In common use, the word *theory* denotes an opinion, conjecture, or speculation. In other words, it represents an unsubstantiated guess or a personal hunch about a phenomenon of interest. In the scientific arena, however, it is important to test a theory so that knowledge moves beyond the stage of mere speculation. A well-developed theory offers an explanation, framework, or model of a natural or social phenomenon or set of phenomena. It enables prediction of future occurrences of, or changes in, the phenomena under certain conditions. If its predictions fail, then the theory may be modified based on the acquisition of new information.

The terms *theory* and *model* are often used interchangeably; however, the terms have slightly different meanings. Whereas a theory is a conceptual system of understanding for the purpose of explaining and/or predicting a phenomenon or phenomena, a model is a representation of the phenomenon in terms of a set of variables and the relationships among them. For example, a model could show the structure of an atom, whereas a theory could explain why some of the parts are more stable than others. Some theories may include a model as a component, but other theories do not. When a *theory* takes the form of a *model,* the two terms may be used interchangeably as referents.

One example of a *model* used to explain stuttering has the acronym DIVA, which stands for "Directions Into Velocities of Articulators" (Civier, Tasko, & Guenther, 2010; Guenther, 2006). In this model, three components are proposed in the regulation of fluent speech production: feedforward control, error monitoring, and feedback control. These components are represented in a diagram with greater detail. Based on the model, a computational formula can describe the relationship of the feedforward and feedback control subsystems to the resultant speech motor act. The model can be used to test predictions about the extent of fluency disruption that arises when sensorimotor errors occur.

An example of a *theory* used to explain stuttering was offered by Travis in 1931. According to his cerebral dominance theory, the right and left brain hemispheres create conflicting neural signals that fail to achieve coordinated control of speech muscle groups in people who stutter. Presumably, this theory is tested based on observations of the status of cerebral dominance in people who stutter: a lack of hemispheric dominance would support the theory.

Although the literature is rich with references to "theories" of stuttering, and, to a lesser degree, "models" of stuttering, it is also true that the majority of proposed explanations were limited to one or a few aspects of the disorder. For example, one notion deals only with why there is a decline in the frequency of stuttering under noise. Another scheme accounts only for the larger incidence of stuttering in boys than in girls. Yet a third belief serves to explain the decline in stuttering across repeated readings of same material. The literature is replete with many similar examples. It is doubtful, therefore, that most would, or should, be regarded as "theories of stuttering" according to the common scientific meaning of the term. At best, some are merely isolated *hypotheses* or *theoretical notions,* whereas others are speculations or guesses. Similarly, few, if any, actual models of stuttering exist because most fail to go beyond hypothetical explanations of the disorder. Still, there are many proposed so-called theories of stuttering and, in turn, various organizational schemes or classifications of those theories. How can the student of stuttering begin to understand the nature of these theories and their contribution to our knowledge of this complicated communication disorder? Following, we suggest a possible approach to this endeavor.

How to Analyze a Stuttering Theory

Prior to the examination of any theory, it is essential to determine what it tries to explain. As discussed in Chapter 1, the term *stuttering* may be constrained in referring only to overt speech disruptions. Or it may be used in a more inclusive fashion with reference to the condition of a speech disorder that grew complicated and includes many associated aspects and effects. It follows, then, that the student should first ask whether the theory under study strives to explain the dynamics of stuttered speech, or stuttering as a complex disorder. Similarly, it should be determined whether an isolated aspect or a subset of stuttering phenomena is being explained, as opposed to a comprehensive account for stuttering.

After determining what a particular theory attempts to explain, the nature of its content should be examined. Such analyses reveal that the field of speech pathology has borrowed from the disciplines of medicine, psychology, and education. Accordingly, some organically based, psychologically based, or learning-based theories of the stuttering disorder have been offered. There are several ways to categorize theories of stuttering. Bloodstein and Bernstein Ratner (2008) distinguished between theories that explain the "moment of stuttering" and those that attempt to explain the etiology of stuttering. With the second group they distinguished three categories: breakdown, repressed need, and anticipatory struggle theories. Guitar (1998) offered another perspective, describing theories in terms of factors that appear to contribute to stuttering. His organically based theories are dealt within the context of *constitutional* factors, and the psychological and learning-based theories are explained on the bases of *developmental* and *environmental* factors. He also offered other possibilities, including motor-based, psycholinguistic-based, or social-based theories. The chapters covering the theories of stuttering in this text, both as abnormal speech events and as a more complex disorder, classify them broadly according to psychological and biological theories.

Science, Superstition, and Stories About Stuttering

Notions of the cause and treatment of stuttering have varied widely over time. In a historical account of speech disorders, Klingbell (1939) noted that several centuries B.C.E., Hippocrates, the "father of modern medicine," thought that stuttering might be due to chronic diarrhea that he observed in people who stutter, the treatment of which resulted in ulcers. One story from ancient Greece proposes that Demosthenes, the statesman, improved his stuttering by the exercise of speaking with pebbles in his mouth. Among many others, Klingbell also lists De Chauliac (1300–1380 C.E.), who ascribed stuttering "to convulsions, ulcers, or other affections of the tongue, to paralysis, or to moisture of the nerves or muscles." Several surgical interventions were performed on the tongues of people who stuttered beginning in 1840 by the German surgeon Deiffenbach and later by others because it was believed that anatomical defects cause stuttering.

According to Klingbell (1939), prosthetic devices were also developed and patented in the 1800s. For example, in 1838 Itard, a French physician, constructed ivory or gold forks attached to the lower jaw, under the tongue, for the purpose of supporting the supposedly weak tongue. Other constructed devices were worn over the tongue to add to its weight, supposedly to improve stuttering. In contrast, in the early 1900s, people who stuttered were given lessons in elocution, reflecting the belief that stuttering is caused by insufficient practice with skills of word usage and pronunciation (Wingate, 1997). It is still true today that, in some cultures, religious ceremonies are conducted to cast out the evil spirits that are thought to cause stuttering (St. Louis, 1986). Although it is understandable why ancient peoples or the contemporary general population may have many diverse ideas and experience confusion over the cause of stuttering, it has been true that also scientists have expressed vastly divergent perspectives on this disorder.

Figure 5.1   The Fable of the Blind Men and the Elephant

A fable from India tells of six blind men who had never met an elephant before visiting the Rajah's palace. The first blind man touched its body and announced, "An elephant is like a wall." The second grasped its ear, and corrected: "An elephant is like a fan." The third man wrapped his arms around a leg, and declared: "The elephant is like a tree." The fourth felt the trunk and countered, "The elephant is more like a snake." The fifth was poked by a tusk, and warned: "The elephant is like a spear!" And the sixth held the tail, and concluded: "The elephant is like a rope." An argument developed as each man insisted on his own perspective. When the Rajah heard them, he instructed: "The elephant is bigger than each part you have touched. Only by putting all your parts together will you understand what the elephant is really like."

The long unresolved search for the cause of stuttering frequently has been compared to the story of the blind men and the elephant (Johnson, 1958) as depicted in Figure 5.1. Unfortunately, this is exactly the kind of problem that has plagued theories of stuttering. Often they have been limited to one, or a select few, of the various facets of stuttering. To date, no one has quite managed to blend the valid elements of the various theories into a single, clear, testable, and, therefore, satisfactory system of explanation. A story could be told about stuttering that parallels that of the six blind men and the elephant, but it would be about six researchers who sought to explain stuttering. Each researcher observed a different stuttering phenomenon (or phenomena), reaching a different conclusion about its cause. The first researcher, after observing that people do not stutter when they sing, concluded that stuttering must be a problem of vocal dysfunction. A second researcher, who observed that people do not stutter when speaking in time to a metronome beat, asserted that stuttering must be a problem of speech rhythm. Yet a third researcher, who experimented with the control of speech fluency using delayed auditory feedback, reasoned that stuttering must be caused by a disorder of the auditory system. A fourth researcher, noting enhanced fluency when people speak in a monotone, decided that stuttering must be caused by deficient skill with suprasegmentals, such as inflection and intonation. The fifth researcher, who observed that in a stuttering block, the speaker stops air from flowing, proposed that stuttering must be a problem of respiration. Finally, the sixth researcher, who found that unison speech is nearly always fluent, argued that stuttering arises from psychological reactions invoked only when talking to other people (i.e., difficulty with communicating meaningful, propositional speech).

If the story actually ended there, the problem might be manageable, but stuttering researchers and clinicians have not limited their perspectives to only six conclusions. Rather, we are faced with a plethora of old, new, and recycled observations and related conclusions about stuttering, each from another point of view. Because researchers struggle with the multiple and inconsistent findings related to stuttering, conflicts regarding interpretation abound. The essential nature of stuttering has been highly controversial. An example of controversy between two opposing views is as follows: "I can find no evidence that the person who stutters is physically different from anyone else, therefore stuttering must be psychological"; the opposite stance may also be asserted: "I can find no convincing evidence that people who stutter are psychologically different from anyone else, therefore stuttering must be physical." Such examples suggest that how we think about stuttering influences our theoretical position. Like the matter of whether the cup is half empty or half full, notions about causality and the nature of stuttering may be different depending on whether, for example, we consider the onset of stuttering to represent the acquisition of new disfluency symptoms or the loss of an already existing fluency. Conflicts among researchers have been common. The literature on stuttering is sprinkled with exchanges in the form of letters to the editor representing the struggle with resolution of differences and communication of diverse perspectives. One example is the series of commentary papers (letters) published by Bloodstein

(1990), Ingham (1990), Smith (1990), and Perkins (1990b) revealing controversy about the nature of stuttering, its perceptual definition, and the conditions for validating when it has occurred.

> In an exchange of commentaries in 1990, diverse views regarding stuttering were expressed. Bloodstein (1990) opined that it is not worth being concerned over precise definitions of stutter events or observer agreement of judgments because the essence of stuttering should be recognized as "a tense and fragmented way of speaking" (p. 393). Ingham (1990) asserted that we need more sophisticated observational measures for stutter events to establish a data-based understanding of the disorder. Smith (1990) said an all-encompassing framework was needed—one that does not take an either/or stance on the question of biological versus behavioral but allows for the contribution of both, among other factors. From still another perspective, Perkins (1990b) insisted on concern with what most distresses the person who stutters—the sense of a loss of control.

The Need for an Integrated Framework

Because ideas about stuttering have been difficult to reconcile, scholars have appreciated the proposal that "workers in the area of stuttering should adopt a multifactorial, nonlinear, and dynamic framework" for the disorder (Smith & Kelly, 1997, p. 205). By multifactorial, it is meant that many variables contribute to the occurrence of stuttering. By nonlinear and dynamic, it is meant that even slight differences may upset the balance of interactions among processes within the complex speech-language production system, yielding disproportionately large disruptions of speech in the form of stuttering. Within the context of a multifactorial model, a wider variety of diverse facts and associated phenomena can be explained. Another potential advantage of multifactorial models is that they may aid in the discovery of how different combinations of variables lead to specific profiles of the stuttering disorder. In this respect, the concept of stuttering subtypes or several different profiles for stuttering is relevant. We discuss the topic of subtypes later in this chapter.

A model of the complex interaction of multiple etiological factors in stuttering can help us examine factors that may need to be integrated into treatment. To illustrate, consider Figure 5.2, in which components that may influence stuttering are presented in a flowchart. The uppermost section represents the various underlying physical constitution factors. The ovals represent language abilities at the top, psychological factors in the middle, and interpersonal and relational dynamics at the bottom. Additional and/or alternative factors could be shown in such a model. The flowchart could also be augmented by including feedback loops, interactions among factors, and by emphasizing the relative influence of various aspects (e.g., by means of size of the font). The specific details of this multifactorial dynamic model would need to be worked out, but the purpose at this point is to grasp the concept for this type of theoretical proposal.

Figure 5.2 Hypothetical Example of a Multifactorial (Multiple-Component) Model of Stuttering

Appreciating the multifactorial nature of stuttering, many researchers prefer to search for causal factors of stuttering, rather than a precise cause. If stuttering had a single cause, would it have evaded detection for so long? If there are multiple, combined agents responsible for stuttering, then it is easier to understand that these factors have been difficult to uncover.

How do we categorize potential causal factors in stuttering? Some find it helpful to differentiate them according to three types: predisposing, precipitating, and perpetuating factors. A *predisposing* factor makes an individual susceptible or vulnerable to having a disease or disorder before that disorder appears. Because genetic factors might predispose a child to develop stuttering, genes could be referred to as a predisposing factor for stuttering. A *precipitating* factor hastens an occurrence or episode of the disease or disorder. To *precipitate* means "to give rise to immediate events." Some parents of CWS report that excitement can trigger moments of stuttering. Thus, excitement could be said to be a precipitating factor for stuttering in some children. A *perpetuating* factor makes the disorder continue even if the original causes no longer exist. A perpetuating factor prolongs, aggravates, or maintains a problem. When a child has siblings who interrupt and compete for the conversational floor, a child who stutters might be prone to attempt speech before being fully ready and this dynamic serves to maintain the disorder. Thus, the social dynamics could be considered to be a perpetuating factor for the stuttering disorder in some children.

Another set of common medical terms used to classify causal factors includes protective factors versus risk factors. Sometimes a factor is not exclusively present when a disorder arises, but a statistical association can be established between that factor and the disorder. By definition, a *risk factor* is a biological condition, substance, or behavior that is often associated with a problem, but does not serve as a *cause* for the event or disorder. Being male can be considered a risk factor for stuttering, although obviously it does not cause stuttering. A *protective factor*, by contrast, is a biological condition, substance, or behavior that is often associated with an absence or alleviation of a problem, but does not serve as a *cure* for the event or disorder. Having a family history of stuttering remission serves as a protective factor, although it is not a cure for stuttering.

Criteria for Strong Theories and Models

Recall that a theory is a scientific framework that accounts for a set of facts or observed phenomena. Scientific theories are based on evidence and lead to predictions about future occurrences that may be observed and tested. Thus when various models and theories of stuttering are presented in the chapters that follow, what criteria should be applied in evaluating their strength? We suggest the following 10 criteria, presented as pairs:

1. **Valid and Predictive.** To be valid, a theory must fit observed phenomena. An etiological theory is predictive when future cases of the disorder develop consistently with the proposed cause. Whether a theory is predictive and valid should be examined from two angles. First, whenever the cause is present, cases of the disorder should occur. One should not find frequent instances in which the causal conditions are present, but the disorder doesn't develop. From the second angle, when the causal conditions are not present, then cases of the disorder should not occur. If the disorder develops in the absence of the proposed cause, then it is not a necessary cause. As an example, let's assess the validity of the theory that excessive tickling causes stuttering. We ask two questions: (1) Do cases of stuttering emerge *in the absence of* excessive tickling? (2) Does excessive tickling often occur *without* triggering cases of stuttering? If the answer is yes to either of these questions, we should infer that tickling does not constitute a valid theory of the cause of stuttering.

2. **Exhaustive and Exclusive.** Theories are most useful when they provide a comprehensive explanation that speaks to all the related observations and phenomena. A theory that can account for all the phenomena associated with a disorder can be considered exhaustive. When only one or a limited number of associated phenomena are explained, it is less than satisfying. As an example, apply this criterion to the theory that "fear causes stuttering." If fear is the reason for stuttering, then how do we account for the fact that people do not stutter when they sing? Why doesn't stuttering occur as a result of stage fright when a person who stutters engages in a vocal (singing) performance? And what does fear have to do with the early age of stuttering onset? Don't all young children have some irrational fears, so why don't all children stutter? Although stuttering might at times appear to occur in moments of fear, this single observation does not fit all the phenomena. Because the "fear theory" cannot adequately explain the related observations and

phenomena of stuttering, it is not exhaustive and it is unsatisfying. A theory also needs to be exclusive. For that, the proposed etiology must be related only to the target disorder, and not also to other potential disorders. Returning to the example of the proposed theory that "fear causes stuttering," one might similarly note that "fear causes psychosomatic illnesses." But for this reason, the "fear theory" is not "exclusive" in relation to stuttering. When a theory is not exclusive, it is a weak because it cannot account for why the one disorder develops rather than the other disorder.

3. **Parsimonious and Elegant.** A theory is parsimonious when it uses the smallest number of variables or components to account for the greatest number of facts. When there are numerous phenomena to explain, as is the case with stuttering with its many ameliorating conditions, varying symptoms, and so on, it is particularly challenging to develop a parsimonious theory. Additionally, the most simple, sufficient theory of a phenomenon is said to be elegant. Can a comprehensive, multifactorial model of stuttering also be parsimonious and elegant? Which components of stuttering theory are truly necessary? For example, suppose a theory were confirmed that stuttering resulted from the simple combination of two mismanaged articulatory elements, speech tension and speech timing, and if this simple combination could account for all the locations of stuttering, all the ameliorating phenomena, age of onset, remission, and so on, such a theory could be regarded as both parsimonious and elegant.

4. **Testable and Flexible.** It is very important for a theory to be testable. If there is no way to disprove the hypotheses generated by the theory, then the theory has no basis in observable facts. Without observable facts to support the theory, it is no better than myth. A theory that proposes stuttering is caused by a speaker's state of mind is problematic because it is so difficult to find an objective means by which to test the theory. Perhaps decades from now there will be measures of brain activity that might provide such a test, but if a speaker's subjective report is the only means to access such data, then the testing of that theory will be weak because human beings are not accurate judges of their own mental status at any given moment. Limits on short-term memory also make it difficult to associate a specific mental state with the exact moment stuttering might have begun. By contrast, a testable theory can be measured by objective data. For example, if it were proposed that tension in the masseter muscle interfered with fluent speech, then it would be possible to actually create some method to insert a probe into the muscle tissue to measure the tension during speech, fluent and stuttered, to compare them. Theories also need to be flexible by permitting modifications as new knowledge is acquired. If a researcher generates a theory that is too narrow or too detailed in scope from the outset, it may not be flexible enough to permit adjustments. To illustrate with the theory about the masseter, it may be too narrowly focused on one vocal tract region. If it is discovered that the masseter muscle is not consistently tense immediately before or during stuttering, then the theory would simply collapse. If the theory proposed that vocal tract tension caused stuttering, then the researchers would be able to keep looking for tension in other regions before the theory was confirmed or dissolved.

Let's say that numerous reports revealed that stuttering continues to occur regardless of variations in the speaking conditions. Someone might generate the idea that stuttering happens in the presence of mystery element Q. According to the scholar who proposed this new theory, element Q has unknown properties except that in its presence, stuttering occurs. Such a theory must be discouraged because there is no way to test it. The theory cannot be proved or disproved until some concrete properties of Q are actually described. It should be clear, therefore, that a theory is not sufficiently credible unless it can be tested.

5. Consistent and Explanatory. It is important for the various components of a theory to agree with one another. Within any proposed theory, there is the possibility of contradictory content. For example, if a theory suggests a motoric cause for stuttering but proposes that motor deficits are not involved, it is unsatisfying inasmuch as it contradicts itself. When components of a theory work together well, without contradicting each other, the theory is more credible because it is internally consistent. Although theories must be sufficiently flexible to permit adjustments, they must not be proposed without enough content to make them useful. If it were proposed that stuttering is caused by a speech system breakdown, the criticism could be made that although the statement uses the terms "caused by," it does not actually explain the phenomenon because a "speech system breakdown" is recognized as the condition created by stuttering. There is a circular logic in proposing that stuttering is caused by a speech breakdown, because stuttering itself is a speech breakdown. A theory, especially of etiology, needs to assert new knowledge to explain the underlying nature of the phenomenon.

Table 5.1 summarizes the 10 criteria just presented and discussed.

Table 5.1	Criteria for Evaluating the Credibility of a Theory or Model
Valid	The model fits the observed phenomena.
Exhaustive	The model explains all associated phenomena.
Elegant	The model is succinct (explains multiple observations with a larger generalization).
Parsimonious	The model uses the smallest number of components to explain the most facts.
Exclusive	The model does not overlap with other explanations.
Testable	The model and its components can be tested and proved or disproved.
Predictive	The model makes predictions about future observations.
Consistent	The model's components do not contradict each other (internal consistency).
Flexible	The model can be expanded or changed with new information.
Explanatory	The model serves the purpose of explaining (i.e., not just describing).

Testing Theories and Models

Having reviewed criteria for a strong theory, what issues need to be considered and what problems are encountered in application? History suggests stuttering has been the topic of more research in the field of communication disorders than any other area. So why is it taking so long to develop a strong theory of stuttering?

Potential problems arise in regard to *observation*. Scientific theories should be supported at least by observed evidence. Unfortunately, it is quite difficult to evaluate the causal nature of particular variables in relation to stuttering. It requires careful consideration of their properties, their timing, and the nature of their association to stuttering. As we alluded to in Chapter 3, it is extremely difficult, almost impossible, for scientists to observe the very first stuttering episode of a 3-year-old to support their theory that parental reaction to normal disfluency has been the cause of stuttering. Those holding to the theory may count on the fact that it is also almost impossible to prove them wrong. Furthermore, to test theories, research must include experimental (dynamic) support and not merely circumstantial evidence. Imagine if, based on circumstantial evidence after observing a number of people who stutter, one proposed that stuttering can be caused by attempts to speak on inspiratory airflow. The speculation is premature until dynamic evidence is obtained through experiments designed to manipulate the variable of inspiratory airflow to observe the resultant effect on stuttering. Only if stuttering responded to the direct manipulation of this variable, would the relationship potentially reveal a causal rather than a circumstantial connection. An association between two or more phenomena or factors is insufficient for demonstrating causal relations. For example, if children who stutter exhibited a low tolerance for physical pain, it would be a mistake to assume that one caused the other. Of course, sometimes the contribution of variables is not simply a matter of yes or no. A factor may contribute to better fluency without directly causing it. Certain variables may improve (e.g., noise) or exacerbate (e.g., fatigue) stuttering, even if they are not directly responsible for it. This is why the separation of circumstantial from dynamic evidence is essential.

Still another issue that poses a challenge to theorizing is the *precision* of the observations made of the phenomena under study. Those seeking to explain stuttering must observe stuttering. If a scientist mistakes another form of nonfluent speech, such as cluttering, for stuttering and then formulates a theory or model based on the results, conclusions may be drawn that are not pertinent to actual stuttering. If scientists do not carefully isolate and define the essential speech characteristics of stuttering to distinguish it from other forms of speech breakdown, erroneous conclusions are likely to result, leading to faulty theories and models.

Several more difficulties arise when scientists attempt to draw causal inferences from observations of any given phenomenon. One is that of co-occurrence. Let's return to the inspiratory airflow hypothesis. Suppose that nearly every time someone stutters, there is evidence of an attempt to speak on inspiration. One possibility is that the inspiratory airflow has a causal connection to the stuttering. It could also be the case, however, that both the inspiratory airflow and the stuttering are separate results of the same underlying, yet unknown, abnormality. Also, factors deemed responsible for a given phenomenon must have unique roles in relation to it. For example, fatigue might be a proposed component in a model of stuttering, but if fatigue leads to the interruption of many kinds of human abilities besides speech fluency, a case may be made that this factor does not play a critical, unique role.

Another issue central to theories concerning living organisms (e.g., humans) is the element of *time and age*. What is meant here is that variables causally related to the phenomenon may not be identical, and/or may not occur in the same proportions or hold the same importance, across its life stages. This is illustrated by analogy: A plant grows underground without light for a while, but later, after it appears above ground, light aids substantially, or may even be necessary, to its growth. That is, the effect of light varies in relation to the stage of the plant's life. The same is apt to be true with respect to stuttering; that is, variables responsible for the onset of stuttering in early childhood may be different (in type and/or degree) from those maintaining it later, as a person ages. Consider the example that anxiety, so common in older children and adults, is seldom an apparent factor at the earliest stage of stuttering in preschool children.

In general, testing theories of stuttering has been remarkably challenging due to (1) inherent difficulties of observing its onset, an important aspect of several theories; (2) its changing characteristics during aging; (3) the inconsistent occurrence of stuttering-related speech events from moment to moment and from situation to situation; (4) technical limitations in testing theories such as the near absence of animal research; (5) ethical problems in setting up scientific experiments including conditions that may induce a person to stutter; and (6) a highly likely possibility that stuttering results from a multiplicity of factors. Further, the relevance of factors may differ depending on the age, development, and experiences of the individual, as well as the number, type, and amount of specific factors.

> A theory is a set of interrelated concepts, principles, and definitions that present a systematic view of a phenomenon, specifying relationships among the relevant variables for purposes of description, explanation, and prediction (Kerlinger, 1986). What must take place in order to arrive at a sound theory? Scientists need to agree on a framework specifying the exogenous (e.g., environmental) and endogenous (e.g., genetic) variables to be studied. Measurement issues must be resolved. Hypotheses must be generated and tested to reveal the systematic relationships among the variables. Confounding factors or control variables must be isolated. Finally, skillful experimentation and multiple observations must be undertaken to refine the range and boundaries of relationships among the variables.

Are There Stuttering Subtypes?

With few exceptions, every entity in the universe can find its place within a system of classification. Systems of classification usually take the form of taxonomies with a hierarchy of divisions and subdivisions. The scientific classification of plants, for example, is based on a hierarchy moving from broad to specific cases according to phylum, class, order, genus, and species. The taxonomic system applied has an important role in the organization and enhancement of knowledge about any particular entity. It is the basis by which we understand which things are similar and which things are different. The question of subtypes is the matter of whether there are subdivisions to be made among people who stutter and/or what form of classification system to apply.

Although certain features of stuttering are relatively consistent, such as the age at onset of the disorder and the presence of certain core speech disfluencies, there are large differences in many aspects of the disorder across people who stutter, including variations in expression of symptoms and their severity. As discussed in Chapter 1, in addition to symptom diversity, in many ways the disorder of stuttering is interwoven with linguistic, phonetic, cognitive, social, emotional, physiological domains, as well as others. Additionally, it has been explained as emerging from a wide range of possible etiologies. A hint of possible taxonomic development for stuttering disorders is evident in literature. For example, a basic division of stuttering disorders has been noted according to age at stuttering onset. Stuttering with an onset in childhood (prior to adolescence) is considered *developmental,* whereas adult onset stuttering is considered to be *acquired.* For a long time within the developmental stuttering framework, there was no division of the two types: *classic stuttering* and *cluttering.* Currently, however, cluttering is viewed as a different disorder. Within the acquired stuttering framework, there also have been two types of cases—*neurogenic* stuttering and *psychogenic* stuttering—distinguished primarily on the basis of etiology.

With these multiple related domains and etiological classes in mind, is it possible that stuttering is not a single disorder? Might different combinations of several or all of the factors just cited create variations that are substantial enough to make clinically meaningful differences? After all, similarly sounding hoarse voices can be a symptom of vastly different disorders: vocal fold cancer, vocal fold infection, or vocal fold paralysis. Alternatively, is it possible that stuttering is a single disorder but contains subtypes of overt variations, such as seen in cleft palate speech that may result from unilateral cleft, bilateral cleft, and other types of clefts? The fact is that for a long time stuttering has been generally considered to be a unitary disorder without an acceptable subclassification system. St. Onge and Calvert's (1964) remark that stuttering has been viewed as a "pathognomonic monolith" (p. 160) nicely summarizes this perspective. The two scholars, however, questioned this view by posing these questions: "What are we studying when we study stuttering? Whatever it is, is it one, several, or many?" (p. 160) and went on to imply that stuttering is not a unitary disorder.

An altogether different view has stipulated that stuttering, at least its overt speech features, is not even a unique disorder but a *quantitative* deviation along the continuum of normal speech disfluency. In other words, stutterers simply do more of the same of what normally fluent speakers do (Bloodstein, 1970). We disagree and posit that stuttering is a unique disorder, qualitatively different from other disfluent speech. Still the question of whether it composes discrete subtypes deserves attention. The implications to the development of theory and related research are obvious. If subtypes exist, do they differ in their etiological components or the relative contributions of other factors? Does the nature of the disorder vary significantly among its subtypes? Do they follow different developmental courses, such as natural recovery or chronic stuttering? Not less important is the question of whether subtypes respond differentially to various treatments.

> The phenomenon of stuttering has perplexed scientists for centuries. Everyone can see or observe that stuttering disrupts the speech of people who stutter, but which characteristics are consistent? Are there features that can be observed over and over again? Often enough, speech disfluencies are not exactly the same from person to person or even identical for the same person at a different time. What does this mean? What does this observation show us? Most researchers would agree that one of the most consistent characteristics of stuttering is its variability, and one of the most consistent conclusions is that people who stutter are heterogeneous! If a system of subtypes is found that better differentiates various groups who stutter and/ or their stutter events, greater research progress may be possible.

Van Riper (1982) noted that that the concept of stuttering subtypes is traceable to at least the 16th century when it was proposed that stuttering is caused by either brain hyperexcitability or by emotionality. New subtype classifications of stuttering have surfaced throughout the modern history of speech pathology as reflected in the writings of Froeschels (1943) and the more current work of Riley and Riley (2000). In a review of the literature, Yairi (2007) suggested that many of the systems offered can be grouped into seven categories based on their frame of reference. These are listed next with an example of a classification under each category.

I. *Etiology*: Brill's (1923) classification based on personality problems (e.g., depressive, psychoneurotic, psychopathic) and stuttering.

II. *Prominent Stuttering Characteristics*: Froeschels (1943) classification of Clonic and Tonic stuttering.

III. *Reaction to drugs*: Alm's (2004b) classification of Type 1 and Type 2 stutterers who, respectively, decrease or increased stuttering in response to dopamine.

IV. *Biological Characteristics*: Hinkle's (1971) classification of right ear preference (RE), left ear preference (LE), and no preference (NE), reflecting hemispheric brain dominance, are also associated with a different stuttering pattern.

V. *Concomitant Disorders*: J. Riley's (1971) distinction between stuttering children exhibiting language deficits and those exhibiting inferior motor skills.

VI. *Developmental Course*: Van Riper's (1971) four distinct developmental courses of stuttering.

VII. *Statistically Generated Models* (multifactorial): Prins and Lohr's (1972) Type I—syllable repetitions/sound prolongations, and Type II—secondary physical movements, word substitutions.

Although ideas have been generated, little research has been conducted in the past that was specifically concerned with stuttering subtype differentiation (e.g., Berlin, 1954; Feinberg, Griffin, & Levey, 2000; Schwartz & Conture, 1988). More typically, researchers have focused on a single dimension of stuttering (e.g., disfluency behaviors, motor skills, language abilities, personality, brain hemispheric lateralization, etc.), thereby overlooking the multifaceted nature of the problem. These studies were also restricted in scope (e.g., small numbers), lacked adequate experimental controls, and were not situated within a clear theoretical framework. Perhaps due to these limitations they have not succeeded in generating strong evidence for straightforward typologies. So far, the scientific activities in this area have not translated meaningfully into the practical levels of either clinical management or the design of studies. None of the proposed classification systems for stuttering as a disorder has been adopted by a significant number of professionals. In spite of more sophisticated recent research (see reviews by Seery, Watkins, Mangelsdorf et al., 2007; and Yairi 2007), it would appear that the inclination to investigate and treat stuttering as a single disorder has generally prevailed. The point most related to this chapter is that if subtypes of stuttering need to be recognized, then our theories and models of stuttering need to be sufficiently dynamic to accommodate the requisite divisions and subdivisions.

Summary

Numerous explanations of the cause of stuttering or its various features have been proposed. Most of them do not qualify to be regarded as theories because they are too narrow to encompass the complex characteristics of the disorder and lack scientific evidence to back them up. Those "theories" or theoretical notions can be generally grouped as those dealing with the cause of stuttering as a disorder and those dealing with the dynamics of its observable features, speech, and so forth. Those that focus on etiology can be distinguished as physiological, psychological, and learning subcategories. The past two decades have seen the emergence of multifactorial models as well as the idea of stuttering subtypes. In this chapter several points were raised regarding the evaluation of theories:

- To be considered credible, a theory of stuttering must (1) fit observed phenomena, make predictions about future observations, and be testable; (2) explain all of the associated phenomena in a succinct way; (3) comprise components that neither contradict each other nor overlap with other possible explanations; and (4) have the potential to be expanded and/or changed with the acquisition of new information.

- Research will add credence to a theory when it reveals dynamic rather than merely circumstantial evidence.

- Stuttering is not apt to be explained by simple principles overgeneralized across the heterogeneous population of people who stutter.

- There is reason to believe that the etiology of a persistent stuttering disorder may be different from the factors that precipitate onset and govern progression.

- Satisfying taxonomies of stuttering disorders and stuttering events have yet to be developed.
- It is not yet clear whether stuttering is better understood as a condition varying along a continuum (dimensional) or as a condition characterized by heterogeneous subtypes. Subtypes may eventually be identified through profiling of multiple etiologic source factors or through more sophisticated models of the systems underlying speech fluency.

As briefly discussed earlier, theories of stuttering have been grouped in several ways. For our purposes, the question of why people stutter is best handled by breaking it down into several subquestions: Is stuttering motor-physiological? Is stuttering psycho-emotional? Is stuttering cognitive-linguistic? Is stuttering developed or learned? Is stuttering genetic? Is stuttering multidimensional? As we explore each of these potential etiologies, it will be important to understand that the answers to these questions are not mutually exclusive. Moreover, it is worth remembering that the various source factors may be differentially relevant for separate subtypes of stuttering disorders.

Study Questions and Discussion Topics

1. What is the difference between a theory and a model?
2. What difficulties are encountered in attempting to provide observational data in support of a theory of stuttering?
3. Generate a theory statement related to stuttering, and answer the following questions:
   a. Is your theory related to the stuttering event or the disorder?
   b. Is your theory about an isolated aspect or a comprehensive explanation?
   c. How well does your theory meet the criteria of being valid, exhaustive, exclusive, predictive, consistent, parsimonious, elegant, testable, and dynamic?
4. Ask a few people from outside the field of communicative disorders whether they believe stuttering is a biologically or psychologically based disorder, and to explain why they think that way. Were you surprised by what they think? Why? Did they use facts as a basis for the belief? Are there facts that you know about stuttering that were not considered in their beliefs?
5. Based on what you know about stuttering, do you think the disorder may be better characterized in terms of subtypes? Why or why not?

Suggested Readings

Packman, A., & Attanasio, J. (2004). What should a theory of stuttering explain? In *Theoretical issues in stuttering* (pp. 55–68). New York, NY: Psychology Press.

Perkins, W. (1999). *Stuttering and science.* San Diego, CA: Singular.

Wingate, M. (1997). *Stuttering: A short history of a curious disorder.* Westport, CT: Bergin & Garvey.

Chapter 6

Is Stuttering Psychological? Theories and Investigations

LEARNER OBJECTIVES

Readers of this chapter will be able to understand and critically evaluate:

- Theories of the psychoemotional contributions to stuttering.
- Theories of the psychobehavioral contributions to stuttering.
- Theories of the psycholinguistic contributions to stuttering.
- The general implications of psychological theories to the treatment of stuttering.

Is Stuttering Psychological?

Many speech-language clinicians, including ourselves, have been asked by people in social situations, or by clients and/or their family members in clinical settings, whether stuttering is "psychological." The typical underlying meaning of the question is whether stuttering is caused by "nerves" or psychological issues. Repeated experience has taught us that most laypeople raising this question already think so; their questions merely seek confirmation of their own beliefs. Furthermore, an old study based on personal interviews of adolescents who stutter regarding their "theory" of stuttering found that they, too, adhere to psychological factors as probable causes (Fraiser, 1955). A national survey of pediatricians revealed a similar set of beliefs (Yairi & Carrico, 1992).

Usually these presumptions treat the concept of "psychological" with a limited perspective confined to the psychoemotional, if not psychopathological, domain. The extent of various psychological dimensions, however, and their potential contributions to stuttering is, in fact, much broader. We recognize three major classes of psychological theories of stuttering: (1) psychoemotional, (2) psychobehavioral, and (3) psycholinguistic. Psychoemotional theories propose that stuttering is based in some psychological maladjustment. Psychobehavioral theories attribute stuttering to learning or conditioning processes. Psycholinguistic theories explain stuttering in terms of cognitive systems underlying the production of speech and language. In the following sections, we explore the essence of these theoretical orientations, related research, their contributions to the understanding of stuttering, and their clinical implications.

Psychoemotional Theories

The general theme of psychoemotional theories is that psychological traumas, emotional disturbances, or personality characteristics cause stuttering. Early written accounts of these models emerged in the 1920s, and investigations of stuttering as a psychopathological disorder reached a peak around the 1950s (see Goodstein's [1958] and Sheehan's [1958] reviews). The early psychoemotional theories of stuttering (e.g., Brill, 1923; Coriat, 1928, 1943b) were influenced by the basic premises of psychoanalytic theory, originally offered by Sigmund Freud (1899, 1901).

Psychoanalytic Theory

A fundamental assumption of psychoanalytic theory was that behaviors and actions could be triggered by earlier traumas to the psyche. The *psyche* was, in essence, the human soul or self, placed in central charge of thoughts and actions. Freud conceived of the psyche as having three parts: the id, the ego, and the superego. The *id* consists of unconscious instinctual drives, the *ego* engages in conscious decisions, and the *superego* is the moral conscience judging the goodness or badness of thoughts and behavior. If the ego experiences a threat or trauma, and the id is inclined toward self-protection through violence, the ego may notice aggressive thoughts surfacing into consciousness. The superego may judge aggressive thoughts and actions as unacceptable, and so in turn, the ego may push the impulses back, deeper into the id's unconscious motivations (i.e., *repressing* them). Thus reactions to trauma within the psyche may be repressed but rise to the surface of ego consciousness as compulsive thoughts or actions, still basically aggressive but having a more acceptable form. So stuttering, for example, might stem from an aggressive or even violent impulse that was repressed and converted into a more acceptable form.

Because stuttering begins in childhood, the early theories were based on Freud's model of child psychosexual development. Freud maintained a child's psyche is developed in response to the id's drive of sexual pleasure, referred to as *libido*. The libido takes on a different character at various stages and/or ages of early childhood. The three psychosexual stages and corresponding ages were the *oral* stage (0 to 18 months); *anal* stage (18 months to 3.5 years), and *phallic-oedipal* stage (3 to 6 years). Emotional problems and conflicts that arise at each stage may end up as a long-term fixation: continuing needs for gratification typical to that stage. The following examples of stuttering theories propose psychoneuroses that vary in relation to the particular stage of its development.

Coriat (1928) opined that stuttering primarily represents a fixation at the oral stage. He explained it was a symptom of an unhealthy solution to the unconscious conflict between a wish for infantile suckling, which is socially unacceptable, and the need for a more appropriate behavior. Summing it up in his own words, Coriat stated that "in the speech of stammerers the illusion of nursing is maintained and the oral gratification continued by this illusory substitution for the maternal nipple, the stammerer thus retaining his mother into adult life" (quoted by Hahn, 1956, p. 29). The symbolic nature of the outward symptom—stuttering, strange as it might be seen—is demonstrated by this example. By contrast, Fenichel (1945) regarded stuttering as a psychoneurosis originating at the anal stage of psychosexual development. Conflicts stemming from ungratified urges toward the retention and expulsion of feces were resolved when the child displaced its expression upward to another sphincter, the mouth. This symbolic symptom, stuttering, was a more acceptable form of "smearing" listeners with aggressiveness and hostility. Such dynamics are buried deep within the unconscious psyche, that is, the person who stutters is not aware of it. The constant neurotic anxiety experienced is general and nonspecific because the source remains unknown to the speaker. Although these early notions of psychological conflicts seem rather peculiar to us now, they represent a more plausible conceptualization of stuttering as a symptom of subconscious psychological dynamics. Several other theories have been based on a similar theme.

> The common theme of the early psychoemotional theories depicts stuttering as a deep-seated neurosis involving a conversion reaction. The unconscious mind converts its hidden, forbidden urges into an open, more acceptable form, even if unpleasant, expressing them as stuttering. Early proponents often debated about whether the stutterer's unmet psychosexual impulses in infancy were oral or anal in nature (Lowinger, 1952; Moskowitz, 1941). Counterintuitively, anal, rather than oral, fixation was the most frequently supported basis for stuttering (Fisher, 1970). These theories were the first among several implicating parent-child interactions in stuttering etiology.

The middle of the 20th century saw other versions of psychoanalytic theories (e.g., Barbara, 1954; Glauber, 1958). Sheehan (1953) proposed that stuttering was a symptom of repressed needs, inhibited aggressions, or other "unspeakable feelings" (an expression used later by Travis, 1957) leading to simultaneous urges to speak and to hold back from speaking. Noting strong rejection of stuttering children by their fathers, Clark and Snyder (1955) contended that stuttering reflects basic disturbances in the child-father relationship, including fear of authority figures and lack of well-defined masculine identification. Similarly centered on parental influence, Murphy and Fitzsimmons (1960) viewed stuttering as a tension-reducing symptom emanating from parents' overprotective attitudes. Travis (1957) explained that the person who stutters is caught in the conflict between repressed urges to suck, eat, evacuate, and explore sexual pleasures, and the parentally induced inhibition of these forbidden needs. The person resents, even hates, these impositions, must abide by them, and has guilt feelings for even harboring such drives. These must be repressed. At the same time, there are mixed feelings of love and guilt toward the parents. Such conflicts are unconsciously resolved through a symbolic symptom: stuttering. It allows the person to express the unspeakable feelings and simultaneously punish themselves for having them without showing what these urges really are.

Weaknesses: The main criticism of these theories is the questionable research-based support. Lee Travis believed that he had greatly helped, if not cured, 11 adult stutterers with 150 hours each of psychotherapy; however, he did not publish actual data by which these subjective impressions could be verified. Despite the popularity of psychoanalysis for many years, the anecdotal stories of success were minimal, and the ideas did not withstand the test of time.

Clinical Implications: Logically, theories that depict stuttering as a psychoneurosis also advocate psychoanalysis as the therapy of choice. This technique is aimed at bringing unconscious desires into conscious awareness so that insight into the real problems will allow the client to deal with them in a healthier manner. Because this approach also traces neurotic parental (especially the mother's) behavior as a factor contributing to the child's neurotic conflicts, some programs also encourage parents to participate in the therapy (see Chapter 10).

Stuttering as a Psychoemotional Disturbance

Even if psychoanalytic theory failed to deliver a satisfactory explanation, a number of researchers wondered whether stuttering represents a psychoemotional disturbance. The most direct form of investigation of this hypothesis is to study whether people who stutter possess similar characteristics to other groups with psychoemotional disturbances. To put this hypothesis to the test, investigators compared people who stutter with psychiatric populations using a variety of methodologies and individuals across age ranges. Goodstein (1958), for example, compared adults who stutter with psychiatric patients. He concluded that the stutterers were not maladjusted by comparison, but found that they were more anxious, tense, and socially withdrawn than the third group, those with no speech or mental disorders. He cautioned, however, that it was impossible to know whether such attributes represented factors influencing the etiology of stuttering or problems that emerged as a consequence of social reactions to stuttering. Sheehan (1958) similarly opined that the absence of a definite personality pattern among those who stutter made them different from populations with emotional disorders, such as hysterical aphonia or depression. Nevertheless, he entertained the possibility that different personality dynamics among PWS may have been obscured in group studies. He went further to support the concept of stuttering subtypes, stating that "it might follow that there are several different kinds of stutterers, psychologically speaking" (p. 24).

Nearly a quarter of a century later, Sermas and Cox (1982) assessed measures of abnormal personality among three groups: patients who stutter, patients with brain dysfunction, and patients with personality disorders without brain dysfunction. To their credit, they employed multiple sources of data: psychiatric interviews, projective tests, and personality tests. The stuttering group scored significantly higher than the other two groups only on the interpersonal sensitivity subscale of one test. This subscale tapped feelings of personal inadequacy, inferiority, and negative expectations during interpersonal interactions. The psychiatric interviews revealed that almost half of the stuttering group displayed noteworthy obsessive-compulsive tendencies, and 25% had experienced some depression. None of the stutterers, however, showed formal neurotic symptoms. The interpretation of this investigation is limited by the absence of a control group of nonstuttering nonpsychiatric participants, the small sample size of 19 per group, and the participants' wide age range, from 16 to 48 years. Nonetheless, it would appear that although PWS are adversely affected by stuttering psychologically, they are not, as a group, evidencing any consistent form of personality disturbance.

Psychoemotional dimensions of stuttering may originate from several planes. As a primary cause, stuttering could be the overt symptom of an underlying psychoneurosis. From this vantage point, the disorder is energized by an unconscious conflict arising between, or among, opposing needs or motives of the psyche. From another angle, psychoemotional factors, such as extremely sensitive temperament traits or anxiety tendencies, may serve in the role as secondary causes, by predisposing the speaker either to start stuttering or to persist in stuttering. Finally, seen from the flip side, people who stutter may be prone to develop psychoemotional disturbances as a result of stuttering.

What potential evidence could lead to acceptance of the commonly held belief that stuttering is rooted in psychoemotional causes and what are the pertinent research findings? Five forms of potential evidence come to mind. First, the onset of stuttering could frequently coincide with psychologically agitating events. What do we know about this possibility? Stuttering onset coincides with emotionally stressful events in approximately 40% of the cases, but these vary in nature and are not typically traumatic. Second, a sudden rather than gradual onset might be seen as more consistent with the premise of a psychologically agitating event. On this point, typical stuttering onset is sudden in about only 40% to 50% of cases (Reilly et al., 2009; Yairi & Ambrose, 2005). Thus, the timing of onset does not offer clear support for this premise, either. Third, the natural recovery from stuttering would be found to co-occur with conditions that improve psychological adjustment. Regarding adjustment, although psychological factors are sometimes important to the amelioration of stuttering for older children and adults undergoing treatment, research has not thus far revealed a noticeable role for these factors in the massive natural recovery experienced by preschool children. Fourth, if psychological (i.e., mental-emotional) states, such as anxiousness, nervousness, or fears, were at the root of stuttering, then age of stuttering onset would be distributed fairly evenly across the life span because people at any age can be vulnerable to such states. Fifth, an especially major prediction is that certain personality characteristics or forms of emotional maladjustments should be consistently noted among those who stutter. The research reveals mixed results with respect to stuttering and personality links, but the bulk of the evidence has not revealed a specific stuttering personality profile or reliable indication of psychological maladjustment (Bloodstein & Bernstein Ratner, 2008).

Thus, the evidence for a psychoemotional problem as the main cause for the onset of childhood stuttering is largely unsupported by research. If this is the case, why should we be interested in psychological theories of stuttering? Several answers come to mind. First, psychological dynamics could be one of several contributing factors responsible for the onset of stuttering in a subset of cases. Second, although psychological factors may not account for stuttering onset, they could contribute to the maintenance and progression of stuttering. Third, even if emotional states and personality traits are insufficient to predict cases of stuttering consistently, such factors could help to explain the timing of occurrence of speech events regarded as stuttering. Fourth, some people who stutter also exhibit emotional problems that, although not the cause of stuttering, complicate the problem and interfere with therapy. The individual's personality and temperament characteristics are also factors that influence the client's responses to therapy, for example, willingness to enter speaking situations with strangers. It is not surprising, therefore, that psychological theories and factors continue to attract interest, and exert influence on stuttering research and intervention. The review of additional research related to these questions appears in the next sections on factors of personality, anxiety, and temperament.

Personality Factors in Stuttering

Even if the evidence does not uphold theories of stuttering as an expression of psychopathology, another factor possibly contributing to stuttering etiology is personality structure. Goodstein (1958) published a review of a large number of personality studies of children who stutter. These investigations employed many kinds of instruments: formal tests of observation, personality inventories completed by parents, and free (word) association tasks. Regardless of methodology, results generally yielded no significant differences between groups of children who stutter and their nonstuttering peers. In the same publication, Goodstein also detailed findings and summarized results of approximately 40 personality studies of adults who stutter. Assessment tools used in this research included projective techniques, clinical interview, paper-and-pencil tests, and a variety of other inventories such as the Minnesota Multiphasic Personality Inventory (Walnut, 1954). A similar conclusion was drawn that no particular personality pattern of PWS could be identified. People who stutter appeared to represent the same broad range of personalities that characterized people who do not stutter.

Also published in 1958, Sheehan reviewed 17 investigations with adults, school-age children, and preschool children who stutter in which projective techniques (e.g., Rorschach inkblot test; Thematic Apperception Test pictures) or scales of aspiration levels were used. About half of these studies reported no significant differences between people who stutter at various ages and control groups on variables, such as morality, aggression, impulsivity, and obsessive-compulsive tendency. A few of these studies, however, suggested that those who stutter have greater tendencies for obsessions, compulsions, aggression, and ego defensiveness. Contradictory findings were also reported regarding levels of aspiration.

Anxiety

Two main aspects of of anxiety related to stuttering have drawn research interest. One explores the potential influence of anxiety on stuttering events and their frequency. The second examines the tendency for people who stutter to experience more general anxiety. Both of these aspects may be relevant to the nature and treatment of the disorder. Regarding the association between specific stuttered events and anxiety, once again, the findings have been inconsistent. In 1972, Gray and England found that the correspondence between stuttering frequency and anxiety was marginal in 15 adults who received deconditioning treatment. Also Wingate (1975) observed that 9 of 10 young adults often failed to predict upcoming stuttering although they claimed that they could do it. He therefore questioned the extent to which emotional responses trigger stutter events. More positive results were reported by other investigators, however. Toomey and Sidman (1970) observed that two of their four stuttering subjects increased and two decreased stuttering with the anxiety of receiving electrical shock. Weber and Smith (1990) found that the timing of elevated autonomic nervous system arousal was strongly associated with stutter events. Blood, Wertz, Blood et al. (1997) noted that the majority of the adults they studied reported increased stuttering on days with increased stress.

Regarding the second aspect of anxiety and stuttering, a number of studies have noted significant differences in anxiety level/type between adults who stutter and normally fluent controls. Greiner, Fitzgerald, Cooke et al. (1985) reported that adults who stuttered scored significantly higher than controls on a measure of anxiety, the Willoughby Personality Schedule (WPS, WPS-R). They suggested that those stutterers may have word-specific anxiety, situation-specific anxiety, and/or general anxiety. Later, Fitzgerald, Djurdjic, and Maguin (1992) used the same instrument (WPS-R) with a group of Yugoslavian participants and essentially replicated the Greiner et al.'s (1985) findings. Specifically, stutterers scored higher on social isolation and social sensitivity, and lower on social confidence compared to control subjects.

Craig (1990) administered Spielberger's State-Trait Anxiety Inventory measure, called the STAI (Spielberger, Gorsuch, Luschene et al., 1983), to a large group of 102 adults who stutter before and after behavioral therapy for stuttering. Anxiety levels were also compared with a control group. Those who stuttered scored significantly higher on *state anxiety* in demanding speech situations, but they also scored higher than the controls on chronic, or *trait,* anxiety. Following treatment, the anxiety levels of PWS were in the normal range, although their scores remained higher than those of the controls. In a more recent investigation, Craig et al. (2003) explored the associations between stuttering and anxiety in 63 PWS, age 15 or older. Using the STAI, the stuttering group was found to have significantly higher anxiety scores than a nonstuttering control group. Thus, more specific research supports the impression that people who stutter tend to experience significant state anxiety as a result of stuttering. Additionally, recent research findings concerning chronic trait anxiety in adults who stutter raise the possibility that personality is a predisposing factor for stuttering persistence.

Temperament

Whereas in the past, many ideas linked the etiology of stuttering to personality, current trends have shifted to the relationship between stuttering and temperament. Whereas research focused on personality intended to reveal the cause of stuttering, temperament research aims to reveal a contributing factor to the complexity of the disorder. Temperament has been considered a subcomponent of personality in some models, but more commonly a developmental distinction has been made between the two concepts. Whereas personality is assumed to take years to develop and be shaped by life experiences, temperament is considered to be evident already in infancy as the product of heredity and in utero experiences. Personality in an adult is influenced by habits; temperament in a child is revealed in dispositions. Both are described in terms of traits. A *trait* is an aspect of an individual's character that is relatively stable, in contrast with a *state,* which is an aspect that fluctuates. A person might possess the trait of being easy-going, but have the temporary state of feeling upset.

Temperament is expressed in constitutionally based individual differences in reactivity and self-regulation (Caprara & Cervone, 2000; Rothbart & Bates, 1998). The term *reactivity* refers to motor, emotional, and attentional responses to internal and external stimuli, while *self-regulation* denotes the processes serving to increase or decrease reactivity. A child who is emotionally reactive cries immediately when a stranger appears, but with high self-regulation, settles down in just a few minutes.

Guitar (2006) suggested that a sensitive (i.e., reactive) temperament may predispose a child to stutter. Similarly, Perkins (1992) proposed that children at risk for persistent stuttering were apt to be those who are more easily intimidated. Some evidence supports these hypotheses. For example, Riley and Riley (2000) found increased sensitivity (reactivity) and higher self-expectations among 50 school-age children who stutter, and Oyler (1996) concluded that school-age children who stutter were significantly more vulnerable and sensitive than children who do not stutter.

As mentioned in earlier chapters, some differences in temperament characteristics have been noted between preschool-age as well as school-age children who stutter and normally fluent children. The CWS were more reactive and more irregular in physiological functions, had less regulation of emotion and attention, were less apt to habituate to their environment or adapt to changes in routine, and were less distractible when engaged in a task (e.g., Karrass et al., 2006; Schwenk, Conture, & Walden, 2007). Significantly less adaptability in children who stutter has been reported in several other studies as well (Embrechts, Ebben, Franke et al., 2000). On the other hand, no differences were found by the Reilly et al. team (2013).

Although it is unclear whether tendencies toward greater sensitivity and reactivity and lower adaptability in children who stutter represent factors contributing to the etiology of stuttering at onset, it appears that personality differences are evident in children who have stuttered for a few years. But these traits may not be specifically related to stuttering. Hauner, Shriberg, Kwiatkowski et al. (2005) reviewed related literature for children with a variety of communication disorders and concluded that they displayed significantly greater sensitivity, anxiety, distractibility, neuroticism, withdrawal, and difficulty in adaptability when compared to typically speaking peers. Hence children who stutter may merely show personality tendencies typical of children with a variety of communication disorders, not specifically linked to stuttering.

Research conducted by a European team (Eggers et al., 2010) compared temperament scales for 58 CWS with matched controls, all from 3 to 8 years of age (mean = 6 years). Parents of CWS assigned lower ratings on inhibitory control and attentional shifting traits, but higher on motor activation (e.g., excessive fidgeting), approach (e.g., excitement about anticipated events), and anger/frustration traits. Although temperament supposedly reflects a constitutionally based construct, the wide age range of participants means it is unclear whether these differences tend to be present at the time of stuttering onset or emerge later developmentally. In 2013, Eggers, De Nil, and Van den Bergh studied 60 children ages 4 to 10 years (mean = 7 years) on tasks of inhibitory control. The responses of the 30 CWS indicated significantly poorer inhibitory control compared to NFC. By contrast, Choi, Conture, Walden et al. (2013) found no significant differences on tasks related to behavioral inhibition comparing nearly the same numbers of children ages 3 to 6 years. Still, the children with the highest stuttering frequency tended to exhibit the lowest inhibitory control.

The dual diathesis-stressor model of stuttering proposes contributions from two major components: linguistic skills and emotional regulation (Walden et al., 2012). The term *diathesis* refers to an inherited predisposition, in this case, to stutter. The term *stressor* refers to environmental events or conditions that cause stress. The premise of this model is that a stable emotional diathesis, such as a child's temperament, interacts with situational stressors, such as emotional states, to effect stuttering. Similarly, the child's language capacities diathesis interacts with the stressor of a child's level of attempted language production to influence stuttering. When these emotional and linguistic contributions combine, they presumably impact the frequency and severity of stuttering.

Weaknesses of Psychoemotional Theories

Research concerning temperament has not established that there is an effect of negative emotion or emotional regulation on stuttering in preschoolers. Stuttering, however, was reportedly higher for children who were described by their parents as having both greater negative emotion and lower emotional regulation than NFC (Walden et al., 2012). Highlighting the inconsistent results of research, Sheehan, like Goldstein (1958), concluded there was very little to show that PWS have a specific personality structure. As mentioned earlier, tendencies toward certain personality characteristics among adults who stutter could represent the impact of stuttering on the person rather than the cause of the stuttering.

Clinical Implications of Psychoemotional Theories

Parents and clinicians can work with young children who stutter to improve adjustment and their responses to stress. During therapy sessions, particular attention should be given to the child's speech responses in relation to language demands. The presence of *general anxiety* in an adult who stutters could be addressed by devoting a portion of therapy to overall relaxation and emotional adjustment. *Event-related anxiety* indicates a need for specific desensitization to experiences with stuttering moments and/or specific speaking situations.

Summary of Psychoemotional Theories

The popular long-standing laypersons' belief that stuttering is caused by emotional problems has also found expression in theoretical notions about this possible etiology of stuttering. Ideas offered during the first third of the 20th century were strongly influenced by Sigmund Freud's psychoanalytic theory of the human psyche with its strong emphasis on deep-seated, unconscious emotional problems and conflicts, which are outwardly expressed in physical symptoms such as stuttering. The stuttering, although unpleasant, serves as symbolic expression of the inner needs. Theories along this line were influenced by later variations of the psychoanalysis framework, and they continued to appear for several decades. For the most part, however, research studies have *not* yielded sufficient evidence to support these theories. Research has failed to show that people who stutter are characterized by abnormal psychology or special personality. Nor has it sufficiently described how such psychopathological factors would contribute to the disorder.

In many of the related studies, psychoemotional characteristics were inconsistent across subjects and across studies. The differences found in emotional-social behavior (e.g., greater withdrawal from social activity), can easily be seen as a normal reaction of the person who stutters to the difficulties experienced with his or her speech problem. Recent studies, however, have provided reasonable evidence for greater levels of trait anxiety in people who stutter as well as hints of possible greater sensitivity in terms of temperament. It is interesting to note here that the diagnosogenic theory of stuttering (discussed in the next section), which is framed primarily within learning perspectives, emphasizes the child's sensitivity to listeners' reactions as an important factor in the onset of stuttering. Perhaps Sheehan's notions of subtypes of stutterers is worth renewed consideration because there may be a subgroup of people who stutter who have at-risk personalities. Further research is needed to examine whether psychoemotional factors (e.g., hypersensitivity) might have a role in the persistence of stuttering.

Psychobehavioral Theories

The basic concept underlying the psychobehavioral theories is that stuttering is a learned behavior, that is, an acquired rather than constitutionally based disorder. This learning may take place in a variety of ways. It may progress slowly as in the formation of a habit, consistent with a gradual onset of stuttering. Gradual learning might suggest that some form of reinforcement is shaping the behavioral response. Or stuttering could result from a very brief motor problem-solving process of learning, consistent with a sudden onset of stuttering. Indeed, as discussed in Chapter 3, both gradual and sudden onsets of stuttering have been reported in the literature.

The foundations for psychobehavioral theory were established by Pavlov (1927) in his work concerning classical conditioning and by B. F. Skinner's (1953) research on operant conditioning. These two modes of behavioral conditioning are quite different. Classical conditioning involves a learning process in which more features in the environment (i.e., stimuli) can elicit the *same* response through a process of association. In the famous example, Pavlov's dog responded at first with saliva when food was presented but later also salivated to the ringing of a bell, after its sound had been paired with food. Next, additional stimuli that were paired with the bell or other already conditioned stimuli also triggered the same response—salivation. In other words, classical conditioning is a process of response generalization in which the subject makes the same response to an ever-growing number of stimuli that occur *before* the behavioral response. In contrast, operant conditioning is aimed at changing the response (behavior), based on events that occur *after* it has taken place. This process can result in a narrowing down (rather than generalization) of the desired response as it is modified by the impact of what follows it (e.g., reinforcement, punishment, or other consequences).

The interest in the application of behavioral principles to stuttering resulted in a host of new theoretical perspectives, some of which are reviewed here, that incorporated one or both of these two types of conditioned learning processes. These, in turn, prompted new research, especially of operant conditions that bring the stuttering response under stimulus control (e.g., Flanagan, Goldiamond, & Azrin, 1958; Martin & Siegel, 1966). For an extensive review of the experimental literature related to the effects of response contingent stimulation on stuttering, see Prins and Hubbard (1988). This group of theories has had a significant impact on stuttering therapy as evidenced in a number of clinical programs that employ conditioning procedures. They will be discussed in Chapter 12.

A professor delivering a lecture paces back and forth in front of the classroom. The students on the left side of the room are showing great interest while those on the right side appear to be disinterested. Reinforced by the interested students, more and more time is spent pacing near them toward the left side. Whenever positioned in front of the students who lack interest, the absence of reinforcement (perhaps punishment) prompts the professor to move away. Gradually the pacing stops altogether and a final stance is established on the left in a position directly in front of the students who are showing great interest. This example of operant conditioning illustrates how human behavior may be modified by its consequences.

Stuttering as a Reactive Avoidance Behavior

One of the earliest theories of stuttering to suggest that a child's speech behavior could be modified by its environmental consequences was developed by Wendell Johnson at the University of Iowa. Although his ideas were not based in behavior modification principles, and he placed a heavy emphasis on emotional reactions to disfluent speech, the theory is being categorized as *psychobehavioral* because it purports that stuttering is a learned response. This well-known view saw its early hints beginning in 1942 when Johnson concluded from his original study of stuttering onset that what parents described as their young child's "first stuttering" was quite similar to what parents of nonstuttering children observed as their child's normal disfluent speech.[1] Johnson's views saw further development when a few years later he elaborated on the early findings, concluding that

---

[1]The study was described in detail by Johnson (1955b).

stuttering, as a clinical problem, was found to occur not before but *after* it was diagnosed. "In order to emphasize these findings, I have coined the term *diagnosogenic*; stuttering is a diagnosogenic disorder in the sense that the diagnosis of stuttering is one of the causes of the disorder" (Johnson, 1944, p. 33). Following additional studies based primarily on parent interviews and some speech samples recorded a while after the time of onset (see Chapter 3), his later publications (Johnson & Associates, 1959) proposed what came to be popularly known as the *diagnosogenic* or *semantogenic* theory concerning the etiology of stuttering. *Diagnosogenic* means that the diagnosis causes the disorder. *Semantogenic* means that the mere labeling of the problem is powerful enough to create the problem.

Relying on data that showed most, if not all, young children exhibit speech disfluency as they develop speaking skills (e.g., Davis, 1939), Johnson felt that stuttering began when overanxious parents erroneously labeled these normal disfluencies as "stuttering." He stated that "stuttering begins not in the speaker's mouth, but in the listener's ear" (1955a, p. 11). His research indicated that the parents of stuttering children tended to be strict, perfectionistic, demanding, anxious, and overprotective. Commensurately, because they held unrealistically high child development standards and expectations they tended to be disappointed in their child's performance. In particular, these parents appeared to be overanxious about speech, and were quick to react negatively to their child's normal disfluencies. Responding to the parents' lead, the child reacted unfavorably to his or her own normal disfluencies, becoming anxious. By actively attempting to avoid these unapproved disfluencies, tension built up that led to a worsening of the disfluency. The child's continued failings invited even stronger parental reactions, leading to further effort on his or her part to avoid disfluencies, resulting in increased tension that eventually spiraled what began as normal disfluency into a real stuttering problem.[2] This view is also reflected in Johnson's (1948) definition of stuttering as "an anticipatory apprehensive hypertonic avoidance reaction" (p. 206). He conceptualized it to be nothing other than what a speaker does trying not to stutter.

Weaknesses: The diagnosogenic theory maintained dominance in the field well into the 1970s, and some scientists and clinicians may still adhere to it. It was attractive in its simplicity and based on premises that are almost impossible to prove wrong. Can anyone prove that the very first disfluencies labeled by parents as "stuttering" were really "normal"? As we discuss in later chapters, it had a profound influence on the treatment of stuttering. With time, the idea that stuttering is caused by listeners' reactions to normal disfluency began to lose ground as contradictory evidence accumulated. Table 6.1 lists the evidence Johnson believed to support his theory as well as our counterevidence that contributed to its fall.

---

[2]Although similar, Johnson's theory predated the well-known Pygmalion (or Rosenthal) effect described in the 1960s, in which a supervisor's or teacher's expectations, either encouraging or discouraging, tend to induce performance outcomes to match.

Table 6.1   Supporting and Counterevidence for Johnson's Diagnosogenic Theory

Supporting Evidence*	Counterevidence
1. Speech data for some stuttering children in the study and their matched nonstuttering controls revealed certain *overlap* in the overall frequency of disfluency.	1. Disfluencies of nonstuttering children are *far less frequent* than what Johnson thought, especially in certain critical types of disfluency (Ambrose & Yairi, 1999; Yairi, 1981, 1982).
2. Parents' descriptions of early stuttering were similar to descriptions of disfluent speech of control children.	2. Many parents have reported that they perceived abnormal speech in their child from the first day of stuttering (Yairi, 1983).
3. Parents overwhelmingly depicted a gradual onset with uneventful circumstances.	3. Sudden onsets of stuttering have been found to comprise nearly 40% of all cases (Yairi & Ambrose, 1992b, 2005).
4. Johnson's speech data showed that every disfluency type found in the speech of the stuttering children was also present in the speech of control children.	4. Critical types of disfluencies near the onset of stuttering are substantially different from normal not only in frequency, but in type, proportions, length, and speed (Ambrose & Yairi, 1999; Throneburg & Yairi, 1994; Yairi & Hall, 1993; Yairi & Lewis, 1984). In fact, Johnson and associates' (1959) own disfluency data do not support the assertions he made (see McDearmon, 1968).
5. Data for normally speaking preschool children revealed that disfluency is a normal phenomenon (Branscom, Hughes, & Oxtoby, 1955; Davis, 1939).	5. Disfluency in normally fluent children is a normal phenomenon but limited in frequency (Yairi, 1981).
6. Parents reported no statistically significant differences between children who stutter and normally fluent controls in many aspects of health and development.	6. Evidence for a strong *genetic component* to stuttering has been growing from several directions, including identification of several chromosomes as likely sites for genes underlying stuttering (Ambrose, Cox, & Yairi, 1997; Suresh, Ambrose, Roe et al., 2006).
7. Children who stutter are often sensitive to negative listener reactions to their disfluent or stuttered speech and seek to avoid reprisal.	7. Experimental studies and surveys revealed that parents' calling attention to their child's stuttering with instructions such as "slow down" and "take a breath and start over" may have contributed to his or her improvement (Martin, Kuhl, & Haroldson, 1972; Wingate, 1976). Although the child may have been destined developmentally to recover, parental instructions did not hinder recovery.

(continued)

Table 6.1   (Continued)

Supporting Evidence*	Counterevidence
8. Reports indicated there were societal/ cultural variations in stuttering prevalence related to the extent of community emphasis on speaking skills. The Shoshone Indians, for example, were reported to have no word for stuttering and no cases of it (Snidecor, 1947). By not labeling or calling any attention to disfluencies, Johnson thought their tribe had successfully prevented stuttering altogether.	8. Revisiting the societal/cultural factor it was discovered Native Americans do have a word for stuttering and did know of individuals who stuttered (Zimmermann, Liljeblad, Frank et al., 1983). It appears that stuttering is found universally.
9. Data showed that listeners might vary greatly in their perceptual judgments of speech as normal or stuttered (Tuthill, 1946; Williams & Kent, 1958).	9. Studies showed that negative verbal responses, mild electrical shock, loud sounds, and other aversive stimuli, administered as the immediate consequence of stuttering moments, often result in substantial declines in stuttering (Costello & Ingham, 1984; Prins & Hubbard, 1988).

*Items without a reference are based on Johnson & associates, 1959.

Clinical Implications: For young children, treatment became largely indirect, keeping the child out of therapy so as to not call attention to his or her speech. Instead, therapy focused on parent counseling, advising them regarding better parent-child interaction. Parents were to reduce communicative pressure, be patient listeners, and accept stuttering without reacting. For adults, an important implication of the theory was a reorientation of the person's perspective on the problem, encouraging the person to view him- or herself as a speaker rather than a "stutterer," with particular emphasis on the use of descriptive language when thinking and talking about stuttering. In other words, assuming responsibility for the behaviors that bring about the stuttering allows the person to change and improve (Johnson, 1961a).

Stuttering as a Conditioned Anxiety Response

The learning-oriented diagnosogenic theory exerted strong and lasting influences but was not firmly linked to learning theory principles. Theoretical as well as clinical questions were left open. For example, why and how does stuttering continue or become reinforced in spite of being so painful? Why is the stuttering block eventually released? Therefore, other investigators stepped in to present stuttering within a more formal behavioral conditioning framework. In 1950 Wischner incorporated principles from the conditioning models of both Pavlov (1927) and Hull (1943) to construct his theory. He pointed out that the stuttering adaptation curve (pattern of decrease in frequency upon successive readings of the same material) is similar to a behavioral extinction curve obtained in animal experiments, and that stuttering increases as the anticipation periods prior to talking get longer. Equating anticipation with anxiety, stuttering was seen to be similar to other behaviors evoked by the avoidance of unpleasant (noxious) stimuli. This is commonly seen in experiments with guinea pigs trapped in a cage, running around frantically to avoid electric shock that is terminated when a certain lever is pressed or floor grid is found.

Imagine learning to walk the tightrope during a circus performance. The rope is high above the ground, without safety nets below. The eyes of all the spectators are glued to your every movement, scrutinizing every bobble. The combination of the fear of falling and a hint of doubt in your ability to perform the task elevates your tension. All effort is concentrated on trying to maintain balance, but the level of mounting anxiety causes you to lose balance over and over again. Each time balance needs to be adjusted, you jerk around in a haphazard array of arm and leg movements until you finally regain composure and prepare to move forward again. You manage to stay on the high wire until reaching the safety of the opposite platform, but your journey there has been filled with a chaotic display of flailing limbs and unusual postures. Perhaps this experience parallels the nature of stuttering as an anxiety response.

Wischner asserted that expressions of parental disapproval of the child's normal disfluency constitute noxious stimuli that create anxiety. The anxiety (anticipation) concerning further painful parental reactions to disfluencies motivates the child to avoid them by changing his or her disfluent speaking behavior. Typically, these attempts end up with mounting tension to the point at which real stuttering ensues. Soon, in a classic Pavlovian manner, other stimuli, such as words, situations, and certain people, are conditioned to become anxiety-provoking stimuli that cause stuttering. Stuttering persists in spite of being painful due to the principle that learning takes place as a result of drive reduction (Hull, 1943). Stuttering is self-reinforcing because the anxiety that builds up prior to talking is greatly relieved when the stuttering finally occurs and is completed. The reinforcing power of the sharp fall in anxiety *immediately* after a stuttering event is greater than the adverse social reactions that follow. The physical behaviors (secondary characteristics) are also reinforced because the person who stutters is convinced that they actually helped "get the word out." Eventually, these tensions and movements become integrated into the stuttering pattern.

Weaknesses: One weakness of Wischner's theory is that many young children do not appear anxious at the time of stuttering onset. Additionally, many children present with sudden onset, which does not support the notion of a gradual learning of behavior.

Clinical Implications: Although extinction of responses set up by avoidance conditioning is difficult, it is still possible if an animal in a cage ignores the danger signal and the expected negative consequences do not materialize. Accordingly, stuttering should diminish if speech disfluency is experienced in the absence of noxious stimuli so that the anxiety is deconfirmed. By inference, remediation for adults is possible through behavioral modification, particularly through the process of *desensitization* that lowers anxiety and sensitivity to listeners' reactions. Practicing easy voluntary disfluencies that, as we know, are not associated with anxiety and do not invite negative reactions, should be helpful. For young children, Wischner's ideas, like Johnson's, imply that parents must be counseled to accept their child's stuttering and stop reacting to it.

The Conflict Theory of Stuttering

Although Wischner's theory provided a better framework for the view that stuttering is an acquired behavior shaped from normal disfluency, additional aspects, such as the initial trigger (is it really normal disfluency?) and the nature of dynamics underlying the moment of stuttering leave room for additional contributions. Sheehan's (1953) conflict theory varies from Johnson's and Wischner's ideas in two respects. First, the underlying cause of stuttering is proposed to stem from various fears, such as fears of specific words or speaking situations, as well as unconscious fears of exposing the ego to the threat of failure, among others. These fears stimulate conflict between any of several pairs of opposing drives, such as the drive to speak and the drive to avoid stuttering, the drive for expression of self versus the drive to avoid exposing oneself, between conscious speech control versus automatic processes, and others. Convolutedly, then, subconscious psychoemotional elements are injected into this primarily psychobehavioral theory.

Second, regarding the dynamics that trigger moments of stuttering, Sheehan used studies of approach-avoidance conflict in animals as the model. In this experimental paradigm, a hunger drive motivates the animal to move toward the food, but when the food is approached, an electric shock is delivered and the animal retreats to avoid pain. Going back and forth, the animal eventually freezes in one place, where the strengths of the opposing drives are equal. This is comparable to the person who stutters who finds himself or herself in a conflict between the urge to speak and drive to avoid speaking and stuttering, regardless of the source of the fear and conflict. Freezing occurs when approach and avoidance drives reach equilibrium, resulting in a stuttering block. Repetition and prolongation would represent oscillating and stopping at the point where the two-drive gradients cross. Stuttering is learned and persists because it is being self-reinforced through reduction in anxiety during the block when the approach drive finally prevails and the word is uttered.

Sheehan (1970) later posited that the central problem with stuttering is another form of conflict: a self-role conflict. Because people who stutter speak fluently at times, they possess two roles: stutterer and fluent speaker. They constantly attempt to embrace the fluent role by hiding/minimizing the stuttering in social contacts, hoping to "pass" as a normal speaker. The guilt feelings about the pretense mount to tension, resulting in stuttered speech.

Weaknesses: Although Sheehan's ideas account well for variations in stuttering frequency with situational factors, such as audience size and identity of the listener, it fails to be exhaustive with respect to explaining the unknown fears underlying stuttering and why singing, which also involves expression of emotion and specific words, is not also stuttered.

Clinical Implications: Accordingly, treatment should be primarily a matter of gaining mastery over fear, decreasing the tendencies for avoidance while increasing the approach drive. Sheehan strongly advocated that the person who stutters should actively accept, rather than hide, the role of the stutterer, by bringing stuttering out into the open. The inclination to hide stuttering creates fears that "it" will be exposed sooner or later. It strengthens the avoidance drive and the related psychoemotional conflicts that are expressed in stuttering moments. Clients should openly talk about their stuttering, even allow for some stuttering on purpose. By being open about stuttering, tension is reduced and stuttering is decreased.

Stuttering as an Operant Behavior

A further significant theoretical development is seen in Shames and Sherrick's (1963) application of a strict operant conditioning frame of reference to stuttering. It is similar to the Johnson and the Wischner notions in that stuttering is said to emerge from normal disfluency. The principal difference from these two, as well as from Sheehan's ideas, lies in their reliance only on observable behaviors and their consequences. There is no allowance for intermediating emotions, such as anxiety or guilt feelings that are prominent in the previous models. Thus, normal disfluencies, probably of physiological origins, are modified through complex interactions among four modes of behavioral learning: (1) positive reinforcement, (2) extinction (nonreinforcement), (3) punishment, and (4) negative reinforcement. Positive reinforcement is said to have taken place when introduction of a stimulus increases a response. Removal of positively reinforcing stimuli reduces the likelihood of the response (extinction). Punishment is said to have taken place when presentation of a stimulus decreases a response. Removal of punishing stimuli increases the likelihood of the response (negative reinforcement). Table 6.2 summarizes the four modes, or principles, of operant learning for purposes of behavior modification (conditioning).

For most children, disfluency is diminished through either extinction, being ignored by parents and others, or through verbal punishment, (e.g., "Stop it!"). In a smaller

Table 6.2	**Description of Various Forms of Behavioral Modification**	
Term	**Stimulus Manipulation**	**Behavioral Outcome**
Positive reinforcement	*Presented* after behavior	Increase
Extinction	*Withheld* after behavior	Decrease
Punishment	*Presented* after behavior	Decrease
Negative reinforcement	*Withheld/removed* after behavior	Increase

number of cases, children's disfluency may draw positive reinforcement if they attract attention of parents or others. When certain disfluency types increase in number, they are likely to be perceived as stuttering, drawing even more attention and being further reinforced.

According to this theory, stuttering persists when environmental consequences continue to reinforce it through multiple complex types and schedules of reinforcement, both positive and negative, punishing and extinguishing. Random reinforcement is particularly effective in shaping behavior that is difficult to extinguish. Also, once established, stuttering provides the child with secondary gains, such as being excused from being called on to recite in class. These add to the mix of reinforcements that shape the behavioral response.

Weaknesses: Although this model of stuttering is powerful in terms of explaining various dynamics of stuttering, especially the triggering of stuttering by neutral stimulus cues, it, too, fails the criterion of being exhaustive in explaining various ameliorating conditions. The precise stimulus-response factors critical to stuttering dynamics have never been uncovered. Also, the model does not explain why stuttering only rarely begins at ages other than childhood.

Clinical Implications: Shames and Sherrick supported behavior modification techniques that employ reinforcement of desired fluent speech and extinction, as well as nonreinforcement of stuttering. In fact, several operant conditioning therapy programs have been developed (e.g., Costello, 1980; Ryan, 2001b). For example, therapy may begin with systematic positive reinforcement of single words uttered fluently, gradually progressing to reinforcement of longer speech segments. Some form of operant conditioning principles can be seen in many therapy programs.

Two-Factor Theory of Stuttering

An outgrowth of behavioral learning was made by Brutten and Shoemaker (1967), who posited that both classical and operant (instrumental) conditioning play major roles in the disorder. This double-pronged approach was motivated by studies that showed conflicting behaviors: Whereas some stuttering behaviors increased when penalized, others decreased. That stuttering could decrease under stimuli regarded as unpleasant negated a widely accepted assumption at the time that predicted it to increase. It also created a challenge concerning the choice of conditioning techniques for therapy. To consolidate the behavior variability and the contradictions, Brutten and Shoemaker suggested that stuttering comprises at least two distinct behavioral phenomena: (1) core stuttering features (prolongations and repetitions) that result from anxiety acquired through classical conditioning, and (2) secondary stuttering characteristics learned via instrumental conditioning. These two processes comprise their "two-factor theory."

Stuttering begins when a child undergoes strong anxieties that naturally result in motor instability, including speech fluency disintegration. This assumption appears reasonable given that many people experience difficulty performing even simple motor tasks, such as sticking a key in the car door lock, when upset or frightened. Next, strong anxiety is paired (conditioned) with many stimuli and situations (e.g., different people), all becoming capable of triggering anxiety that induces stuttering-type fluency failures. A parallel instrumental learning takes place when the person who stutters attempts to cope with in-progress stutter events (to get the word out) or prevent anticipated stuttering. These attempts involve secondary characteristics, such as swaying of the head or arms. When successful, they are strongly reinforced as well.

Weaknesses: Like its predecessors, the theory fails to be exhaustive. It is not clear why some individuals develop a stuttering problem related to experiencing negative emotion whereas other individuals do not. It does not explain why stuttering is a disorder primarily of early childhood, especially because most onsets of stuttering do not appear to be associated with indications of anxiety. Its premises conflict with evidence that the "classically conditioned" disfluency types can be decreased when time-out periods are delivered as their consequence (e.g., James, 1981). Moreover, other phenomena, such as the consistency of stuttering loci (see Chapter 4), suggest that other factors besides negative emotion and conditioned associations contribute to fluency failure.

Clinical Implications: The fears and anxieties that prompted initial disintegration of fluency must be lessened through therapy that addresses emotions and attitudes. Hence, a logical result of the theory has been the application of the technique known as systematic desensitization. As will be detailed in a later chapter, this is done by having the client imagine going through a hierarchy of anxiety-provoking situations, learning to reduce the anxiety. Finally, the stuttering behavior itself is decreased through extinction (removal of reinforcers) and positive reinforcement of desired behaviors.

The Anticipatory-Struggle Hypothesis

Yet another angle within the learning domain of stuttering theory is evident in Bloodstein's (1997) *anticipatory-struggle hypothesis.* The theory suggests that for some children, the complex, automatic, serially ordered motor activity required for speech is overwhelming, causing them to initiate it with excessive tension and fragmentation— stuttering. They are thus prone to experience failure and frustration when speech develops. Any kind of difficulty or pressure involving speech during childhood might lead to stuttering. For example, phonological and articulation problems could cause frustration when a child attempts to communicate but is not always understood. Out of that frustration, the child soon believes that speaking is difficult and learns to struggle when stuttering is anticipated. As supporting evidence, Bloodstein pointed to research that has shown stuttering can be eliminated for short periods by the power of suggestion, highlighting the impact of an individual's beliefs about stuttering on its perpetuation. Also, stuttering is governed by self-fulfilling prophecies, for example, words, sounds, or letters stuttered once and noticed by the speaker, are more likely to be stuttered again. Similarly, the longer a person must wait before talking, the speaker's anticipation grows stronger and stuttering becomes more likely.

Weaknesses: Like the previous theories, the *anticipatory-struggle hypothesis* fails to account exhaustively for ameliorating conditions (e.g., rhythm and singing). It is also not clear how its concepts should be tested. Even if it were determined that "speech is hard" for children, why do they develop a debilitating belief about speech difficulty instead of displaying symptoms (as some children do) of more frequent phonological, semantic, or syntactic errors without stuttering? Although the hypothesis aptly describes the nature of stuttering in its advanced form, it is less clear that it fits stuttering close to onset. Children are less accurate than adults at predicting their stuttering; about half predict less than 50% (Avari & Bloodstein, 1974). In our experience, some young children do not display either anxiety or tension when stuttering begins. Also, a number of adults have reported feeling perfectly relaxed yet still stuttering. The model further does not fully explain why or how there is a shift from a "speech is difficult" belief into an overwhelming experience of a "block" that entirely prevents speech from happening.

Clinical Implications: If people who stutter could forget that they stutter, they would have "no further difficulty with speech" (Bloodstein, 1997, p. 170). Similarly, parents can best support recovery in their children by preventing the belief that talking is difficult. They need to inspire the child's confidence in his or her speaking abilities. Adults should be encouraged to take any steps that could change their self-image as a speaker. For example, an adult could join the Toastmasters organization to become knowledgeable and proficient at giving speeches, thereby substantially altering his beliefs about the difficulty of speaking.

The Demands-Capacities Model

Included among the psychobehavioral theories is the *demands-capacities model* of stuttering (Adams, 1990; Starkweather & Gottwald, 1990). Although some researchers have also considered it a multifactorial model, it is primarily a theory of behavioral responses or capacities in relation to stimulus demands. In simple terms, stuttering arises when a child attempts speech performance beyond his or her abilities. Adequate capacities, especially in four domains (cognitive, linguistic, motor, emotional maturity) are needed to withstand corresponding environmental demands and still produce fluent speech. No deficits are implied in this model; if the conditions exist in which demands (e.g., expectations to use new and complex language structures) exceed capacities, fluency can be expected to fail.

A high level of multitasking is required by the stay-at-home mother of a toddler. Within the same 10 minutes, Mom may need to juggle such activities as preparing a cake for a party, cleaning dishes, adding softener to the laundry, keeping the baby out of the garbage can, answering the phone, and so on. As the number of demands increases, and she reaches the limits of her capacities to give each task the time and attention it requires, there is a greater likelihood of a mishap (e.g., an egg dropped on the floor). Mom's weakened performance is not due to any inadequacy on her part. The multiple demands simply overloaded her attentional capacities. In a similar manner, the demands-capacities model proposes that various demands of communication (e.g., figuring out which words to say, selecting the desired intonation, time pressure to say it quickly, etc.) can overwhelm the child's speech system—and disfluent events occur as the result.

As evidence for the *demands-capacities model,* nearly all speakers find that speech fluency tends to break down in highly demanding situations, such as speaking publicly, conveying complicated concepts, reciting tongue twisters, and feeling threatened for accountability. With respect to children who stutter, this model accommodates well the research findings that many who persist remain above average in language skills (Watkins, 2005; Watkins & Yairi, 1997). Cyclical patterns of stuttering during the early developmental period also can be explained by this model. If the rate of various developing capacities does not keep pace meeting the demands, greater disfluency ensues. As capacities meet or surpass demands, fluent speech is recovered once again.

Weaknesses: In terms of the limitations, the theory does not fit the facts on all accounts because there are occasions when some children stutter in what appear to be low-demand situations. On the flip side, this model does not explain why sometimes high-demand situations do not result in moments of stuttering. For example, some people who stutter can be very fluent when speaking to large audiences.

Clinical Implications: The theory stresses the importance of addressing any imbalances among demands and capacities, and especially working with parents to alter environmental demands on children's speech performance (Starkweather & Givens-Ackerman, 1997). A thorough assessment of a child's linguistic, motor, cognitive, and social skills could serve as the starting point to identify the potential areas needing compensatory adjustments. Subsequent observation of the child in various settings would reveal behavioral and environmental demands to be adjusted as well. Cooperation among clinicians, parents, teachers, as well as the child, would be important to implementing adjustments.

Summary of Psychobehavioral Theories

Psychobehavioral theories view stuttering not as what a person is, or what is wrong with him or her, but as a behavior that can be acquired by means of various and complex processes under various conditions. The review of a range of theories has demonstrated this point. In principle, the learning point of view assumes that just about everyone may acquire stuttering given the proper circumstances. Once acquired, many stimuli can trigger stuttered speech that may be reinforced and modified by its consequences, either internal (e.g., anxiety reduction) or external (listener's reactions). Quite different in orientation from psychoemotional theories, psychobehavioral theories offer considerable insight into the dynamics of stuttering moments, but the reasons for initial onset are often obscure. These theories are concerned with observable phenomena, however, and therefore lend themselves more readily to scientific experimentation. From a clinical viewpoint, they have supported several general therapy approaches and specific programs, and are by nature optimistic because, supposedly, whatever is learned can be unlearned.

Psycholinguistic Theories

Psycholinguistics is the study of the psychological processes (*psycho-*) underlying language use (*-linguistic*). A speaker can sometimes be disfluent in the process of correcting an error in selection of word stress. For example, after uttering a syllable repetition of "re-re-re-relative," a normally fluent speaker was retrospectively aware that during the "re-re-re," the word *related* (with second syllable stress) was just under the surface, ready to come out by mistake, until finally the intended stress pattern for *relative* (first syllable stress) was ready and produced for the intended word. This is an example of a disfluency resulting from a failed psycholinguistic process. A number of researchers have proposed that the occurrence of some stuttered speech may result from subtle aberrancies or deficiencies in the underlying psychological processes responsible for transforming selected words into integrated patterns of segmental (phonemic) and suprasegmental (voice inflection) speech gestures. Theories that explain stuttering in terms of these dynamics are considered *psycholinguistic* theories.

We must clarify what the psycholinguistic domain *is* in contrast to what it *is not*. Psycholinguistic processes are primarily responsible for the retrieval and assembly of language elements. A "disorder of phonology" or "a disorder of language," however, does not necessarily imply a disorder of retrieval and assembly. They do imply impaired knowledge of the elements and/or rules governing the use of phonemes, or limited vocabulary to convey meaning. A child may adopt an erroneous set of phonemes (deficient in number or features in his or her language) or apply unusual rules for their combination. Still, the child may have no trouble using that set of deficient phonemes in the way they intend, although it is difficult for listeners to understand. Likewise, a child may lack vocabulary (lexical) items or generate unique words or word combinations that are erroneous in the target language but still select and order these words as intended and in a timely fashion. Psycholinguistic theories of stuttering do *not* propose that people who stutter are lacking in their knowledge of the phonology or vocabulary of their language. What they do propose is that the processes or systems responsible for the retrieval and integration of those elements are failing to operate smoothly.

A psycholinguistic theory might assert that stuttering is a "disorder of phonological *encoding*." Encoding refers to the subconscious cognitive activity of generating the elements of the code. Therefore a *phonological encoding disorder* refers to an impairment of a system or process responsible for the timely and precise retrieval of phonological elements, primarily phonemes. As an analogy, imagine a manufacturing plant. The parts (phonemes) are available in their storage area, and even the procedures (phonological rules) for putting the parts together are established, but the manufacturer's mechanical systems for the assembly of the parts into a product are malfunctioning and/or breaking down, resulting in a faulty product. Similarly, a *disorder of lexical (word) encoding* indicates that the speaker, even if he or she has an ample vocabulary (lexicon) and well-developed morphosyntactic knowledge, has a problem, or weak mechanism, within the systems responsible to retrieve and assemble those words into an utterance. The distinction between systems responsible for psycholinguistic processing versus those responsible for knowledge of the linguistic elements is an important one because they may break down independently. A speaker can have problems with the cognitive systems that handle the assembly of the language regardless of sufficient knowledge related to the phoneme or word elements and rules for combining those elements for the language itself.

Psycholinguistic Processes Resulting in Fluent Speech

Before examining psycholinguistic theories of stuttering, it is important to consider a model of the processes underlying normally fluent speech production. Based on experimental research, Levelt (1989) proposed that the processes for generating fluent speech consist of three major phases: conceptualization, formulation, and articulation. Each phase receives the by-product of the previous phase in sequential order. During conceptualization, the speaker conceives the message. In formulation, its grammatical and phonological representations are generated. Finally, in the articulation phase, the representations are transformed into motor programs that reach the peripheral speech musculature so that actions achieve the desired acoustic outcomes of speech. Figure 6.1 shows these phases in sequence.

The assembly of speech is handled during the formulation phase, which is further divided into two sequential subphases: grammatical encoding and phonological encoding. In grammatical encoding, the underlying semantic and syntactic representation is prepared; in phonological encoding, the syllable and sound (phoneme) specifications are made. Finally, when the idea, word selection, and structural form have been retrieved, then the movements of speech (e.g., articulation) can be generated and produced. If the speaker needs to hold up the initiation of articulation, for example, while chewing and swallowing food, then the retrieved thoughts and word forms can be held temporarily in a short-term memory storage (referred to as the buffer) until the vocal tract structures are available.

The psycholinguistic processes of speech production mostly take place without conscious awareness on the part of the speaker (Levelt, 1989). Retrieval of words, grammatical structures, intonational patterns, and phonemic elements are achieved with operations that are fully "automatic." The speaker does not have to devote attentional resources to these activities; therefore they occur in parallel without mutual interference. Even more important, they operate simultaneously with the actual act of speaking. Simultaneous psycholinguistic processes make it possible for articulation to follow conceptualization almost immediately. The implication of simultaneous speech-encoding processes that do not need conscious attention is that the latter parts of an utterance can be planned while the earlier parts are being articulated. The fact that early products of speech planning usually are immediately delivered while subsequent sections are being prepared is referred to as a "staged and feedforward" process (Howell, 2002; Levelt, Roelofs, & Meyer, 1999).

Figure 6.1   Model of Psycholinguistic Processes Underlying Speech

Psycholinguistic Factors in Stuttering

What do simultaneous word retrieval processes mean for stuttering? It has long been suspected that when someone stutters on a particular word, the word being uttered might not be the problem at all. It may be another word that is being retrieved simultaneously that has not even been uttered yet. Or the words being stuttered may also hold clues to underlying processes related to stuttering. Might the locations of stuttering within and/or between words in connected speech tell us something about its nature? There are still many questions to answer regarding the relationship of stuttering to psycholinguistic processes. Why are people who stutter unable to move past the sound or syllable fragments to complete their utterances? When and how is the word assembly process breaking down? Several researchers have offered possible theories.

The Covert-Repair Hypothesis

One theoretical perspective that received considerable attention during the past two decades is the *covert-repair hypothesis*. This model explains stuttering as an outcome of hyperactive self-monitoring of inner speech (Postma & Kolk, 1993; Postma, Kolk, & Povel, 1991). An error in the centrally devised speech plan (e.g., in the phonetic plan) is detected subconsciously and because the speaker's system attempts correction before it reaches the surface, he or she stutters. Restated in another way, disfluencies occur when the speaker is late repairing errors in the phonological system that arise during their formulation. The term *covert* refers to things hidden or unseen, and the term *repair* refers to the speaker's attempt to correct the original formulation and replan the intended speech. An underlying assumption is that people who stutter may have some form of deficit with phonological encoding. At typical rates of speech, their process of generating the phonological elements does not keep up well. Alternatively, perhaps their tendency to talk too fast makes it difficult to correct errors in a timely fashion, leading to disfluencies (and the need for slower speech). Some supportive evidence takes several forms. First, stuttering appears to be a moment in which speech is held back. Second, most fluency breakdown appears to occur at points of transition between sounds within words. Third, people who stutter have been observed to be slower with silent reading (i.e., a "covert" process).

Weaknesses: The counterevidence for this theory has been noted in two ways. First, research (Postma & Kolk, 1992) shows that people who stutter do not make more speech errors than those who do not stutter, and second, a subgroup of children who stutter have no difficulty with complicated phonological sequences (Seery, Watkins, Ambrose et al., 2006). Also, phonologically difficult words, or words that followed them, did not draw more instances of stuttering than other words (Howell & Au-Yeung, 1995; Throneburg et al., 1994).

Clinical Implications: People who stutter should take more time (slow down) to initiate and do talking that would thereby permit time for their systems to plan the correct speech sounds. They may benefit by production practice of speech sound combinations to increase speed and accuracy. Young children would be expected to benefit from phonological awareness activities.

The nature of psycholinguistic processes is illustrated by "tip of the tongue" and "slip of the tongue" phenomena, common to all speakers. When a speaker has an idea (perhaps envisioning the flowers in the garden) but cannot find the right descriptive word, then the conceptualization stage was accomplished, but formulation failed. If the wrong grammatical form is selected, the result may be a *semantic* slip of the tongue, such as the error of saying "pansies" instead of "violets." Although conceptualization was accurate (envisioning the violets), the word-generating (formulation) process has failed at the grammatical encoding level. Similarly, phonological encoding can break down when a speaker knows the word he or she wants to say (grammatical content was retrieved) but has trouble finding the sound and syllable sequences for it. Partially successful phonological encoding may retrieve the initial sound (e.g., 'v') but not the rest of the sounds in the word. The speaker senses the word is near and expresses, "It is on the tip of my tongue." If phonological encoding fails, however, the error could result in a "slip of the tongue," such as saying "violence" for "violets."

The Fault Line Hypothesis

Wingate hypothesized that stuttering is a defect in the language production system, an indication of a lack of synchrony in the assembly of linguistic elements. He explained that stuttering occurs at the "fault line" of phonological formulation where initial consonant and vowel are joined. These elements are "unitized" by the generation of syllable stress. Thus stuttering represents a failure to merge the prosodic and phonologic aspects of speech (Perkins, Kent, & Curlee, 1991; Wingate, 1988). Wingate reasoned that because the specific sounds that are the loci of repetitions or hesitations are usually recognizable and appropriately articulated, the difficulty is not with the production of those sounds but with moving past the sound to the production of the next phonetic element. He conceptualized stuttering as a *phonetic transition defect* in which the speaker has trouble connecting the speech elements rather than with producing the elements themselves. This means that the difficulty is not with the articulatory act of speaking, but with psycholinguistic processes that must act to synchronize word assembly.

Wingate observed that the common element describing the loci of most stutter events is that they occur on stressed syllables. The linguistic factors associated with the loci of stuttering as described by Brown (1945): word length, initial sounds, content words, initial words, and so on—were explained as all sharing the common element of stress. He reasoned that the execution of stress is primarily a phonatory function requiring laryngeal adjustments for pitch and loudness. This inference, combined with the view of stuttering as a transition defect, led Wingate to conclude that stutterers have central processing sources of failure with the neurophysiological adjustments to produce stressed vowels.

Weaknesses: Even if stuttering occurs predominantly on stressed syllables, the fact remains that not all stressed syllables are stuttered. In some languages, such as Hebrew, the stress occurs on the last syllable of most words. In addition, in a variety of speaking conditions, stressed syllables are not stuttered at all (e.g., talking to one's self, etc.). Thus, it would appear there is more to stuttering than a phonatory transition defect for the execution of stressed syllables. It is also not clear that stressed syllables are the primary locus of stuttering in young children, and the course of stuttering development was not addressed directly by Wingate's theory. The correspondence of stuttering and early pro-sodic development warrants further research. Before children develop contrastive word stress in their multiword utterances, there appears to be a tendency to give each word emphasis (no contrast). Use of intonational contrasts appears to develop separately from durational contrasts (Patel & Brayton, 2009; Snow, 1994). Investigations are needed to explore whether stuttering onset (or significant increase in disfluent speech) coincides with some form of transition between stages of prosodic development.

Clinical Implications: These are similar to those of the previous psycholinguistic hypothesis. That is, people who stutter may benefit by speaking slower to allow the additional time needed for their linguistic assembly processes. Because stressed syllables are particularly vulnerable to stuttering, these locations may especially need a slower, easier approach. Finally, given the speaker's difficulty with phonatory transitions, another clinical target would be the management of voicing for speech.

The Neuropsycholinguistic Theory

The essence of Perkins et al.'s (1991) proposal is that stuttering results when the syllable framework is not ready at the same time as the speech sounds (segments). They assert that fluency is interrupted by asynchronies between the arrival of syllable frames and segmental fillers and that time pressure to continue the attempt to speak ultimately precipitates the stutter event. The concepts of syllable frames and segmental fillers are explained in a box at the end of this section. Basic to their neuropsycholinguistic theory of stuttering is the understanding that speech is planned hierarchically as well as sequentially. Sequentially, speech sounds must be ordered within words, and words must be ordered within sentences. Hierarchically, however, the initial sound (onset) and final vowel-consonant ending unit (coda) must be inserted within the syllables, and syllables must be inserted within the intonational phrase. When the various compo-nents of the speech plan, both sequential and hierarchical, are being generated, they must all be ready at the necessary time for speech to move forward smoothly. If the syllable frames are ready, and the onset retrieved, a speaker may initiate talking under time pressure even if the coda or pattern of the rest of the intonational phrase has not been resolved. When the rest of the pattern is not forthcoming, the asynchrony in the delivery of the syllable components for production is evidenced as stuttering. Stuttering is the speaker's time- and place-holding activity until all of the speech components are properly arranged and ready for final execution.

Weaknesses: Although this hypothesis offers a suitably complex account for why speech breaks down in the form of disfluency, it does not offer any further insight into why children are prone to this breakdown rather than adults. Moreover, it has offered little insight into why the conditions such as singing, delayed auditory feedback (DAF), choral reading (unison), and so on, facilitate the synchronization of these components.

   Clinical Implications: Like the other psycholinguistic theories, the present one also offers a model that suggests people who stutter should approach speech more slowly. They must develop resistance to time pressures. In addition, the speaker should self-monitor the moments of speech difficulty so that these may be met with an easing strategy to counter the tendency to press onward forcefully.

The way freight trains are loaded may help to illustrate the concepts of syllable frames and sound fillers central to the neuropsycholinguistic theory of stuttering. As train cars are moved along the track, the freight must be loaded into each car. Each car must wait for its freight before it can move forward and let the next car be filled. In speech, each syllable is like a train car that must be loaded with the sound segments, like the freight. If the freight (sounds) arrives before the train car (syllable) arrives, then the freight (sounds) may spill out (and repeat). Alternatively, if the train cars (syllables) move forward, but the freight (sounds) are not ready, then the position of the car may be fixed (and be prolonged) waiting for the sounds to arrive.

Related Areas of Research

Stuttering Loci

In Chapter 4 we explained that the loci of stuttering coincide with specific elements and structures of spoken language. The more factors may congregate in a single word (e.g., unfamiliar, longer, content word, etc.), the higher its chance to be stuttered. These loci have led to the question of whether there are significant links between stuttering and language. Are these loci special for stuttering? Evidence suggests that stuttering locations may merely reflect the nature of underlying psycholinguistic processes in general, rather than the specific nature of stuttering. Research shows that these loci are vulnerable locations of disruption for all speakers, whether they stutter or not. The initial sounds of words often attract stutter events, but these same locations also attract slips of the tongue by all speakers. When speech sound transpositions occur, they are most often on the initial sounds of words (MacKay, 1970). For example, a common form of speech error occurs if a speaker says "fog dude" for "dog food," switching the initial sounds of the words. It would be highly unusual, however, for a speaker to switch the final sounds of the words to produce the error "fod doog." Interesting in this respect is the fact that stuttering rarely occurs on the last sounds or syllables of words.

Conditions of Psycholinguistic Interference

The multilevel parallel system of speech planning and production raises questions as to how each subsystem can be protected from interfering influences by other parts of the system. Bosshardt (2002) examined the effect of concurrent psycholinguistic processing activities on the speech of adults who stuttered and normally fluent individuals. The experiment consisted of the primary task of repeating words continuously and secondary tasks, either silent reading or word memorization, to be accomplished simultaneously.

In addition, two conditions related to phonemic content were compared. In one, the phonemic content of words was similar between the primary and secondary tasks. In the second, the phonemic content was dissimilar. Speech fluency analysis revealed that those who stutter were significantly more disfluent when similar words were read or memorized concurrently with the word repetition task than when dissimilar words were involved. By contrast, there was no significant difference in disfluency between these stimulus conditions for those who do not stutter. Bosshardt concluded that people who stutter are more sensitive to interference from concurrent cognitive processing tasks compared to people who do not stutter and that their phonological and articulatory systems are not efficiently protected from interference by attention-demanding processes. Thus, when a person who stutters encounters challenging phonological patterns, the weight of these demands would be expected to interfere with speech fluency. This raises the question of whether the phonological systems of individuals who stutter are more error prone than for people who do not stutter.

Stuttering and Phonologic Complexity

The notion that stuttering is linked to speech sound production has been around for many years. When Johnson and Brown (1935) analyzed several hundred thousand words spoken by adults who stuttered, they found that certain sounds (e.g., /d, z, g/) were the most frequently stuttered. Shortly after, Fairbanks (1937) showed that the frequency of stuttering on those sounds was positively related to their developmental difficulties in young children, and offered that the occurrence of stuttering is determined by physiological factors involved in sound production. Decades later, Postma and Kolk (1993) shifted the theoretical focus from peripheral difficulties to central speech sound planning. Whether true for adults and whether peripheral or central, an important question here is whether the covert articulation or phonological deficiencies are present at the time of stuttering onset or shortly thereafter.

Throneburg et al. (1994) studied children who stuttered at ages 29 to 59 months, selected to represent four conditions: severe stuttering/good phonology, severe stuttering/poor phonology, mild stuttering/good phonology, and mild stuttering/poor phonology. Words were classified according to seven possible types of phonological difficulty: consonant clusters, multiple syllables, late-developing sounds, and the four possible combinations of these three. Words that were not phonologically difficult (i.e., none of those just listed) constituted an eighth category.

A conversational speech sample with approximately 1,000 words was recorded for each child near stuttering onset, and the frequencies of words in the eight categories were analyzed. Also, stuttered words were identified, and the proportion of these in each of the eight categories was determined. Results showed that the largest proportion of stuttered words (about 50%) used by each of the four groups of children were "not phonologically difficult." That is, they fit none of the seven categories of phonological difficulty. The proportion of stuttered words among each of the seven categories of difficulty was small, and no category was more prevalent than any of the rest for any of the four participant groups. The investigators concluded that phonological difficulty was not associated with the locations of stuttering in young children. More specifically, the phonologic difficulty (complexity) of a word does not predict the occurrence of fluency breakdown regardless of a child's stuttering severity or phonologic ability. An almost identical conclusion was reached by Howell and Au-Yeung (1995).

Although phonologic ability level does not appear to predict the coincidence of stutter events with phonologically difficult words, the Throneburg et al. (1994) investigation did not address whether stuttering tends to coincide with phonological errors irrespective of word difficulty. A later investigation by Wolk et al. (2000) analyzed the frequency of simultaneous disfluency and phonological errors in 4- to 5-year-olds, with coexisting stuttering and phonological disorders. The overall analysis revealed that the occurrence of stuttering was not more frequent on syllables with phonological errors than on syllables without phonological errors. There was, however, a significantly higher stuttering frequency on word-initial consonant clusters with phonological errors than on word-initial consonant clusters without phonological errors. These results suggest most stuttering is not associated with phonological production demands, but some stuttering is.

Priming of Linguistic Structures

Priming studies are another means of exploring whether stuttering is a symptom of failed phonological encoding processes. In an auditory priming paradigm, the participant is presented with an auditory stimulus, such as a word that sounds like the name of the picture they will see, prior to being shown the picture to be named. The experimenter can then examine whether primed conditions yield faster or slower response latencies and thereby assess the function of psycholinguistic processes.

Using this paradigm, Byrd et al. (2007) compared picture-naming performance between young children who stutter and normally fluent children. Three auditory priming conditions were created to test neutral, holistic, and incremental phonological encoding processes. For example, if the target word was *book,* a neutral prime might have sounded like "d," a holistic prime would have sounded like "ook," and an incremental prime would have sounded like "b." The children's speech reaction times (response latencies) were measured from the onset of picture presentation to the onset of participant response. The investigators observed that as NFC grew older from 3 to 5 years of age, there was a shift from being significantly faster in the holistic priming condition to being significantly faster in the incremental priming condition. By contrast, the majority of both 3- and 5-year-old CWS exhibited faster reaction times in the holistic than the incremental condition. It was inferred that children who stutter tend to be delayed in making the developmental shift in phonological encoding from holistic to incremental processing, and that such a delay may contribute to their difficulties generating fluent speech.

Summary of Psycholinguistic Theories

Psycholinguistic theories of stuttering are not concerned with environmental factors or emotional responses. Unlike motoric perspectives of stuttering (see Chapter 7) that emphasize dynamics of speech execution, psycholinguistic viewpoints shift the focus to central cognitive processes involved in the planning of speech. Psycholinguistic theories provide us with insight into the nature of disfluent speech, but they generally do not offer the breadth of explanation necessary to understand the full picture of stuttering etiology and onset. They also have fallen short of accounting for all the phenomena related to stuttering (e.g., ameliorating conditions). They do help to account for the various loci of stuttering and illuminate the associations of speech and language assembly processes and stuttering.

Summary

Is it possible that psychoemotional, psychobehavioral, and psycholinguistic factors all contribute to stuttering? The answer is undoubtedly "yes." Familiarity with them enhances clinicians' insight into their therapeutic regimens. These classes of theories substantially influence clinical management with rationale for reducing anxiety and the power of stimulus cues that trigger stuttering. They also reinforce the old intuitive advice given to people who stutter to slow down their speech. There were several points raised in this chapter:

- Theories that present emotional/personality problems as the cause of stuttering have not received research support. There is no evidence that people who stutter, as a group, especially young children, are emotionally maladjusted.
- Although stuttering does not originate from some form of deep psychoemotional disturbance, it remains possible that temperament has a role in the persistence of stuttering and the person's handling of the problems it presents.
- Stuttering and anxiety are related; however, more evidence suggests that stuttering leads to anxiety rather than the other way around.
- The diagnosogenic theory, placing the blame for stuttering on parents' behavior, has lost credibility.
- Regarding other psychobehavioral contributions, research has demonstrated that the frequency of stuttering can be manipulated by delivery of contingent reinforcements. This fact alone is not sufficient to prove that stuttering is a learned behavior, but it does imply that, once stuttering begins, environmental factors influence it, at least by triggering moments of stuttering.
- Psycholinguistic theories of stuttering support the hypothesis that speech fluency may be interrupted by processes that govern the assembly of sounds and words into connected speech, but future research is needed to reveal the exact nature of their role in the occurrence of stuttering.

Study Questions and Discussion Topics

1. Paradoxically, stuttering has been described as both tension-provoking and tension-reducing. Compare and contrast the psychoemotional versus psychobehavioral views of this paradox.

2. Provide a psychobehavioral explanation for the acquisition of secondary behaviors of stuttering.
3. Describe the tendency for a person to stutter on his or her own name from a classical conditioning perspective. Is this psychobehavioral view sufficient, or might psychoemotional factors play a role in this tendency? Explain.
4. How would the persistence versus recovery of stuttering be explained in terms of operant conditioning? Is this view of stuttering progression sufficient? If not, what facts regarding recovery and persistence of stuttering are *not* explained by psychobehavioral dynamics?
5. A child is heard to stutter on the initial word *Mommy* of a multiword utterance. Is it appropriate to conclude that the word *Mommy* is difficult for the child to say? Why or why not? Offer an explanation for this location of fluency breakdown based on psycholinguistic processes underlying speech production.

Suggested Readings

Bernstein Ratner, N. (1997a). Stuttering: A psycholinguistic perspective. In R. Curlee & G. Siegel (Eds.), *Nature and treatment of stuttering* (2nd ed., pp. 99–127). Boston, MA: Allyn & Bacon.

Costello, J. (1980). Operant conditioning and the treatment of stuttering. In W. H. Perkins (Ed.), Strategies in stuttering therapy. In J. L. Northern (Series Ed.), *Seminars in speech, language, and hearing.* New York, NY: Thieme-Stratton.

Ezrati-Vinacour, R., & Levin, I. (2004). The relationship between anxiety and stuttering: A multidimensional approach. *Journal of Fluency Disorders, 29*(2), 135–148.

Koedoot, C., Bouwmans, C., Franken, M-C., & Stolk, E. (2011). Quality of life in adults who stutter. *Journal of Communication Disorders, 44,* 429–443.

Chapter 7

Is Stuttering Biological? Theories and Investigations

LEARNER OBJECTIVES

Readers of this chapter will be familiar with:

- Evidence related to genetic bases of stuttering.
- Theories and research concerning the association between stuttering and brain anatomy and physiology.
- Theories and research concerning the association between stuttering and motor dysfunction.
- Theories and research concerning the association between stuttering and auditory processes.
- Multidimensional theories and models of stuttering.

Introduction

During the 18th century, it was suggested that an abnormally large tongue causes stuttering by interfering with its mobility and proper positioning. This is a prime example of a belief in an anatomical basis for stuttering. Another idea circulating many years ago was that the tongue of a person who stutters is too weak, incapable of moving sufficiently fast or far enough in the oral cavity. This is an example of a belief in an abnormal function, or physiological basis, for stuttering. Might stuttering have biological bases, such as physical and/or physiological abnormalities (e.g., a thick tongue or a shallow breathing pattern)? Is stuttering the symptom of an underlying neurophysiological impairment? Is stuttering caused by a structural abnormality? Is there a genetic basis for it? These are the types of questions that have led to several so-called *organic* theories of stuttering. Scientists have speculated that stuttering could be the result of a variety of physically based limitations, such as inadequate neural structure and organization, deficient capacities to regulate speech timing, weak sensorimotor integration for speech targets, and impaired self-monitoring processes. Again, could stuttering be related to any or all of these conditions? Familiarity with past and current theories of stuttering, as well as with research findings, provides clinicians with the underlying rationale for various therapeutic approaches and equips them to answer questions raised by apprehensive parents of young children who stutter, as well as inquisitive older children and adults who stutter.

It seems reasonable to hypothesize that at least some cases of stuttering may have a neurophysiological basis. Neurophysiology refers to the function of the nervous system. Perhaps the most apparent signs are the hypertonicity associated with stuttered speech (often affecting the entire body), some uncontrolled movements, respiratory irregularities such as gasping, and tremors associated with stuttering events (see Chapter 4 for a review of secondary characteristics). Observing these, West (1958) wrote that "if a specialist in convulsive disorders, without any previous experience with, or knowledge of stuttering, came upon a stutterer, he might at once label the disorder a seizure" (p. 175). In fact, he hypothesized that "stuttering is primarily an epileptic disorder that manifests itself in dyssynergies of neuromotor mechanism for oral language" (p. 197).

A second phenomenon that prompts the idea of a neurophysiological component to stuttering is the variety of stuttering characteristics witnessed as a result of neurological damage secondary to strokes, head injuries, and so on (e.g., De Nil et al., 2007). In a number of these patients, the stuttering symptoms ceased with natural recovery or after medical treatment for the neurological lesions. Third, the vulnerability for stuttering of certain groups, such as males, identical twins, and families with stuttering histories, suggests a genetic component to stuttering. Fourth, the remarkable way in which stuttering subsides under conditions of altered phonation (e.g., unison singing, whispering) or alterations in auditory feedback (e.g., loud noise, delayed auditory feedback [DAF]) suggests the possibility of underlying failed neurobiological systems. Finally, when the stuttering of some individuals is particularly chronic and unyielding, even to conditions that often ameliorate stuttering, such symptomatology is more consistent with what could be expected from a physically based disorder.

An important question in regard to the preceding is: What evidence would be needed to establish a physically based stuttering disorder? In Chapter 5, we pointed out several challenges to be addressed by research in order to identify potential physical bases for stuttering. It was suggested that evidence should be found in children who stutter close to the onset of stuttering. If research only examines evidence in adult populations, the physical conditions could have developed secondary to stuttering, perhaps as a response to the disorder over many years. These conditions may not be the cause but rather the result of stuttering. Also, organically oriented theories must account for why the stuttering symptoms generally are not constant but so highly variable.

Another question is relevant to clinical implications: What would it mean to intervention approaches if stuttering was caused by some deficiency in the individual's physical constitution? One obvious conclusion would be that our interventions and expectations of clients' progress must be altered accordingly. On one hand, psychological and behavioral approaches to modification would have to be understood as compensatory rather than remedial measures. On the other hand, efforts to discover/develop medical treatments (drugs, electrical stimulation, surgeries, etc.) would probably receive greater attention.

Genetic Perspectives

Although the idea of multiple etiologies of stuttering has been frequently expressed in the literature, so far not a single cause of developmental stuttering has been unequivocally identified. One thing we know with increasing certainty, whatever the cause of stuttering, it is in large part genetically transmitted. This may involve structural brain features, functional brain features, motor abnormality, personality or temperament characteristics, or others. But which one (or ones) is still unknown. Furthermore, a particular characteristic that increases the susceptibility for stuttering may not, by itself, cause the stuttering. But, when it co-occurs with certain other characteristics, stuttering may be expressed. It is possible, then, that something is inherited that only under certain conditions causes stuttering. It is interesting to note that quite frequently a child with a nonstuttering parent inherits stuttering from a grandfather who stutters. Is it possible that the parent carries certain traits conducive to stuttering that are not overtly expressed in him/her? (See data/discussion in Subramanian & Yairi, 2006.)

To be sure, genetics may be relevant to various theories of stuttering so that when some time in the future we know what is being transmitted, a particular theory will receive strong support, even confirmation. Nevertheless, the body of data that supports genetic transmission of stuttering, and the models that depict the kind of transmission, should not be construed as a theory of stuttering because it does not attempt to suggest the cause of stuttering, the dynamics of stuttered speech, or rules that govern stuttering. It is likely, however, that when more specific information about genes underlying stuttering becomes available, it will influence theories of stuttering. Evidence for genetic factors for stuttering from different types of data is briefly described next.

Familial Incidence

For many years, clinicians working with children and adults who stutter have noticed that the disorder runs in families. One of the authors (Yairi) has had an extensive familial history of stuttering on the paternal side, including his grandfather, father, two uncles, one aunt, a cousin, a brother, a son, and a grandson. A letter from a father of a child who began stuttering reflects this common situation. It also suggests the possibility that, at times, stuttering may be linked with other inherited conditions and disorders.

> I have read several articles you've authored and beg your indulgence on behalf of my 3 1/2-year-old son. He suddenly began stuttering a few weeks ago. . . . There is a strong history of both motor and vocal tics in my family. I have three children. My oldest daughter, 9, was diagnosed with Tourette's syndrome[1] at age 6. She still has excessive eye blinking (more like eye squinching). My second daughter, now 7, has a throat-clearing tic and some obvious OCD[2]-type behaviors and sensitivity issues, mostly related to food and eating. And, of course, I am writing you regarding my youngest, our son, who has recently developed a severe stutter.

---

[1] It is regarded as a genetically inherited disorder with onset in childhood, characterized by the presence of multiple motor tics. These include facial movements, eye blinking, throat clearing, and/or sniffing. Tics of the vocal folds result in uncontrolled random phonation. Some exhibit tics as well as characteristics of other conditions, such as obsessions, compulsions.

[2] OCD refers to obsessive-compulsive disorder.

Moving up the family tree, I have four siblings and we ALL have various motor and vocal tics, though none of us were ever diagnosed with Tourette's, autism, ADHD, ADD, OCD, etc. However, we're all aware that we're "different." We're all functioning, well-adjusted adults (for the most part), and most would say, I think, that we're "normal"; but we know better. I, too, struggled with a stutter as an adolescent, but seem to have developed sufficient compensatory mechanisms to have buried the issue—until my son started stuttering! Now, my own stuttering seems to be returning—and I'm 45.

Still further up the tree, my father was diagnosed, at age 7, with Sydenham's chorea in 19XX. He had a neck and eye twitch, which he recalls as being stress-related. A year off from school seemed to have "cured" him, though he still displays several vocal tics. Tourette's syndrome didn't come to be called such until the 1970s, I believe. Dad is now 70 and recently retired after a successful business career. He had two brothers, at least one of which had many motor and vocal tics—deep knee bends, throat clearing, and foot shaking. . . . That individual, my late uncle, had two daughters (now middle-aged) who freely engage in laughter with me and my siblings, all being first cousins, about how strange it is that we all have such strikingly similar behaviors, especially that we did not all grow up together. We'd all be open to participating in a three-generation genetic study. The genetics are remarkable to all of us, especially from my wife's perspective [because she] sees most of this much more clearly than even we do.

Clinicians' observations have been substantiated in a good number of studies. One of the first surveys found that 46% of the probands who stuttered (in the genetic literature, the person whose relatives are surveyed is referred to as the *proband*) had a family history of stuttering compared with only 18% in probands who did not stutter (Bryngelson & Rutherford, 1937). A review of 28 studies concluded that the majority of them yielded familial stuttering in 30% to 60% of those who stutter as compared with less than 10% for families of normally fluent controls (Yairi, Ambrose, & Cox, 1996). In their own research, these investigators found 71% of stuttering children had stuttering histories in the immediate (parents and siblings) or extended family. About 43% had stuttering in their immediate family only, and 28% had at least one parent with such history. This type of information, however, is insufficient to reach conclusions about the genetic nature of stuttering because it failed to take into account size of family and the specific familial class of the relatives who stuttered. For example, a person may report one stuttering relative in a family of only 4 members, whereas another person reports one relative who stutters in a family of 16. Or one person may report a father who stutters, whereas another person reports a second cousin who stutters. Still, the information provided a strong motive for better research approaches.

Twin Studies

Twin research compares the similarity, referred to as the *concordance,* of the two members of a pair of identical twins in relation to a particular trait such as stuttering. Identical twins develop from a single fertilized egg (which is why they are also called maternal or monozygotic twins) and, therefore, share 100% of their genes. Hence, close similarity for the trait is expected. The level of similarity is then compared to that of nonidentical (fraternal or dizygotic) twins, who develop from two fertilized eggs and therefore share only 50% of their genes like any non-twin siblings.

Clearly, the approach highlights the relative role of genetic versus environmental effects underlying the trait or behavior under study. Specific to our topic, the question is if one member of a twin pair stutters, does the second member stutter too? The answer tends to be positive. Several investigations reported a much higher concordance for stuttering in monozygotic than in dizygotic twins (Andrews, Morris-Yates, Howie et al., 1991; Godai, Tatarelli, & Bonanni, 1976). In one study (Howie, 1981), two thirds of identical twin pairs in whom stuttering was found, both members of a pair stuttered. If stuttering was purely genetic, then all pairs with one stutterer would have concordance. But in a third of identical twin pairs in which stuttering occurred in one member, the other member was not affected. Therefore, although the findings strengthened the evidence for genetic components to stuttering, they also indicated some environmental influences.

Refreshing the reader's familiarity with genetics, the nucleus of each living cell contains a DNA molecule. A *gene* is a section of a DNA molecule that serves as a recipe or code for various regulatory functions. Importantly, many sections provide codes for diverse proteins that serve as building blocks for various parts of the body. There are approximately 20,000 genes in a single DNA molecule. The DNA molecules are coiled up tightly into compact bundles with an X-shaped appearance called *chromosomes*. Human cells typically contain 46 chromosomes (pairs of 23 chromosomes). Certain chromosomes contain the genes that are responsible for such features as a person's gender, eye color, hair color, and so on. Monozygotic (identical) twins have the same DNA, while dizygotic (fraternal) twins have different DNA. Despite their identical DNA, some physical features of identical twins are not the same, for example fingerprints. Differences in the uterine environment experienced by each twin are believed to influence such characteristics.

Four additional twin studies carried out during the first decade of the current century continued to provide strong support for genetic factors to stuttering. Felsenfeld et al. (2000) surveyed 1,567 Australian pairs and 634 singles to identify those with stuttering history. They concluded that approximately 70% of the variance in liability to stuttering was attributable to genetic effects. In Japan, Ooki (2005) investigated 1,896 twin pairs. Concordance for stuttering in monozygotic pairs was 52% but only 12% in dizygotic pairs. Their estimate of the genetic contribution to stuttering was also high, at 80% to 85%. In the UK twin study conducted by Dworzynski et al. (2007), concordance rates were consistently higher for monozygotic than dizygotic twin pairs. Finally, a questionnaire-based study was conducted in the Netherlands with parents of 10,500 five-year old twins. Among pairs described by parents as "probable stuttering," concordance for stuttering was 57% in monozygotic versus 31% for dizygotic pairs (van Beijsterveldt, Felsenfeld, & Boomsma; 2010).

Family Aggregation

Unlike surveys of the percentage of people who stutter having familial history of stuttering, aggregation studies analyze the detailed distribution patterns of stuttering in familial pedigrees (trees), accounting for gender, family size, and degree of relatedness (e.g., first degree = siblings; second degree = cousins). The most important feature of these studies is that statistical methods, such as *segregation analysis,* allow investigators to determine the most likely mode of genetic transmission by matching the familial distributions of stuttering against several possible genetic models:

- No genetic components
- Multifactorial polygenic (MFP: environmental factors + many genes)
- Single major locus (SML: one or a few main genes are involved)
- Mixed (both MFP and SML components)

First to carry out an aggregation study were Kay and Garside in the United Kingdom. It was published as part of the Andrews and Harris (1964) report. They concluded that the familial distribution of stuttering had the best fit with a model that depicted a disorder controlled by a primary gene (SML) with contributions from other genes. Their data, however, also allowed for the possibility of a purely polygenic inheritance (MFP). Over the next several decades, other researchers proposed and tested genetic models to explain the transmission of stuttering as a family trait. Large-scale investigations at Yale University concluded that the data could fit any of three models: multifactorial polygenic, single major locus, and mixed (e.g., Cox, Kramer, & Kidd, 1984; Kidd, Heimbuch, & Records, 1981). Two later reports came from the University of Illinois Stuttering Research Program where all families were identified through young children shortly after stuttering onset. Their samples provided a considerably more complete representation of the population of people who stutter. This team was the first to report statistically significant evidence for both a single major locus and a polygenic transmission of stuttering (Ambrose, Yairi, & Cox, 1993). The finding is particularly encouraging because it should be easier to isolate one or several primary genes than to identify many genes. Major gene involvement was also found in a segregation analysis of 56 pedigrees of PWS performed by Viswanath, Lee, and Chakraborty (2004).

The Illinois team also compared the genetic bases of two subpopulations: children who recovered spontaneously from stuttering and those with persistent (chronic) stuttering. They concluded that the divergent pathways of these subgroups were related to differences in genetic factors. Specifically, both forms of stuttering share a common major gene (or genes), but persistent stuttering involves additional genes (Ambrose et al., 1997). In 2005 Yairi and Ambrose reinforced their earlier findings, reporting that whereas 88% of children who persisted had a positive familial history of stuttering, only 65% of children who recovered naturally had such a history. Nevertheless, the British twin study (Dworzynski et al., 2007) that included a focus on the phenomena of recovery/persistency (950 CWS recovered and 150 persisted) found no difference in the best-fitting genetic model for persistent versus recovered stuttering.

> Regardless of the research progress concerned with *how* stuttering is propagated, it is still unclear *what* is being transmitted genetically that contributes to the cause of stuttering. The "what" could be related to personality traits, speech motor skills, sensory feedback character-istics, neural timing properties, or other constitutionally based abilities or features impacting fluency. Because a combination of factors may interact to cause susceptibility, even nonstuttering family members can transmit genetic characteristics that could lead to the disorder. The good news is that if major genes are involved, there is a high chance of eventually locating them.

Biological Genetics

The strong evidence for major genetic components to stuttering accumulated through behavioral/statistical genetics, provided the necessary impetus for progressing into the next research sphere: biological genetics. That is, analyzing DNA materials to locate candidate genes that underlie the disorder. Typically, the first phase in such genotyping research is known as *linkage analysis*. It uses body materials, such as blood or saliva, to identify chromosomes, and the region(s) within each one of them, where genes under-lying a disorder (stuttering in our case) are located. It relies on DNA segments pre-viously identified for their chromosomal locations and genetic properties. These are called "markers" because they serve as points of reference. We know that genes that are physically close tend to be inherited together (they are said to be "linked"). It is assumed, therefore, that genes close to a marker will be co-inherited. Linkage analysis identifies DNA segments that are close to markers found to be inherited by family mem-bers who stutter but *not* by those who do not stutter. This, then, provides clues as to the possible locations of the target genes.

Early findings have been promising. Four linkage studies are listed in the upper part of Table 7.1 showing the chromosomes on which the strongest evidence for a candidate gene, or genes, underlying stuttering were found. The largest of these was conducted by the Illinois Stuttering Research Program, which extracted DNA from blood samples of 585 individuals (Suresh et al., 2006). In addition to the overall strongest support for the evidence as listed, they found the strongest linkage signal for males on chromo-some 13 and for females on chromosome 21. The latter one had the strongest signal. Additionally, their findings indicated the possibility that genes from three different chro-mosome combinations: numbers 2 and 9; 7 and 12; 7 and 18, may result in stuttering.

Advancing biological genetic research to the next stage, scientists have pursued techniques aimed at identifying specific genes underlying stuttering (see Kraft & Yairi, 2012, for a comprehensive review). Employing a technique known as *candidate gene analysis,* a team from China (Lan et al., 2009) relied on some reports that children who stutter tend to also suffer ADHD problems. Hence, they searched specific regions on

Table 7.1   Summary of Genotyping Studies of Stuttering

Linkage Studies		Chromosome with Most Significant Signal
*Shugart et al. (2004)		18
*Riaz et al. (2005)		12
**Suresh et al. (2006)		9
**Wittke-Thompson et al. (2007)		13
SPECIFIC GENE STUDIES	**GENES**	**CHROMOSOMAL LOCATION**
Lan et al. (2009)	DRD2	11
* Kang et al. (2010)	GNPTAB	12
**Kraft (2010)	N/A2	2
	PLXMNA4	7
	PCSK5	9
	CTNNA3; ADARB2	10
	FADS2	11
	ARNT2; FMN1	15
	EYA2; SLC24A	20
**Kraft, Cox, Evans et al. (2012)	11 genes	

* NIH team led by Dr. D. Drayna.
** University of Illinois/University of Chicago team led by Drs. N. Cox, N. Ambrose, and E. Yairi.

chromosome 5 and 11, looking for genes designated as SLC6A3 and DRD2, respectively, both associated with ADHD and involve dopamine control in the brain. Only one significant variation within the DRD2 gene was found in stutterers, supporting the notion that dopamine excess might be involved. We note, however, that the notion of high incidence of ADHD among people who stutter has been reported by only one study (Donaher & Richels, 2012).

More well-known is the NIH study (Kang et al., 2010) that focused on a single, highly inbred, Pakistani family. The team identified a mutation in gene GNPTAB (chromosome 12) in most of the family members who stuttered. The gene has a metabolic function. Additionally, mutations on a gene NAGPA (chromosome 12) were identified in six American-British persons who stuttered. These genes have certain functions in brain and body metabolism. Although Kang et al.'s findings were initially celebrated as the first discovered "stuttering genes," the study was severely criticized by several scholars. Among them, Kraft and Yairi (2012) noted that the study offers little information that can be generalized to the larger population of people who stutter.

Employing the method known as *genome-wide association study* (GWAS), Kraft (2010) analyzed DNA from 88 Americans and Europeans who stutter and from that of 107 controls. Her preliminary report indicated 10 genes significantly associated with persistent stuttering. Interestingly, eight are critical to many developmental or neurological functions related to speech production, and two others with behavioral functions. These genes and those identified in the studies cited above are listed in the lower part of Table 7.1. Lastly, using an even more sophisticated technique, *functional genome-wide association* (fGWAS), Kraft, Cox, Evans et al. (2012) extended the research just described. In a preliminary report, they identified an additional 12 genes that prompted the conclusion that the pathology underlying stuttering may involve zinc- and/or glucose-mitigated neurological functions. Findings of the last two studies, however, have not yet been published in peer-reviewed journals.

Summary of Genetic Perspectives

A growing body of evidence supports the existence of a genetic basis for stuttering. The incidence of stuttering among family members of those who stutter is significantly higher than among family members of those who do not. It is more likely for both members of an identical twin pair to stutter compared to both members of a fraternal twin pair. Family aggregation studies indicate there might be a single major locus for the genes underlying stuttering, and that a polygenic transmission could also be responsible. As we have gradually moved from the crude method of family incidence into the most advanced genotyping techniques, evidence for a strong genetics factor in stuttering has become unquestionable. Genotyping research has revealed chromosomes with the greatest linkage signal for stuttering and the most recent studies have pointed out (tentatively) several specific candidate genes. It is, however, too soon to declare that specific genes underlying stuttering in the population at large have been isolated. Nevertheless, it appears that scientists have come close to identifying such genes, perhaps even gaining some understanding of how some of them function. Still, there is a long way to go before we know what exactly is being transmitted, whether genetic differences are primarily affecting aspects of motor, linguistic, temperamental, or other factors in speech development. Because multiple genes appear to underlie stuttering, understanding of their complex interaction remains difficult. Undoubtedly, future research will reveal which factors are the major players and whether there are subtypes influenced by different sets of factors.

Current knowledge about genetics and stuttering is useful for diagnosis, prognosis, treatment, and counseling. For example, if a child who begins to stutter has a family history of persistent stuttering, it raises a red flag of a higher risk that he or she will follow the familial pattern of persistent stuttering. Alternatively, if the child has a family history of recovered stuttering, there is a much better chance for natural recovery. Inasmuch as there are several genetic pathways leading to stuttering, the prospect for improved future identification of subtypes is reinforced.

Neurological Perspectives

Insofar as genetics plays a major role in the causation of stuttering, one reasonable hypothesis is that responsible genes seed an atypical development of brain structure and function. Several points of evidence lend support to this idea. First, individuals with brain damage often exhibit fluency problems. Although overall their disfluent speech differs from that exhibited by people who stutter (Yairi, Gintautas, & Avent, 1981), some patients reveal remarkable similarity to developmental stuttering. Second, a growing number of studies report brain structure differences between people who stutter and normally fluent speakers (e.g., Chang, Erickson, Ambrose et al., 2008; Sommer, Koch, Paulus et al., 2002; Watkins, Smith, Davis et al., 2008). Third, other biophysiological differences in adults who stutter have been documented, such as atypical cerebral blood flow during speech and stuttering (Watson & Freeman, 1997). Fourth, brain activation patterns in adults who stutter are different from normal (Beal, Gracco, Lafaille et al., 2007; Brown, Ingham, Ingham et al., 2005). Fifth, reduced stuttering as a result of therapy is associated with changes in patterns of brain activity (e.g., De Nil, Kroll, Lafaille et al., 2003). It is not surprising, then, that theories proposing brain-related causes of stuttering would attract interest. Several are briefly reviewed here.

Cerebral Hemispheric Dominance

One of the earliest theories of stuttering published in the modern era of speech pathology upholds that it arises from an improper balance of control between the two cerebral hemispheres. A pioneer of 20th-century stuttering research, Lee Travis (1931) proposed that stuttering is caused by a *lack* of hemispheric dominance, more commonly referred to as the *cerebral dominance theory*. The theory rests on the nature of hemispheric innervations as relay centers of neural signals to the opposite (contralateral) side of the body. To accomplish simultaneous movement of both sides of the body working together toward a common goal (e.g., oral postures for speech), each brain hemisphere must participate in a carefully orchestrated set of neural signals. If the hemispheres operated independently, then there would be no predicting whether their signals to musculature on opposite sides would be coordinated. For example, both left and right *masseters*, muscles on the opposite sides of the face, must be activated concurrently to move the jaw up and down. Similarly, both sides of the tongue, a single muscle structure, must act together to change position from one vowel gesture to the next, across syllables.

The cerebral dominance theory assumes that to accomplish simultaneous movement, one brain hemisphere must take the lead in establishing the movement pattern while the other hemisphere follows to match it. But, according to the theory, the brains of people who stutter lack the necessary dominance. The result is an asynchrony (mistiming) of neural impulses from both sides of the brain being transmitted to the speech musculature, creating disruptions to the fluent execution of speech. In other words, overt stuttering events are the result of something akin to neurological blocks.

In its time, the cerebral dominance theory gained strength that was derived from a combination of facts. For one, hemispheric functions indeed exert contralateral control, being responsible for muscles on the opposite side of the body. Second, the notion of cerebral dominance and body-side preferences for various motor activities was recognized. And third, it was known that oral language expression in right-handed people, the majority of the population, arises mainly from left-hemisphere regions (Broca's and Wernicke's areas). It is not surprising, therefore, that the cerebral dominance theory attracted considerable attention and influence, even among the general public. Consequently, parents and schoolteachers were blamed for stuttering because they had shifted a child's handedness for writing, supposedly causing hemispheric conflict. Even at the time of writing this textbook, an elderly man who stuttered told one of us he was still inclined to believe what he had been told as a child, that he stuttered because his writing handedness had been switched in elementary school.

> To explain the lack of cerebral dominance for speech in people who stutter, it was suggested that they were naturally left-handed with a right-hemisphere dominance for speech. Their handedness, however, had been changed, perhaps through adult pressure to do so. The shift from left- to right-handedness led to an underused, weakened right hemisphere that was losing its dominance for the person's speech. The result: lack of cerebral dominance with confusion and conflict over which hemisphere should take the lead. Stuttering presumably occurred as the hemispheres struggled over which side should dominate control of the act of speech.

Early support for the theory came from several directions. For example, in a survey conducted by one of Travis's students, a majority of 13 children trained to change handedness developed stuttering within 1 year (Fagan, 1931). A number of studies measured electrical activity in the speech musculature using electromyography (EMG). One EMG investigation revealed that the action potentials from right and left masseter muscles, responsible for lower jaw movement, were unequal during stuttering, unlike those measured in fluent speakers (Travis, 1934). Several investigators used an electroencephalograph (EEG) to record cortical electrical activity. They found that the alpha brain waves during fluent speech of people who stutter were larger and slower than those of normal speakers during fluent speech (Travis & Knott, 1936; Travis & Malamud, 1937).

Interestingly, for a period Travis abandoned his brain-related theory, shifting his attention to psychoanalytical perspectives on the disorder (Travis, 1957). Some research activity concerned with brain function and structure of people who stutter continued at low levels for about 25 years before a new surge of interest emerged in the 1970s. Lee Travis (1978a, 1978b) himself contributed to promoting this renewed trend when he published two articles in which he asserted he had never disavowed the cerebral dominance theory. He summarized relevant research related to the Wada test,[3] auditory

---

[3]In the Wada test, sodium amobarbital is injected into one of the internal carotid arteries to temporarily shut down the function of the associated cerebral hemisphere for several minutes. This is done to evaluate the functions of the opposite hemisphere. The patient is asked to talk, respond to questions, engage in memory tasks, and so on. The test was named after Juhn Wada, the Japanese-Canadian neurologist who invented it.

evoked potentials, and dichotic listening studies in PWS and NFS, proposing that the resultant differences still supported interhemispheric problems.

Weaknesses: From the mid-1940s to the beginning of the 1970s, the cerebral dominance theory lost ground for several reasons. Brainwaves research (e.g., Rheinberger, Karlin, & Berman, 1943; Scarbrough, 1943) failed to provide support. An EMG study of the masseter muscles found that the same anomalous activity observed in stutterers was also seen in normal controls when they faked stuttering (Williams, 1955). It was concluded that the specific jaw movement involved in stuttering caused the abnormal signals, not necessarily abnormal brain and muscle activity. Additional counterevidence surfaced regarding handedness, showing that the majority of left-handers were left-hemisphere dominant for speech, not right dominant as previously assumed. Rather than being an "all or none" phenomenon, handedness was shown to be a continuum of varying degrees of ambidexterity across the human population, with the more adept hand varying across different skills (Daniels, 1940). Also, even earlier research revealed that shifting handedness for writing in 23 children did not cause stuttering (Ojemann, 1931).

Clinical Implications: The cerebral dominance theory had several consequences. For a while, some clinicians retrained people who stutter in shifting from their right to the left hand, aiming to return them to the supposedly original handedness. It was believed that the increased left-hand usage would also strengthen their right cerebral hemisphere to the point of retaking its dominance and restoring fluency (Williams, 1955). With the hope that cerebral dominance might be influenced and improve speech, both Wendell Johnson and Charles Van Riper participated in the act of constraining their right forearms and hands in plaster casts for a year. Neither, however, found this process afforded any relief for their speech (Travis, 1978a). A much greater influence spawned by this theory is seen in the advocacy of procedures that encourage the stutterer to remain "objective" during stuttering as suggested by Bryngelson in 1931. Inasmuch as the cause is organic, went the logic, the best the client can do is accept the stuttering and reduce emotional reaction to minimize further aggravation of the neurologically-based affliction.

The Modern Era of Brain Research

As knowledge of the neurological underpinnings for fluent speech expands, it serves as a foundation for revealing the brain regions and processes potentially responsible for stuttering. For normal speech, a sequenced chain of commands originates at the anterior frontal region of the cortex where action is planned, and projects through the cingulate, supplementary motor area, and premotor area, and then to the primary motor area. This hierarchical activation pattern is enhanced by tandem connections of these areas with other cortical areas so parallel activations can take place as well. For example, action may be influenced by sensory feedback, as well as being enhanced by information from other brain areas. Table 7.2 and Figure 7.1 (see p. 179) illustrate the brain regions involved in these functions.

Table 7.2 Brain Regions and Their Functions for Movements

Speech Function	Brain Region
1. Decisions are made about the type and characteristics of actions to be taken (e.g., lift tongue blade to touch alveolar ridge).	Parietal lobes and prefrontal motor areas
2. Anticipatory planning and initiation of movement based on past experience (e.g., start contracting muscles to raise tongue).	Primary motor area and supplementary motor area
3. Integration of sensory and spatial information used to guide movements (e.g., tongue is short distance from center).	Posterior parietal cortex and premotor area
4. Specifications for the sequence and duration (timing) of movements: Activities of each body part are coordinated with precision (e.g., open lips and raise tongue, then exhale air).	Cerebellum
5. Movements are inhibited until time for their delivery (e.g., wait to breathe until tongue is ready).	Basal ganglia indirectly involved with the thalamus

Although currently there is no formal theory of how brain structure and function may cause and sustain stuttering, the resurgence of interest in the relations between stuttering and the brain has expanded in two directions, brain anatomy (structure) and brain physiology (function), yielding a growing body of supportive evidence.

Brain Structure

Among the most interesting findings, adults who stutter were found to have:

- Atypical brain asymmetry with the left planum temporale (PT) smaller than the right. In normal speakers the left planum temporale was larger than the right. People who stuttered also had extra gyri (convolutions) on the left PT. The structure is located in Wernicke's area, which is critical for auditory processing of speech/language. Hence, these observations led to the hypothesis that perhaps auditory processing of speech and language is different in people who stutter (Foundas, Bollich, Corey et al., 2001; Foundas, Bollich, Feldman et al., 2004).

- Increased *volume* of white matter within a right-hemispheric network, including brain structures relevant for language and speech such as auditory areas and Broca's right-sided homologue where the face and mouth are represented. The findings suggest an increased, possibly atypical, intrahemispheric communication, as well different processing strategies in the right hemisphere (Jancke, Hanggi, & Steinmetz, 2004).

- Reduced white matter integrity in the brain, that is, lower fiber density, deficiencies in the myelin covering, and/or tract disorganization. This was first found by

Sommer et al. (2002) in the left hemisphere linking the temporal and frontal areas. More recently, Watkins et al. (2008) found that regions involved in speech production and sensorimotor integration in both hemispheres featured lower white matter integrity. They too found that tracts linking the temporal and frontal (sensorimotor) areas were characterized by lower integrity. The finding indicates that the speech motor and the auditory cortex are not well connected. Structural anomalies of the left inferior frontal region were also reported by Kell et al. (2009).

- Larger corpus callosum, the structure connecting the two hemispheres. It was suggested that the larger callosum may have developed due to left hemisphere dysfunction. A larger callosum allows for greater participation of, or greater interference from, the right hemisphere in activities that are typically left lateralized (Choo et al., 2011).

- Reduction of gray matter volume in the bilateral cerebellum and medulla regions. This was assumed to be related to the neural mechanisms controlling speech production and may be the essential cause of the stuttering disorder. Also, there were clusters of increased gray matter in the temporal, parietal, and frontal lobes, perhaps the result of functional compensation for the cerebellar and medullary function deficiencies (Song, Peng, Jin et al. (2007).

Gray matter is a major component of the central nervous system found in the brain and the spinal cord. It consists mainly of neural cell bodies. In the brain, the gray matter is distributed at the surface of the cerebral hemispheres known as the cortex but also in lower brain structures, such as the thalamus and basal ganglia. The gray-brown color reflects the minute blood vessels and the cell bodies themselves. The gray matter brain involves muscle control, sensory perception, cognitive and emotional processes. White matter mostly contains myelinated nerve fibers (axons) and tracts of fibers. The nerve fibers transmit signals among various gray areas of the brain as well as neural commands to muscle and sensory signals from the periphery to the brain. The whiteness results from the myelin sheath covering the neural fibers. Myelin acts as an insulator, increasing the speed of transmission of nerve signals. The left hemisphere has a proportionately greater volume of gray matter, while the right hemisphere has proportionately more white matter.

A very recent study by the Watkins group at Oxford University, which included 29 adult PWS, replicated previous findings that showed reduced integrity in white matter underlying cortical areas, as well as in the cerebellum and corpus callosum, relative to NFS controls. Within the PWS, the higher the stuttering severity, the lower the white matter integrity within the left parietal lobe region associated with language. On the other hand, there was greater white matter integrity in the left corticobulbar tract (Connally, Ward, Howell et al., 2013).

As for children who stutter, only three brain imaging studies have been reported. The first was conducted at the University of Illinois with 9- to 12-year-olds. The 15 CWS had less gray matter volume in speech-relevant regions in both hemispheres as compared

Figure 7.1   Lateral (A) and Medial (B) Views of a Left Cerebral Hemisphere

(A) Left hemisphere, front on the left, viewed from outside

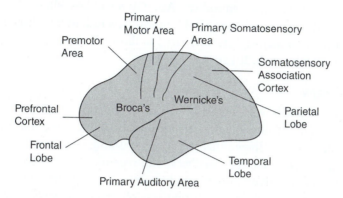

(B) Left hemisphere, front on the right, viewed from inside, zoom in

to the 7 NFC. Within the stuttering group, the 8 children with persistent problems had reduced white matter fibers in the left hemisphere, just under the cortical areas responsible for speech and facial muscles as compared to the 7 children who recovered (Chang et al., 2008). This decrease was in the same location found by Sommer et al. (2002) in adults who stutter as described above. A follow-up study with the same participants, plus one additional participant, focused on the corpus callosum. It indicated no differences among children with persistent stuttering, those who recovered, and normally fluent peers in the volume and integrity of white matter of this structure (Choo, Loucks, Chang et al., 2012).

Finally a study carried out in Canada with 11 CWS and 11 NFC, ages 6 to 12 years, found the former group had reduced gray matter volume in both hemispheres in locations serving speech-language functions, such as Broca's area but had more gray matter in other areas of the right hemisphere. Also CWS had less white matter volume in certain areas of the corpus callosum. Children with severe stuttering had less gray matter volume in the right hemisphere compared to those who stutter less severely (Beal, Gracco, Brettschneider et al., 2012).

Brain Physiology

Brain imaging of people who stutter by means of functional MRI (fMRI) has been applied in the study of physiological characteristics. With some differences among studies, the findings have shown that in various speaking conditions, such as with or without several types of auditory feedback, and regardless of the fluency level, PWS demonstrated greater activity in the right hemisphere cortex (gray matter) than NFS (Watkins et al., 2008). Such overactivation was observed particularly in an area on the right frontal lobe which is homologous (having the same relative position) to the Broca's area in the left hemisphere. Their report also indicated reduced bilateral activity in the auditory cortex. Generally, these findings were labeled as the "neural signatures" of stuttering (Brown et al., 2005). Two other studies reported reduced auditory cortex (right hemisphere) activity in association with greater stuttering regardless of the different technologies applied: fMRI (Giraud et al., 2008) and PET scans (Fox, Ingham, Ingham et al., 2000). Interestingly, abnormal activation is not limited to the cortex but also observed in lower levels in the brain, such as the basal ganglia (Kell et al; 2009; Ludlow & Loucks, 2003) and the cerebellum, which is an important part of the brain for sensory-motor integration (De Nil, Kroll, & Houle, 2001; Lu, Chen, Ning et al., 2011; Watkins et al., 2008).

Although many modern brain studies used fMRI, several employed electrophysiologic (QTE) and metabolic regional cerebral blood flow (rCBF) to measure brain function. Investigators reported a tendency of a subgroup of PWS with below normal right-left asymmetry of blood flow in the temporal lobe to exhibit longer laryngeal reaction times (LRT) than NFS (Watson, Pool, Devous et al., 1992). In another study, adults who stuttered and also exhibited language deficiencies had significant blood flow asymmetry (left < right) in the temporal and frontal lobes compared to those without language deficits (Watson, Freeman, Devous et al., 1994). More recently, brain blood flow measures obtained by means of PET were applied for comparisons of males and females who stutter. Differences were found, although interestingly, not in brain regions correlated with variations in stuttering (Ingham, R., Fox, Ingham, J., Xiong et al., 2004).

Modern brain research has continued to generate interest in the possible role of hemispheric function in stuttering. Based on studies that used positron emission tomography (PET), an imaging technique that produces a three-dimensional map of the functional processes in the body region being scanned, the idea emerged that rather than a lack of cerebral dominance, the overactivation of the right hemisphere during speech leads to stuttering. Recall that normally, brain activity during speech is greatest in Broca's and Wernicke's speech-language centers in the left hemisphere. Studies that employed the technique revealed different brain activity patterns for stutterers in both oral and silent reading conditions compared to baseline levels. The focal area of excess activation was the right frontal motor cortex, just behind the central sulcus (e.g., De Nil, Kroll, Kapur et al., 2000). They proposed that people who stutter may have innate, or early acquired, excessive right hemisphere activity. Supporting data were reported by Preibisch et al. (2003). Again, in both speech and nonspeech tasks, greater right hemisphere activation was demonstrated by participants who stuttered.

Weaknesses: The theory for the role of excessive right hemisphere activation has been challenged by others who offer alternate explanations. They argued that because these studies were conducted only with adults, excessive right hemisphere activation could be the result, rather than the cause, of stuttering or other developmental domains (Buchel et al., 2004). It has also been pointed out that right hemisphere activity could represent compensation for other brain differences that cause stuttering (Fox et al., 2000; Ludlow, 2000). Alm (2004b) explained that if the basal ganglia (deep brain structures) were not providing adequate timing information to the supplementary motor area (SMA), its activation with increased right-side dominance would show up as compensatory processes during stuttering. This explanation is consistent with findings by Fox, Ingham, Ingham et al. (1996) and Ingham, Fox, Ingham, and Zamarripa (2000). As mentioned earlier, however, other recent research has revealed additional brain areas involved with stuttering, not necessarily situated in the right hemisphere.

Clinical Implications: Are there at the present clinical implications of all these findings? Kell et al. (2009) reported differences between naturally recovered adults who stuttered and those who persisted. Unassisted recovery was underpinned by overactivated left motor cortex in the vicinity of white matter anomaly. The investigators entertained the idea that therapy methods capable of inducing similar compensatory activation may induce fluency in PWS. Indeed, several studies have compared brain activities in pre- and post-fluency-inducing therapy, reporting that improvement is associated with normalized brain activation patterns, including more pronounced left hemisphere activity in the frontal and temporal cortex, and reduced activity in the right auditory cortex. Left-sided activation increases were located close to the area where white matter anomalies were reported in the past (De Nil et al., 2003; Giraud et al., 2008; Neumann et al., 2005; Preisbisch et al., 2003).

Summary of Neurological Perspectives

There have been several theoretical points of view regarding stuttering as a function of abnormal brain activity. These have hypothesized that stuttering occurs secondary to a lack of cerebral dominance, or from a hypersensitive brainstem reflex response. Although the results of reported studies may be confusing in their specifics, overall the relevant findings just described support the notion of brain differences between people who stutter and normally fluent speakers. Research conducted during the past 20 years has provided sufficient data demonstrating both structural and functional abnormalities. The most consistent findings have indicated:

- Abnormality in left hemisphere white matter in terms of reduced volume, organization, and myelin covering of fibers
- Right hemisphere hyperactivity
- Indications for reduced gray matter in subcortical centers

As Watkins (2011) pointed out, the deficient neural tracks are located just under the cortical sensorimotor area (gray matter) where the speech articulators are represented in the left hemisphere. They connect the cortical areas above them, as well as cortical with subcortical structures, some of which also have speech functions. Hence, one reasonable interpretation is that stuttering is the result of poor connection between these regions. Perhaps the right hyperactivity is generated to compensate for the deficient structural connectivity in the left hemisphere. Other potentially very important findings indicate that (1) brain abnormalities are also found in children who stutter, (2) stuttering subgroups might be identified by the relative magnitude of blood flow abnormality in the brain, and (3) gender differences in susceptibility and recovery may be related to brain differences between males and females who stutter.

Auditory Perspectives

The Role of Audition

It is well recognized that normal speech development relies heavily on the close relation between speech control and audition. Adequate sensory-to-motor integration processes between hearing and speech are essential to its production. Deaf children do not develop normally sounding speech because they lack auditory feedback about their speech output. Other evidence for the interactive relation between audition and speech is the *Lombard sign* (*Lombard effect*), observed when people automatically raise their voices by a predictable amount when speaking in noise. It is of interest, therefore, to note several potential connections between hearing acuity and stuttering. For example, there is a very low incidence of the disorder in the deaf population (see Chapter 2). Also, as seen in Chapter 4, when people who stutter speak in the presence of a sufficiently high noise level, their stuttering is substantially reduced. Similarly, amelioration of stuttering is seen when PWS hear their own speech through delayed auditory feedback, or DAF, instruments or other form of altered auditory feedback, such as frequency-shifted auditory feedback (Stuart, Kalinowski, Rastatter et al., 2004). In contrast, it has been shown that DAF can induce disfluencies and speech errors in normally fluent people (e.g., Chon, Kraft, Ambrose et al., 2013; Jones & Striemer, 2007). Finally, several scholars have suggested classifications of people who stutter based on their dichotic listening, which is an indirect method of probing auditory processing (see review by Yairi, 2007).

The relation between stuttering and audition was heavily researched by Cherry, Sayers, and Marland (1955) and Cherry and Sayers (1956). These investigators conducted a series of experiments on the effect of loud sounds on stuttering using tonal and noise stimuli in selective frequency bands, all delivered either via air or bone conduction. They concluded that the largest reduction in stuttering, nearly to elimination, occurred under low-frequency, bone-conducted noise. They proposed that people who stutter suffer from a *perceptual* defect. The defective auditory feedback loop interferes with accurate speech motor activity, causing disfluent speech. By overriding the reliance on one's own feedback, for example by means of noise, stuttering can be averted.

Several alternative explanations have been proposed for the stuttering-audition link. In the first experiment of noise effects on stuttering, Shane (1955) proposed a *psychological* explanation. Adhering to the Johnsonian ideas that stuttering results from people's anxiety about their own stuttered speech, Shane postulated that because people talking in noise cannot hear their own speech, they cannot be critical of it, become apprehensive, and consequently stutter. Another plausible explanation based on *motoric* factors was offered by Wingate (1976). He pointed out that a person's manner of speaking changes in conditions of altered auditory stimulation. For example, under masking noise, speech becomes louder, slower, and the vowels are longer.

A somewhat more specific "theory" of stuttering as an auditory perceptual disorder was developed by Harrington (1988), who suggested that people who stutter experience a defect in the timing of auditory feedback. The lagging auditory feedback causes a speaker to expect to hear sound earlier than the system feeds it back. The speaker therefore waits (prolongs) or repeats the speech segment in an effort to correct the mismatch of information about speech timing. Observations that stuttering is frequently ameliorated in conditions of DAF or under loud noise were taken as supportive evidence. Also, PWS appear to need more time to speak fluently, as if they are permitting their auditory system sufficient time to feed back the sound of speech.

A combination of changes in articulation and vocalization could be the mechanism responsible for the increased fluency when auditory stimulation is introduced. Max, Guenther, Gracco et al. (2004) considered the possibility that people who stutter may be overly dependent on afferent, including auditory, feedback. They hypothesized that an external auditory signal (e.g., noise) reduces stuttering because it facilitates activation of the auditory cortex. But it is not the heightened monitoring of auditory feedback that supports fluency; instead they suggest that the extra cortical activation improves the speaker's feedforward regulation of speech by enhancing predictions of the acoustic outcomes of their speech motor planning.

Auditory characteristics of people who stutter have continued to attract research interest over the years. Children whose stuttering persisted had a larger overall threshold variance and poorer backward masking thresholds than peers whose stuttering recovered (Howell, Davis, & Williams, 2006). Adults who stutter performed significantly less well at discriminating voicing contrasts in stop consonants compared to fluent controls (Neef et al., 2012). Additionally, evidence is emerging from studies of latencies in vocal response to pitch-shift stimuli that neural processing of auditory feedback for speech may deviate in adults who stutter (Bauer, Seery, LaBonte et al., 2008; Loucks, Chon, & Han, 2012). Deficient utilization of real-time auditory feedback for short-latency (feedback delay of 40 ms) articulatory adjustments has been noted in adults who stutter during both vowel productions and connected speech (Tourville, Cai, & Guenther, 2013).

> Conditions of delayed feedback and masking noise often generate fluency in people who stutter. By contrast, fluent speakers in the same conditions often find their disfluencies increase. These observations lend support to the hypothesis that auditory attention is important to the delivery of fluent speech. To what aspect of the speech signal do fluent speakers typically direct their auditory attention when talking? Do fluent speakers find this attention disrupted by the conditions of competing auditory stimuli? By contrast, do people who stutter shift their attention over to that aspect of the speech signal when competing auditory stimuli are present, which they otherwise tend to ignore in the ordinary circumstances of talking? Perhaps research will eventually reveal where the focus of auditory attention needs to be for fluent speech, so we can assist those who stutter to direct their attention to it.

Weaknesses: A major limitation of defective audition theory is that it does not account for the fact that people sometimes begin stuttering, as seen in their facial and oral tension and apparent attempt to speak, before they have uttered any vocal sound. How, then, can stuttering occur if there is no sound fed back through the defective auditory system? Additional questions stem from research that demonstrated reduction in stuttering when noise was presented only during nonphonated periods of speech (Sutton & Chase, 1961) or in only one ear when self-hearing is still preserved in the other ear (Yairi, 1976). Finally, it is also a fact that not all individuals who stutter respond with more fluency in the conditions of either noise or delayed auditory feedback.

Clinical Implications: Some treatment programs had people who stutter engage in *shadowing* speech, instructing them to closely mimic a clinician's speech, almost simultaneously. This was quite effective in reducing stuttering because, according to the program, the stutterers relied on external feedback rather than on their own defective system. More popular, however, have been miniature instruments that generate masking noise or deliver DAF or other altered auditory feedback signals to the ears that have been employed in the treatment of stuttering. These are discussed in Chapter 12.

Summary of Auditory Perspectives

Evidence from multiple sources suggests a relation between audition and stuttering, particularly as evidenced in the effect of noise and DAF on diminishing overt stuttering. If the auditory defect theory holds, however, it may only be relevant for a subgroup of individuals who stutter. Initial support for this possibility was provided by Chon et al. (2013) who found three subgroups, *low, middle*, and *high responders* based on normally fluent speakers responses to DAF.

The audition-stuttering link has also been highlighted by brain imaging research that reported reduced brain activity in the temporal region known to be responsible for auditory functions during stuttering (Fox et al., 2000; Watkins et al., 2008). Such observations add to the concern with whether people who stutter process auditory stimuli in the same way as those who do not stutter. Regardless of a tenuous understanding of the underlying mechanisms, auditory feedback in various forms has already been exploited for therapeutic purposes.

Motor Perspectives

Earlier in this chapter, we pointed out that various ideas about motor factors contributing to stuttering have been entertained for hundreds of years. During the first third of the 20th century, motor abilities of people who stutter began to be researched in controlled laboratory studies. Among early investigators, West and Nusbaum (1929) compared PWS and NFS on their speed of jaw and facial muscle contraction. The slowness exhibited by the stutterers in the action of these muscles was interpreted as a cause, or related to the cause, of stuttering. Others who looked at breathing found general malfunctioning of its mechanism during stuttering (e.g., Fletcher, 1914; Fossler, 1930). Cross (1936) reported that although PWS were not inferior to NFS in unimanual (use of a single hand) tasks, they were significantly inferior to them in bimanual tasks. Much later, some studies found slower manual reaction times of PWS compared to NFS (Till, Goldsmith, & Reich, 1981).

One of the challenges to the study of potential motor sources of stuttering is determining the most pertinent questions to address. What kind of a breakdown and in what system(s) is evidenced as stuttering? Is stuttering but one symptom of a general, extensive motor disorder that might have additional, apparently unrelated symptoms? Does the underlying problem, whatever it is, exist during nonstuttered speech? In nonspeech systems? On a broad level, three types of movement-related systems could play a role in breakdown of speech fluency: executive (central) decisions, motor actions, and sensory perceptions. In combination, they aid the speaker's control of motor speech.

The diagram in Figure 7.2 can be used to illustrate these three systems. Regarding movement decisions, there must be instructions from brain centers to the speech structures as to (1) whether to move, (2) when to move, (3) where to move, (4) what distance to move, and (5) what speed to move. With respect to actual movement or action, the structures (e.g., the tongue) must both respond to command and achieve the target parameters. Sensory perceptions (feedback) are essential for generating instructions for the movement in progress because they are the source of information about the structures' position (e.g., spatial location of the tongue), size/weight (e.g., how heavy is the tongue?), activity (e.g., is the tongue moving already?), contact (e.g., is the tongue touching something?), and elasticity (e.g., is the tongue resistant/stiff?). Research could be conducted to reveal which of these dimensions are most important where stuttering is concerned.

Figure 7.2 Three Systems Involved in the Regulation of Movement

Motor Learning Theories of Stuttering

The theory of motor learning in general deals with the science of how skilled actions are developed, how practice and its associated variables influence permanent changes in performance, and how trial-and-error processes are involved in learning. Because speech is a motor act, we can expect its acquisition and refinement to be governed by motor learning principles, a number of which can be examined relative to stuttering. One principle is that movement skills can be improved with practice. It has been suggested that adaptation, the decline of stuttering with multiple readings of the same passage, may reflect the benefit of practice or *motor rehearsal* (Max & Caruso, 1998). Experienced clinicians are well aware that when a person who stutters repeats the same word or phrase over and over, the word or phrase soon becomes fluent. In motor learning terms, *massed* practice saying each word over multiple times can be as effective at improving speech motor performance as *distributed* practice, saying the whole passage or paragraph over multiple times (Schmidt & Lee, 2005). The greatest challenge to the application of the motor rehearsal hypothesis to stuttering, however, is that the fluency gains do not readily generalize. Thus, another motor learning principle, *generalization* after rehearsal, does not hold up in stuttering. But the limitation is not just for generalization. People who stutter also seem to be less able to *maintain* learned skills when asked to apply them later in the same motor task. In one study participants practiced 100 repetitions of a single, monosyllabic, nonsense word sequence, returning after 24 hours to perform an additional 50 repetitions. PWS had significantly slower sequence durations as compared to NFS. The difference, however, indicated a subgroup effect among the stutterers in that several participants failed to show any improvement (Bauerly & De Nil, 2011).

Another potential motor learning principle is that rehearsing an action in slow motion generalizes to sped-up actions. There is no need to relearn the motor act just because a different speed is used (Schmidt & Lee, 2005). In theory, then, the practice of a slow rate of fluent speech in therapy should carry over to conditions when a faster rate is used. In reality, however, stutterers must be careful not to attempt speaking rates beyond their capacity to sustain the desired fluent speech. Another motor principle is Fitts's law of speed-accuracy trade-off: The precision of a motor act will deteriorate if the attempted rate is too fast. Fitts's law reminds us that there is an inverse relationship between the difficulty of a movement and the speed with which it can be performed.

Dynamics of motor learning may eventually be important to our understanding of stuttering. Consider the child who discovers a button to push, and does it over and over again, just exploring it. Perhaps there are young children who, by chance, find and explore the means of triggering stuttering, exploring it over and over again without being able to help themselves from it. Impulse control and the refined regulation of action take some time to develop. In the meantime, the child may often trigger stuttering, making it an unintentionally practiced habit. These motor learning principles lead us to next consider two concepts of stuttering that possibly qualify as motor theories.

Brainstem Reflexes: A Disorder of Movement

Kinematics, the study of how things move, has been applied quite extensively in stuttering research. In 1980 Zimmermann conducted a series of kinematic investigations using cinefluorography, a method of producing X-ray motion images. These were used to measure movements of the lower jaw and lip of adults who stuttered during fluent speech. He found that PWS produced slower oral movements, such as transitions between consonants and vowels or when building up movement speed, than did NFS. He conjectured that stuttering should be considered a disorder of movement triggered by brainstem reflex responses. When speech movements deviate from the typical range in both space and time, when movements either overshoot or undershoot the speaker's intended targets, they trigger conflicting afferent (sensory) and efferent (motor) brainstem reflexes to correct the movement. The struggle between the original movement and the reflex corrective response could be abnormal oscillatory movements (repetitions), frozen postures (silent blocks or voiced prolongations), or something else that constitutes stuttering (Zimmermann, 1980b). Upon analyzing stutter events Zimmermann (1980c) made an observation of potential clinical significance: that just prior to terminating blocks, PWS often repositioned their oral structures, lowering the jaw and changing the lip and/or tongue shape. Since that time, investigators have paid particular attention to the jaw, gaining insights about its movement associated with stuttering. One team found that although both PWS and NFS employed the same control strategies for the jaw when speaking fluently, the stutterers' opening and closing jaw movements were more restricted as well as slower to build up speed (Jäncke, Bauer, Kaiser et al. 1997).

Weaknesses: Although recent research of the jaw uncovered significantly greater target errors and spatial variability in PWS than in NFS, there were no differences in the velocities and durations of movements (Loucks, De Nil, & Sasisekaran, 2007). The researchers suggested that the jaw-phonatory discoordination of their stuttering participants indicated either an oral proprioceptive or a motor control deficit. Despite basic agreement with the conclusions regarding speech motor instability in PWS, they reported their observations had failed to support Zimmermann's hypothesized reflex function differences.

Another challenge to these conclusions is that they fail to explain why such limitations seem not to be imposed during singing, choral speech, rhythmic metronome speech, and so on, that, in general, tend to be fluent. It can be argued, though speculatively, that the fluency-enhancing conditions provide a scaffold for the sensory-motor deficit. Conditions such as rhythmic motor movements (during singing, metronome, etc.) are known to assist in movement execution.

Clinical Implications: Based on this theory, people who stutter need to speak more slowly so as to move the articulators within the allowable range of space and time to avoid triggering brainstem reflex interference. It also implied they should learn to assume new articulatory postures (e.g., lowering the jaw) to release blocks.

Sensorimotor Dysfunction

Earlier we reviewed studies that found differences in brain structure and processes associated with motor and somatosensory functions in people who stutter. Hence one of the possibilities is that PWS inherits a sensorimotor system that is insufficient to support fluent speech. If the sensorimotor systems of PWS do not offer timely or otherwise sufficient information related to the speech musculature, fluency breakdown might occur. This proposition provides a context for the sensorimotor model of stuttering known as DIVA (directions into velocities of articulators) proposed by Guenther (1995) for normal speech and adopted for stuttering by Max et al. (2004). It depicts PWS as having trouble acquiring or activating the internal schemes necessary to integrate feedforward and feedback aspects of speech motor control. The planning of movement is *feedforward motor control*. The feedforward system generates instructions that specify which articulatory structures will move, the distances to be traversed, the level of force needed over what duration of time, and more. The precision of feedforward instructions depends on accurate sensory knowledge about the preliminary conditions of the structures. After movement has begun, the result can be adjusted based on the *feedback system*. The information and controls however, are generated at a point in time too late to alter the initial movement. Corrections can take any of several forms: changes in speed and/or force, interrupting the movement, and/or reinitiating the movement.

Proponents of the DIVA model hypothesize that people who stutter have impaired (unreliable) feedforward systems so that they rely excessively on controlling speech via the feedback system instead (Civier et al., 2010). The overreliance on feedback control supposedly leads to an escalated amount of repair information tending to prompt a "reset" or restart of the speech motor act (e.g., a sound/syllable repetition). We may add here that a role for motor programming factors underlying stuttering is supported by findings of hyperactivation of right hemisphere motor and premotor areas in people who stutter reviewed earlier in this chapter. A tendency for deficient auditory sensory feedback is also supported by the many findings reviewed earlier, indicating that people who stutter exhibit abnormal cortical, subcortical, and connecting neural pathways that are related to auditory processing of speech and language.

> Speech, among other physical movements, is potentially controlled or regulated with a combination of feedforward and feedback processes. Feedback occurs when a person receives information about the outcome of movement *after* it has occurred (e.g., was the intended sound spoken?). In feedforward, the parameters of movement are established *before* the action, and no attention is given to tracking or checking on the result of the movement that takes place (as is often the case when swearing or yelling). Feedforward processes are considered *open loop* because they consist only of the instructions and the actions. Sensory information is used prior to the initial decision for action but is not consulted while action is in progress. Feedback processes, by contrast, are *closed loop* in that during the action, sensory information is consulted and used to adjust and refine the movement.

Weaknesses: One of the challenges for any sensory feedback theory of stuttering arises from the observation that people who stutter often block before they have uttered any speech. If a speaker is overrelying on feedback to manage the speech act, one should expect some speech to escape prior to attempts by the speaker to make alterations. Similarly, such theories do not explain why stutterers are slower or activate the brain differently even during silent reading.

Clinical Implications: Similar to other theories mentioned, the DIVA model favors the use of slow, prolonged speech by people who stutter to compensate for their self-monitoring tendencies. The theory also supports the clinical application of the various forms of altered auditory feedback (e.g., masking, DAF, etc.).

Evidence of Motor Differences

Regardless of etiology, it is clear that stuttering manifests itself as a breakdown of speech movements. Motor involvement is apparent from the observable physical tension in various parts of the body, especially in abnormal articulatory movements and postures during the disfluent speech events. The gross secondary characteristics add to the general impression of motor involvement. Some of the ways that people who stutter differ in motor system function, however, are detected only through instruments that provide data about fine abnormal patterns of activation of muscle groups in the lip, jaw, tongue, or larynx, as well as in nonspeech systems. The past several decades of stuttering research have seen a wealth of studies that employed acoustic, kinematic, electromyographic, and other methodologies. Measures have included reaction time; various kinematic and temporal parameters of speech; spatial dimensions of articulation; dynamics of respiratory, phonatory, and articulatory aspects of speech production; finger-tapping and hand-clapping patterns; and more. Examples of the relevant research findings involving different anatomical areas and functions are presented next.

Respiration

Early investigators found general malfunctioning of the breathing mechanism during stuttering (e.g., Fletcher, 1914). Recent research by Raczek and Adamczyk (2004) also yielded evidence of less effective breathing. Carbon dioxide (CO_2) concentrations in exhaled air during stuttering were one-fifth lower than during fluent speech. In a study of respiration during fluent speech, PWS tended to display substantially higher or lower lung volumes than NFS (Johnston, Watkin, & Macklem, 1993) and poor timing of breath patterns have been observed by Williams and Brutten (1994). Denny and Smith (2000) found atypical respiratory control during speech and nonspeech activities of PWS, particularly in tasks that required fast-paced, precisely timed, or highly rhythmic breathing.

Although various associations are observed between respiration and stuttering, no etiological connections have been found between respiratory diseases and stuttering. With respect to clinical strategies, attention to regulation of breath support and timing is usually helpful. It is an important component of a good number of stuttering therapy programs (Conelea, Rice & Woods, 2006; Webster, 1980a; b). Research is needed to reveal whether the benefits are related to specific patterns of breath control or the potential effect of relaxation enhanced by the attention to breathing.

Laryngeal Physiology

There is a long history to the idea that the larynx is responsible for, or an important contributor to, stuttering. This can be seen in the early 19th-century notion relating stuttering to a spasm of the larynx (e.g., Arnott, 1828). Some research is cited here according to type:

Vocal Pitch. Reduced range was reported for adults who stutter (Bryngelson, 1932), and a tendency for reduced prosody in imitated utterances (Bosshardt, Sappok, Knipschild et al., 1997). No significant differences were evident between PWS and NFS in fundamental frequency in vowel onsets, average level during vowels, speed of change, or range of change (Healey & Gutkin, 1984).

Laryngeal Reaction Time (LRT). The time it takes to phonate in response to a stimulus. PWS had slower laryngeal reaction times than NFS (Watson & Alfonso, 1987). An association between LRT and stuttering severity was indicated in one study (Dembowski & Watson, 1991) but not in another (Watson et al., 1992).

Laryngeal Muscles. Electromyography (EMG) showed that stutter events were associated with greater levels of laryngeal muscle activity and disruption of normal reciprocity between abductor and adductor muscles (Freeman & Ushijima, 1978). In contrast to excessive force, Smith et al. (1996) detected insufficient force. Measures of intrinsic laryngeal muscles revealed that periods of disfluent speech were not typically characterized by higher levels of activity than periods of fluency. Adults displayed a lower operating range of muscle activity during speech that could interfere with performance.

Vocal Fold Function. Video photography showed that stutter events involved simultaneous contractions of antagonistic vocal fold abductor and adductor muscles (Conture et al., 1977). Also, the vocal folds were more likely to be inappropriately adducted during sound prolongation than during sound/syllable repetition. These two disfluency types influenced differently the fold movement as well as the position of the larynx in the throat (Conture, Schwartz, & Brewer, 1985). Only a few studies with preschool children related to vocal fold function were reported. For example, no differences in fundamental frequency between the stuttering and normally fluent groups were reported by Healey and Bernstein (1991), but significant differences were found in shimmer (cycle-to-cycle amplitude perturbations), although not in jitter (cycle-to-cycle frequency perturbations) during fluent speech (Hall & Yairi, 1992).

Oral Motor and Articulatory Differences

Normal speech presumably depends on carefully orchestrated activation of the various muscle groups—jaw, lip, tongue, and so on—that could fail by being inappropriately timed for coordination, level of force, or order of activation. Such problems have been documented in both stuttered and fluent speech.

Articulatory Acoustics. Acoustic data must be interpreted cautiously as an indirect representation of articulatory movement. The voice onset time (VOT) measure indicates time elapsed between the release of a stop-plosive consonant and the beginning of vocal fold vibration for the subsequent voiced sound. Results have been inconsistent. Agnello and Wingate (1972) reported longer VOT for PWS than for NFS, while Jäncke (1994) found no differences. Max and Gracco (2005) measured the correlation between the gap in the stop consonant /p/ in fluent utterances and the voice onset time (VOT) of the following sound. The PWS had longer durations for the consonant gaps and the VOT, as well as greater variability. Stopgap and vowel durations in the speech of severe stutterers were longer than those of NFS (Borden, Kim, and Spiegler, 1987). Acoustic studies with children close to stuttering onset, have measured articulatory speaking rates (Hall, Amir, & Yairi, 1999) and changes in the second formant (F2) transition in fluent speech to reflect tongue movement (Subramanian, Yairi, & Amir, 2003). Both studies revealed few differences between CWS and NFC.

Oral Muscles. Slower rate and slower acceleration speed of the lower lip and jaw in the fluent speech of PWS were found by means of high-speed cineradiography (Zimmermann, 1980a). EMG studies revealed PWS applied a reversed order of lip muscle activation (depressor anguli oris vs. depressor labii inferioris) on fluent single words, but particularly so during stuttering (Guitar, Guitar, Neilson et al., 1988). Significantly greater lower lip EMG peak latencies were measured in the fluent speech of PWS compared to NFS (van Lieshout, Peters, Starkweather et al. 1993).

Articulatory Coordination. Applying an index of motor stability, PWS were much less consistent in their coordinative patterns over repeated productions of nonwords (meaningless utterances). As length and complexity of the utterances increased, group differences in coordinative consistency were even more pronounced (e.g., Smith, Sadagopan, Walsh et. al., 2010). Of particular interest were data reported in several studies showing the relationship between motor instability and language and phonological complexity in children who stutter (e.g., Smith et al., 2010). MacPherson and Smith (2013) reported more variable motor coordination of lip and jaw movement during fluent speech in many of their 4- to 6-year-old CWS as compared with NFC.

> Some studies derived their data from the fluent speech of persons who stutter. Atypical or abnormal movement patterns in the *fluent* speech of people who stutter could indicate that their physical systems carry the seeds of stuttering moments constantly, just under the surface. The physical system is thus vulnerable to produce the stutter, whereas other factors (e.g., environment, emotion, attention, etc.) play a role in precipitating it. The finding of atypical physiological dynamics beneath the surface of fluent speech in people who stutter would lend support to the view that stuttering is not just a more severe form of normal disfluency. The physiological vulnerability to stutter is something that normally fluent people presumably do not have.

General Motor Skills

Some investigators have proposed that speech motor system insufficiencies of people who stutter may reflect a general motor system problem affecting other physical abilities as well (Max, Caruso, & Gracco, 2003). Indeed, several studies of nonspeech systems have documented that adults who stutter show different patterns of adaptation for novel motor tasks than NFS. Motor limitations are more evident when task complexity is increased. Significant differences between PWS and controls were found in finger-tapping skills and in improved speed and/or accuracy of tapping sequencing with practice (Smits-Bandstra, De Nil & Rochon, 2006; Smits-Bandstra, De Nil & Saint Cyr, 2006). People who stutter revealed significantly more difficulties than NFS with a bimanual dual task of finger tapping with one hand while turning a knob with the other one (Forster & Webster, 2001). Olander, Smith, and Zelaznik (2010) employed a hand-clapping task in which CWS produced remarkably higher variability levels of their interclap intervals than control peers. This finding led to the suggestion that in early years, stuttering is associated with a fundamental deficit in a child's ability to generate consistent, rhythmic motor behaviors.

Multifactorial Theory from a Motor Perspective

In Chapter 5 we mentioned the dynamic, multifactorial, nonlinear model offered by Smith and Kelly (1997) and Smith (1999). It is based on the idea that complex systems and factors, such as central speech programming, language, emotions, cognition, and genetics, interact in both the causation and further development of stuttering and in the overt breakdowns in speech motor control perceived as stuttering. When the disorder exists, such interaction intermittently affects the motor function necessary for speech production. Nonlinearity suggests that even small changes in one system may have a significant impact on the overall course of speech production. In general, perceptible disfluencies are hypothesized to reflect underlying instabilities in the speech motor system of individuals who stutter, the system being particularly vulnerable to changes in the organism. Although the model is not "purely" motoric, we believe it is important to mention here for two reasons. First, it serves to remind students the reality that the human organism is not a collection of separate organs or systems and that everything influences everything. Second, of the rich body of experimental data that support the model, most notable are the findings demonstrating how alterations in language and phonology complexity affect speech motor instability in people who stutter. We asked Anne Smith, a renowned speech scientist, to elaborate on her team's research concerned with the motor aspect of stuttering. Her account in a personal communication follows.

Anne Smith's Speech Motor Perspective on Stuttering

Stuttering is clearly a motor disorder. During disfluent speech events, the central nervous system of the person who stutters fails to generate the correct signals to control muscle activity for ongoing fluent speech. Indeed, early research focused on the motor characteristics of people who stutter. As stuttering theories shifted to the learning and/or personality domains, work on the physiological bases of stuttering was largely abandoned. The 1980s saw a resurgence of experimental work aimed at clarifying the physiological concomitants of stuttering (McClean, Goldsmith, & Cerf, 1984; McClean, Kroll, Loftus, 1990; Peters & Boves, 1988; Zimmermann, 1980 a; b). It revealed that, even when adult PWS speak fluently, their speech motor systems show signs of underlying instabilities not present in normally fluent speakers. Thus we can think of PWS as continuously operating with unstable speech production systems that sometimes overtly fail to operate within the bounds perceived as fluency; these breakdowns are the "moments of stuttering" that listeners perceive.

A large-scale project on the physiological correlates of stuttering funded by the National Institutes of Health began at Purdue University in the late 1980s. In its early phases, my colleagues and I sought to understand what "went wrong" with the command signals to speech muscles during moments of stuttering. Based on earlier experimental work (Freeman & Ushijima, 1978) and the general clinical impression that stuttering is associated with excessive muscle activity, we recorded electromyographic (EMG) activity from lip, jaw, chest wall, and intrinsic laryngeal muscles during stuttered and fluent speech (e.g., Denny & Smith, 1992; Smith et al., 1996). We found that moments of stuttering, including tense, silent blocks and long sound/syllable repetitions, are not associated with high levels of muscle activity. Rather, each PWS showed a stereotypical pattern that was repeated across disfluencies. In some cases this could be a relative decrease in muscle activity compared to the fluent surrounding speech, a slight increase in activity, or no change in EMG amplitude. This was true in all systems examined, including the intrinsic laryngeal muscles (Smith et al., 1996). The only frankly abnormal muscle activation pattern observed was tremor, a repetitive discharge of the muscle at a frequency beyond voluntary control, 5 to 15 Hz, also observed by earlier investigators (Fibiger, 1971; McClean et al. 1984). Tremor was observed in all of the subsystems examined, but only in a subgroup, about two-thirds, of the adults who stutter, especially on more severe disfluencies.

The "take-home" message from these studies is that stuttering is not "caused" by excessive muscle activation levels as some have proposed (Freeman & Ushijima, 1978; Starkweather, 1995). This result often surprises students, because PWS often complain of feelings of tension, especially in the "throat." Whereas perceived excess tension in the speech musculature is frequently associated with stuttering, its physiological basis is not high levels of muscle activation. In fact, individuals can perceive muscle tension even when the level of background activation of the muscle is quite low. For example, no systematic relationship has been observed between the perception of high levels of muscle tension and higher EMG activity in facial, neck, and shoulder muscles in individuals who suffer from headaches and myalgia (Bansevicius et al., 1997; Nilsen et al., 2006).

In later phases of the Purdue Stuttering Project, Smith, Weber-Fox, and colleagues turned to examining the interaction between the speech motor system and factors extrinsic to that system, such as the linguistic complexity of the utterance to be spoken. An extremely important finding was that the linguistic complexity of utterances influences the motor stability of the speaker. Adults who stutter were more destabilized by increasing linguistic demands, syntactic and phonological, compared to their fluent controls (Kleinow & Smith, 2000; Smith et al., 2010). The results reveal a vulnerability of the speech motor system in PWS to increasing speaking demands. This provides strong evidence that over the course of maturation from childhood to the adult years, PWS do not develop stable speech motor systems that are resistant to breakdown in the face of increased demands (Smith et al., 2010; Max et al. 2004). Interestingly, a large-scale developmental study by Smith and Zelaznik (2004) conducted with groups of 30 typically developing children aged 4, 5, 7, 9, 12 years, and young adults revealed that the maturational process for speech motor systems is quite protracted and adultlike stability is not present until after 14 years of age (Walsh & Smith, 2002). This is important because stuttering is a developmental disorder, and the typical, protracted development of speech motor systems suggests that even in the teenage years, treatment for fluency disorders is still operating on a fairly flexible system, one that has not yet settled into fixed motor patterns. Another finding was that boys age 4 to 5 years lag girls in developing consistent patterns of speech motor coordination. The fact that preschool boys mature more slowly than girls in speech motor control processes may contribute to their lower probability of natural recovery from stuttering compared to preschool girls.

Given the results of our studies of adults who stutter, an important next step was to determine when abnormalities in speech motor characteristics can be detected in PWS. Are relatively high levels of instability present at the onset of stuttering? Or, are the destabilized speech motor systems of adults who stutter a result of their long stuttering experience? To this end, our team at the Purdue Stuttering Project has adapted methods for recording physiological activity during speech that can be employed with children as young as four years of age. Results of these recent experiments have very significant implications because they revealed that instabilities in the speech motor systems of preschool children who stutter can be greater than that of their normally fluent controls. Comparing these two child groups in a sentence production task, we (MacPherson & Smith, 2013) reported that already at this early age the preschoolers who stutter showed greater instability in their speech motor coordination patterns compared to their fluent peers.

It should be emphasized that in all of these studies, remarkable heterogeneity has been observed in preschoolers who stutter in terms of their speech motor system function (just as there is in adults who stutter). Such heterogeneity in motor abilities also has been observed for manual tasks. Olander et al. (2010) tested groups of preschoolers abilities to "keep the beat" in a clapping task. They found that a significant subset of the CWS performed very poorly, well outside the normal range for timing control in clapping. Our laboratory also recently completed a large-scale electromyographic (EMG) study of 64 preschool CWS and 40 NFCs (Walsh & Smith, 2013). Consistent with the studies of adults, there was no evidence of higher levels of lip muscle activity during stuttering events, nor were there differences between CWS and NFCs in EMG activation levels, right/left bilateral synchrony, or any other measured pattern of EMG activity during speech. As in an earlier study of preschool and school-age children who stutter (Kelly, Smith, & Goffman, 1995), Walsh and Smith found no evidence of tremor in the muscle activity of the preschoolers who were stuttering. This suggests that tremor, the abnormal, uncontrolled oscillation of muscle activity sometimes observed in adults who stutter, is a symptom that develops later in the school-age and teenage years. Finally, important insights about motor aspects of stuttering also have been gained by investigations of the anatomy and physiology of the brains of individuals who stutter. These studies reveal both abnormal structure and function of brain regions involved in premotor and motor processes for speech in PWS.

In summary, the past three decades have produced remarkable progress in our understanding of stuttering as a problem in speech motor development. A critical question for the future is to understand what enables some children to recover from a period of vulnerability of the speech motor system to stuttering-like disfluency and become normally fluent speakers, and why other children develop a chronic stuttering. At present, the Purdue Stuttering Project is focused on longitudinal studies, expanding previous research by Yairi and colleagues at the University of Illinois, with the overall objective of identifying early predictors for persistence or recovery from stuttering with special emphases on motor, linguistic, and emotional domains.

Summary of Motor Perspectives

Motor inadequacies have long been suspected as the cause of stuttering. The motor breakdown of speech fluency could arise from one of the three major systems involved in movement: sensory perception, motor action, or central decision/instruction. Motor learning theories, brainstem reflex models, and sensorimotor dysfunction have also been proposed to explain stuttering. Early laboratory studies focused on a wide range of gross motor skills, such as unimanual and bimanual skills (e.g., finger-tapping studies). Later research focused on the three parts of the speech production apparatus, looking both at stuttered and fluent speech for possible seeds of the stuttering disorder. Abnormal functions of the respiratory, phonatory, and articulatory systems, or movement coordination among them, have been documented in PWS, both in stuttered and fluent speech. Differences from normally fluent speakers have been documented even in nonspeech movements. Overall, in spite of some contradictory findings or evidence of small differences, it appears that slight motor abnormalities, such as some instability of movement, are involved in stuttering. These appear to be influenced by factors outside the motor system, such as language complexity. Small as they may be, they are sufficient to cause significant disruption in a delicate system. Still, speech is a complicated motor act, and much more research is needed to understand the related factors underlying stuttering and fluency.

Summary

Various characteristics of stuttering and of the population of people who stutter make it reasonable to hypothesize that the disorder has neurophysiological bases. Robust evidence for strong genetic components of stuttering reinforces this view. Nevertheless, whatever is being transmitted genetically remains unknown. Several theoretical notions stemming from the neurophysiological orientation present a wide range of concepts, such as lack of cerebral dominance, abnormal brain morphology, excessive right brain hemisphere activity, abnormal auditory processing, deficient brainstem reflexes, motor learning, or sensorimotor integration. Regardless of the particular theory, a growing body of positive findings has emerged concerning differences in brain structures and processes between people who stutter and people who do not stutter. Much of it, however, has been acquired from adults who stuttered for years or children 6 years and older, leaving somewhat open the question of whether these deviations were present at the onset of stuttering. Inasmuch as brain differences are the results of the genetic factor, there is good reason to believe they are present from the beginning. It is possible, however, that, with time, they become increasingly pronounced in cases of more pathological persistent stuttering. Certainly, much more research with increasing focus on young children soon after stuttering onset is warranted.

Already a decade ago, one speech scientist asserted that when relevant research with adults is examined, on balance it would appear to suggest that the speech production processes of those who stutter are somewhat different from those of normally fluent individuals (Kent, 2000). Such conclusions, however, would be more constrained in regard to young children who stutter for whom limited research has shown small differences from normally fluent peers. Inasmuch as there is a biological basis for stuttering, it is reasonable to assume that motor problems are present from the beginning, though perhaps to a milder degree. These children may initially exhibit different thresholds for sensorimotor perturbation. Here too, an alternative explanation is that the reported dysfunctions in adults may represent compensations or anticipations for the possibility of stuttering. If a theory of motor dysfunction underlying stuttering is to be validated, considerably more research is needed to uncover the nature of the dysfunction. We conclude that the current state of the art in genetics, brain anatomy and physiology, and motor dysfunctions of people who stutter reveals growing evidence for a generally unstable/unreliable neuromotor system for speech.

Among the key points made in this chapter are the following:

- Familial incidence, twin studies, and gene analysis research has provided strong evidence for genetic contributions to the etiology of stuttering.

- Both the structure and function of the brains of PWS are different from those of NFS. It is not clear, however, whether or not these are the result of stuttering.

- Differences in motor activity during stuttering have been found in nearly every region of the vocal tract (lips, jaw, vocal folds, and respiration) but no particular dysfunction is common to all people who stutter.

- Recent research suggests neuromotor differences in children who stutter compared to their fluent peers.

- Differences in muscle activation sequencing and slower rate of movements during fluent speech reinforce the possibility of motor dysfunction underlying stuttering.

- The apparent loss of motor speech control experienced by PWS provides the necessary background for motor theories of stuttering.

- Models of motor learning and tests of related principles could be helpful in understanding the nature of stuttering and fluent speech change.

Study Questions and Discussion Topics

1. What observations about stuttering would seem to make it reasonable to hypothesize that stuttering may have a neurophysiological basis?
2. Why study the fluent speech of people who stutter?
3. What kinds of evidence have supported genetic components to stuttering? Explain.
4. What kinds of evidence have supported brain structure and function as factors underlying stuttering?
5. What evidence has supported a relationship between stuttering and audition?
6. Explain Zimmermann's theory of stuttering as a motor disorder.
7. Explain how it can be that stuttering is associated with so many different dimensions of the physical and neurophysiological system.
8. How would treatment for stuttering differ if research were to reveal that the specific cause of stuttering was:
   a. a genetic defect?
   b. a brain abnormality?
   c. an auditory processing dysfunction?
   d. a motor system deviance?
   e. a respiratory system dysfunction?

Suggested Readings

De Nil, L. F. (1997). Stuttering: A neurophysiological perspective. In N. Bernstein Ratner & C. Healey (Eds.), *Current perspectives in stuttering: Nature and treatment.* Hillsdale, NJ: Erlbaum.

Kraft, S., & Yairi, E. (2012). Genetic bases of stuttering: The state of the art, 2011. *Folia Phoniatrica and Logopaedica, 64,* 34–47.

Ludlow, C., & Loucks, T. (2003). Stuttering: A dynamic motor control disorder. *Journal of Fluency Disorders, 28,* 273–295.

MacPherson, M., & Smith, A. (2013). Influences of sentence length and syntactic complexity on the speech motor control of children who stutter. *Journal of Speech, Language, and Hearing Research, 56,* 89–102.

Watkins, K., Smith, S., Davis, S., & Howell, P. (2008). Structural and functional abnormalities of the motor system in developmental stuttering. *Brain, 131,* 50–59.

Chapter 8

Assessment of Adults and School-Age Children

LEARNER OBJECTIVES

Readers of this chapter will understand:

- The purposes and rationale for the initial evaluation of stuttering and its components.
- Appropriate stuttering evaluation procedures.
- Specific procedures for recording speech and the various methods of disfluency analyses and measures available.
- How stuttering severity is evaluated.
- Administration and scoring of different available scales/checklists/assessment protocols for stuttering.
- How to interpret comprehensive evaluation data, make recommendations for therapy based on assessment results, and prepare professional clinical reports.

General Considerations

Assessment of Stuttering

There is wisdom in the maxim attributed to Charles Kettering that "a problem well-stated is a problem half-solved." The goal of assessment is to articulate an understanding of the nature of a presenting disorder and associated communication difficulties, so that appropriate treatment objectives and activities may be pursued. One end result of an assessment is a *diagnosis*, which refers to the identification of a specific condition usually not apparent at the beginning. For example, in medicine, when a patient complains about abdominal pain, the underlying problem must be isolated from the range of possible ailments, such as food poisoning, ulcers, ruptured appendix, cancer, and so on. This is not the case with advanced stuttering, where just about all those who seek professional help state the correct diagnosis, *stuttering*, when they first contact the clinician. Given this reality, with some qualifications to be addressed next, *the main assessment task is that of characterization and quantification of the client's stuttering and related factors,* not the search for an unconfirmed diagnosis.

Differentiation

As stated, a classic diagnostic objective is the differentiation of a client's problem from other possible clinical entities. For a long time, stuttering has been viewed as a single disorder. Delineation and application of meaningful clinical subtypes began to be examined more closely only recently. It has been suggested that stuttering subtype distinctions could be based on etiological factors, gender, personality, stuttering characteristics, language abilities, concomitant disorders, among other things (Seery et al., 2007; Yairi, 2007). Although an acceptable subtype system for stuttering is not currently available, a few distinctions can be made. For example, diagnoses may differentiate psychogenic versus neurogenic stuttering or developmental versus acquired disorders (Seery, 2005). Therefore, clinicians engaged in assessment should be aware of the fine details of fluency disorders and be prepared to differentiate possible subtypes of stuttering, as well as stuttering from other fluency disorders, such as cluttering and language-based disfluency. Although false diagnoses of stuttering in school-age children and adults are not common, there are times when teachers, parents, and pediatricians refer children to speech-language clinicians because they diagnosed the problem as stuttering when the issue is actually another fluency problem, such as cluttering, or not even a fluency issue. Clinicians need to listen closely to their clients' concerns, carefully observe structure and function of the speech and hearing mechanism, appraise normal and abnormal communication characteristics, and recognize the barriers that prevent clients from speaking normally. More about assessment of fluency disorders other than stuttering is covered in Chapter 15.

The general components of a stuttering assessment are not substantially different from those applied in the evaluation of other communicative disorders. They include:

- Gathering background and case history information
- Observing speech production in multiple, controlled speaking contexts
- Assessing the severity of the overt stuttered speech as well as that of the overall disorder
- Assessing other communication problems as well as motor and health issues
- Discerning factors contributing to the communication difficulties.

Where assessment of stuttering differs, however, is the relatively large variability in the disorder and the special concern given to evaluating the client's emotional reactions associated with the speaking difficulties, as well as his or her attitudes about speaking. This difference reflects the often large emotional component of advanced stuttering. As we explained in Chapter 4, this component can be more of a problem to the client than the core overt stuttering by itself.

Multidimensionality

One reason why it is especially important to expand the evaluation beyond the speech domain is the multidimensionality of the stuttering disorder. Consistent with ASHA's knowledge competency standards for the assessment of communication disorders, speech-language clinicians must be prepared to consider the "etiologies, characteristics, anatomical/physiological, acoustic, psychological, developmental, and linguistic and cultural correlates" (ASHA, 2008b) of fluency disorders. In the case of stuttering, although assessment of these correlates do not typically lead to the identification of the direct etiology of the disorder, it does help to reveal how individual abilities and characteristics in these correlates (domains) contribute to the complex picture of what triggers stutter events and why the disorder persists.

Several commercial instruments are available to guide the clinician through a comprehensive fluency assessment. One example is the Overall Assessment of the Speaker's Experience of Stuttering (OASES; see Yaruss & Quesal, 2006). With this protocol, the clinician analyzes information about the total stuttering disorder, including the client's (1) broad views of stuttering; (2) affective, behavioral, and cognitive reactions to stuttering; (3) functional communication difficulties; and (4) the impact of stuttering on the quality of life. Speech is addressed in section 3 related to communication difficulties. Another instrument, the CALMS, addresses five key components believed to be central to maintaining stuttering: (1) cognitive, (2) affective, (3) linguistic, (4) motor, and (5) social factors (Healey, Scott-Trautman, & Susca, 2004). The model is intended to highlight the individual differences among those who stutter as well as relative strengths and weaknesses among the five CALMS components.

Variability

One of the hallmarks of stuttering is its variability. Rarely does a person who stutters produce all the possible stuttering behaviors, yet some who stutter may not even demonstrate the usual features (Barr, 1940). Stutter events vary both across and within individuals who stutter. Within the same individual, the severity and types of stutter events can vary considerably at different times and in different situations. As described in Chapter 4, certain situational contexts (e.g., talking with an infant, saying typically automatic phrases) can be ameliorating conditions, whereas others can be aggravating conditions (e.g., saying one's name, talking on the telephone). Although there are trends of stuttering variability that are similar across clients, such as the contexts just mentioned, responses to speaking conditions are different across individuals. One client may seldom stutter during interpersonal conversation but have severe stuttering events during oral reading or talking over the telephone. Another client may rarely stutter in oral reading but exhibit severe stuttering during conversation. Hence it is desirable to obtain speech samples in a variety of conditions so that the range of variability and the influence of different contexts for a particular client are appreciated by the clinician.

Special Considerations for School-Age Children

For the sake of minimizing unnecessary repetition, this chapter addresses the initial evaluation of both adults and schoolchildren. Although there are several important procedural modifications necessitated by age differences, the commonalities, such as the kind of information sought or the specific procedures of analyzing speech samples, prevail. Thus when a clinician applies the information presented here, the procedures should be adapted flexibly to suit adults, high school students, or children in elementary school.

Typically, an initial evaluation of adults involves only the client who provides the history background, fills out questionnaires, and offers a relatively mature level of self-awareness of emotions and attitudes. Most high school students are able to function similarly but may lack information pertaining to their history. They should be able to respond to most of the case history questions listed later in the chapter. It is obvious, however, that a question about the person's wife or children's reactions to stuttering should be skipped or reworded to fit the particular individual's circumstances. For many children, asking about parents' and siblings' reactions would be more appropriate. The presence of one or both parents is welcome and may be helpful, but it is not essential for the narrow purpose of the evaluation. Relevant missing information may be secured at a later time.

By contrast, a full evaluation of a third grader would greatly benefit from a parent's participation. Many of the case history questions can be answered more surely by the parent, not only regarding the stuttering history but regarding emotional reactions, social impact, and so on. It is wise to interview the parent alone before talking with the child to be aware of potential problems and behaviors, and to be able to more effectively direct the interview with the child. Again, a good number of questions from the list can be presented but with wording altered to suit the child's age, apparent behavior, maturity, and intellectual aptitude. It is also important to examine the complete profile of the child's communication abilities (i.e., articulation and language testing), as well as the academic impact of stuttering. In addition to parents, the clinician may need to interview other persons important to the client, such as teachers and professionals who have evaluated or treated the child for stuttering or other communication disorders. In the table of case history questions, presented later, the last section contains extra questions that may be especially relevant for school-age children. The Communication Attitude Test (CAT) and Self-Efficacy for Adolescents Scale (SEA Scale) are additional tools designed specifically for this age group. As mentioned, procedures for recording and analyzing speech samples are similar to those used with adults. Some children, however, are less verbal or cannot read well enough, requiring more flexibility in obtaining sufficient speech samples, using passages appropriate to the child's ability level. Finding topics of special interest to the child can be particularly important to enhancing the client's motivation and receptivity.

Assessment Objectives

Based on the previous discussion points, we propose a set of eight evaluation objectives for the adult/adolescent/school-age child fluency assessment. Specifically those aims are designed to:

1. Establish rapport with the client.
2. Obtain background and case history information.
3. Describe the client's speech characteristics.
4. Understand the client's home, social, and work environment.

5. Identify conditions and variables affecting the client's speech.
6. Understand the impact of the communication disorder on the individual's life.
7. Provide information about the nature of fluency/stuttering and its treatment.
8. Recommend a plan of action for the client.

Background and Case History

The purpose of the case history portion of a clinical evaluation is to provide an *organized record* of all the relevant information concerning the client's condition, problem, or disorder that might be useful in its treatment and related counseling. This may encompass a detailed account of factors ranging from the initial onset and development, to the current status of the stuttering. In the case of children, the history includes such details as the home environment and family background (e.g., genetic factors, family dynamics, and attitudes), parental and/or caregiver legal rights over the client, and whether stuttering varies predictably in any conditions (e.g., emotional responses, certain settings/people, time of day). Also very important is information about the nature and effects of present or past treatment. Although not all of the data collected may eventually prove useful, the case history provides clinicians with an overall picture of the problem at hand, sometimes with critical information as to what direction to pursue in treatment or which ones to avoid.

The initial contact with the client and the circumstances surrounding the referral for services are important foundations for the entire assessment and remediation process. During the first moments of interaction with the client, the clinician begins to establish the rapport and trust that will open the lines of communication between them. In Chapter 10 we elaborate on the clinician's qualities that underlie an ideal client-clinician relationship, so critical for successful therapeutic processes. For now, let it just be said that clinicians need to develop and express genuine interest in their clients as people, and have the strength of courage and understanding to journey along with clients on the ups and downs of their path to improved speech.

The circumstances of referral can make a major difference in the trajectory of the treatment process. If a client is self-referred, has individually reached a point of courage and resolve to enter into the treatment process, then foundations for change have already been established. In contrast, if an employer, professor, or family member has urged the client to seek help, and the client is undertaking the therapy mainly to please others, then the process could already be jeopardized. In the latter case, the clinician will need to devote time to educating both the client and those who referred him or her about the nature of treatment and the critical matter of the client's independent motivation and readiness to undertake the difficult, sometimes arduous, process of change.

Table 8.1 lists a set of potential case history questions to be included during the initial interview with the client. The question "What do you do when you stutter?" is particularly important because it begins the process of examining the stuttering as a behavior on the part of the client. It also reveals the client's understanding of stuttering and whether there is readiness to discuss it in terms of his or her own initiated speech

---

Table 8.1   Case History Topic Areas and Potential Interview Questions

I. Stuttering History

a. Do you remember, or have you been told about, when you began stuttering?
b. From how far back do you remember stuttering?
c. Are you aware of any factors/events surrounding the time of on-set? Do you think any of these was the cause of the stuttering?
d. How has stuttering progressed over time? Has it been up and down? Only gone up? Only down? About the same all the time?
e. Have there ever been time periods, for example, several weeks, when you hardly stuttered at all?
f. Have any other relatives stuttered? Who? When? Did any of them stop stuttering? Who? When?

II. Treatment History

a. Who referred you to us?
b. Have you received any treatment? When? Where?
c. How long did each treatment last? Frequency of sessions?
d. What were the therapy approaches?
e. What were the results for each treatment?
f. What technique has helped you the most? And the least?
g. What led you to seek help at the time(s) you did?
h. What led to your interest in therapy right now?

III. Current Speech Description

a. Currently, what are your main problems related to your speech?
b. How would you describe your speech and your stuttering?
c. What do you do when you stutter? (Show me.)
d. What is the severity range of your stuttering—is it mild, moderate, or severe? What is the most common severity? In what situations?
e. Do you know when you are going to stutter?
f. Describe what you experience/feel/think just *before* you stutter.
g. What do you experience/feel/think *during* stuttering?
h. How do you react/feel *after* you have stuttered?
i. What kinds of things do you do to cope with stuttering moments? (Clinicians should probe for avoidance/postponement methods and speech modifications.)

IV. Environmental Variables Affecting Speech

a. What increases your stuttering? (e.g., places, situations, friends, other people, sounds, words)
b. What decreases your stuttering? When is speech easier for you?
c. When do you stutter the most? The least?
d. How much talking do you do each day? In what settings?
e. With whom do you usually talk (family, friends, colleagues, superiors, strangers)?
f. How do others respond to your stuttering (friends, teachers, strangers)?
g. What are your plans related to school? Are you attending school now? If not, when did you last attend school? Has your school situation been comfortable regarding your speech?
h. What are your plans related to work? Are you working now? Part or full time? Where? If not, when did you last work? Where? Is your work situation comfortable in regard to your speech?

V. Impact of Stuttering on Quality of Life

a. Does stuttering affect your relationships with family? With whom? How? (If married, with spouse and/or children? If young, with parents and/or siblings?)
b. Does stuttering affect your social life? How?
c. Do you ever talk about stuttering? If so, with whom?
d. Has stuttering affected your school achievements?
e. Has stuttering affected your choice (or plans) of career or job/vocation?
f. Does stuttering affect you in any way we haven't mentioned?
g. If you didn't stutter, how do you think life would change?

VI. Other Relevant Case History

a. Have you ever had any other speech or language difficulty?
b. Any difficulty reading or writing?
c. Is English your first and only language?
d. Have you tended to move a lot or live mostly in one location? Has moving been associated with changes in the stuttering? How?
e. Are you currently taking medication that could affect speech? If so, what medication? For what health condition? Does this health condition affect your speech in general? The stuttering? How?
f. Have you ever had difficulty hearing? When was your last hearing test?

(continued)

Table 8.1   (Continued)

VII. Client's Perspective	a. Do your feelings and mood affect your speech? How?
	b. How would you describe yourself as a person? For example, easygoing, serious, ambitious, good-humored, energetic/calm, persistent/easily gives up, self-confident or unsure, enjoys people, afraid of new situations.
	c. During this interview, has your speech/stuttering been typical? Better or worse than usual? How?
	d. What do you know about stuttering?
	e. What do you believe causes stuttering?
	f. How important is your speech therapy goal? (Relative to other goals?)
	g. What do you hope/expect to gain from speech therapy?
	h. What do you think you will need to do to change your speech?
	i. Are you ready to make those changes?
	j. Do you have any questions?
VIII. Identifying Information	a. Who referred you?
	b. Check spelling of name, correct birth date, current address, phones, and so on. Where/how do you wish to be contacted?
	c. Are there others (doctor, family, caseworkers) with whom you would like for us to share information regarding your speech services? (Be sure to fill out proper consent forms.)
	d. Do you wish for a copy of our evaluation report to be sent to your home? And/or reviewed with you, in person?
IX. Additional Questions for School-Age Children	**For interviewing children:**
	a. Do you go to school? What grade are you in?
	b. What subjects do you like most? Least?
	c. Are you in any after-school activities? Sports? Music? Hobbies?
	d. What do you like to do best? Why?
	e. Tell me about some things you do well.
	f. Do you like talking? How much talking do you do each day? Where? With whom?
	g. Do you participate in class discussions? Answer questions?
	h. Do other children make fun of your stuttering?
	i. Are your teachers understanding of your stuttering problem?

For interviewing parents:

a. Does stuttering affect how [child's name] does in school?

b. Does [child's name] stutter the same at school and at home?

c. Aside from speech, does [child's name] struggle with any other areas (for example, in school or with developing other skills)?

d. Is a typical day for [child's name] fairly calm or busy? How/Why?

e. Are there frequent big family gatherings?

f. Does he or she play with neighborhood children? Do they get along? Has teasing been an issue? How has it been handled?

g. Does [child's name] prefer to play alone? or with others? Has stuttering appeared to affect play or socializing?

h. Does stuttering affect your family or you in any way(s) we haven't mentioned?

i. How important do you think speech is to [child's name]?

movements and consequent emotional reactions, or just how much it is ascribed to a mysterious extraneous force or impulse that arises out of nowhere, over which the client has no control (Williams, 1957). Later on, in therapy, the clinician will strive to have the client develop a point of view of stuttering in which his or her own doing is a big part of the disorder. Finally, even if the client is able to discuss stuttering in terms of self-initiated behaviors, there can be a certain amount of mismatch between the characterization of stuttering events and reactions described by the client and what the clinician observes. In some cases, the clinician will need to observe much more in order to develop an understanding of what the client is experiencing. In other cases, the clinician will need to guide the client toward an improved level of self-awareness to promote therapeutic change.

Another important question centers on the client's attitudes and expectations. Is the client expecting that the clinician will impart a treatment, for example, sets of prescribed exercises, a powerful electrical stimulation, hypnosis, or all sorts of other treatments that should do the job of removing the stuttering? Or does the client understand that she or he will have to work diligently toward a process of multiple changes, keep practicing new speaking behaviors, altered emotional reactions and social interaction, and move out of his or her comfort zones to accomplish the various therapy objectives? If the client expects the former, then the clinician will need to devote time to educating the client about the nature of speech therapy for stuttering, the essential approach, and the work to be done to accomplish change. That is, therapy is not about "fixing" stuttering for the client but is aimed at providing the client with skills and abilities that will have to be practiced to deal effectively with stuttering and improve communication. *Clients ought to realize that stuttering therapy often requires doing the very things that they least like to do,* such as speak on the telephone, talk to strangers, make oral presentations to groups, and so on.

Each individual will have his or her own painful memories and strong emotions related to stuttering that may need to be released. The clinician must be ready to listen closely to the expressed feelings, appreciate the client's perspective, and offer reassurance that it is safe to expose those feelings and experiences in the clinician's presence. The clinician's acceptance of the client's feelings and experiences, just as they are, is apt to go far in promoting progress. Because the client may need to enhance skills of self-comfort in the wake of emotional distress, the clinician can note and validate such skills of self-understanding as the client may already evidence.

Observations and Examinations: Speech

Speech Sample Context

Inasmuch as disfluent speech is the cardinal feature of stuttering, analyses of speech samples typically play a central role in the assessment of the disorder. They are the means by which fluency, disfluency, and associated conditions are observed and quantified for the sake of diagnosis and treatment decisions. Due to the variability of stuttering across situations, at least two, ideally three, separate speech sample contexts are recommended for a reliable and valid evaluation (Gregory, 2003; Riley, 2009). With adolescents and adults, those usually consist of a spontaneous speech sample, such as conversation or monologue, oral reading, and another speaking context with individual relevance (e.g., classroom, group discussion, phone call, etc.).

A conversation and monologue are different in that there is frequent turn taking during conversation. In contrast, a relatively continuous stream of speech is delivered during a monologue. If the clinician speaks as little as possible to encourage a monologue, the collection of a large sample can be accomplished more quickly than if there is an exchange of conversational speaking turns. Hence a monologue is a more efficient means to reach the goal of quickly obtaining a large speech sample for type/frequency analysis of disfluencies. A monologue, however, is not the most common form of daily speaking context; if a primarily valid and representative sample of speech is desired, conversation may be a better choice. Conversation, with its many shifting topics and potential interruptions, may also exert more pressure on the client, thus providing more examples of stuttering events.

To elicit a spontaneous monologue, the examiner prompts with requests such as "Tell me about your hobbies/interests," or "Tell me about the work you do." A standard monologue elicitation procedure known as the *job task* (Johnson, 1961a) is conducted by asking the client to talk for 3 minutes about a current job or vocation, future jobs or those held in the past, or current school classes and other activities to prepare for employment. To secure continuous speech, the client should also be asked to talk about why she or he chose the job, as well as anything else about it that would be interesting to discuss. The client is given a minute or so to prepare before starting. If the client stops talking too soon, the clinician prompts with additional questions to elicit more talking. For a monologue sample, the clinician should note whether any adaptation occurs with continued talking, that is, some speakers tend to become more fluent as they keep talking. Such adaptation may suggest a milder or more readily modified form of stuttering.

Sometimes, for efficiency, a clinician might choose to record the initial interview as a form of conversational speech sample. If this context is selected, considerations may be given to whether the sample is representative of daily conversations. The topics discussed in the initial interview could elicit either more mild or more severe forms of stuttering than are typically encountered. There is an argument to be made in favor of obtaining a speech sample that reveals the full extent of the client's stuttering severity rather than just the average level. It is important to obtain information about the client's level of education and reading ability prior to selection of the reading passage. This will prevent the uncomfortable experience of asking a client to read material that is either way beyond or way below his or her abilities. An important factor in deciding the sample context is whether the clinician will compare the client's disfluency in terms of type and frequency or any other measure of stuttering, only to other speech samples generated by the client (relational assessment), or to published reference data (normative assessment). If the latter is the goal, a valid comparison depends on selection of a sample context that reasonably matches the one(s) used to generate the normative data set.

Other Speaking Conditions

There are many other possible speaking conditions and factors related to a client's stuttering that the clinician may wish to observe and evaluate. Because often people who stutter are relatively more fluent on shorter, less complex utterances, it may be useful to observe speech on a set of sentences that are systematically increased in length and linguistic complexity. Similarly, the clinician may want to observe the client's speech in tasks such as picture naming, automatic series, imitation and unison, to appreciate which demands and conditions aid or stress fluency. If a client's stuttering tends to be mild, the client may agree that the clinician should observe speech under added stress factors such as speaking on the telephone, time pressure, interruptions, with groups, and so on. Therapeutic probes may be employed to observe how well the client responds to various fluency-enhancing techniques or to identification and modification instructions.

As with any speech-language assessment, the examiner should not neglect to note other possible disabilities or factors that may influence the client's speech and communication skills. These may be in areas of articulation, phonology, vocabulary, syntax, semantics, pragmatics, attention, cognition, word-finding, fine/gross motor skills, oral-peripheral/oral-motor skills, voice/resonance, intonation/prosody, respiration, and hearing/auditory processing.

Speech Sample Size

How long should a speech sample be to obtain valid and reliable data for analysis of stuttering? This is not an easy question to answer. So far, only two studies have compared disfluency data from different sample sizes: one with adults who stutter and one with adults who do not stutter. Both reported nonsignificant differences for the number of disfluencies more typical of stuttering among speech samples ranging from 300 to 1,800 syllables (Logan & Haj Tas, 2007; Roberts, Meltzer, & Wilding, 2009). Some sources suggest a modest 200 syllables for each situation or speaking mode: conversation and oral reading (Riley, 1994), or 300 to 400 words (Shapiro, 1999). Others recommended an amount of speaking time, such as 3 or 5 minutes (Roberts et al., 2009; Ward, 2006). Several sources addressing evaluation do not specify speech sample size (e.g., Manning, 2001). Initial information directly relevant to the effect of speech sample size was provided by Sawyer and Yairi (2006) based on samples of speech from preschool CWS. They reported that longer samples, upward of 1,200 syllables, were necessary to capture all the relevant disfluent speech behaviors and especially for differentiating cases near borderline stuttering. It is unjustified at the present, however, to generalize this finding to adolescents and adults.

One of us (Seery) requires at least 300 words or syllables for the adult spontaneous speech sample, either conversation or monologue. She reasons that if the measure will be per 100 units, then 300 will be 3 times greater than the sampling unit basis. When evaluating baseline measures, at least three data points are required to establish a trend (Barlow, Hayes, & Nelson, 1984). In contrast, a minimum standard of 600 syllables was advocated by Yairi and Ambrose (2005). They argue that the larger sample size is necessary to sample certain disfluency types adequately, for example, disrhythmic phonations or repetitions of four or more units (e.g., "Bu-bu-bu-bu-but"), which generally occur at a much lower frequency than other disfluencies, especially in mild to moderate stuttering, but yet are very important contributors to the overall impression of stuttering and its severity. They assert that "it is advisable to have at least three tokens for any given type of disfluency. Just one could be random, two are insufficient to identify a pattern or obtain a mean, but three indicate that the behavior is more than a fluke, presenting some semblance of pattern or typicality" (p. 106). Again, although their comments were made in regard to young children, it may be even more critical for older children who may have found ways to suppress their stuttering-like disfluencies and be at risk for under detection of their speech problem.

For the oral reading context, longer samples are usually not necessary to find out whether this condition differs from spontaneous speech samples. Although the "per 100 unit" basis will be applied in measurements, a paragraph of oral reading is often enough to reveal the severity of stuttering in that context. If the examiner is looking for adaptation or wants to establish a baseline frequency measure, then a passage of least 200 syllables would offer more representative data. The issue of sample size is important for the purpose of counting the frequency of specific disfluency types. This, however, is not the case if the clinician is interested only in assigning an overall rating of stuttering severity.

> The severity of stuttering can affect the decision about the size of the speech sample to collect. When stuttering appears to be severe, a short sample can suffice. The milder the stuttering, the longer the sample size necessary to rate severity with confidence. Severity also affects which measurement basis, time or syllable/word counts, is the meaningful denominator. When stuttering is quite severe, time is a more meaningful basis, for example, how much speech is produced in 3 minutes? Whether fluent or disfluent segments are measured can also be decided based on severity. For example, if blocks are many seconds long, the number of fluent words or syllables spoken could be more representative than the number of disfluencies per 100 words.

Measures of Stuttering or Disfluency

A variety of systems of analysis have been employed to measure and report the amount of stuttering in speech samples. Although they appear similar, important differences exist. For example, the frequency of stuttering per 100 words is quite different from the percentage of stuttered words. Both measures are based on the clinician's perception that some instances of stuttering occurred. The first measure, however, provides more accurate information in that it allows for counting more than one stuttering event on the same word (e.g., "A-a-ari-zo-zo-zo-na" has two events). The second measure allows for counting only one stuttering instance per word. Thus "A-a-ari-zo-zo-zo-na" is counted as only one stuttered word. As you can see, the first method reports twice as much stuttering for the same amount of speech. These measures of perceived stuttering events, however, do not provide information about the *kind* of stuttering that took place. They only reveal the *total number* of the events. A third measure, the objectively counted frequency of various disfluency types per 100 syllables or words, yields much more information on the specific characteristics of the client's speech. It not only reveals how many interruptions are contained in the speech but also *provides specific descriptions of them, discriminating among repetitions, sound prolongations, interjections, and other types or forms.* How the person stutters is meaningful information to have.

In 1988, Kully and Boberg sent an identical set of speech samples to multiple clinical sites to be analyzed for stuttering frequency, and they discovered that the approaches and the actual event counts differed substantially across sites. Although their specific procedures and findings have been seriously questioned (Ryan, 1997; Yairi, 1997[1]), such disagreement can be understood given the fact that there are many ways in which stuttering has been quantified. The major differences among metrics of stuttering come from two parameters: (1) the target characteristics of interest and, (2) the units over which they are measured. The target(s) of interest, that is, what is being measured[2] may

---

[1]Yairi (1997, p. 54) stated that "although Kully and Boberg (1988) emphasized the disagreement among clinics in identifying stuttering and disfluencies, an inspection of their Table 2 reveals that the average agreement between the two clinics which counted 'percent disfluency' was 81.7%, a respectable level that was considerably better than agreement among clinics which counted 'percent stuttering.'"

[2]See discussions by Yairi (1997) and Yairi & Ambrose (2005).

be any of the following: perceived stuttering events also referred to as "moments," or "instances," of stuttering; descriptive disfluency types; or perceptually fluent speech. The sampling units may be syllables, words, or time intervals.

A variety of measurements are possible based on different combinations of the target event (e.g., disfluencies, stutters) and sampling units (e.g., syllables, words, utterances, time intervals). The *frequency of disfluencies* represents the average number of disfluencies per 100 sampling units in connected speech. To calculate this measure, *all* disfluent instances (more than one per word or syllable) are counted and the total sampling units (e.g., words or syllables) actually spoken are counted. For example, if the speaker displayed 20 disfluencies during 400 words, then the frequency is 5 per 100 words. Several considerations are important to the application of this measurement:

- The result should not be worded as a *percent* of sampling units because some words may contain several disfluencies.
- Only the actual number of syllables or words spoken should be counted as sampling units. If a client read a passage composed of 200 syllables, but omitted several words so the syllables spoken were actually 175, then the actual number 175, not 200, should be used in the calculation to represent the total sampling units.
- This type of metric is not valid when the sample size is substantially less than 100 words. If the client produced 10 disfluencies in only 20 spoken words, it is not appropriate to convert the frequency of disfluencies to 50 per 100 words. The examiner cannot presume to know that this many disfluencies would have occurred in a larger sample in which the speaker may have acclimated to the speaking task to experience more fluency.
- The formula to calculate the frequency of disfluency: Divide the total disfluencies by the total syllables (or words) spoken, and multiply the outcome by 100.
- An alternative shortcut to the calculation formula: Multiply the total number of disfluencies in the sample by 100 (just add two zeros), and then divide by the total number of syllables (or words).

Another type of measure is *percent syllables or words stuttered*. To obtain this metric, each sampling unit (i.e., word or syllable) is examined for whether stuttering is present. For example the number of stuttered words could be 25 among 250 total words, or 10 percent words stuttered. Table 8.2 shows the formulas for several types of speech behavior analyses.

A clinician who specializes in stuttering will want to shift flexibly among these methods, depending on the assessment needs. If a clinician wants to obtain a severity rating using the Stuttering Severity Instrument (SSI-4) by Riley (2009), then the percentage of syllables (not words) stuttered metric would be applied. If, however, there is an interest in analyzing the specific types of disfluent characteristics displayed by the client, then a calculation of disfluencies per 100 words (or syllables) could be used. Both of these methods of analysis are based on the clinician's careful review of previously recorded

Table 8.2 The Target Behaviors, Sampling Units, and Formulas for the Various Measures of Stuttering from Speech Sample

Type of Measure	Target Feature	Sampling Unit	Formula
Disfluency frequency per 100 syllables or words	Descriptive disfluencies according to type	Syllables or words	$\dfrac{\text{No. disfluencies} \times 100}{\text{No. syllables or No. words}}$
Percentage of words stuttered	Perceived stuttering	Words	$\dfrac{\text{No. stuttered words} \times 100}{\text{No. words}}$
Fluency frequency index	Perceived fluency	Words	$\dfrac{\text{No. fluent words} \times 100}{\text{No. words}}$
Frequency of stuttered intervals	Perceived stuttering	5-s intervals (or shorter) of speech	$\dfrac{\text{No. stuttered intervals} \times 100}{\text{No. intervals}}$

audiovisual speech samples and are referred to as *offline* analysis. Alternatively, if during a clinical session, a reliable live (*online*)[3] method of stuttering data collection is desired, judgments of whether 3- to 5-second time intervals in the sample contain stuttering might be helpful (Cordes & Ingham, 1994, 1999). There are some handheld devices and smartphone applications that a clinician might use to collect these data. When this method is used, the step of transcription of the words spoken by the client is typically bypassed. A simple calculation of the percentage of stuttered syllables to total syllables is made to complete the analysis.

Another measure that may be useful to assess progress in stuttering treatment is the fluency frequency index (FFI), based on the number of fluent words per total words (Shapiro, 1999). Of course, this is not a direct measure of the stuttering per se. It provides information about the amount of speech not affected by the disorder and may help focus the client's attention on fluent rather than disfluent speech. In sum, there is no universally adopted system of speech sample analysis for purposes of evaluation of stuttering and fluency. Clinicians may opt to employ a single method with which they feel comfortable or train themselves in several methods that they are capable of using as the need arises.

Several additional methods have been proposed for measuring fluent, also called *stutter-free*, periods of speech. Costello and Ingham (1984) offered the following two measures, among several more: the average *duration* of the three longest nonstuttered intervals measured in seconds and/or minutes, and the average *length* of the

---

[3]Note that the term *online* here is synonymous with "live" and must not be confused with the common but entirely different meaning of "being connected to the Internet."

three longest nonstuttered intervals measured in numbers of syllables. An alternative to measuring fluent time periods is the measurement of disfluent time. Starkweather, Gottwald, and Halfond (1990) suggested the percent time disfluent (PTD) measure. PTD is derived by summing up the duration of all disfluencies in a sample, then calculating its percentage of the total duration of the sample. In a later publication, Starkweather and Givens-Ackerman (1997) referred to this same measure as the percentage of discontinuous speech time (PDST). Although sometimes measures like these are useful for showing progress with treatment, *they do not reflect the client's specific stuttering pattern.*

> Another train car analogy (see Chapter 6) may help illustrate the different ways speech samples may be analyzed. The general question is: How much cargo is there? One way to find an answer is to look in each train car for whether it contains boxes of cargo, count the cars with cargo in them, and divide by the total number of train cars to arrive at the percentage of train cars with cargo. This method is like measuring percentage syllables (or words) stuttered. Another way to find an answer is to count all the boxes of cargo in the entire train, then divide by the total number of train cars. This calculation yields the number of cargo boxes per train car. By multiplying that number by 100, the number (frequency) of cargo boxes per 100 train cars is estimated. This latter method is like measuring the frequency of stuttering (or disfluencies) per 100 syllables (or words). The information yielded by the two ways of obtaining measures is different.

Speech Recordings and Transcription

Audiovisually recorded samples are more desirable than audio samples alone because visual information aids in the interpretation of an obscure disfluent event that is difficult to classify. For example, a silent pause may represent a type of disfluency, such as a static oral posture, or it could simply be a moment when the client stopped talking to think about something. An audio-recorded sample, however, may be a useful backup if the video technology fails. The recording system should be checked in advance for sound clarity and unwanted noise. The gain control switch should be turned off in recorders that have this feature to avoid variations in loudness and loss of some speech, especially at the beginning of utterances. Another decision regarding *video* recordings has to do with what view of the client to frame (e.g., full face, full body, upper body, etc.). Because it is of interest to capture potential secondary behaviors that can involve arm movements as well as upper body posturing, it is desirable to obtain a video image that includes the upper body from the waist to the head, at a distance close enough to reveal oral postures and facial expressions.

Once a speech sample is recorded, the next step is making a written transcription of it to facilitate detailed analyses. For this task, it is usually best to start by transcribing only the client's words in an utterance without noting the disfluencies. The next step, disfluency analysis, will be easier as each spoken utterance is distinguished in the transcript by starting it on the next line. Knowledge of the context of the words beforehand aids in resolving challenging questions, such as whether an utterance was a word "a" or an interjection "uh." In our practice, we review (listen to) the recorded speech sample as many times as necessary to ensure the most valid and reliable transcript as the basis for the analysis.

Procedures for Speech Sample Analysis

After all the words in the speech sample have been determined, the examiner can then listen again to the utterances, marking the location of the specific target according to the clinician's preferred measure or the particular need. It is also helpful to add in the transcript any comments or behavioral observations that could aid interpretation later (e.g., "started to speak before examiner finished" or "coughed and scratched his head"). Notes about secondary behaviors (e.g., "looks away," "gasped," "head jerk," "lip tension," etc.) are also useful to include where applicable in the transcript. Braces can be used to set these apart from the spoken words.

If *percentage of stuttered words* is the desired measure, each word perceived with confidence as stuttered is marked. As explained earlier, the stuttered words are then counted and their percentage in the total number of words in the speech sample is calculated. Example: In a 369-word sample containing 23 stuttered words, the percentage of words stuttered is $23/369 \times 100 = 6.23\%$.

If *percentage of stuttered syllables*[4] is the desired measure, the procedure is very similar. Each syllable perceived as stuttered is marked, the total number of syllables in the sample is counted, and the percentage of stuttered syllables is calculated. Example: In a speech sample of 443 syllables containing 65 stuttered syllables, the familiar math involved is as follows: $65/443 \times 100 = 14.67\%$.

When specific disfluency analysis is desired, the clinician indicates on the transcript each of several disfluency types (e.g., syllable repetition, interjection, sound prolongation), using a simple marking code. This can be aided by applying a different color highlighter for each type of disfluency where it occurs.

After the transcript is completely marked, the occurrence of each type in the sample is counted and its frequency per 100 syllables is calculated and tabulated. Then, the total frequency per 100 syllable of *all* types combined is derived. The clinician may also wish to derive subtotals of these disfluency types grouped as Stuttering-Like Disfluency (SLD) and Other Disfluency (OD), or other desired categories. A display of this type of analysis in a 566-word speech sample, in which a total of 147 disfluencies (25.97 per 100 words) were identified, is illustrated here (Table 8.3):

---

[4]In published literature, "percent syllables stuttered," "percent stuttered syllables," "percentage of stuttered syllables," and "percentage of syllables stuttered" are synonymous, as are parallel measures in which "words" is used in place of "syllables."

Table 8.3

Disfluency Type	Per 100 words
Part-word repetitions (45)	7.95
Whole-word repetitions (19)	3.36
Disrhythmic phonation (33)	5.83
SLD Subtotal (97)	**17.14**
Phrase repetitions (12)	2.12
Interjections (34)	6.01
Revisions (4)	0.71
OD Subtotal (50)	**8.83**
Disfluency Total (147)	**25.97**

Selection of Sampling Units

Prior to the analysis, the examiner must decide what sampling unit to apply, usually words or syllables. Several considerations are necessary. First, if comparisons will be made to published data sets, then the same constituents, words or syllables, must be applied in the analysis. If a direct match is not possible, adult sample estimates may be made by converting the word count to a syllable count (or vice versa), applying a 1.5:1 syllables-to-words ratio, whereas young children's speech, characterized by a larger percentage of monosyllabic words, is converted with a smaller ratio of approximately 1.15:1 (Yaruss, 2000).

> The following example illustrates the conversion of a syllable metric to a word metric: Suppose a 600-syllable speech sample was collected with 60 disfluencies. The frequency of disfluency is 10 per 100 syllables. If the clinician wants to compare this value to the norm, which is about 7 disfluencies per 100 words for adult spontaneous speech, then a conversion is needed. By applying the ratio of 1.5 syllables per word, the number of words is estimated by dividing 600 syllables by 1.5, yielding 400 words. The disfluency frequency can then be recalculated based on 60 disfluencies per 400 words, which would be 15 per 100 words. The result turns out to be considerably higher than the normative standard.

Second, there may be practical factors in the choice of unit applied. If word or syllable information is already available to the examiner (e.g., a reading paragraph), then time can be saved by moving directly to the analysis process. Third, there may be an interest in the nature of the disfluent speech relative to language or speech planning.

Conceptually, the number of words would better reflect the amount of language produced, whereas the number of syllables better reflects the amount of speech produced. The more multisyllabic words used by a speaker, the less the word count reflects the speech motor demands of the utterances because a word such as *aluminum* is reflected in the count just the same as the word *go*. Syllable counts are apt to capture such demands more closely. Finally, the total counts of either words or syllables tend to be more accurate when smaller sections of the speech sample are summed first. For example, next to each line in the transcript, the examiner would record the count of words or syllables, then for each section or page subtotals are derived, and finally the subtotals are added to arrive at the grand total of words or syllables.

Rules for Syllable or Word Counts

An essential rule for counting words or syllables in the speech samples of people who stutter is that the count should be based on the number of words or syllables that would have been spoken had there been no disfluent speech. For example, "bu-bu-bu-but" counts as one spoken syllable. Additionally, standard rules for what should, and should not, be counted as a word or syllable have been offered (Brown, 1973; Guitar, 2006; Retherford, 2000). We suggest the following three conventions, adapted from those sources:

1. Repeated, interjected word or phrase segments are not included in the counts.

   Thus "The ba-ba-ba-baby is uh uh crying" has 6 syllables, 4 words.

2. Words that precede or follow revisions *are* included in the word count.

   Thus "The infant—the baby is—has been crying" has 11 syllables, 8 words.

3. The following are considered to be one word:
   a. Expressions like "Oh boy" (2 syllables)
   b. Acronyms like "MTV"
   c. Proper names like "Mary Kay"
   d. Catenative forms such as "gonna" or "hafta"
   e. Ritualized reduplications such as "bye-bye" or "so-so"

Although some clinicians may prefer to exclude unfinished or abandoned words, we usually include any partial words that are still intelligible, counting only the portion that was actually uttered (e.g., "bana-" and "stra-" would be 2 syllables + 1 syllable = 3 syllables).

Additional rules ensure that word or syllable counts are not artificially inflated with a preponderance of utterance types that are either atypical, exceedingly short, or a known fluency-enhancing condition. Rules for the types of utterances to exclude from the analysis set are as follows:

- Direct quotes (precise imitation) of another person
- Words spoken or listed in a series ("One, two, three . . . A, B, C, D . . .")

- Words that are sung or automatically recited
- Isolated single-word utterances indicating yes or no
- Unintelligible words or syllables

Disfluency Reference Data

Appendix 8.1 (see end of this chapter) offers a reference for disfluency type/frequency data per 100 words for nonstuttering speakers based on two sources. Participants in the Yairi and Clifton (1972) study were younger and older adults, both males and females, who produced narrative speech samples of unspecified length in response to three picture cards. Participants in the White (2002) study were 30 men and women who produced narrative samples on four topics: a typical day in their life, how to drive a car, how to make a favorite meal, and how to change a car tire. Speech sample sizes ranged from 300 to 363 words. Note that, except for the category of interjection, the two studies provide reasonably similar data for the young adults. Disfluency data for reading (see Appendix 8.2) are based on the same set of participants in the White (2002) study, who read the 331-word Rainbow Passage (Fairbanks, 1960).

The reference data shown in appendices (8.1 and 8.2) reveal that among NFS disfluency frequency in oral reading is typically much less than in narrative tasks. For this reason, if an adult who stutters is prone to stutter when she or he reads aloud, it may be particularly noticeable in contrast to what a normally fluent speaker would do. Additional disfluency reference data are offered in Appendix 8.3. Here we selected a few data (rounded) from two studies and arranged them according to our system. The first, by Roberts, Meltzer, Wilding (2009), is the only source that provides information for normally fluent adults employing the per 100 syllables metric. It is based on spontaneous speech tasks of 30 men ages 20 to 51 years telling about their jobs and, hobbies, and explaining how a sport is played. No significant differences in overall disfluency frequency were found among the three topics or across three sample lengths, 300, 500, and 900 syllables. The second study by Conture and Brayton (1975) reported disfluency data in oral reading of 17 adults (13 men and 4 women) based on a 500-word sample. Note that the reference data shown in appendices (8.3 and 8.4) reveal inconsistency in the amount of disfluency by PWS generated by spontaneous speech and reading tasks. Individual clients are indeed different in this respect. Hence, clinicians should obtain data for both tasks.

Appendix 8.4 presents data reported by Silverman and Zimmer (1979), who recorded spontaneous speech samples from 20 participants (10 men, 10 women) with a mean of 965 words for the women and 882 words for the men. Although females produced significantly more part-word repetitions, word repetitions, and disrhythmic phonations statistically, the investigators concluded that women do not tend to have more severe stuttering than men. Also here note the inconsistency with the White (2002) study with NFS that found significantly higher disfluency frequency for men than for women.

There are surprisingly few disfluency type/frequency data reports for school-age children. Overall disfluency and within-word disfluency (similar to SLD) for 14 children (11 boys; 3 girls) who stutter, ages 5.5 to 11.5 years, based on 300-word conversation samples, were reported by Zebrowski (1994). Overall frequency of disfluency per 100 words ranged from 10 to 49 with a median of 16. Within-word (core) disfluency ranged from 4 to 36 with a median of 12 per 100 words.

Silverman (1974) published disfluency data according to frequency/type distribution for 56 school-age children who stutter and 56 normally fluent controls. Comparing oral reading and a story narrative, he concluded that the latter material provided better differentiation of the two groups. As reported by Silverman, the data presented in Appendix 8.5 are in the form of quartiles. The appendix displays figures for only the first three quartiles (Q1 = lowest 25% of subjects; Q2 = the second 25% of subjects; Q3 = the third 25% of subjects). We suggest that the 50% (Q2) figures may be applied clinically for a diagnostic reference (comparing the child's data to the stuttering group) or for establishing a therapy target for a child who stutters (reaching the nonstuttering group).[5]

Overall, the important observation to make from the various sources is the large differences between those who stutter and those who do not stutter in the critical subset of disfluencies referred to as within-word, core, or SLD. These are the most characteristic of stuttered speech and also tend to be perceived by listeners as stuttering. Note that the total mean for this subset of disfluencies for the normally fluent speakers in oral reading is less than 1. It is about 10 for those who stutter. Typically, at least three SLDs or core disfluencies is seen as the minimum required to classify speech as stuttering.

Stuttering Severity

In its most frequent usage, the term *stuttering severity* refers to the level of disruption in the delivery of continuous speech. There is a high correlation between the objective quantity of stuttered speech and listeners' ratings of stuttering severity (Young, 1961). The number of times speech is disrupted, the specific characteristics of the disfluent speech, and the duration/length of the disruptions usually affect judgments of the level of breakdown that has occurred.

Overt stuttering severity, however, does not necessarily reflect the impact of the total stuttering disorder. Some speakers do plenty of stuttering but experience minimal emotional reactions, and others have no disabilities or difficulties in social or

---

[5]It should be noted that Silverman's data were based only on male school-age children in second through sixth grades. As discussed in Chapter 9, preschool data yielded no significant differences between genders (Ambrose & Yairi, 1999). Some adolescent data revealed no significant differences between genders (De Oliveira Martins & Furquim de Andrade, 2008; Furquim de Andrade & De Oliveira Martins, 2007). We therefore suggest that the Silverman data are apt to be relatively applicable with either gender for children in elementary school.

vocational realms. Other speakers stutter mildly but experience intense disorder. The occasional overt instances of stuttering cause enough emotional distress to result in serious social or vocational debilitation. Although the impact of the disorder is ultimately important, this discussion is meant to highlight the point that the term *stuttering severity* is reserved for a description of the overt speech aspects rather than the disorder as a whole.

Clinicians may estimate the severity of stuttering in several ways. The simplest, devoid of any actual measurement or counting, is based on observing a client speak or read and then assigning a global rating on a subjective perceptual scale of stuttering severity. Clinicians seem to favor a 3-point scale with the most popular ratings being *mild, moderate,* and *severe.* Yairi and Ambrose (2005) used an 8-point perceptual scale, ranging from normal fluency (rated 0) to most severe stuttering (rated 7). They reported that some experience should yield high agreement with other clinicians. Clinicians, however, have been provided with several more analytical methods that take into account several factors in the assignment of a severity rating. For diagnostic purposes, Wingate (1976) recommended a 5-point scale (very mild, mild, moderate, severe, and very severe) that considers the frequency of stuttered events, the effort involved, and the presence of concomitant behaviors. An example of a similar Severity Rating scale is presented in Table 8.4.

Two of the more well-known stuttering severity scales are the Iowa Scale of Severity of Stuttering (Sherman, 1952), and the more recent Stuttering Severity Instrument, also known as the SSI-4, by Riley (1994, 2009). Both are based on three components: (1) frequency of stuttering events, (2) duration of events, and (3) intensity of concomitant

Table 8.4   Severity Rating Scale

Overall Rating	Descriptive Assessment		
	Stuttering Frequency (per words)	Effort	Secondary Behaviors
Very mild	3/100 (3%)	No visible tension	No noticeable movements
Mild	1/20 (5%)	Minimal visible tension	Barely noticeable movements
Moderate	1/10 (10%)	Moderate visible tension	Noticeable movements
Severe	1/5 (20%)	Severe visible tension	Very distracting movements
Very severe	1/4 (25%)	Very severe visible tension	Painfully agitated movements

characteristics. The SSI-4, one of the most popular instruments, employs separate ratings of each of the three components to arrive at an overall score. The examiner must obtain at least two speech samples, from spontaneous speech and oral reading contexts. Samples beyond the clinic setting are also encouraged. These samples are then analyzed in terms of the percentage of syllables stuttered, the average duration of the three longest stuttering moments, and the perceived level of distraction presented by any concomitant physical behaviors associated with stuttering. The total score summed across the three areas is then converted to a severity rating at one of the five levels: very mild, mild, moderate, severe, or very severe. The SSI-4 also includes a naturalness rating guide (Martin, Haroldson, & Triden, 1984) as well as a set of self-reported rating scales for clinical purposes. The Iowa Scale of Severity of Stuttering expands the ratings of severity to seven levels: very mild, mild, mild-moderate, moderate, moderate-severe, severe, and very severe. The larger range of ratings suggests increased discernment. Application of this scale can be challenging, however, because the descriptions may not fit clients' features too well. The scale presupposes that dimensions of frequency and duration of stuttering moments always increase together. If this is not the case, the clinician is forced to base the rating on only one of the two dimensions. No guidance is offered regarding the prioritization of the various dimensions.

Physical Concomitants

Various movements and postures can occur in the head and neck areas, and at times also in other parts of the body, in association with stuttering events. The terms *concomitant, secondary,* and *accessory characteristics* have been commonly used as referents to this dimension of stuttering. As we discussed in Chapter 4, they contribute to the impression of tense, struggled speech and to the overall perception of stuttering severity and abnormality.

To be considered "secondary behaviors," the movements must be associated with speaking and stuttering. Some people who do not stutter close their eyes or blink frequently when talking. An observer must appreciate the range of what is normal. If an extraneous movement is present at times when the client does not speak or stutter, then it would not appropriately be considered "secondary" to stuttering. Impulsive jerking movements, such as tics associated with Tourette's syndrome, are differentiated in part by being present even though a person is not engaged in speaking.

The number of variations in secondary characteristics is almost limitless among and within individuals who stutter. To review, the list of the most common observable characteristics, taken from Chapter 4, are shown on the next page (p. 222).

During the interview, occurrence of these may be specified in the clinician's notes. Or they may be more carefully reviewed later from the recorded videotape. Prins and Lohr (1972), who studied physical concomitants in detail, reported that the number of areas within the head and neck region involved in stutter events had a significant weight on the severity factor. The clinician should consider secondary characteristics when assigning the overall severity rating of the observed stuttered speech. As already

Table 8.5 Physical Concomitants (Secondary or Accessory Characteristics)	
Head jerks	Head turns (side; down)
Forehead tension	Nostrils flaring/constricted
Eyes closed; squinting	Eyes widely open
Facial contortions	Lips pressured
Jaw closed tightly	Teeth grinding
Jaw wide open	Rotational or sideways jaw movement
Tongue protrusion	Throat tightened
Body swaying	Hand and/or arm movements
Stepping sideways or backward	Clenching hands
Raising shoulder	
Irregular exhalation (blowing) during speech	
Irregular inhalations (gasping) in the midst of speaking	

mentioned, the Stuttering Severity Instrument-4 (Riley, 2009) includes this factor in the final score. The information is also relevant for those clinicians who prefer specifically to target secondary characteristics in therapy. Certainly, it is also a good variable to include for assessing progress in subsequent evaluations.

Speaking Rates

A slower than normal speaking rate was pointed out in Chapter 4 as one characteristic of advanced stuttering. Rather obviously, this results directly from the extra time consumed by the stuttered portion of speech. The higher the frequency of disfluencies and the longer their duration, the slower the speaking rate. Hence, it may serve as one indicator of therapeutic progress (Tomblin, Morris, & Spriestersbach, 2000). Slower rate is a common target in fluency intervention, as we discuss in Chapter 12, and influences perceptual judgments of speech naturalness (St. Louis, Myers, Faragasso et al. 2004). It is reasonable, therefore, to assess speaking rate as part of the initial evaluation of stuttering. Furthermore, it is a key element in the diagnosis of cluttering (see Chapter 15).

When measuring rate, clinicians should keep in mind that variations are expected with speech context. Speech rates in the following contexts were found to differ significantly, in decreasing order: oral reading, conversation, and picture description (Duchin & Mysak, 1987, p. 256). Compared to general discussion topics, contexts involving storytelling and content sequencing may require greater language formulation processes, and therefore take more time. Two measures have been employed for this domain: The first, *overall speech rate,* refers to how many words (or syllables) were spoken in the time needed to deliver an entire message or read a complete passage. It includes any pauses, disfluencies, or other variable dimensions of speech production. Syllables per minute is the preferred metric because the words per minute metric does not account for speaker differences in the numbers of multisyllabic words produced (Guitar, 1998; Pindzola, Jenkins, & Lokken, 1989). The second measurement, *articulatory rate,* refers to the speed of perceptually fluent utterances free of all disfluencies, hesitations, breaks, and detectible pauses longer than 250 milliseconds (Yaruss 1997a). The typical metric for articulatory rate is either syllables per second or phones per second (Hall et al., 1999; Pindzola et al., 1989). Articulatory rates do not directly reflect oral movements for speech, but they do reflect those movements better than overall speech rates.

Rate Measurement Procedures

Begin with recording a speech sample, transcribing the words, and counting words/ syllables as described earlier. For most clinical purposes, the time taken for the speech sample, or segments of interest, may be measured in minutes and seconds using a stopwatch. If measures will be compared with published data, the clinician must ensure that methods and standards of measurement match what was applied. For *overall speech rate,* the time from beginning to end of the sample is clocked. The clock should not keep running when the conversational partner talks or during periods of 2 seconds or more of silence while thinking about what to say or while yawning, coughing, sneezing, or similar. To ensure accuracy, re-clock the sample twice, or even three times, find the mean, then calculate the rate by dividing the number of words or syllables spoken by the amount of time. The examiner must remember that calculations are based on a 60:1 system when decimal figures are converted. For example, 1.25 minutes is the same as 60 + 15 (75 seconds), not 60 + 25 (85 seconds). As stated in Chapter 4, Fairbanks (1960) reported that a satisfactory range of oral reading rate by more than 200 college students for a 300-word passage was 150 to 180 words per minute (wpm). A later study by Walker (1988) reported the mean oral reading rate for 120 young adults was 188.4 wpm (SD = 19.7); for conversational speech it was 172.6 wpm (SD = 33.4).

For making *articulatory rate* measures, because the human ear is capable of detecting short silent intervals (e.g., 65 ms), even the slightest perceptible break should disqualify an utterance from analysis (Prins & Hubbard, 1990). Also disqualified should be utterances bounded by any disfluency either just before it begins or after it ends. For this measure, select from the speech sample three perceptually fluent, uninterrupted utterances. An example of the calculation is presented in Table 8.6.

The clinician should bear in mind that articulatory rate measures are sensitive to factors such as utterance length, word lengths, and location within utterance. Longer stretches of continuous speech (e.g., 15 syllables) are apt to yield faster rates than shorter utterances (e.g., 5 syllables). If only partial segments of utterances are measured, rate will be affected by location of the segment because utterances are started quickly and

---

Table 8.6 An Example of Measuring Articulatory Rate

1. Count the number of spoken syllables in each utterance:

   Utterance A: "Can you find the answer for me" 8 syllables

   Utterance B: "Was on the old table over there" 9 syllables

   Utterance C: "Remembered to go the grocery store" 9 syllables

   (expected word "to" before "the" was not uttered; grocery said as: "gros-ry")

2. Measure the duration of each entire utterance 3 times and find the average duration for *each* of the utterances. For example:

Utterance A	Utterance B	Utterance C
1.60	1.72	1.67
1.58	1.75	1.65
1.57	1.72	1.68
Averages: 4.75 / 3 = 1.58	5.19 / 3 = 1.73	5.00 / 3 = 1.67

3. Find the articulatory rate for each utterance by dividing the number of syllables by the time. Next average the values from each utterance to arrive at the overall rate measure. For example:

   Articulatory Rate

   Utterance A: 8 syllables / 1.58 s = 5.06 syl/sec

   Utterance B: 9 syllables / 1.73 s = 5.20 syl/sec

   Utterance C: 9 syllables / 1.67 s = 5.38 syl/sec

   Overall Rate   15.64 / 3 = **5.21**

---

ended slowly (Lehiste, 1972). Articulatory rates from spontaneous monologue contexts for nonstuttering adults for utterances of 7 to 8 words (8 syllables) typically range from 4 to 8 syllables/second (syl/sec; unpublished research by Seery; also consistent with converted data from Tsao & Weismer, 1997). Some evidence suggests articulatory rates in oral reading tend to be on the slower end (approximately 4.35 syl/sec) of this range (Logan et al., 2002). In contrast, other reports (Johnson, 1961) showed oral reading to be faster than spontaneous speech, probably because pauses are shorter and less frequent in oral reading: In school-age children ages 9 and 11, articulatory rates ranged from 4 to 6 syllables per second, and children age 7 years produced significantly slower rates from 3 to 5 syllables per second (Sturm & Seery, 2007).

If a client's speech rate is perceived to be faster or slower than expected, the clinician must consider what is leading to that impression. Naturally, when a speaker is disfluent, speech takes additional time and seems slower. Without disfluency, however, the perception of speech as fast or slow results largely from the placement and timing of pauses

(Goldman-Eisler, 1961). The clinician would do well to consider factors that could affect the types of utterances that are apparently faster or slower. Overlearned and previously prepared automatic sequences of spontaneous speech can be delivered at much faster rates than unrehearsed statements, especially those composed of new thoughts, unfamiliar words, or novel phrases (Levelt, 1989). The impression of a rapid and irregular rate of speech is also common symptom of cluttering (see Chapter 15).

Voice and Other Communication Skills

Speech samples afford an opportunity for the clinician to screen other domains of communication besides fluency: articulation, language (syntax, semantics, pragmatics), and voice. The domain of voice requires particular attention in the evaluation of stuttering but is too often neglected or minimized because of the great concentration on the client's disfluency. The examination of voice (and other domains) can be made during the interview and later listening to the recorded speech. The clinician should remember to make note of such domains both in fluent and disfluent speech. Is the voice quality normal and relaxed, or is it tight or harsh? Are there notable changes during stuttering (e.g., vocal fry, sharp upward pitch breaks)? This is also the time to observe intonational variations: inflections and prosodic contours. A reduced range of these variations, in addition to the stuttering, may significantly affect the speaker's communicative effectiveness and the overall listener's impression of the disorder. This type of information is useful in planning goals for therapy.

Another aspect of evaluation not to be overlooked is the appraisal of the client's communication strengths. Perhaps the client does well with nonverbal behaviors such as eye contact, facial expression, body postures and gesturing, and such. Voice and intonational patterns may be particularly pleasant, stuttering aside. The client may do well with appropriate pragmatic uses of language compared to most speakers, have a strong vocabulary, pronunciation mastery, or display above-average command of grammatical constructions. The clinician should make a point to look for the client's strengths, being sure to discuss them in postassessment counseling. An awareness of these areas is important to enhance the client's self-understanding of his or her overall effectiveness as a communicator. Self-perceptions can often be distorted by a speaker's emotional frustration with stuttering.

Speech naturalness and speech quality have been common concerns about the outcome of stuttering treatment programs (Martin et al., 1984; Onslow & Ingham, 1987). Speech naturalness is usually measured on either a 9-point or 7-point scale, where 1 represents highly natural-sounding speech, and 9 (or 7), highly unnatural-sounding speech. These ratings may be made by listeners such as the clinician or peers, or by the speaker in the form of self-ratings of naturalness. Ingham, Ingham, Onslow et al. (1989) demonstrated that adult clients can both rate and modify their speech based on the application of such scales. A later study revealed that speech quality could also be assessed through self-ratings of speech effort on a 9-point scale, where 9 is most effortful and 1 is least effortful (Ingham, Warner, Byrd et al., 2006).

Observations and Examinations: Other Domains

Having obtained speech samples for the multiple analyses just described, the focus of the initial evaluation shifts to other domains of the complex stuttering, those involving affective reactions. As discussed in Chapter 4, affective reactions become increasingly important with more years of experience with stuttering. Fear and discomfort may develop for specific types of social settings or in relation to speaking and stuttering, more generally. Following we present two classes of protocols, those related to (1) speaking situations and (2) more general attitudes and reactions to stuttering.

Situational Rating Protocols

The variability of stuttering across individuals and contexts is the main reason why clinicians seek information regarding a client's difficulties in different speaking contexts. It is first gained during the case history interview but can be greatly enhanced through the administration of one or more available protocols. Several are briefly discussed below. These protocols are similar in that they use lists of situations, such as talking on the phone, introducing oneself, and so on, to which the client is to respond. What differs among them are the ways in which the client is to evaluate each situation. The knowledge gained provides for better insight into the client's difficulties and may also be utilized in constructing therapy programs aimed at alleviating these difficulties.

Stutterers' Self-Ratings of Reactions to Speech Situations (SSR; Darley & Spriestersbach, 1978): The instrument's 40 situations are each rated by the client on a 5-point scale corresponding to various descriptive statements for the following dimensions: (1) frequency—how frequently the situation is met, (2) stuttering—how much stuttering occurs in it, (3) avoidance—how much the client tries to avoid the situation, and (4) reaction—how much the client likes/dislikes speaking in the situation. An advantage to this scale is that a good amount of important information is obtained from the client. Also available are reference data (p. 314) for the scores in each of the four areas. A disadvantage is that some terms and expressions used in the situation list have become antiquated. For example, the descriptions refer to "parlor games," "a bull session," and "taking leave of a hostess."

Southern Illinois University Speech Situation Checklist (Hanson, Gronhovd, & Rice, 1981): The original version assessed 51 situation items. Its much shorter version is composed of only 21 items. In either version, situations are rated on a 5-point scale in only one dimension: how much it disturbs the client to speak in it. Clearly, the shortened version with fewer situations and only one area to rate offers greater efficiency. Another advantage is the research support for the item selection process for the shortened version. There are, however, no reference data against which scores can be compared, and a few items are worded in antiquated language. For example, there is a reference to "talking when high." In the past, it meant being very excited but because these words later became associated with intoxication from drugs, clients may find the item offensive or confusing.

Reactions to Selected Speaking Situations (Prins, 1993, p. 138): The original version includes 25 situational items, each of which is evaluated on a 5-point scale for three dimensions: (1) frequency—how frequently the situation is met, (2) level of difficulty—how much trouble speaking in it, and (3) level of confidence—how confident the client is in the situation. Like the previous protocol, the small number of items makes for a more efficient use of time. In addition, none of the situation descriptions is worded in a way that is antiquated or ambiguous. A possible disadvantage is that clients might find it harder to evaluate levels of confidence than levels of disturbance, avoidance, or like/dislike of a situation. There also are no reference data for the scores obtained, but this should not necessarily detract from its clinical value.

An informal, non-scaled protocol to evaluate the difficulty and importance of situations based on conversational partners and purposes is shown in Table 8.7. The information obtained from the client aids the preparation of situational hierarchies to be applied during intervention. These protocols simply add more organization and detail to the information obtained in the interview. They also best serve for comparing a client's baseline ratings (pretreatment) with later progress (posttreatment) and not primarily as a differential diagnostic tool to distinguish the stuttering disorder.

Another meaningful way to engage in evaluating a client's concern about various speaking situations is devising an individualized situation hierarchy. Its advantage is that the client only has to deal with the situations that are personally meaningful, with immediate implications to his or her own treatment. The client is first asked to list and describe as many situations as are meaningfully relevant to his or her life. The list should not be lengthy, and the clinician can offer suggestions of types of situations or permit the client to look at a list from a protocol for suggestions. After the list is constructed, the client ranks the situations in order from least to most difficult. Such a list is valuable when subsequent therapy is focused on desensitization. It is advisable to check in with the client later on, and on multiple occasions as necessary, to find out whether the sense of difficulty and ranking of the situations has changed.

The previous protocols evaluating the difficulty of speaking situations might also be viewed as assessments of client attitudes about speaking situations. In that light, two additional protocols also can be used. These are the Self-Efficacy Scale for Adult Stutterers (SESAS; Ornstein & Manning, 1985) and the SEA Scale: Self-Efficacy Scaling for Adolescents Who Stutter (Manning, 2001). The SESAS has the client rate the same 50 speaking situations on two dimensions: (1) approach attitude and (2) fluency performance. For either dimension, clients apply a 10-point scale from 10 to 100, where 10 is "quite uncertain" and 100 is "very certain." To assess approach attitudes, clients answer whether they would (1) enter the situation, and (2) how much confidence they have with their response. To assess fluency performance, clients answer whether (1) they would be able to achieve fluency in that situation, and (2) how much confidence they have with this response. Advantages of this protocol are that the descriptions use current terminology and the contexts are familiar, such as McDonald's, the shopping mall, or ordering a pizza. Also, rating confidence in a response could be easier than

Table 8.7   Evaluation of Talking to Various Partners for Various Purposes

Conversational Partner	Importance Rating *	Difficulty Rating *
1. Talking to my father.		
2. Talking to my mother.		
3. Talking to my siblings.		
4. Talking to other family relatives.		
5. Talking to my spouse/significant other.		
6. Talking to my date/someone attractive.		
7. Talking to a good friend.		
8. Talking to an unfamiliar person.		
9. Talking to a teacher.		
10. Talking to a classmate/colleague.		
11. Talking to a small informal group.		
12. Talking to a large formal group.		
CONVERSATIONAL PURPOSE		
13. Introducing myself.		
14. Ordering food.		
15. Reading aloud.		
16. Talking in a classroom.		
17. Phone calls.		
18. Asking a question.		
19. Giving direct information.		
20. Explaining something or sharing ideas.		
21. Interviewing for a job.		
22. Delivering a formal spoken presentation.		

* Importance Rating	* Difficulty Rating
This is:	This is:
Q. Quite important	Q. Quite easy
R. Relatively important	R. Relatively easy
S. Somewhat important	S. Somewhat difficult
T. Trivial importance	T. Tough
U. Unimportant or N/A	U. Utterly impossible

evaluating self-confidence, and reference data for stuttering and nonstuttering populations are available.

The SEA Scale requires adolescents to rate 100 situations on a scale from 1 to 10 to indicate confidence in the ability to enter and speak in each situation. All situational descriptions are worded with current and unambiguous statements. Responses can be evaluated with respect to 13 subscales related to telephone, arguments with familiar people, arguments with strangers, conversing with a family member, conversing with an authority figure, conversing with a familiar group, conversing with an unfamiliar group, formal presentations, making requests of a stranger, making requests of an authority figure, time-pressure contexts, and memorized or unchangeable texts. Although making estimations of self-confidence can be challenging, the authors have provided clear descriptive statements to apply when using the scale. A disadvantage could be the time required for responding as well as for scoring the numerous responses.

Listed here are several possible choices of a method for assessing reactions to speaking situations. As we explained previously, the first two in this list address many situations but may use wording that confuses some clients. The next two offer relevant situations but still involve making a sizable number of ratings. An individualized hierarchy is quite functional but may pose the risk of overlooking some common situations. When one of these tools is chosen, many other factors (e.g., time, cost, client age, etc.) must also be considered.

Tools for Assessing Speaking Situations

- Stutterer's Self-Ratings of Reactions to Speech Situations (SSR; Darley & Spriestersbach, 1978)
- Southern Illinois University Speech Situation Checklist (Hanson et al., 1981)
- Reactions to Selected Speaking Situations (Prins, 1993, p. 138)
- Self-Efficacy Scale for Adult Stutterers (SESAS) and SEA Scale: Self-Efficacy Scaling for Adolescents Who Stutter (Manning, 2001)
- Individualized situation hierarchy

It cannot be emphasized enough that whether the assessment is of reactions to speaking situations or of attitudes about stuttering, the clinician must have established a relationship of trust with the client prior to their administration. The clinician should judge whether a client is ready to disclose this kind of information, or if it would be better to wait until the client is more comfortable trusting the clinician. One of us (Seery) has seen multiple instances in which clients have filled in responses according to what they believed they *should* answer, rather than what they actually experienced. In another occasion, a client marked all 25 situations with midscale ratings of 3 on the 5-point scale rather than reveal specific troubles. Rather than admitting limitations, clients may also provide a rating for a situation despite insufficient basis for self-evaluation after years of avoidance of speaking in it. For this reason, the SESAS would be a preferable instrument to elicit informative responses. In some cases, it may be wise for a clinician to postpone administration to a later time when sufficient rapport has been established.

Attitude Rating Scales

Attitudes are one of the most important variables related to disfluent speech but are quite challenging to assess. Part of the challenge comes from the many attitudes that may be relevant and the large range of individual differences in their extent. Clinicians should consider attitudes about stuttering, speaking, self, other people, and more. Naturally, the clinician's understanding of the client's needs begins with the dialogue that takes place during the case history interview. Attitudes need to be explored in a manner that is both respectful and sensitive to the feelings that may be close to the surface. It can be difficult for a client to review the impact of stuttering and their attitudes about it. Several formal instruments have been published for the purpose of assessing attitudes related to stuttering. A few of these will be described next.

Modified Erickson Scale (Andrews & Cutler, 1974): The origin of this instrument was the S Scale (Erickson, 1969) that consisted of 39 items in the form of statements to which clients must respond as true/false about whether they agree with it. For example, "I find it easy to talk with almost anyone." Reference data are available to interpret the extent to which the score is more similar to those who stutter or who do not. The Modified Erickson Scale (S-24) has only 24 items, and it also comes with reference data for comparing responses for those who stutter or who do not. In scoring either scale, each item's response is compared with a key of expected answers established during the construction of the instrument. Agreement receives a score of 1 point; disagreement is scored as 0 points. The number of agreements is then totaled to compare with the scale scores. The closer a score is to the maximum of 24, the stronger is the negative emotionality associated with stuttering. The 24-item version is a relatively efficient tool, with the exception of one item with such antiquated wording that people might not know what it means (i.e., "I am a good mixer.")

Communication Attitude Test (Brutten, 1985; Brutten & Dunham, 1989): This instrument should be administered to adolescents, not adults. Appropriate for school-age children, 8 of the 35 statements make reference to "other children," "other kids," or being "in class" or with "classmates." Clients must answer true/false about their agreement with each of 35 statements. A revised version, the CAT-R with 32 items (De Nil & Brutten, 1991; Vanryckeghem, & Brutten, 1992), yields reliable results with reference data for both stuttering and nonstuttering children, ages 7 to 14.

Overall Assessment of the Speaker's Experience of Stuttering, OASES (Yaruss & Quesal, 2006) is designed for adults who stutter, ages 18 and older, to assess the comprehensive impact of stuttering on the person's life. Clients respond to 100 items in four sections (General Information, Reactions to Stuttering, Communication in Daily Situations, and Quality of Life) using a 5-point scale that differs in meaning across sections. In the General Information section, 20 items address a broad overview of perceptions of speaking ability, knowledge about stuttering, and feelings about speaking and stuttering. In the Reactions section, 30 items address specific stuttering-related emotions, experiences, and attitudes. In the Daily Situations section, 25 speaking situations are rated for level of difficulty. The Quality of Life section contains 25 items about how much stuttering negatively impacts or interferes with the client's life, personally, socially, and vocationally. The scores for each section on the OASES are converted to Impact Ratings interpreted on a 5-level scale, ranging from mild to severe. There is also a Total Impact Score that is interpreted similarly. Score interpretation is based on published research and reference data. The questions and situation descriptions in the OASES are clearly worded, and its content has current relevance. Because the instrument is meant to be comprehensive, it is also lengthier than the rest. One limitation may be that, unlike the SESAS, clients do not indicate how certain they are of their responses.

To assess the quality of the instruments, Franic and Bothe (2008) reviewed 17 attitude and situation assessment instruments for psychometric properties. Ten of the 17 were evaluated in detail with respect to 15 measurement criteria. These criteria included conceptual model, validity, reliability, responsiveness, interpretability (reference data), burden (client respondent and examiner administrative), depth, and versatility. Of the instruments discussed, only the CAT/CAT-R and Modified Erickson Scale (S-24) met at least half of the standard criteria for application as a diagnostic tool. These were criticized for their low test-retest reliability, lack of being based on clear constructs, and insufficient research on their responsiveness to clinical change. The SSR and OASES met fewer criteria. The authors expressed concern that the OASES may overidentify problems. The SSR has not received adequate testing for validity and reliability. These four tests were the only instruments reviewed among those that we have discussed in this chapter.

Like the assessment of speaking situations, rapport must be established first to ensure the client is ready to trust the clinician with the information prompted by attitude scales. Some scales are best suited to serve as pre- and posttherapy surveys with clients who have had previous experience with therapy. Some surveys, like the OASES, are best applied in the context of an interpersonal interview and not as a self-administered questionnaire given to the client to fill out. Because such scales prompt the sharing of highly personal emotional information, they may not be best to administer during the very first encounter with a client or in the context of a diagnostic clinic where the examiner will not be the one who is later administering the therapy. The following is a list of the attitude assessment options:

- Modified Erickson Scale (S-24; Andrews & Cutler, 1974)
- Communication Attitude Test (CAT-R; Brutten, 1985; Brutten & Dunham, 1989)
- Overall Assessment of the Speaker's Experience of Stuttering (OASES; Yaruss & Quesal, 2006)
- Individualized interview regarding attitudes and emotional reactions

Interpretations and Treatment Recommendations

Diagnosis

As explained at the beginning of the chapter, a classic diagnosis of stuttering in adolescents or adults is not apt to present much of a challenge. In the great majority of cases, the correct diagnosis has been made by the client. The clinician's main goal is to describe, quantify, and assess the various aspects of the stuttering disorder and determine its overall severity and impact. In some cases, differential diagnosis from other fluency disorders (see Chapter 15), or faked stuttering, is called for. Other problems of communication or different suspected health issues may be revealed or just suspected. All these should be reflected in the final evaluation report. On occasion, when individuals with very mild stuttering seek intervention, the inexperienced clinician may be inclined to question whether the speaker's perception of the disorder is valid or out of proportion with the actual difficulty. The reality of the stuttering disorder in such cases should be apparent by means of the following analogy. Imagine that your knees suddenly and unexpectedly buckled under you about twice each week. Wouldn't it be enough to make you seek out a doctor? Similarly, even occasional stuttering episodes can be sufficient to generate a sense of great vulnerability for a speaker. It is precisely because these moments occur infrequently and surface when least expected that they pose such an insidious threat. The client with mild stuttering can still benefit from intervention strategies and counseling.

A related issue is how much of a client's stuttering is hidden or suppressed compared to what would be observed without the client's coping mechanisms. The evaluation may also attempt to find out the nature of a client's coping mechanisms. How well is the client able to describe and discuss characteristics of his or her coping mechanisms? Which coping mechanisms might best be left alone at this time, and which ones is the client most needing or wanting to change?

Treatment Recommendations

When all assessment results are analyzed, clinicians should first determine if therapy is warranted and, if positive, how will they be useful in selecting, or recommending, appropriate treatment. One of the most important considerations is what the client envisions as his or her goals in treatment. Are those goals realistic? How will the client's vision of the clinical intervention process need to be brought into alignment with how the clinician understands that process? The stuttering assessment should inform the clinician about how the client views the stuttering so that these questions can be addressed.

How do speech characteristics guide the planning of treatment? In addition to providing a pretherapy baseline to evaluate progress, the clinician should have observed the speech characteristics in terms of the patterns of movement of various anatomical structures (i.e., lips, tongue, jaw, neck/larynx, and chest). How does their positioning, timing, and tenseness differ from what is associated with typically fluent speech?

Does stuttering tend to occur at the most common location of utterance initiation? Then a slower, easier approach to starting to talk may be an appropriate strategy to develop. Does the speaker have a high level of tension in the articulators? Then a gentler, relaxed approach to their movement and contacts may be needed. Does the speaker hold his or her breath when starting to talk? Instruction for appropriate breath support may help. Are reactions and attitudes toward speech and stuttering preventing progress with speech change? Then these fears and avoidances may need to be addressed through counseling and desensitization activities. Do nonverbal behaviors or suprasegmental speech characteristics (e.g., irregular rate patterns, awkward phrasing, lack of eye contact, etc.) interfere with communication? Then these may need attention in therapy. How big is the factor of secondary characteristics? Although these tend to lessen or disappear of their own accord as the core stuttering and avoidance behaviors are decreased, occasionally secondary characteristics may need to be dealt with directly through awareness and self-monitoring. Additionally, each individual will have specific situations to address depending on their life roles (e.g., student, family relations, etc.), vocation, and recreational/social interests and needs. Finally, information obtained regarding past therapy experiences should be taken into consideration in deciding the future course of therapy.

The Diagnostic Report

The example of a speech evaluation report in Table 8.8 reveals the types of information obtained from a stuttering assessment. It also offers a model of possible wording and content organization for professionals who are new to reporting in this area.

Table 8.8   Sample Diagnostic Report

The Greater Midwest	1818 Midcontinent Blvd.
Speech & Hearing Center	Chatter City, USA 77778

SPEECH EVALUATION REPORT

Name: Basil Karger	Date of Evaluation: 01/01/14
Birth Date: 01/01/14	Informant for History: Self
Age: 23	Clinic File No.: 1111112
Gender: Male	Diagnostic Code No.: 333
Address: 510 Snow Rd.	Diagnosis: Stuttering
Chatter City, USA, 77778	

COMPLAINT AND REFERRAL

Basil, a 23-year-old male, was seen at his request at the Greater Midwest Speech and Hearing Center for evaluation of his stuttering. Basil, a college graduate who works in the receiving department of a major furniture store, feels the stuttering is distracting to other workers in the facilities, delivery drivers, and personal friends, and interferes in his career development.

(continued)

Table 8.8   (Continued)

HISTORY

Basil was raised on a farm near Chatter City. He is the youngest of four siblings, with only one of them being a full-blooded sib. He is the only one of the four who has ever stuttered. Basil did state, however, that his father had a stuttering problem that he overcame on his own after college. No other relatives were known to stutter.

Basil could not recall exactly when he began stuttering, but said he was aware of it at approximately 8 years of age. There was no recollection or knowledge of any medical or traumatic experience that precipitated the onset of stuttering. He also related that his family has always accepted his speech problem and that rarely have there been comments made on it.

During high school years, tension was intensified due to meeting new teachers and peers, as well as increased academic responsibilities, resulting in Basil's stuttering becoming more severe. In college, familiar speaking situations and speaking with friends were thought by him to be relatively easy, whereas speaking to professors and in front of classes posed more difficulties.

Basil received previous speech therapy at another clinic for approximately 2.5 years during his high school senior year and his undergraduate years at a community college. He recalled "cancellations" and "pull-outs" as the major therapeutic techniques and felt that they were effective. Therapy was terminated by mutual decision of the clinician and client after they felt sufficient progress had been made. Recently, however, stuttering had increased.

EXAMINATIONS AND OBSERVATIONS

Disfluent Speech: An analysis of a 566-word sample of Basil's conversational speech revealed a total of 147 disfluencies, an average of 25.97 per 100 words. The breakdown of this figure according to specific disfluency types and categories is shown in the chart:

	Conversation	Reading
	(566 wds.)	(463 wds.)
Part-word repetitions	7.95 (45)	1.94 (9)
Whole-word repetitions	3.36 (19)	0.65 (3)
Disrhythmic Phonation	5.83 (33)	0.65 (3)
SLD Subtotal	**17.14 (97)**	**3.24 (15)**
Phrase repetitions	2.12 (12)	1.51 (7)
Interjections	6.01 (34)	4.31 (20)
Revisions	0.71 (4)	0.04 (2)
Other Disfluency Subtotal	**8.83 (50)**	**6.26 (29)**
Disfluency Total	**25.97 (147)**	**9.50 (44)**

As can be seen, the predominant types of disfluencies in Basil's speech were part-word repetitions and disrhythmic phonation (sound prolongations and blockages). The clinician estimated the average repetition contained two additional units (e.g., bu-bu-but), although sometimes three and four extra units were produced. Sound prolongations often lasted 2 sec or more. Although Basil indicated no specific phonemes on which he had more disfluencies, it was noted that they occurred quite consistently on words or syllables beginning with the vowel /a/. Basil exhibited relatively fluent speech in reading both the Rainbow Passage and My Grandfather, a 463-word combined sample. The total SLD in this task was 3.24 per 100 words. Postponement behaviors observed were primarily in terms of interjections that tended to precede instances of severe stuttering. His disfluency in reading was less severe than in conversation.

Secondary Characteristics: Physically tense movements that typically accompany stutter events were observable as Basil spoke. Eye blinking, poor eye contact, and neck and facial muscle tension occurred quite consistently during moments of disfluency. He was often observed wringing his hands and fingers while he held the rest of his body rather still.

Severity: Judging the impact of both the disfluency and the secondary characteristics on a 7-point scale for an overall rating severity of stuttering, with 1 being very mild stuttering and 7 being very severe stuttering, Basil's speech was rated by the clinician at 5, although moments of more severe stuttering did occur.

Speaking Rate: Basil's conversational speech was timed. His average overall speaking rate, 132.5 words per minute, was below normal range.

Voice: During testing, Basil's voice quality was characterized by glottal fry and voice breaks. His optimal pitch was assessed by estimating the pitch level approximately a fourth from the bottom of his total pitch range. In conversational speech, Basil spoke at a lower pitch than the estimated optimal. Indeed, when asked to read in a monotone, the pitch he used was the same estimated as the optimal.

Speech Mechanism: The speech mechanism appeared both structurally and functionally adequate for speech.

Language: Although no formal language assessment was done, Basil used both vocabulary and syntax appropriate for his age and education level.

Hearing Screening: An audiometric screening was administered at both 25 dB HTL and 15 db HTL (re: ANSI 1969) with a portable Beltone audiometer. The following frequencies were tested bilaterally: 250, 500, 1,000, 2,000, 4,000, 8,000 Hz. Responses to all stimuli were consistent.

Client's View: Asked to describe the experience of a stuttering block, Basil said he felt "tension and inability to speak." He felt like "a hundred things were going on in his mind at once." After the moment had ended, he experienced a great relief, "like a weight off his chest." Basil stated that he felt the cause of his stuttering was nervousness. Asked what he does to change his stuttering, he said, "Trying to relax, slow down, and sometimes take aspirin hoping it would calm me down." Basil felt that some situations increase the severity of his stuttering.

(continued)

Table 8.8 (Continued)

It is more difficult for him speaking to a group than to individuals, also speaking to strangers (e.g., various people with whom he has to communicate on the job) than to familiar people. He added, however, that he feels most people generally ignore his stuttering, although some former colleagues in college expressed difficulty in listening to, and understanding him, at times. He is often afraid to talk when expected to. On a 9-point scale of speech naturalness, Basil self-rated his speech as 7, which is rather unnatural. Among anxiety-producing situations he also listed speaking with people having authority, such as former professors and current superiors at his work environment; having to talk after arriving late to a meeting; and some phone conversations. It was also mentioned that Basil's stuttering seems to increase when he does not sleep enough.

Attitudes: Basil was administered the Modified Erickson Scale (S-Scale) and received a score of 37 points out of a possible 39, which would seem to reflect a very low attitude toward speaking when compared with normal speakers.

Social Effects: Asked about how stuttering influences his life, Basil replied that he feels avoidance reactions to various situations. In discussing plans for the future, he stated that he would prefer jobs that required less frequent speaking then his current one. He felt it would be unrealistic to do otherwise because the stuttering would always be there. As far as dealing with current social situations, Basil did not feel that his stuttering keeps him much from being more socially active than he currently is. Still, he is rather comfortable with a number of his friends, and stutters less when he is talking with people he knows. Although he dates women, he admits to some obstacles in this domain.

CLINICAL IMPRESSION

Throughout the diagnostic session, Basil exhibited moderate to severe stuttering in terms of the frequency, types, and length of disfluencies that were accompanied by several secondary characteristics and the usage of an inappropriately low voice pitch and significant components of glottal fry. His stuttering during oral reading was less severe in frequency and intensity than in conversation. The affective reactions to the stuttering are strong. Basil's stuttering clearly interferes with his personal life and professional career aspirations. Although the speech therapy he received 2.5 years ago provided improvement, it is apparent that Basil needs additional therapy that will target the overt stuttering, voice, and affective reaction. Basil has expressed a desire to begin speech therapy, and stated his main goal to accomplish is to be able to go before a group of people without stuttering much and be able to handle it better.

RECOMMENDATIONS

It is recommended that Basil Karger be enrolled in therapy for remediation of stuttering, voice, and affective reactions.

Student Clinicians _____

_____

Supervising Clinician _____

Summary

Stuttering assessment typically involves the major components of case history and client interview, speech sampling and analysis, supplemental speech tasks, emotions related to speaking and stuttering, and other factors impacting a client's personal, social, and professional life. A thorough assessment involves informal screenings, such as of the parameter of voice, and an appraisal of the client's overall profile of communication abilities, especially his or her strengths. An in-depth assessment provides an essential foundation for the selection of treatment goals and objectives. The clinician has considerable choices of procedures and measures of the various aspects of the overt stuttering as well as an array of instruments to evaluate the emotional component. To individualize assessment appropriately, the clinician considers multiple options related to:

- Selection of speech sample contexts
- Speech characteristics and nonverbal concomitants to be analyzed
- Frequency measures
- Severity scales
- Speaking rate measures
- Protocols for the examination of attitudes and/or reactions to speech and stuttering
- Variability of difficulty across situations

Study Questions and Discussion Topics

1. Which assessment procedures help clinicians discover the extent of a client's stuttering variability?
2. Pretend you are administering the stuttering evaluation, and explain to your client the reason for including each of the components in your assessment: speech samples, attitude protocols, and so on.
3. In what ways is a client required to engage in self-assessment during the clinical evaluation? How can clinicians help to ensure that clients use that self-assessment constructively?
4. Compare and contrast the two measures: percentage of syllables stuttered and frequency of disfluency per 100 syllables.
5. Clinicians sometimes adopt an alternative reporting format showing the relative proportions of the various disfluency types as in the following chart. Note the absence of any information about the size of the speech sample. Why is it important to report the disfluency frequency relative to the size of the speech sample, as demonstrated in the chapter? Explain how this alternative format may enhance some specifics but lacks the contextual information necessary for an appropriate interpretation of the data.

Disfluency Type	Percentage
Part-word repetitions (45/147)	30.6%
Whole-word repetitions (19/147)	12.9%
Disrhythmic phonation (33/147)	22.4%
SLD Subtotal (97/147)	**66.0%**
Phrase repetitions (12/147)	8.1%
Interjections (34/147)	23.1%
Revisions (4/147)	2.7%
Other Disfluency Subtotal (50/147)	**34.0%**
Disfluency Total (147/147)	**100.0%**

Suggested Readings

Hillis, J. (1993). On-going assessment in the management of stuttering: A clinical perspective. *American Journal of Speech-Language Pathology, 2,* 24–37.

Manning, W. (2001). Assessing adolescents and adults. In *Clinical decision making in fluency disorders* (2nd ed., pp. 113–184). San Diego, CA: Singular (Thomson).

Riley, G. (2009). Manual for the *Stuttering Severity Instrument for children and adults* (4th ed.). Austin, TX: Pro-Ed.

Yaruss, S., & Quesal, R. (2006). Overall Assessment of the Speaker's Experience of Stuttering (OASES): Documenting multiple outcomes in stuttering treatment. *Journal of Fluency Disorders, 31,* 90–115.

Appendixes

Appendix 8.1

Frequency of Disfluency Types per 100 Words in Narrative Contexts for Younger and Older Adults Who Do Not Stutter

Disfluency Type	White, 2002 Ages 20–22 (N = 30)		Yairi and Clifton, 1972 Ages 17–18 years (N = 15)		Ages 69–87 (N = 15)	
Part-Word Repetition	0.06		0.18		0.39	
Whole-Word Repetition	0.56		0.41		0.81	
Disrhythmic Phonation	0.03		0.15		0.28	
Tense Pause	NA		0.04		0.02	
CORE Subtotals		0.65		0.78		1.50
Interjections	4.69		1.66		2.92	
Phrase Repetitions	0.21		0.30		0.30	
Revisions	1.13		1.10		1.47	
ACCESSORY Subtotals		6.03		3.06		4.69
OVERALL Totals		6.68		3.84		6.19

Reprinted with permission from "Disfluent speech behavior of preschool children, high school seniors, and geriatric persons" by E. Yairi and N. Clifton, *Journal of Speech and Hearing Research, 15,* 714–719. Copyright 1972 by American Speech-Language-Hearing Association. All rights reserved. Adapted from E. White, 2002, *Normal disfluency in young adults across three speech tasks,* unpublished master's thesis, University of Wisconsin-Milwaukee, Milwaukee, WI.

Appendix 8.2

Frequency of Disfluency Types per 100 Words in an Oral Reading Context for 15 Male and 15 Female Adults Who Do Not Stutter, Age 20–22 Years

Disfluency Type	Males		Females	
Part-Word Repetition	0.40 (0.45)		0.16 (0.19)	
Whole-Word Repetition	0.34 (0.37)		0.22 (0.35)	
Disrhythmic Phonation	0.06 (0.12)		0.04 (0.11)	
Tense Pause	NA			
CORE Subtotals		0.80		0.42

(continued)

Disfluency Type	Males	Females
Interjections	0.41 (0.60)	0.20 (0.27)
Phrase Repetitions	0.56 (.0.57)	0.52 (0.45)
Revisions	0.56 (.0.58)	0.68 (0.47)
ACCESSORY Subtotals	1.43	1.40
OVERALL Totals	2.23	1.82

Standard deviations are in parentheses.

Adapted from E. White, 2002, *Normal disfluency in young adults across three speech tasks*, unpublished master's thesis, University of Wisconsin-Milwaukee, Milwaukee, WI.

Appendix 8.3

Mean Frequency of Disfluency Types per 100 Syllables for Adults: In Monologue (Job Task) for Normally Fluent Speakers (NFS) and in Oral Reading for People Who Stutter (PWS)

Disfluency Type	Mean NFS	Mean PWS
Part-Word Repetition	0.25	5.00
Whole-Word Repetition	0.60	0.40
Disrhythmic Phonation	0.25	5.00
CORE Subtotal	1.10	10.50
Interjection	4.00	0.60
Phrase Repetition	0.25	0.60
Revision	1.00	0.70
ACCESSORY Subtotal	5.25	1.90
Grand Total	6.35	12.40

Appendix 8.4

Frequency of Disfluency Types per 100 Words in Spontaneous Speech for 10 Male and 10 Female Adults Who Stutter, Ages 19–48 Years

Disfluency Type	Males	Females
Part-Word Repetition	3.08 (2.74)	4.50 (7.23)
Whole-Word Repetition	1.89 (0.75)	2.85 (3.24)
Disrhythmic Phonation	2.70 (2.07)	4.42 (6.03)
Tense Pause	0.22 (0.25)	0.29 (0.87)
CORE Subtotals	7.89	12.06

Disfluency Type	Males	Females
Interjections	4.29 (1.93)	5.47 (8.45)
Phrase Repetitions	0.66 (0.35)	0.46 (0.37)
Revisions	4.43 (2.38)	2.52 (1.77)
ACCESSORY Subtotals	9.38	8.45
OVERALL Totals	17.27	20.51

Standard deviations are in parentheses.

Appendix 8.5

Frequency of Disfluency and Types per 100 Words in Story Narratives for 56 Male Children Who Stutter and 56 Male Children Who Do Not Stutter

Disfluency Type	Stuttering Males			Nonstuttering Males		
	Q1	Q2	Q3	Q1	Q2	Q3
Part-Word Repetition	1.2	3.0	6.8	0.3	0.8	1.2
Whole-Word Repetition	1.3	2.5	4.4	0.4	0.8	1.3
Disrhythmic Phonation	0.2	0.6	2.6	0.0	0.1	0.3
Tense Pause	0.0	0.0	0.4	0.0	0.0	0.0
Interjections	0.2	0.8	1.9	0.3	0.5	1.5
Phrase Repetitions	0.2	0.5	1.3	0.0	0.3	0.9
Revision-Incomplete Phrases	1.5	1.9	2.7	1.7	2.8	4.2
All Categories	6.9	11.3	21.4	3.6	5.8	9.5

Figures are for the first (Q1), second (Q2), and third (Q3) quartiles.

Chapter 9

Assessment of Preschool-Age Children

LEARNER OBJECTIVES

Readers of this chapter will understand:

- Differences between the initial evaluation of a preschool child and that of older children and adults who stutter.
- Objectives and rationales for the initial evaluation of preschool children who stutter.
- Structure and content of the parent interview.
- Procedures and formal instruments for measuring stuttered speech in young children.
- Criteria for differentiating early stuttering from normal disfluency.
- Criteria for making early prediction of persistent stuttering and natural recovery.
- How to offer parent counseling in conjunction with the evaluation.

Challenges, Objectives, and Settings for the Initial Evaluation

In Chapter 8 we stated that in health fields, a typical diagnostic evaluation involves an analysis of presenting symptoms, both objectively observed and reported by the patient. It is a process that eventually leads to the diagnostic finding: the identification of a disease or a disorder that often is not apparent at the beginning of the process. Sometimes the diagnosis is substantiated by a single sign; in other cases there may be a pattern of signs. The primary motivation for isolating the condition or disorder from other alternatives is to facilitate decisions concerning suitable treatment. It was suggested that because the majority of adults who stutter correctly diagnose their own speech problem, the main purpose of initial evaluation for adults is to understand, describe, and measure the various dimensions of the disorder, rather than to identify it. Is this also true for preschool age children? Frequently, the answer is positive. By the time the speech-language pathologist is consulted, typically more than one caretaker has noticed the appearance of excessive and unusual disfluencies in the child's speech and correctly diagnosed it as "stuttering." Occasionally disorders of phonology and/or language may be called "stuttering" by individuals unaware of the distinctions. At other times parents who expected greater fluency proficiency during the language learning process may express concern about a child's repetitions, not sure if it is stuttering. In our experience, however, these are the minority of cases.

Stuttering versus Normal Disfluency: A Diagnostic Challenge

The literature reflects a common opinion that it is, or may be, difficult to distinguish early stuttering from normal disfluencies (e.g., Conture, 2001; Manning, 2001). Evaluating hundreds of preschool children, however, Yairi and Ambrose (2005) stated that rarely did they have occasions to question parents' diagnoses of their child's speech as stuttering. They also cited studies showing close agreement between the parents' and clinician's diagnosis of stuttering in preschool age children. Similarly, Curlee (1999, p. 3), stated that "I can recall only a handful of parental misdiagnoses of stuttering in over 25 years of clinical practice."

Yet there can be exceptions to agreement as well as to clear evidence for a diagnosis. Disagreements arise primarily when parents have had opportunities to observe more pronounced stuttering episodes that never occur even during two or three visits to the clinic. Overly anxious parents may take normal childhood speech characteristics, such as "placeholder" word and phrase repetitions, as signs of stuttering. Also, in isolated instances children are brought in because of parental concern about "stuttering," when they exhibit another communication disorder. Of course, for some children the objective evidence indicates a borderline case. These few cases do present the classic challenges of the diagnostic process in determining whether a disorder of clinical significance exists, and which one.

How do we explain Curlee's and our observations? Suppose investigators conducting a field survey of stuttering prevalence screen a random sample of 1,000 preschool children. In this situation, they will encounter each child once and for only for a few minutes. The investigators are likely to find the vast majority of the children as falling within a range varying from low to medium to high normal disfluency levels. They will probably judge 10 to 20 children (1%–2%) as exhibiting beyond normal disfluency (stuttering) and perhaps wrestle with the uncertain classification of an additional 5 children.

The clinical setting, however, presents an altogether different situation. There, preschoolers referred for evaluation constitute a very narrow, highly selected sample, not at all similar to a random sample of the population at large with a wide range of disfluent speech. Why? Because the parents of all 1,000 children have actually acted as screeners and have "screened" their children not once for a few minutes but for many days. Furthermore, those few who thought that their children began stuttering still waited several weeks, if not months or longer, until their observations were self-confirmed. No wonder that after such an intense screening process borderline cases seen for evaluation are infrequent and instances of clinician-parent agreement are frequent. Figure 9.1 illustrates the highly selective clinical group within the population distribution of disfluent speech.

According to a recent study, a substantial majority of preschoolers seen for initial stuttering evaluation exhibit moderate or severe stuttering that makes for unmistakable diagnoses (Yairi & Ambrose, 2005). Regardless, several disfluency measures, to be discussed later in the chapter, may be applied to make reasonably clear differentiation between normal fluency and stuttering.

Figure 9.1   Proportions of Children Who "Pass" Their Parents' Screenings

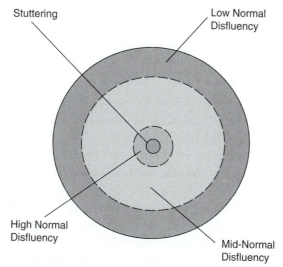

Other Key Diagnostic Issues

The initial evaluation of preschoolers who stutter is different in several significant aspects from that of adults who stutter. Key aspects include the role of parents, the accuracy of stuttering history information, the lack of clarity regarding emotional factors, the possibility of concomitant disorders, and the challenge of eliciting representative speech samples to observe the stuttering.

The Role of Parents

Whereas adults are typically self-referred for consultation and therapy and are the main source of information about themselves, parents are the ones who bring the child to the clinician out of their own worries, and the role of informant falls to them, typically the mother. Not only do they provide the background information, they also collect important data from the child. Being so close to the problem, parents become a second major focus of the evaluation. Their own background or family's experience with stuttering, their personality, the atmosphere they create at home, and their attitude and reaction to the child's stuttering are important for an understanding of the child's problem and factors that may aggravate it. Of course, potential positive parental resources also can be revealed and tapped for more effective handling of the problem. Finally, it is the parents who ultimately make the decision about the nature and timing of clinical intervention.

Accuracy of Information

Because of the short history of the disorder, information about onset and surrounding circumstances should be accessible from parents in greater detail and better validity than what typically is obtained for older clients. For some children such information may be only a few days or a few weeks old. Additionally, in the early years of life, most of a child's relatives are alive and available to provide extra information, greatly enhancing the accuracy of the history and familial incidence of stuttering that are important details for prognostic purposes.

The Emotional Domain

Whereas most adults are willing to share and verbalize their feelings about stuttering, assessing the emotional reactions of young children is difficult. On the one hand, children may not have such reactions. On the other hand, if emotional reactions do exist, preschoolers are often incapable of verbalizing them. True, some children clearly express their awareness and frustration. For many others, however, we simply do not know what goes on inside their minds. Age is a factor in the domain of emotional reactions. The percentage of children 4 to 5 years of age who appear to be aware of their stuttering is certainly greater than among 2-year-olds (Ambrose & Yairi, 1994). Other factors, such as severity of stuttering or environmental reactions to the child's speech, probably play a role. We may logically assume that the more severe the stuttering and the stronger are the environmental reactions, the higher the likelihood for the child to respond emotionally. Unfortunately, the information available for this domain is very limited.

Concomitant Disorders

All children in the preschool age range undergo fast developmental growth in multiple domains. An appreciable number of them may exhibit either slowness or more serious problems in one or more of these domains. Therefore, the initial evaluation of a young child who stutters must also include comprehensive testing of hearing, language, phonology, motor, and cognitive skills that constitute an integral part of standard speech-language-hearing evaluations of children. This point is particularly important in light of information suggesting that various disorders, especially those of phonology and language, are present concomitantly with childhood stuttering more frequently than in children who do not stutter (e.g., Arndt & Healey, 2001; Blood et al., 2003; Ntourou et al., 2011). Some of this information, however, has been contested (e.g., Nippold, 2012a).

Speech Elicitation and Stuttering

Not infrequently, eliciting an adequate speech sample from young children is not a simple matter. Children may remain quiet during the first visit or two, speak little, and be uncooperative during the administration of various tests. Hence several visits are sometimes required to accomplish a comprehensive evaluation. Even if a child is cooperative, on a "good day" he or she may exhibit little stuttering, way below the typical level as described by parents. Thus at least two or three speech samples may be necessary, including one at home.

Objectives of the Initial Evaluation

We turn now to the specific objectives of the initial evaluation. These are as follows:

1. Obtain from parents a thorough history of the disorder: (a) exact time, circumstances, and type of onset (sudden, gradual, etc.); (b) description of the initial stuttering characteristics, including speech, physical behaviors, and emotional reactions; and (c) description of changes in the stuttering characteristics and severity from onset to date.

2. Identify other factors relevant to the stuttering (e.g., familial history of stuttering and current home environment conditions).

3. Identify other factors that may be relevant to the stuttering, such as health issues.

4. Describe/quantify the various aspects of the child's disfluency and other features of stuttering, including their fluctuation in response to various conditions.

5. Examine the child's language, phonology, motor skills, and hearing.

6. Assess the current stuttering in light of its history and the potential risk factors in order to reach a prognosis and suggested course of action.

7. Share findings and recommendations with parents.

8. Provide parents with information about stuttering and guidance for handling it at home, day care, and in other settings.

Setting and Preparations

In our experience, a comprehensive evaluation of a preschool child may require two or three sessions, depending on the child's cooperation and availability of a second clinician to assist with the testing. Keep in mind that it is necessary to record speech samples over at least two different days, and administer language, phonology, motor, and other tests in addition to the evaluation of stuttering. Also, the initial parent interview may require a whole session, and, similarly, the parent conference at the completion of the evaluation. As with the evaluation with adults, both audio and video recording are desirable. Special attention should be paid to the child's typical daily schedule, especially in regard to naps, snacks, or other routines. Having the child scheduled for the evaluation at the time when he or she is most alert during the day can make an appreciable difference. Parents should be advised to bring with them notes about their child's developmental progress, birth and health history, the incidence and course of stuttering among the extended family, and, if possible, a recorded speech sample of the child. They may also bring along favorite quiet toys and/or books that the child would be inclined to want to talk about.

The evaluation is structured in three parts: the case history interview with parents, observing and testing the child, and a concluding conference with parents. These are detailed in the next section.

The Case History

The initial case interview with one or both parents is conducted without the child present so that the parents and clinician can focus on an open and comfortable sharing of information. The case history includes four components: (1) personal and family information, (2) time and circumstances of onset, (3) symptomatology at onset and at the present, and (4) general child development and health. Specific information items and interview questions are presented in our Case History Form. Comments on specific items are inserted at the end of each section.

Case History Form: Preschool Children

Part I: Client and Family Information

Client Information

Child's Name _____ _____   File # _____
               Last   First

Address _____

Home Phone (____) _____   Parent's Work Phone (____) _____

E-mail _____

Child's Date of Birth _____   Age _____   Gender _____

Race/Ethnicity _____

Informant _____   Relation to child _____

Referral _____

Date of Evaluation _____   Clinician _____

Family Information

Parents Married _____   Divorced _____   If yes, child lives with _____

Language(s) at Home _____

Mother: Name _____   Age _____   Education Level _____

Occupation _____

Stuttering History: No _____   Yes _____   When/How long _____

Relatives on mother's side (her parents, siblings, nieces, and nephews) who have had stuttering history. For each one who stuttered, indicate if/when recovered or if it persists:

_____

_____

Father: Name _____   Age _____   Education Level _____

Occupation _____

Stuttering History: No _____   Yes _____   If yes, when/how long?

_____

Relatives on father's side (his parents, siblings, nieces, and nephews) who have had stuttering history. For each one who stuttered, indicate if/when recovered or if it persists:

_____

_____

Siblings: List siblings by gender and age. Indicate if sibling has had a stuttering history.

_____

_____

_____

Comments on Part I

Items referring to familial history of stuttering serve two purposes. First, they are critical in relation to the child's prognosis. As explained in earlier chapters, a child has about a 65% chance of matching the pattern of family history for stuttering. If there is a family history of recovered stuttering, there is about a 65% chance the child will follow the same pattern; if there is a family history of persistent stuttering, there is about 65% chance of following that pattern. Hence both parents should be urged to check with the relatives of their respective families about stuttering history: Who had it, when, and for how long? Questions about familial history should be raised in subsequent opportunities because new information may surface. Telephone calls to these relatives may add significantly to the reliability of claims. A helpful means for tracking familial history of stuttering is to draw a pedigree (a family tree) that includes the relatives of both parents. A second purpose for pursuing this topic is that it may shed light on the feelings and attitudes toward stuttering at home.

The importance of urging parents to ask questions of their relatives about stuttering must be underscored. It should not be assumed that stuttering would have been mentioned had it occurred. In our experience, relatives often do not offer the information until someone else raises the topic. For example, one young mother, who herself stuttered, was surprised when she learned that her own grandmother, with whom she was close, was someone in the family who had stuttered. She remarked how she might never have known this fact if she had not initiated a discussion of the topic.

Part II: Time and Circumstances of Onset

1. When was the stuttering first noticed? Probe for an accurate date through surrounding circumstances.

   Approximate date of onset _____   Child's age at onset _____

   Child's current age _____   Time since stuttering onset _____

   Notes regarding parent's estimation of date of onset: _____

   _____

   _____

2. Who first noticed the child's stuttering? _____

3. Was the onset sudden or gradual?

   _____ Sudden: 1 day   _____ Gradual: 2 weeks
   _____ Sudden: 2–3 days   _____ Gradual: 3–4 weeks
   _____ Sudden: 1 week   _____ Gradual: 6 weeks or more

4. Were there any illnesses, accidents, or physical traumas when he/she began stuttering or shortly (2–3 weeks) before that time?

   No _____   Yes _____   Which/When _____

5. Were there any identifiable emotionally upsetting events in the child's or the family's life just prior to or at the time of the stuttering onset?

   No _____   Yes _____   Which/When/ Explain _____

   _____

6. Did the time when the child began stuttering coincide with the arrival of a new baby, pregnancy of the mother, or other sibling rivalry?

   No _____   Yes _____   Explain _____

7. Was the child undergoing toilet training, giving up thumb sucking, or changing other habits at the time?

   No _____   Yes _____   Explain _____

8. In general, was the child under some pressure/stress during the period when he/she began stuttering?

   No _____   Yes _____   Explain _____

9. Generally, based on the above, the clinician estimates the manner of stuttering onset as:

   _____ Sudden, following emotionally stressful event
   _____ Sudden, following physical illness
   _____ Sudden, uneventful
   _____ Gradual, following emotionally stressful events
   _____ Gradual, following physical illness
   _____ Gradual, uneventful

10. Was the onset of stuttering associated with noticeable changes or development in the child's general speech and language skills?

    No _____ Yes _____ Explain _____

11. In your opinion, what was the most important cause of the stuttering? What other factors contributed?

    _____

    _____

Comments on Part II

Question 1 "When was the stuttering first noticed?" is the most important item because it provides the estimated time elapsed from onset to the date of the evaluation. This information is critical to determining the current status of the disorder and its prognosis, and considering possible intervention. If the post-onset interval is short, say less than 6 months, and stuttering has slightly declined, an additional waiting period is a reasonable option in light of the possibility of natural recovery. The shorter the interval, the more additional waiting is justified. As the post-onset interval increases, particularly when it is 9 months or longer, the chance is smaller for natural recovery, and intervention may be given greater consideration. Also, there is a trend for children who had onset at an early age to have a greater chance for recovery as compared to those who reported late onset (mentioned in Chapter 3, Buck et al., 2002; Yairi & Ambrose, 2005). Clinicians should guide parents to identify the time of onset with questions that systematically narrow the possible time window. To this end, encourage parents to recall the onset in reference to other events, such as birthdays, holidays, trips, or illnesses. For example, if the child began stuttering in the winter, urge parents to recall whether the child had already stuttered during the December holidays or was it closer to the end of February. Or, if the child began stuttering during summer, was it before or after the Fourth of July, or around the time of a birthday or other significant events such as a vacation.

Question 3 "Was the onset sudden or gradual?" is pertinent in revealing the circumstances and the degree of parents' confidence in their diagnosis. It is not surprising that our data show that stuttering associated with sudden onsets tends to be perceived as more severe. Perhaps it is the severity that calls it more immediately to the parents' attention. Also, some significant differences have been found between children who experienced sudden and those who experienced gradual onset, such as a tendency for parents of the latter group to report recent spurts of language growth (Watkins, 2005). As we discuss later in the chapter, rapidly emerging or precocious language skills is a potential risk factor for persistent stuttering.

Questions 4 through 8 are straightforward, helping the clinician assess physical health and emotional factors possibly contributing to the stuttering. The clinician asks questions that may lead parents to recall and consider stressors that either facilitated or complicated the onset. At the very least, the answers may shed light on the child's home environment and parents' evaluation of, and reaction to, the events that are discussed.

Question 11 is a broad, open-ended invitation for parents to present their point of view and look at parameters that have not been discussed. Conditions, processes, and behaviors such as advanced language skills, nutrition, apparently unrelated medical issues, and other life factors, might surface. Although many of these explanations are typically rejected by most scientists, they should be evaluated for their merit in each case.

Overall, the very task of parents analyzing a child's stuttering and its background might produce secondary therapeutic values, helping them take a good look and reassess their home environment and family style. Johnson and associates (1959) were convinced that the lengthy parent interviews they conducted for their study of stuttering onset were instrumental in the eventual improvement reported for many of the children.

Part III: Symptomatology at Onset and at Present

12. Describe and demonstrate the child's speech when he/she first began stuttering:

_____

_____

13. Indicate which of the following speech disfluencies were observed near onset and now:

Disfluency	Onset	Now
Repeating sound/syllable (ba-ba-baby)	_____	_____
Repeating short words (and-and)	_____	_____
Repeating phrases or longer words (going to-going to)	_____	_____
Prolonging vowels (aaaall)	_____	_____
Prolonging consonants (sssso, mmmy)	_____	_____
Silent blocks (b-aby)	_____	_____
Incomplete words (ba-)	_____	_____
Revisions (it was it went)	_____	_____
Interjecting (ah, um)	_____	_____
Other _____	_____	_____

14. Classify the main disfluency type at the time of onset and now:

Onset: __ Repetitions __ Prolongations __ Blocks __ Interjections

Now: __ Repetitions __ Prolongations __ Blocks __ Interjections

15. Were there secondary characteristics associated with the stuttered speech?

Secondary Characteristics	Onset	Now
Facial grimaces	_____	_____
Eyes closing/blinking	_____	_____
Eyes wide open	_____	_____
Lip tension (e.g., on /p, b, m/)	_____	_____
Lip tremor	_____	_____
Tongue tension (e.g., on /t, d, s, z, l, n/)	_____	_____
Mouth wide open	_____	_____

Secondary Characteristics	**Onset**	**Now**
Jaw tremor	_____	_____
Throat tension	_____	_____
Respiratory irregularities	_____	_____
Upward swings in vocal pitch	_____	_____
Head tilting	_____	_____
Arm/leg movement/tension	_____	_____
Other _____	_____	_____

Parent Scale of Stuttering Severity

16. Rate the severity of the **earliest** stuttering at onset (may select midpoints):

0   I   2   3   4   5   6   7

Normal   Mild   Moderate   Very Severe

17. Rate the **current** severity of the stuttering (may select midpoints):

0   I   2   3   4   5   6   7

Normal   Mild   Moderate   Very Severe

18. Where in the speech stream did the stuttering occurred at onset? Now?

At onset: ___ First word primarily ___ Words throughout the sentences

Now: ___ First word primarily ___ Words throughout the sentences

19. Were there indications of the child being aware or reacting negatively to the stuttering soon after onset? Currently?

At onset: _____ Not aware _____ Somewhat aware _____ Clearly aware and bothered

Describe: _____

Now: _____ Not aware _____ Somewhat aware _____ Clearly aware and bothered

Describe: _____

Comments on Part III

Questions 12 through 19 are designed to provide detailed information about the stuttering characteristics both at onset and at present. Requesting an imitation of the child's stuttering is a good way to obtain a more valid description. The direct comparison of past and present characteristics is an excellent way to evaluate the child's progress in relation to the length of the stuttering history. This is important: Neither the initial stuttering nor the present stuttering, each in and of itself, is as meaningful as the comparison of the type, amount, and direction of the differences that have taken place over time. *The disorder's progression over time is a key component in the assessment and prognosis.* For example, a current severity rating of 5 (on our 8-point 0 to 7 scale) should be alarming if the case history reveals that when stuttering began it was rated by the parent as 2. The same rating of 5, however, would be viewed as a positive sign, if the stuttering severity at onset was rated by the parent as 7 because of the apparent progress. Having this information may have a significant impact on the prognosis for the child and the counseling given to parents concerning decisions for intervention.

Although parents are initially encouraged to describe in their own words the general course of stuttering and changes they have observed in overt stuttering characteristics as well as the child's reactions, checklists of speech and secondary characteristics are used because many parents often are unable either to recall or express all the details. The clinician should carefully differentiate between parent descriptions of stuttering at onset and at the present time, and repeatedly remind parents to do so. When rating the severity of stuttering on the 8-point scale, parents should be instructed to evaluate their overall impression. The clinician makes sure to define 0 as normal speech, 1 as borderline stuttering, 2 as definite but mild stuttering, 3 as mild+, 4 to 5 as a range of moderate, 6 as severe, and 7 as very severe. Parents are allowed to choose points halfway between numbered intervals. Comparison can also be made with the clinician's rating.

Part IV: General Development and Health History

20. Were there physical illnesses or emotional problems that the mother experienced during pregnancy that caused concern or required treatment?

    _____

    _____

21. What medications, drugs, and other medical treatments did the mother have during pregnancy with this child? _____

22. Were there any problems related to delivery?

    No _____   Yes _____   Explain _____

23. Did the child require special medical attention at or immediately after birth?

    No _____   Yes _____   Explain _____

24. Were there any medical problems noted in the child, at birth or shortly after, at a level to cause concern?

    No _____   Yes _____   Explain _____

25. Has the child had any serious health problems since birth?

    Yes _____   No _____   Explain _____

26. Has the child ever had any facial tics, jerks of other body parts, or any other type of involuntary muscle movements?

    No _____   Yes _____   Explain _____

27. Is the child on any medication now?

    No _____   Yes _____   Explain _____

28. In general do you regard the child's health now as:

    _____ Good   _____ Fair   _____ Poor

29. Has the child ever had a behavioral or psychological problem? (ADHD, ADD, depression, Behavioral Disorder, others)

    No _____   Yes _____   Explain _____

30. Indicate age in months when the child acquired the following skills:

    Sat without support _____   Crawled _____   Walked without support _____

31. Overall, how do you regard the child's motor development?

    Below average_____   Average _____   Above average _____

32. Child's handedness:

    Right _____   Left _____   Mixed _____   Undetermined _____

33. In terms of speech, at what age did the following occur?

    Babbling _____   First word _____   Combined 2 or 3 words _____

34. Overall, would you say that the child's speech development was:

    Below average _____   Average _____   Above average _____

35. Aside from stuttering, has the child ever had any speech/language problem? If so, describe.

    No _____   Yes _____   Explain _____

36. Has the child ever had hearing problems? If yes, describe.

    No _____   Yes _____   Explain _____

37. Has the child ever received any treatment for speech, language, or hearing disorders?

    No _____   Yes _____   Explain _____

38. Has the child ever exhibited any of the following at a level to cause concern, or at age-inappropriate levels?

    _____ Sleeping problems   _____ Separation anxiety
    _____ Eating difficulties   _____ Excessive crying
    _____ Unusual fears   _____ Refusal to talk
    _____ Destructiveness   _____ Withdrawn behavior
    _____ Temper tantrums   _____ Restlessness
    _____ Excessive shyness   _____ None of the above

39. In comparison to other children, how much energy does the child have?

    _____ Below average   _____ Average   _____ Above average

40. In terms of overall maturity is this child:

    _____ Below average   _____ Average   _____ Above average

Comments on Part IV

Research has not found any consistent medical problem, or a tendency for having medical issues in general, to be present in the health histories of children who stutter. Yairi and Ambrose (2005) reported that only 14% of cases reported any physical stress associated with stuttering onset. Sometimes stuttering does coexist with other developmental or health problems that should be considered in the clinical recommendations and intervention planning. The clinician, therefore, must discuss and consider the medical and health history. But clinicians should realize there are many variations in pregnancy, delivery, and health histories that occur in the general population without any resultant stuttering. If, in one case, a mother had 2 weeks of confinement to bed rest during pregnancy, or, in another case, there was jaundice at delivery, there should be no assumption these were causes of the child's speech problem. The health history helps the clinician understand the client and the speech difficulty in the larger context of the whole person's individual issues and needs.

Collecting Clinical Data

Obtaining Speech Samples

After obtaining a comprehensive case history of the onset and development of stuttering, as well parental description of the stuttering and judgment of its severity, the clinician proceeds to observe and test the child to obtain more objective as well as quantifiable data. A considerable portion of this part of the evaluation is similar to typical speech-language-hearing evaluations of preschool children seen for other communication problems in that standard tests of phonology, language skills, hearing, motor, and other domains are administered. The main difference is the need to obtain recorded speech samples to quantify the stuttered speech. A few opportunities to observe the child talking may arise in the waiting room and hallways when the child talks to the parents or responds to the clinician's greetings. Hence, having a small handheld tape recorder is advisable to secure these brief moments of spontaneous speech before entering the examination facility. Permissions for audiovisual recording are obtained beforehand.

The more formal recording procedures for young children require similar equipment as specified in Chapter 8 for adults but call for extra flexibility. For example, some children may respond well when sitting at a small table in the recording room; others do better sitting on the floor, interacting with the clinician or parent. This condition, however, makes it difficult to adapt video recordings, resulting in a loss of useful information. To be effective, the camera should be focused on the child's head and upper body. We have had excellent experience obtaining speech samples with the child "confined" to a chair-table setting in a small test room yielding both good speech output and high-quality video and audio recordings. A small lavalier microphone attached to the child's shirt is ideal. But if the child will be free to move, an inexpensive, omnidirectional boundary microphone can detect speech quite well.

For practicality sake, quiet play materials, such as plastic clay or interesting action pictures, are preferable. Plastic and wooden toys generate noise that interferes with the quality of the recording. The clinician or parent initiates conversation about what the child is making with clay, then moves on to open-ended questions regarding the child's favorite toys or TV shows. Find out from parents about topics that particularly excite the child, such as certain pets, toys, TV programs, or events. Stuttering increases with heightening emotion, such as excitement or frustration and these topics also often stimulate longer responses that are also more likely to trigger stuttering. Avoid/minimize questions that invite "yes" or "no" answers or other single-word responses because they stop the conversation and typically are not stuttered as often as words in phrases. After the child says something, questions such as "What happened next?" and prompts such as "Tell me more about it" are quite useful to get the child going.

Preschool age children who stutter, especially in early stages of the disorder, tend to exhibit considerable fluctuations in their stuttering (Yaruss, 1997b). An evaluation that happens to be conducted on a "good day" could underestimate the magnitude of the problem. Therefore, as mentioned earlier, two or three speech samples recorded on different days should be the target, especially when the stuttering is seen as mild. If the child exhibits severe stuttering, a single sample provides much of the needed information because, and this is significant, there is more interest in the potential severity than in how mild it may be at times. Also, due to expected fluctuations, home speech samples are particularly desirable for the young child who stutters. We provide parents with a handheld recorder and ask for 15 to 20 minutes of speech recorded in three to four brief (e.g., 5-minute) segments.

Recording in the clinical setting, the goal is to obtain at least 500 to 600 syllables and ideally close to 1,000 syllables of conversational speech. The higher figure can often be achieved over two recording sessions, 15 to 20 minutes each, separated by a few days. As already explained, larger samples are necessary to capture certain disfluency types or lengths.

As indicated in Chapter 8, data by Sawyer and Yairi (2006) show that in four consecutive 300-syllable segments taken from continuous 1,200-syllable speech samples of 20 children who stutter, the greatest amount of disfluency tended to occur in the last two segments, especially the fourth one. Had they used only the first 300 syllables, some or much of the children's disfluency would not have been reflected in the data. Several disfluency types, such as sound prolongations/blocks or complex disfluent events (e.g., those containing four or more repetition units), might occur in low frequency and cannot be adequately evaluated in short samples, if at all. In other words, the validity and reliability of the data may be questioned. The risk with short speech samples is greater when the stuttering appears to be mild or mild to moderate.

It is desirable to record one of the sessions when the child interacts with a parent and another one with the clinician. Of course, the interaction during the recording of longer samples also provides more time to observe the child's behavior, reaction, and interaction.

Other Related Assessments

Two other aspects of stuttering—secondary body movement and tensions involved with disfluencies, and the child's awareness and emotional reactions—should be included in the direct initial evaluation of preschoolers. In our experience, too often these do not receive sufficient attention. The child should also be assessed for the possibility of other concomitant speech, language, or hearing problems.

Secondary Characteristics

For a long time these were regarded as late phenomena, emerging in late developmental stages of stuttering. During the past 25 years, however, research that employed videotape analyses of young stuttering children's speech demonstrated head and neck movements near the onset of stuttering (Conture & Kelly, 1991; Throneburg, 1997; Yairi et al., 1993). Additionally, direct observation of nearly 150 children near stuttering onset revealed secondary characteristics, such as head turn, lip pursing, and eye blinking, in 75% of the children (Yairi & Ambrose, 2005). Hence, clinicians should look for, and note, the type and severity of secondary characteristics. The same list of secondary characteristics that appears in Chapter 8 is reproduced below. The clinician indicates which ones are observed. At the end, assign a severity rating based on the global impression of these secondary behaviors (mild, moderate, or severe).

Secondary Characteristics Checklist

_____ Head jerks	_____ Head turns (side; up; down)
_____ Forehead tension	_____ Nostrils flaring/constricted
_____ Eyes closed; squinting	_____ Eyes widely open
_____ Facial contortions	_____ Lips pressured
_____ Lip tremor	_____ Jaw tremor
_____ Jaw closed tightly	_____ Teeth grinding
_____ Jaw wide open	_____ Rotational or sideways jaw movement
_____ Tongue protrusion	_____ Throat tightened
_____ Body swaying	_____ Hand and/or arm movements

Estimated Severity: _____

Awareness and Emotional Reactions

This aspect of the initial evaluation of preschool-age children who stutter is quite different than it is with older children or adults. As we discussed in Chapter 3, recent experimental data, clinical observations, and parental reports, have indicated that some children do project various levels of awareness. Thus, it may be possible to obtain important information for those children. Toward this end, we suggest three procedures:

1. **Parental report:** Simply ask parents if they have noticed any indication that the child is aware of the stuttering and/or visibly reacting to it emotionally. If positive, pursue in more detail: What is the evidence? Let the parents respond first, and note whether they refer to a clear verbal expression, such as "I cannot talk," or a nonverbal display of frustration during stuttering events. Also ask them to evaluate the frequency and strength of the child's expressions of awareness and affective reactions.

2. **Direct questioning:** Ask the child if he or she is a good talker or ever makes mistakes when talking. Perhaps better, the clinician may stutter on purpose (e.g., "Do you like i-i-i-i-ice cream?") and then proceed to ask the child, "Who else talks like that?" and "Do you sometimes talk like that?" Note the verbal reply and other possible reactions.

3. **The puppet test (see Ambrose & Yairi, 1994):** The clinician holds two identical puppets, one on each hand. Each puppet says an identical sentence, with one speaking fluently and the second one stuttering. The child is then asked, "Which puppet talks the way you talk?" This should be repeated several times, changing the order and hand of the stuttering and the fluent puppets. The level of accuracy and consistency provides some information. A discussion of the methods with the parents beforehand may help to ensure that they will be comfortable with the method used by the clinician to explore awareness.

Anxiety, Temperament, and Personality

Recent research by Karass et al. (2006) has implicated a role for temperament in the disorder of stuttering (see discussion in Seery et al., 2007). They found that compared to nonstuttering children, a significant proportion of preschool children who stutter tended to (1) become more emotionally aroused, (2) settle down less easily after arousal, and (3) show less emotional control during everyday stressful and challenging situations. If these initial observations are valid, then an evaluation of temperament may aid intervention planning. Instruments of assessment include the Children's Behavior Questionnaire (CBQ; Rothbart, Ahadi, Hershey et al., 2001) and the Behavioral Style Questionnaire (BSQ; McDevitt & Carey, 1978), which have been used in research with children who stutter (Anderson, Pellowski, Conture et al., 2003). Considering typical results of a temperament assessment, clinicians might work together with parents to discourage overly exciting environmental conditions for their child to talk in, provide more reassurances and calming encouragements to their child, and/or make a special point of preparing the child for what to expect before new or potentially fear-evoking situations (e.g., medical exams, fire drills, sitters, travel, etc.).

Language, Phonology, Motor, and Hearing

The initial evaluation of CWS, like that of other children, should include comprehensive screening of the speech mechanism, phonology, language, voice and hearing domains. Motor and other skills may be added according to case needs. Standard tests or tape-recorded conversational speech samples can be used for phonological and language analyses. Because deficits in these domains may impact decisions of whether to initiate therapy, and what approach is selected (Byrd, Wolk et al., 2007), careful assessment must be pursued in addition to the primary focus on stuttering. These aspects of the evaluation, however, are not discussed in this book.

Analyzing Clinical Data

Disfluency Frequency and Types

After securing a tape-recorded speech sample, the next task is to quantify the characteristics of stuttering. In most respects, the parameters and procedures involved are identical to those employed in the initial evaluation of adults as described in Chapter 8. Again, clinicians are faced with the choice of metric. Some clinicians prefer making categorical judgments of each word or syllable as either stuttered or not, and then calculate the percentage of stuttered words or syllables. This is the easiest method of quantifying stuttering that provides general information. It is also the method used in the Stuttering Severity Instrument (SSI-4; Riley, 2008). The disfluencies that are considered to be "stuttering" for the previous measures are the core types.

As we already explained, however, these metrics do not yield specific descriptive data about the characteristics of the person's stuttering: How did he or she stutter? Did the stuttering contain repetitions, prolonged sounds, blocks, or other behaviors? If the client repeated a word, how many times was the word repeated: one, four, or seven times? Measures of percentage of stuttered words or syllables simply do not address such questions because they report a single number of "stutterings." Because there is a growing body of information showing the significance of specific disfluency types, as well as the length of disfluency in terms of the range and mean number of repetition units[1] in differential diagnosis and prognosis of stuttering (e.g., Ambrose & Yairi, 1999; Schwartz & Conture, 1988; Throneburg & Yairi, 2001), we believe that reporting the frequency-type-length of specific disfluency types is a preferred method even though it requires more analysis time. Furthermore, changes over time in the specific disfluency types and their extent or length, rather than just changes in the percent of stuttering events, is of great value in monitoring important aspects of the child's progress.

---

[1]As we discussed in Chapter 8, repetition units refer to the number of extra productions of a syllable or a word. For example, in "bu-but," the number of repetition units is one. In "bu-bu-but" there are two units, and in "bu-bu-bu- bu-but" there are four. To calculate the range and mean of the number of repetition units, data for monosyllabic part-word and whole-word repetitions are combined.

The importance of specific disfluency data is illustrated with the following example. Suppose one clinician counted 15% stuttered syllables at the initial evaluation of a child. Three months later, the child again scored 15% stuttered syllables, leading to the conclusion that no change had occurred. Consider a second clinician who saw the same child at each of those same times but analyzed sample data differently. She noted 20 stuttering-like disfluencies (SLD) per 100 syllables at the initial evaluation (more than one disfluency, e.g., repetition followed by prolongation, may occur on the same syllable). Among these, 5 were sound prolongations and 15 were part-word or word repetitions. The mean number of repetition units was two (e.g., bu-bu-but). At the 3-month follow-up, the child again scored 20 SLDs per 100 syllables, however, 15 were sound prolongations and only 5 were part-word repetitions. Furthermore, the mean number of repetition units was four (bu-bu-bu-bu-but). In contrast with the first clinician, she infers that the child's speech is worsening, not stable. In conclusion, when total SLD or overall disfluency remains constant, there may still be significant changes in the stuttering characteristics both in type and length of the disfluent events. These could show a significant worsening or improvement of the problem. Such information is missed by the counting methods employed by the first clinician.

The same procedures for disfluency analysis described in Chapter 8 for adult speech samples should be followed when analyzing the samples of little children:

1. Transcribe the recorded speech sample(s), replaying the audio or video-material phrase by phrase or word by word, one line per phrase.

2. Identify and classify each disfluent event according to the six disfluency types listed in the chart below using a symbol for each type.

3. Calculate the respective frequencies of each type per 100 syllables.

4. Add up the three SLD types and the 3 OD types as indicated in the chart:

Disfluency Type	Number in Sample	Per 100 Syllables
Part-Word Repetition	_____	_____
Monosyllabic Word Repetition	_____	_____
Disrhythmic Phonation	_____	_____
SLD Subtotal	_____	_____
Interjection	_____	_____
Revision	_____	_____
Phrase Repetition	_____	_____
Other Disfluency Subtotal	_____	_____
Overall Disfluency Total	_____	_____

Disfluency Length

The following three measures of the extent, or length, of disfluencies are worth consideration for inclusion.

Repetition Units

In addition to estimating the mean repetition unit, it is quite important to keep track of the number of word or part-word repetitions (per 100 words or syllables) that contain three or more units. It is perhaps the most powerful information for differentiating early stuttering from normal disfluency (Ambrose & Yairi, 1999). Repetitions of this size are extremely rare in the speech of normally fluent children. In fact, these authors found that even instances of two repetition units are infrequent in normally fluent children. Hence their conspicuous presence in a speech sample is a strong diagnostic sign of stuttering.

Rate of Repetitions

The temporal characteristics of the child's repetitions also provide diagnostic clues because children who stutter tend to repeat syllables and words considerably faster than normally fluent children. The repetitions are faster because the intervals between the iterations are shorter. Conversely, the repetitions of normally fluent children are slower because the intervals between their iterations are about twice as long as those of children who stutter. Investigators have reported that interval duration alone was sufficient to differentiate children who stutter from normally fluent peers with 72% to 87% accuracy (Throneburg & Yairi, 1994). Such measurements may be too difficult to execute in a clinical setting. Nevertheless, clinicians should make a point to note the tempo with informal observations.

Sound Prolongations

The length of sound prolongations is measured in terms of time duration. Because most of these disfluencies are sustained only up to 1 second (Bloodstein & Bernstein Ratner, 2008), it is useful to obtain and document the mean of only the three longest prolongations. The presence of prolongations longer than 1 second is also a strong sign of stuttering (Zebrowski & Conture, 1989). A few such events can easily increase the overall severity rating.

Speech Rate

Speaking rate is of diagnostic interest because of its negative correlation with the amount of disfluent speech. It is, however, often difficult to assess with reasonable accuracy in young children in the clinical setting because of their high frequency of both short utterances and long silences. Thus some clinicians may opt to spend more of their assessment time on other measures. Regardless, if deemed desirable, speech rate data can be extracted from the spontaneous speech sample. Reasonable estimates of *overall speech rate* can be obtained by measuring several minutes of conversational speech using a stopwatch. As explained in Chapter 8, it is considerably more complicated to accurately measure *articulatory rate,* which is based only on fluent portions of the speech sample, and it is more reliably obtained with sophisticated equipment for acoustic analysis. An illustration comparing the relative nature of overall speech rate and articulatory rate is shown in Figure 9.2. The limited research with preschool

Figure 9.2   Illustration of Overall Speech Rate and Articulatory Rate

Overall speech rate is based on the time used for the entire sample (words, pauses, disfluency). For example, the time measure would include the whole quote spoken below.		
"I-I-I thhhink like the quick **brown fox jumped over** the lazy, you know, lazy dog."		
Articulatory rate excludes words with disfluencies, like the quote starting above.	Articulatory rate is based only on truly *continuous spoken words (underlined, bolded in the quote above).*	Articulatory rate excludes mazes and words separated by brief pauses, like the quote ending above.

children has shown that close to stuttering onset, children who stutter tend to exhibit somewhat slower articulatory rates than normally fluent peers. The respective means were 8.43 and 11.42 phones per second (Hall, Amir, & Yairi, 1999) for children 3 and 4 years of age. In another study conducted by Meyers and Freeman (1985), 4- and 5-year-old CWS had a mean articulatory rate of 3.5 syllables per second compared to the NFC's rate of 4.04 syllables per second.

Interpreting Clinical Data

Although a subjective determination of stuttering can probably be made during the examination, and it will most likely be correct and in agreement with the parents' diagnosis, the clinician should apply a careful evaluation of all the information gathered, starting with the speech data, comparing the client with other children who stutter and with normally fluent children. As we stated earlier, in most cases of stuttering, the purpose of the initial evaluation is to describe/quantify the problem and understand all contributing and complicating factors. At completion, the clinician should be able to provide a rather comprehensive description of the problem, determine its severity, assess prognosis, formulate recommendations, and counsel the parents.

Disfluency Status

As in other standard speech-language evaluations, the client's performance is compared against available data starting with those pertaining specifically to stuttering: percentage of stuttered words or syllables, or the type/frequency of disfluency, the extent and/or duration of disfluency, and secondary characteristics. For comparison, Table 9.1 displays disfluency data for large groups of stuttering and normally fluent preschoolers.

   As you can see, there are large differences between children who stutter and normally fluent children both in absolute and relative measures of each of the three SLD components. It is very important to examine the total SLD. Note that it is almost 10 times larger for CWS than for NFC. Also note that whereas the total SLD constitutes approximately 66% of the CWS's *overall disfluency* (10.37/15.78 per 100 syllables), it is only 24% (1.33/5.65) for NFC. When you subtract the one standard deviation of 6.42 from the mean SLD of 10.37 the resultant value of 3.90 SLD (per 100 syllables)

Table 9.1   Mean and Standard Deviations of Stuttering-Like Disfluencies, Other Disfluencies, and Number of Repetition Units per Repetition per 100 Syllables*

Type	CWS *Stutter*		CWNS *Normal*	
	Mean (SD)	Proportion	Mean (SD)	Proportion
SLD				
Part-Word Repetition	5.29 (4.20)	0.34	0.56 (0.40)	0.10
Single-Syllable Word Repetition	3.34 (2.14)	0.21	0.69 (0.60)	0.12
Disrhythmic Phonation	1.75 (2.00)	0.11	0.09 (0.12)	0.02
TOTAL SLD	**10.37 (6.42)**	**0.66**	**1.33 (0.83)**	**0.24**
Repetition Units	1.54 (0.39)		1.10 (0.12)	
OD				
Interjection	2.55 (2.20)	0.16	2.08 (1.89)	0.37
Revision	1.97 (1.09)	0.12	1.80 (0.85)	0.32
Multisyllable/Phrase Repetition	0.89 (0.63)	0.06	0.44 (0.44)	0.08
TOTAL OD	**5.41 (2.75)**	**0.34**	**4.32 (2.28)**	**0.76**
OVERALL DISFLUENCY	**15.78**			**5.65**

*Also, the proportion of each disfluency type in the overall number of disfluencies for children who stutter and normally fluent children ages 2 to 4. CWS, children who stutter; CWNS, children who do not stutter; OD, other disfluencies; SD, standard deviation; SLD, stuttering-like disfluencies.

Source: Reprinted with permission from "Normative Disfluency Data for Early Childhood Stuttering," by N. Ambrose and E. Yairi, *Journal of Speech, Language, and Hearing Research, 42,* 895–909. Copyright 1999 by American Speech-Language-Hearing Association. All rights reserved.

is approximately the low level for stuttered speech. The data for the NFC controls support this. Adding even 2 standard deviations of 0.83 to their SLD mean of 1.33 yields the figure of 2.99. *Generally then, 3 or 4 SLD seems to be the lowest level for stuttering.* Interestingly, several older differentiating protocols arrived at a similar conclusion. For example, Van Riper (1971) required at least (a) two syllable repetitions and/or (b) one sound prolongation of 1second or longer per 100 words. His concept of minimal three stuttered events is similar to 3 SLDs per 100 words except that we prefer the per 100 syllables measure. This figure seems to be consistent with what often has been applied in clinical and research matters (e.g., Conture 2001; J. Ingham, 1999).

Next, look at the line for repetition units. The numbers are small yet extremely revealing. The mean of 1.10 for the NFC tells us that these children mostly repeat once per instance ("bu-but"). By contrast, the mean of 1.54 tells us that most repetitions by CWS contain two or more units ("bu-bu-but"). Matching the client's data against these published normative values, and by adding observations on the presence of secondary characteristics, the disfluency analysis provides an anchor for the diagnosis and offers a clear picture of the essential features of the child's stuttering. The clinician is then in a position to also estimate the severity of the stuttering.

Stuttering Severity

Having observed, recorded, described, and quantified the child's speech and associated behaviors, a general overall rating of the severity of stuttering is in order. As we discussed in Chapter 8, there are several ways to do so, the simplest being a perceptual rating scale. This may be the same 8-point scale used earlier to obtain the parent's rating and is displayed again below. Or, it may be another scale with a different interval range, such as those discussed in relation to the evaluation of adults and school-age children who stutter. When a perceptual scale is employed for assigning a global severity rating, the rater presumably takes into account all the parameters that are typically analyzed in the evaluation of stuttering: frequency and length of disfluent events, the degree of muscular tension and effort involved, and the type and number of secondary characteristics. Either a specific scale number or an in-between number (e.g., 4.5) may be selected. Using the identical scale and method as the parent has the advantage of allowing direct comparison between the clinician's and the parent's perception.

Rating Scale of Stuttering Severity

0	1	2	3	4	5	6	7
Normal		Mild		Moderate			Very Severe

A subjective severity rating can be made online, that is, while the clinician watches and listens to the child talking with the parent. Severity can also be evaluated during the face-to-face interaction by the clinician with the child. It would be wise to assign a separate rating for the two speaking situations. Another option is to delay the rating until after completing the quantified analysis of the recorded speech sample. If desired, a formal instrument can be used, such as the Stuttering Severity Instrument-4 (Riley, 2009) or the University of Illinois Stuttering Severity Scale (Yairi & Ambrose, 2005). The Illinois scale scores four components of disfluency. The first three, frequency, duration, and tension, are rated from 0 to 6 where 0 = normal, 1 = borderline, 2 = mild stuttering, and 6 = severe stuttering. These three scores are added and averaged (a maximal mean of 6). The fourth component, accessory characteristics, is rated only from 0 to 1, and this number is added to the mean of the first three. Thus, in total, the maximum score is 7 (very severe stuttering).

Borderline Cases

The real diagnostic challenges in identifying early childhood stuttering are a very small number of children, in our extensive experience, who present too few disfluencies in their speech sample. Group means and standard deviations are not too useful in such cases. The clinician should again review parents' detailed descriptions and their imitations of the child's stuttering at home, which can provide very useful hints. If parents report and imitate occasional daily stuttering such as "whe-whe-whe-when," or /a-a-a-ai/ ("I"), the case should not be dismissed even if the speech sample recorded in the clinic contained only isolated disfluent events that could have been perceived as stuttering.

> The differential diagnosis of stuttering from normal disfluency requires familiarity with the nature of speech characteristics at the margins of both. No single speech characteristic, observed only once, is sufficient to confirm stuttering. Such a basis could cause mistakes of over diagnosis. Requiring validation from too many instances or types of speech characteristics, however, could lead to an under identification of cases. Adopting a careful approach, clinicians should look for data at the very low end of the range of children who stutter where there is still no, or only minimal, overlap with normally fluent children. There are two questions: (1) What are the minimal disfluent speech characteristics associated with very mild stuttering? and (2) What are the upper limits for normal?

Based on a careful analysis of a large body of data, Yairi and Ambrose (2005) also offered a set of seven minimal diagnostic criteria specifically for young children (ages 2 to 5 years) who appear to be borderline cases. Examining a young child's speech sample data, each of the following is assessed at its occurrence per 100 syllables. The child's results are then compared with the values in the list below to determine if any meet (or exceed) the criterion values. Among these seven items, if *at least three* meet (or exceed) the values, the results are sufficient to establish stuttering:

1. Part-word repetition (PW)   1.5
2. Single-syllable word repetition (SSW)   2.5
3. Disrhythmic phonation   0.5
4. Total SLD   3.0
5. Weighted SLD[2]   4.0
6. Mean repetition units   1.5
7. (PW + SSW) with 2 or more extra units   2.0

Finally, the parents' description and rating of stuttering severity should be considered. If the child does not exhibit stuttering in the clinic but parents describe speech characteristics at home that raise suspicion of stuttering, home speech samples should be secured for further analysis.

---

[2]Weighted SLD is a measure that reflects three dimensions of disfluency—frequency, type, and extent—in a single score. It is calculated by adding together the frequency of part- and single-syllable word repetitions per 100 syllables (PW + SS) and multiplying that sum by the mean number of repetition units (RU), and then adding twice the frequency of disrhythmic phonation (DP; blocks and prolongations) per 100 syllables. See Ambrose and Yairi (1999, 2005).

Making Prognosis

Having completed the data-gathering, analysis, and diagnosis steps of the initial evaluation, the clinician is faced with the challenge of assessing the likely future development of the child's stuttering, that is, making a prognosis. It should first be understood that a diagnosis of stuttering based on the characteristics described previously does not imply an unfavorable prognosis, particularly when the identification is made soon after stuttering onset. Thus, data have shown that soon after onset the initial severity of stuttering does not predict the outcome for the child (Yairi & Ambrose, 2005). However, when a child has been stuttering without any indication of a decline for at least a year, the chances for recovery without treatment are reduced, and prognosis becomes more guarded or negative. Once a child has stuttered for 3 or 4 years, the prognosis is "persistent" or "chronic" stuttering.

With strong evidence that approximately 75% or more of children who begin stuttering can be expected to exhibit natural recovery (e.g., Andrews & Harris, 1964; Månsson, 2005; Ryan, 2001a), the ability to make early predictions as to who will recover and who will develop persistent stuttering could be a tremendous asset to clinicians and a major factor in the clinical strategy recommended to parents. It also raises several serious ethical and practical issues.

The challenge of prognosis is highlighted by the example of a clinician who assesses a child as having good chances for natural recovery and recommends a waiting period rather than immediate intervention. What level of accuracy in prediction should be acceptable, and how long should the waiting period be, if the child continues to stutter 3, 6, 9, 12 months, or even longer? Placing a child in unnecessary therapy poses a burden to the family, in terms of time, cost, and concern. Additionally, it unjustifiably places a strain on professional and public resources while children with other pressing needs compete for the same opportunity. It should be obvious that if all 5% or more of the preschool children who begin stuttering are in line for treatment, resources could quickly be exhausted. Health insurance companies, too, would probably resist footing the bill for this high proportion of controversial cases.

Some have argued that unnecessary treatment may be ethically questionable as seen in the following quotation: "[w]e should candidly entertain the proposition that it might be ethically *inappropriate* to categorically direct all cases of early childhood stuttering for treatment, as has been advocated by other clinicians. It seems that, intentionally or unintentionally, clinicians do tend to scare parents into submitting their child to treatment by presenting a bleak picture of what might happen to the child and his/her speech if therapy is not immediately initiated. Typically, they press the point that, if left untreated, stuttering will grow in severity and will acquire many additional unpleasant characteristics, such as strong fears of talking, social withdrawal, etc. Statistically, however, the reverse is true." (Yairi & Ambrose, 2005, p. 416)

Past Prediction Guidelines

Over the years, several clinicians have offered lists of danger signs and criteria for predicting persistent (chronic) stuttering in children; others published more elaborated guidelines and formal instruments. The list below presents the main criteria of either general suggestions or more organized clinical tools.

Stromsta (1965)—Based the second formant (F2) transition in the acoustic waveforms of disfluencies recorded from children after they began stuttering, Stromsta found that 89% of children whose disfluencies lacked F2 transition and/or had irregular termination of phonations continue to stutter 10 years later. Conversely, 91% of children whose disfluencies contained normal F2 transitions and terminations of phonation recovered. Yaruss and Conture (1993), however, were unable to corroborate these findings.

Van Riper (1971)—A review of his four subgroups (tracks) yields several danger signs for persistency: (1) blocks as the early dominant disfluency, (2) late onset, (3) sudden onset, (4) a lack of episodic cycles of stuttering, and (5) poor articulation skills.

Curlee (1980)—Risk increases with (1) part-word repetitions of two or more units on >2% of the words, (2) prolongations longer than 1 second, (3) blocks longer than 2 seconds, (4) secondary characteristics, (5) noticeable emotional reaction, (6) complaints of not being able to function satisfactorily, and (7) marked variation in frequency/severity of stuttering.

Conture (1990)—Two or more of the following: (1) prolongations or blocks constitute more than 25% of the total disfluencies; (2) lack of eye contact; (3) frequent and/or unusual use of phonological processes; (4) prolongations, blocks, or part-word repetitions on the first production of diadochokinetic tasks; and (5) delayed neuromotor development.[3]

Riley (1981)—Based on the Stuttering Prediction Instrument for Young Children (SPI) that gathers information from parents and observing the child: (1) secondary characteristics, (2) frustration with disfluencies, (3) parents' reactions (4) part-word repetitions with more than 3 units, (5) part-word repetitions appearing "abnormal," (6) prolongations and blocks, and (7) frequency of disfluencies per 100 words. Each item is scored within a range of possible points (e.g., 0 to 4). A total score of 10 or higher out of a possible 40 suggests a risk.

Cooper and Cooper (1985)—The Chronicity Prediction Checklist, suggests any of the following: (1) 5% disfluency over 6 months, (2) duration of disfluencies greater than 2 seconds , (3) blocks and articulatory struggle, (4) secondary characteristics, (5) child reacts negatively to stuttering, or (6) parents react negatively to stuttering. Possible scores range from 0 to 27, with 7 to 15 indicating a need for monitoring and a score above 16 predicting chronic stuttering.

---

[3]Conture also believed that the use of fast speaking rate or complex vocabulary by the parents might aggravate the child's stuttering, making it more difficult to become fluent.

Review and Summary

We note with interest that the top criteria listed in these sources refer to stuttered speech: type or frequency of disfluency, acoustic features, or secondary characteristics. Overall, the main focus is on the severity of overt stuttering with some consideration of the emotional reaction to it. Van Riper also considered some information regarding onset. Unfortunately, these indicators were not accompanied by strong scientific data. For example, in the Stuttering Prediction Instrument (SPI) some data were collected from children who were nearly 9 years old. Hence their predictive value for children near the onset of stuttering, ages 2 to 4, when the prognosis is most needed, is substantially diminished. Also, the sample consisted of 75% persisting and 25% recovered children, just the reverse of the expected proportion. Similarly, several items on the Chronicity Prediction Checklist assume the child has already stuttered for 2 years, too long for "early" prediction.

In reviewing past criteria and the way they were derived, Yairi and Ambrose (2005) pointed out two fundamental requirements essential for establishing criteria for early prediction of the course of stuttering. First, data should be collected from *unbiased, representative samples* of many stuttering children over several years. Second, children must be observed and followed from a time as *close to onset* as possible, so that those who exhibit early natural recovery are taken into account. They emphasized the second point, stating, "It goes without saying that the longer the stuttering history is at the point when data are collected, the less applicable they are to predicting the course of very early stuttering, when prognosis is needed the most" (Yairi & Ambrose, 2005, p. 346).

Recent Developments: The Illinois Prediction Criteria

The large-scale longitudinal study conducted at the University of Illinois mentioned in Chapter 3 identified a substantial number of children close to the time of stuttering onset and followed them for several years. A wide range of aspects of the disorder were examined, such as type of onset, characteristics of early stuttering, language and phonology, motor skills, cognition, affective reactions, genetics, and many others (Yairi & Ambrose, 2005). Because changes over time were measured for children who eventually recovered without treatment, as well as for those who persisted in stuttering, the study is unique in its wealth of information pertaining to clinical assessment of a child's risks for persistent stuttering or the chance for natural recovery. These authors distinguished three levels of prognostic criteria according to their strength. These are listed here followed by explanations. Primary factors are arranged in an approximate order of importance. There is no particular order within the secondary and tertiary factors. Also, see Chapter 3, the section on predictive factors, for additional information.

Predictive Factors

Primary Factors	Secondary Factors	Tertiary Factors
Family history	Stuttering severity	Concomitant disorders
Gender	Head and neck movement	Awareness and affective reactions
Stuttering (SLD) trends	Phonological skills	
Duration of stuttering	Expressive language	
Age at onset	Acoustic features	
Disfluency length		
Sound prolongations/blocks		

Comments on Primary Factors

Familial History   Currently, this is the strongest as well as earliest predictor. A history of familial stuttering, however, is not sufficient information. What counts is the *pattern* of the history. If the child has relatives who recovered from stuttering, he or she has a 65% chance for natural recovery. Conversely, a familial history of persistent stuttering gives the child a 65% chance for persistent stuttering. A pattern of familial persistence is apt to reduce the amount of waiting time prior to intervention.

Gender   Boys have greater risk for persistency than girls. Girls also tend to recover sooner. If a girl fails to improve within a year, then her risk for persistent stuttering increases.

SLD Trends   The change over time in the frequency of SLD provides a critical clue. A *downward* trend during the first year, even if the frequency remains high, is a strong sign for recovery. A decline from 20 to 12 SLDs over 3 months is good whereas a stable number of 12 SLDs over the same period is not. In most children who show such decline, however, full recovery will take 2 to 3 years post-onset. By contrast, a child who exhibits a flat or an upward trend of stuttering by the end of 1 year is at risk for persistency. Children should be recorded every 3 months to obtain data. Severity ratings made by the parents may also be used to evaluate the trend. Figure 9.3 provides an illustration.

Duration of Stuttering History (Time Since Onset)   If stuttering has continued for 1 year, the risk for persistency increases. The longer the history, the higher is the risk. Soon after onset, the chance for recovery is at least 75%. A year later, it is down to 63%, declining to 47% at 2 years post-onset, dropping to 16% at 3 years, and to only 5% at 4 years after onset. This critical information has been overlooked in the prognostic schemes reviewed. For example, if the prognostic criteria include a certain level of stuttering as a risk factor, it has no practical meaning without reference to the duration of the stuttering history.

Figure 9.3   **SLD Frequency (vertical axis) over time (horizontal axis) illustrates that a child with a higher SLD level (squares) has a good prognosis for recovery if the line is declining with time whereas a child who exhibits a lower SLD level (diamonds) has a poor prognosis if the line remains flat over time. The expected trends (dashed lines) differ.**

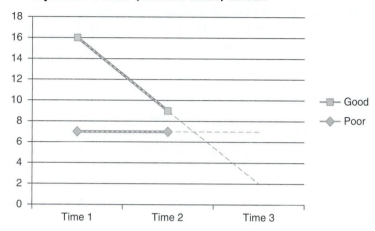

Age at Onset   Late age at onset, for example, 50 to 60 months (4 to 5 years), tends to be associated with persistency. Also, the older the child is at onset, the higher is the awareness of stuttering and the consequent emotional reactions. Additionally, the child's friends are older, and they too are more likely to react negatively to the stuttering.

Disfluency Length and Tempo   During the first year of stuttering, the continuing presence of disfluencies with two, three or more repetition units (e.g., "bu-bu-bu-but") is a sign of risk. Reduction of the repetition units typically coincides with a diminution in the frequency of stuttering as a sign of possible recovery. A slower tempo of the repetitions favors recovery as well. Duration of blocks and prolongations early on is *not* a predictive factor.

Sound Prolongation/Blocks   A substantial number of sound prolongations or blocks pose a possible risk, although *not* during the first few months of the disorder. When the percentage of sound prolongations in the total disfluency declines over time, it signals recovery. Conversely, when the percentage grows, so does the risk for persistency.

Comments on Secondary and Tertiary Factors

Stuttering Severity   Stuttering severity during the early stage of the disorder (6 months or so) is *not* a predictive sign. One year after onset, however, severe stuttering does become a risk signal.

Head and Neck Movement   Secondary characteristics are *not* an early danger sign. They become a sign of risk if, after 1 year, there is no substantial decline in their number and severity.

Phonology   During the early phase of stuttering, phonology skills below norms might be a risk. In isolation, however, phonology is not a strong factor. It serves to reinforce other indicators. Poor phonology, however, should alert the clinician to look for other possible risk signs. After one year of stuttering, phonological skills are not a predictive factor.

Expressive Language   The value of language skills in predicting the course of stuttering is questionable. If at all, *advanced* skills may be a danger sign, especially if they remain ahead of normative expectations across time (Watkins, 2005). Combined with other signs of persistence however, weak language skills could add risk rather than being a neutral factor.

Acoustic Features   F2 transition data are not useful at the present for making early predictions.

Concomitant Disorders   The predictive value of other disorders associated with stuttering (not including language and phonology) is unknown. Their presence and the medications used for treatment may exacerbate stuttering, indirectly increasing the risk for persistency.

Awareness and Affective Reactions   There is no evidence that a young child's awareness of, and emotional reaction to, stuttering predict persistency. However, temperament characteristics such as nonadaptability and high reactivity could add risk in combination with other factors. It is possible that either the child's or a parent's strong negative reactions to stuttering may negate potential recovery factors.

When making a prognosis regarding risk of persistence, clinicians should evaluate the combined weight of (a) the strength (rank order within the primary factors, as well as primary versus secondary factors), and (b) the numbers of risk factors present. For example, a family history of persistent stuttering is considerably more important than the length of disfluencies (average number of repetition units). The predictive power of the Illinois criteria varies greatly, and no single characteristic is sufficient for valid estimates of the chances for persistence or recovery. It is the converging of several factors that clinicians must look for. Below are several hypothetical combinations:

Combination I. Child age 3 years. Family History—has a blood related uncle (alive or dead) who stuttered for 20 years. This factor alone is sufficient to raise a red flag. Add two more factors: (1) Gender—male, and (2) Duration of Stuttering History—has stuttered for 8 months, the risk of persistence is very high.

Combination II. Same child in terms of Family History and Gender, but in terms of Duration of Stuttering History—has stuttered for only 4 months. Although this post-onset duration is too short to raise a concern, if the SLD Trend factor indicates no reduction in the frequency of SLD over the past 3 months, then the risk is still high.

Combination III. Another 3-year-old child. Family History—none. Gender—female; Duration of Stuttering History—8 months post-onset; SLD Trend—the frequency of SLD has continued to increase. Sound Prolongations—increased proportion. Secondary Risk Factors include concomitant disorders of asthma and moderate language delay. The upward disfluency trend after 8 months is a major risk even for a girl. The presence of two secondary factors strengthen a prognosis for persistence.

Combination IV. A 5 year, 10 months-old child. Family History—none; Gender—female; Duration History—15 months post-onset; Sound prolongations—increased proportion; SLD Trend—No change over the past 6 months; Stuttering Severity—Moderate. This child has a relatively late onset age, has stuttered for a relatively long period, exhibits numerous sound prolongations, and has shown no signs of improvement. All these suggest a high risk for persistence in spite of the fact that the child is a girl without a familial stuttering history.

Combination V. A 2-year old child. Family History—none; Gender—male. Duration—2 months; SLD Trend—has increased; Prolongations—relatively frequent; Disfluency Length—4-5 repetition units per instance; Secondary Risk Factors include Stuttering Severity—high; Head & Neck Movement—yes. Because of the very short post-onset duration and the absence of a persistent familial history of stuttering, the combined factors do not yet indicate a substantial risk of persistence. It is still too early to interpret this SLD Trend as a higher risk. If no change occurs within 4-6 months, a risk emerges.

Case Studies

A few cases will illustrate the point.

Case 1

Julie was first evaluated at 29 months of age, 4 months after onset. At the time she exhibited severe stuttering, about 18 SLD per 100 syllables, mostly repetitions of two to four units with moderate tension. Being so young with a brief stuttering history and no apparent danger signs, waiting and reevaluation in 3 months was recommended in spite of the severe stuttering. At the second visit, the frequency of SLD dropped to 13 per 100 syllables and repetition units to only 2 per instance. Her mother reported similar observations. Although the stuttering was still moderate in severity, being a girl, the clear decline in frequency and length of disfluency, and the continuing lack of other danger signs indicated high chances for recovery. Again, a waiting period and another reevaluation were recommended. Three months later, stuttering was mild. By 1 year post-onset, she displayed completely normally fluent speech without intervention.

Case 2

Matthew was evaluated at 34 months of age, 2 months after stuttering onset. He exhibited low-moderate stuttering, about 8 SLD per 100 syllables composed mainly of repetitions of two extra units. The boy's father had a history of stuttering and still exhibited mild-to-moderate stuttering. No other danger signs were identified. In spite of the family history of persistent stuttering, because of the very short history of the problem and the moderate stuttering, it was decided to recommend a 3-month waiting period under close monitoring. At the reevaluation, the frequency of SLD rose to 11 SLD per 100 syllables, and a few sound prolongations were observed. Hence because of the three danger signs—being a boy, family history of persistent stuttering, and the increase in the level of stuttering over time—immediate therapy was recommended.

Case 3

Todd was evaluated at 58 months of age, 6 months after a sudden onset. At that time he exhibited moderate stuttering, about 12 SLD per 100 syllables, consisting of about 50% sound prolongations and 50% repetitions, mostly of two to three units, all associated with moderate tension and some secondary characteristics. Language tests indicated precocious skills, but a few age-inappropriate phonological errors were noticed. There were also indications of frustration associated with stuttering episodes. No history of stuttering was recalled by parents. The mother reported essentially consistent amount and pattern of stuttering over the past several months. In view of the multiple danger signs: being a boy, sudden and late onset, a large percentage of sound prolongations, precocious language, phonological delay, and apparently consistent, unabated stuttering patterns, Todd was viewed as having a high risk for persistent stuttering. Therapy was recommended.

Concluding Parent Conference

Having taken part in providing the background information at the beginning of the evaluation, the parents, most often only the mother, are brought back into the process for the conclusion that includes two distinct parts: (1) receiving feedback about the clinician's findings and recommendations, and (2) having an opportunity to ask questions and receive information and guidance regarding stuttering.

Diagnosis, Prognosis, and Recommendations

As in any other speech-language evaluation, the clinician should state the main finding, confirming or contradicting the parent's diagnosis of stuttering, as well findings concerning problems in other areas covered in the evaluation. The clinician then outlines the main characteristics of the stuttering, such as the dominant disfluency type(s), typical length of the disfluencies, (e.g., "He tends to repeat three extra times"), secondary characteristics, tension, variations in the level of stuttering when talking to parent and clinician, the overall stuttering severity rating, indications of awareness or emotional reactions, and whether the stuttering seems to be at an early or a more advanced stage. Of course, when warranted, parents might instead be informed that the child exhibits normal disfluency. Next, specific results of language, phonology, motor, hearing, and any other tests and observations are presented with explanations and comparisons to the normative range.

The focus then shifts to discussion of the possible future course (prognosis) of the disorder. The clinician should inform parents that about 5% or more of all children experience stuttering for some period during the preschool years but that at least 75% of them stop stuttering on their own, a phenomenon referred to as *natural recovery*. Some experience natural recovery rather quickly, within a few months to 1 year after onset. For most children, however, although signs of improvement begin during the first year, complete recovery takes 2 to 3 years. Whereas the outlook for positive development is statistically good, parents should keep in mind that some children do not recover and develop chronic stuttering that lasts for several or many years.

The clinician should clearly caution parents that, at the present state of knowledge, it is not possible to make an accurate prediction about a specific child's eventual course of stuttering. Nevertheless, given what we do know, reasonable estimates of the relative chances of change in the near future are possible and can be helpful in making clinical recommendations and decisions. Therefore the clinician proceeds to review for the parents their child's standing in relation to the various risk factors listed and discussed earlier. An example of information explained to parents is presented next:

> "Boys have a poorer chance for recovery than girls, which is a negative point. Your son's grandfather, however, stuttered when he was very young but stopped after 3 years. This is a favorable sign because your son has a good chance of following the same pattern. Still, many of the child's disfluencies are sound prolongations at half a year post-onset, another negative point. But although you have expressed concerns that your son has stuttered for 6 months, you have noticed an overall improvement during the last 2 months from a stuttering severity rating of 6 (severe) to a rating of 4 (moderate). This is a positive point." Given the family history and the signs of improvement, the clinician would be in a position to support an additional waiting period with continued monitoring over the next 2 to 3 months. A decision to initiate intervention is appropriate, however, when the parents prefer it.

Having considered all factors with due regard to their importance, the clinician has the responsibility of either recommending a waiting period of 2 to 3 months followed by reevaluation or urging the parents to seek an immediate intervention program. When a waiting period is recommended, the child can be monitored for the prescribed duration, allowing the clinician to compare his or her own data over that time period. If the improvement endures, the monitoring will continue. If the stuttering does not improve, intervention options will be considered in due time. If therapy is recommended, parents should be provided with a list of local providers. The clinician may explain that whereas in the past, intervention was conducted mostly in the form of parent counseling, the past 25 years have seen a growing trend of providing direct therapy to the child while keeping the parents in the picture too. Now the clinician can proceed by pointing out the rationale for the traditional and the current approaches, explaining essential features of the four major types of therapies, as follows:

1. Having the child practice slow speech or other voluntary speech movement.
2. Reinforcing fluency and discouraging speech behavior that triggers disfluencies.
3. Improving parent-child relations and the child's interpersonal skills.
4. Participating in psychological play therapy.

A review of several specific therapy programs representing these approaches is presented in Chapter 14. The clinician explains that practitioners use different specific techniques under each of the categories just listed. For example, slow speech may be practiced using stretched speech or a metronome-paced speech. Reinforcing fluency can be done by praising each instance of fluent speech (e.g., the Lidcombe method; Harrison, Onslow, & Rousseau, 2007) or by reinforcing a gradually increased length of fluent utterances (e.g., the ELU; J. Ingham, 1999). Parents, however, should be informed that although therapies sometimes appear to help either directly to reduce stuttering or indirectly to create a more favorable home environment for fluency, only a few reasonably-controlled studies confirming the clinical effectiveness of treatment programs have been conducted.

Parent Counseling

Limited immediate parent counseling in conjunction with the initial evaluation of the preschool child who stutters has been a standard practice for a long time. Already several decades ago, many authors wrote on this subject, offering general and specific advice (e.g., Brown, 1949; Johnson, 1961b; Sander, 1959; Schuell, 1949). Not knowing what action parents will take or when, or in response to their queries about stuttering, the clinician should impart:

- Essential information about the disorder
- Advice about the desired home environment
- Advice concerning responding to the child's stuttering
- Follow-up contacts

It is important, however, for the clinician and parents to understand that much of the commonly given advice lacks sufficient scientific evidence for the sake of realistic expectations. Nevertheless, much of it reflects common sense and clinical experience. A special visit without the child affords a more relaxed and open discussion. The main points, to convey to parents, based on a review of the rich literature, focus on providing answers to four questions: (1) What causes stuttering? (2) What can be done at home? (3) What to do when the child stutters? What's next? A verbatim example of the feedback provided to parent follows.

Feedback to Parents: General Outline

"Based on our observations and speech analysis, your son exhibits a moderate degree of stuttering which is clinically significant. Although sometimes he may be completely fluent, the stuttering reappears rather consistently. The stuttering we observed consists mainly of syllable and short word repetitions, 2 to 4 times per event on about 9% of the words. There are also some sound prolongations as well as a few instances of facial tension and occasional eye closing. He shows some indications of awareness of the stuttering. His language development, hearing, and motor skills are age-appropriate. There are some difficulties in the correct pronunciation of several sounds although it is not much of a concern right now.

"Let me provide some information about stuttering. It is a problem that typically begins before age 5, after the child already has had normal fluency. It afflicts about 5% or more children in this age range. No exact cause has been identified but we do know that strong genetic factors are involved although the familial transmission is not always easily seen. Recent findings suggest that perhaps the genetic factors are associated with some minute brain differences that, at a certain developmental point, may result in disfluent speech. This information, however, is only in its initial stage and much more research is needed.

"There have been numerous explanations of stuttering that you should not buy. For example, many people think it is a reflection of some emotional problem. Extensive research suggests this is not true. The reverse appears to be more valid, that is, the stuttering is the cause of some distress for the person who stutters. Another popular idea is that parents' behavior has caused the stuttering. Again, this is not true according to research. But, once the child stutters, the parents' reaction can have a significant influence.

"Most encouraging is scientific information strongly suggesting that most children (75% and likely even more) who begin stuttering will stop on their own without treatment. Scientists call this *natural recovery*. Also a good number among those who persist eventually show improvement. Only a minority develop severe chronic stuttering. So, your child's average chance of stopping his stuttering is good. Or, he might at least get much better. Although recovery time can be short, only a few months, most children take a longer time, up to 3 years from the time of onset. Signs of recovery typically begin within 9 months or so. Still, remember that 15% to 25% of children continue to develop persistent stuttering.

"In spite of good average chances for recovery, an accurate prognosis is not possible to make at the present. We can, however, estimate relative chances of risks. For example, we consider gender, type of family history, time from onset, changes in severity over several weeks or a few months, types of disfluency, and more. The initial severity, however, is not a factor during the first few months. Because your child is a boy, is now a 4-year old, has stuttered for more than 9 months, has a grandfather who stuttered for many years, and has shown little improvement in his stuttering according to your rating, and is still presenting a moderate degree of stuttering according to our evaluation, we consider him as having more than the average risk for continuing to stutter. Although natural recovery is still a possibility, we recommend clinical intervention now. In this clinic, the general approach for intervention with preschool children is based on encouraging the child to use slow speech through modeling and practice, including training the parents to talk slowly at home and provide a model. Other centers or clinicians may employ other methods, such as discouraging and correcting instances of stuttering while also reinforcing instances of fluent speech, improving the child's interpersonal communication skills, play therapy, and two or so other methods.

"Regardless, here is some advice to follow at home. These recommendations have not been examined scientifically but they do represent cumulative clinical experience. The advice is focused on two areas, the *home environment* and *listeners' responses*.

"In the *home environment*, several strategies can be used to create a more comfortable situation of communication for a child who stutters and thereby reduce the intensity of stuttering. Three such strategies are:

1. Decrease excessive pressure. Because stuttering increases under pressure, examine various home situations that create pressure, and alleviate these situations. Examples include easing the demands to speak quickly and precisely, replacing rigid rules with simpler expectations, and having fewer conflicts with the child.
2. Minimize physical and emotional excitement and irritations. The resulting faster speech yields more stuttering. Instead, encourage slow play activities and avoid rushing the child. Small changes may have significant effects.
3. Talk slowly to the child when he/she is around. Slow down your pace when you read a book aloud. A slow speaking rate also reduces the intensity of stuttering. Parents' slower speech may serve as a model of an easier, relaxed approach to talking. Slow speech is associated with slower, more relaxed behavior and activity, in general."

"In terms of listeners' responses, especially as parents deal with stuttering, keep in mind that a child will tend to react to stuttering the ways that others do. If others become uptight and uncomfortable with moments of stuttering, the child will learn to get uptight and uncomfortable, too. But this will tend to make the child uncomfortable with the whole act of talking, not just stuttering. So we want to prevent this result by listening in ways that place the child at ease, even when there is stuttering and provide a model of a relaxed way to modify stuttering:

1. In instances of mild stuttering, just wait patiently. Regardless of stuttering, listen and respond to the child's intended message, not how the speech is coming out.

2. When stuttering is moderate, you may wish to reflect back or *echo* the message calmly. This involves a slow, easy, restatement of the words spoken by the child. No further comment about how speech came out is needed.

3. When stuttering is severe, gently suggest to the child that there is time to say the words again to say them more easily or suggest that the words can be repeated again more easily with you ("e.g., let's say this easily together).

4. If the child appears to be upset or frustrated by the experience of stuttering, provide empathy and encouragement. For example, a parent can say, "Sometimes talking is hard."

"Whether you want to begin therapy immediately or elect to wait a while, you should closely monitor the child's speech, other behaviors, and reactions. Schedule a follow-up visit within a few weeks. If possible, obtain audio or video speech samples and keep detailed notes concerning variations in the features and severity of the stuttering. These will be very helpful in assessing your son's progress and reevaluating treatment decisions. Use all opportunities to secure missing information about your extended family's family history of stuttering."

Clinicians may explain to parents that children often react to stuttering in whatever way listeners/parents react. If listeners convey concerns, or if the child's speech is frequently and rudely interrupted because of stuttering, he or she will sooner or later learn that it is not okay to say something if it might come out with "bumpy" stuttering. This can lead to more hesitation over talking and interfere with the learning process for smoothing out speech. Parents should strive to find a balance between being patient with the child's stuttering on one hand and helping the child cope with the stuttering, learning to modify it in a calm manner on the other one.

Summary

The initial evaluation of the preschool-age child who stutters is typically initiated by concerned parents. In the great majority of cases, the evaluation ends up as a systematic process of information gathering about the various aspects or dimensions of the disorder rather than a classic diagnostic search for an unknown condition. This is so because most often parental diagnosis of a child's speech impediment as "stuttering" is shared by the speech-language clinician who backs up his or her subjective perception with objective data. The major parts of the evaluation include an extensive parent interview; audiovisual recording of speech; analyses of disfluency and secondary characteristics; probing into awareness, emotional reactions, and temperament; and testing for language, phonology, hearing, and motor skills. Early childhood fluency assessments are different from the assessments of school-age and adult clients in several ways:

- The young age of the child necessitates greater involvement of the parents at several points throughout the evaluation.
- The brief history of the disorder in young children allows for the collection of more reliable information, some of which, such as the familial history of stuttering, may be particularly useful for prognosis and clinical recommendations.
- Specialized interview materials, normative disfluency data, and stuttering severity scales aid in the identification of the stuttering disorder.
- Questionable, borderline cases in the gray area between normal disfluency and stuttering are few, but clinicians are provided with diagnostic procedures and criteria for such cases.
- Because children at this early stage of the disorder have a good chance for natural recovery, the weighing of these chances for prediction purposes is an important element of the evaluation. The knowledge that most children will outgrow the disorder without intervention presents clinicians with questions: Should children who are good candidates for recovery be directed to receive therapy or wait awhile? If waiting is recommended, for how long?
- Clinicians and parents should bear in mind that the prognostic criteria reviewed here are tools for making reasonable risk assessments. They are not, however, powerful enough for making accurate predictions. Their review is a matter of assessing probabilities and risks. Children who appear to be at low risk and are recommended for waiting should continue to be closely monitored.
- The evaluation concludes with parent counseling, which, among other objectives, focuses on providing information about stuttering, risk assessment, suggestions for modifying general home environment, and advice concerning handling stuttering. Specifics were provided.

Study Questions and Discussion Topics

1. What are the main differences between the initial evaluation of preschool-age children and adult or school-age children who stutter?
2. Why it is important to determine accurately the time of stuttering onset?
3. Why it is important to ask parents to compare the various characteristics and severity of stuttering at the time of onset and at the time of the evaluation.
4. What are the minimally sufficient disfluent speech characteristics required for the classification of a child as exhibiting mild stuttering?
5. What dimension and characteristics of stuttered speech are typically used in rating its overall severity?
6. Is it necessary to include speech and nonspeech domains other than fluency in the evaluation of stuttering in preschool children? Defend your answer.

7. What are the main criteria for assessing a child's chance for natural recovery or persistent stuttering? Briefly explain each one.
8. What are the main objectives of parent counseling at the conclusion of the initial evaluation? Explain.

Suggested Readings

Dillolo, A., & Manning, W. (2007). Counseling children who stutter and their children. In E. Conture & R. Curlee (Eds.), *Stuttering and related disorders* (3rd ed., Chapter 7). New York, NY: Thieme.

Gregory, H., & Hill, D. (1999). Differential evaluation—differential therapy for stuttering children. In R. Curlee (Ed.), *Stuttering and related disorders of fluency* (2nd ed.). New York, NY: Thieme.

Richels, C. & Conture, E. (2010). Indirect treatment of childhood stuttering: Diagnostic predictors of treatment outcome. In B. Guitar & R. McCauley (Eds.). *Treatment of stuttering: Established and emerging interventions.* Baltimore, MD: Lippincott Williams & Wilkins

Riley, G. (1984). *Stuttering prediction instrument for young children.* Austin, TX: Pro-Ed.

Yairi, E., & Ambrose, N. (2005). *Early childhood stuttering: For clinicians by clinicians.* Austin, TX: Pro-Ed. See Chapters 10 and 11.

Chapter 10

Stuttering Therapy Overview: Issues and Directions

LEARNER OBJECTIVES

Readers of this chapter will be able to:

- Analyze issues related to the therapy-theory connection.
- Distinguish potential long-term goals of stuttering treatment.
- Examine and categorize various treatment approaches.
- Reflect on clinician qualities that enhance clinician-client rapport.
- Contemplate issues concerned with clinical ethics.
- List issues of evidence-based practice, clinical efficacy, and clinical research related to stuttering.

Introduction

The earlier parts of this book dealt with the definition of stuttering, its nature as event and as disorder, prevalence, onset and progression, variations and unique phenomena, the characteristics of advanced stuttering, and the various theories about it. Whereas this knowledge is interesting in itself, it fulfills a greater purpose when integrated and applied to decisions concerning treatment. The realm of knowledge related to the clinical management of stuttering encompasses a host of aspects all on its own. The literature, however, reveals that often this enterprise has had little connection to the breadth of the knowledge previously described. Prior to reviewing the relevant clinical literature, several questions are worth considering: Is it important for treatment to be theory-based? What are the possible aims of treatment? How do we make order out of the variety of treatment approaches available? What are the objectives of evidence-based practice? How can we meet the challenges associated with clinical efficacy research? What qualities are desired in clinicians? What are the essential ethical considerations? This chapter addresses these issues as underpinnings to the general topic of the clinical aspects of stuttering.

Theoretical Considerations

We propose that treatment of stuttering should emanate logically from theory, formal or informal, about the causes and factors that influence stuttering. Because it is likely that multiple factors contribute to the disorder varying across clients, clinicians may need multiple techniques to individualize treatment appropriately. A sensible clinician can be expected to practice intervention approaches consistent with either a known theory or his or her own set of beliefs and associated rationales. In either case, an evidence-supported theory and rationale are ideal.

Despite the importance of theoretical foundations, history suggests that a number of therapies, some of which are currently practiced, originated from layperson or clinician hunches. A few were later recognized for their beneficial effects and received experimental support. A classic example is the technique of rate control. For generations, parents and friends have implored people who stutter to talk slower. In his youth, one of us had been so advised by relatives and neighbors. At the time, no particular rationale was provided. The approach originated from "gut-level" instincts. By now, many clinicians incorporate different versions of slow speech practice into their therapeutic regimens; furthermore, the method has been backed by both theoretical rationale (e.g., psycholinguistic theories) and research data (Curlee & Perkins, 1973; Onslow, Costa, Andrews et al., 1996).

> Conditions found to ameliorate stuttering (see Chapter 4) have been adapted for formal therapy. For example, long ago it was noticed that when people who stutter talk in noisy environments, their stuttering may be substantially reduced as long as the noise continues. Although this phenomenon is not understood, it has been adopted in treatment regimens incorporating portable miniature noise-making instruments such as the Edinburgh Masker (Dewar, Dewar, Austin et al., 1979). The therapeutic rationale is simply based on the obvious reason that it works, not because of any theory about the cause and nature of stuttering.

As Van Riper (1973) noted, there have been a number of therapies grounded only in the principle that if the treatment works, it does not matter much why. This is known as the *pragmatic* approach, sometimes combining procedures into an *eclectic* program representing different philosophies and methods. The effectiveness of some pragmatic stuttering therapies has been supported by research, for example, the noise application program (MacCulloch, Eaton, & Long, 1970) and the Lidcombe Program, which targets speech disfluencies in children who stutter (Onslow, Packman, & Harrison, 2003). Admittedly, then, in spite of our advocacy, therapy-theory links are not always essential for clinical success. If certain procedures are found to yield reliable positive outcomes independent of any theory, or without a complete understanding of why they work, it makes sense that they should be used providing there is research evidence to support the effectiveness of the applied practice.

Still, we have several reservations about the preceding statement. Although picking and choosing procedures from diverse approaches appears to yield more efficacious individualized therapies, there is a downside. A single clinician cannot be an expert in every method. Perhaps more importantly, if clinicians do not understand or cannot explain why their treatment works, it is difficult, if not impossible, to provide clients with a rationale. This handicap interferes with therapy because the rationale, as presented to the client, can greatly influence the therapeutic process. According to Yairi and Ambrose (2005):

> When identical procedures are presented to the client with different rationales, it results in different understanding, responses, and learning. When a person who stutters is told to speak slowly so that (a) he can better attend to and analyze what he does in speaking, or (b) he can better cope with neurological spasms, or (c) he can better control his hostile reaction to the listener, very different learning takes place. (p. 409)

Without a theoretical framework, it is difficult to determine what needs to be done if the therapy fails.

The preceding examples of pragmatic therapies for stuttering notwithstanding, there is ample evidence that from early on, discernible links between clinicians' theories of stuttering and the prescribed treatment were the rule rather than the exception (see reviews by Klingbell, 1939; Sheehan, 1970; Wingate, 1997). Centuries ago, when the cause of stuttering was believed to reside in the tongue, caused by either its oversized or weak musculature (Brosch & Pirsig, 2001), treatment was prescribed accordingly: Size was reduced by removing pieces from the tongue; weak movement was enhanced with hot spices, supporting prosthetic devices elevated it, and so on. Obviously if the theory itself is not well founded, a strong theory-therapy link is not enough to yield the best treatment approach.

The therapies for stuttering have only been as comprehensive as the theories supporting them. Theories of stuttering thus far have been limited in scope. For example, the psychoanalytic theory was narrowly focused on the emotional etiology of stuttering and on psychoanalysis as its treatment. It neglects the potential impact of stuttering on a person's behavioral reactions and how these can be handled. It has nothing to say about the speech aspects of stuttering and what can be done about changing them.

Other interesting illustrations abound. When Friedrich Otto, in the 19th century, regarded stuttering as a problem of transitions between speech sounds, he recommended phonetic drills and a conscious effort to integrate articulatory transitions as the logical treatment (see Sheehan, 1970, p. 40). Similarly, relegating the cause of stuttering to muscular spasms of the larynx, several clinicians, including Ssikorski (1891), Sandow (1898), and Makuen (1941), offered vocal exercises as well as maneuvers for repositioning certain laryngeal muscles to prevent spasm. When stuttering was explained as an outward symptom of deep-seated emotional conflicts, it was treated with psychotherapy (e.g., Brill, 1923).

These examples also remind us that the theory-therapy link is only as good as the theory itself. Furthermore, theories may have negative influences on whether intervention is viewed as beneficial. In the extreme case, certain religions object to all treatments, leaving the remedy entirely in God's hands. Another example is the far-reaching influence of the diagnosogenic theory of stuttering (see Chapter 6). Because of the theory's claim that calling attention to the child's disfluency causes and sustains stuttering, direct speech therapy for young children was avoided for more than three decades, especially in the United States. The theory, which has lost much credibility over the years, also inflicted undue pain on many parents by assigning the cause of stuttering to their behavior.

In spite of the qualifications just described, we adhere to our proposition that the theory-therapy link is advantageous. A theory-driven therapy provides clinicians with a frame of reference. If clinicians believe stuttering is a symptom of a psychological prob-lem, then they should not be applying an oral motor treatment. A theory also provides the rationale for the therapeutic approach, an understanding of why specific procedures are applied, and a logical basis for sensible alternatives when progress fails to occur, rather than yielding a haphazard trial and error strategy. Theories, however, need to be tested, refined or modified and thus give rise to better treatment methods.

Unfortunately, the field suffers from large gaps between stuttering therapies and theories, mainly because of the narrowness of the theories. For example, the covert repair hypothesis (Postma & Kolk, 1993) proposes that disfluencies result from prob-lems in premotor phonological encoding in which a speaker attempts to correct speech errors before they are uttered. The theory seems to provide a rationale for therapies that emphasize slower speaking rate. It does not, however, offer any guidance for intervening with a client's psychological attitudes, an important domain within the grand scope of the disorder of stuttering.

There is also the phenomenon of therapies that originate from a certain theoreti-cal position and then spread out, incorporating procedures that are not rooted in the theory. For example, a clinician may counsel parents against calling attention to stutter-ing, based on Johnson's diagnosogenic theory. She may also advise that parents model slow speech and use simple language. In this case, a theoretical connection for the latter advice (simple language) does not exist and the experimental evidence to support the procedure is scant. If a clinician believes persistent stuttering is ultimately genetic, she should be able to explain why success is being expected from a behavioral reinforce-ment treatment approach. Perhaps the weak theory-therapy connection in stuttering during the past 30 years reflects the absence of a strong theory accepted by scientists and understood by the public (Siegel, 1998).

The Objectives of Therapy

Knowing that the vast majority of people who stutter begin by age 4 and certainly by age 6 (see Chapter 3), preschool children present a brief history and little experience with the disorder. By contrast, it can be assumed that the great majority of afflicted school-age children have been stuttering for a good number of years whereas adults have stuttered for many more years. Naturally, the longer their stuttering history, the greater is their experience with the disorder. Having missed the best opportunity for natural recovery, on one hand, and having formed strong associated emotional reactions and habits of dealing with stuttering, on the other, the question arises as to what are the realistic goals of treatment for them? Are the same goals applicable to school-age and preschool-age children alike? With respect to the latter question, increased knowledge in the future concerning stuttering subtypes may lead to differential treatments. At the present, however, while recognizing that some distinction should be made between preschool children and older people who stutter, from our perspective there is substantial commonality among all age groups in respect to the general therapeutic aims. The three major alternatives to consider in setting up long-term therapeutic goals for people who stutter are increased fluency, reduced the severity stuttering events, and improved emotional adjustment.

Increased Fluency

Naturally Fluent Speech

Naturally fluent speech is produced by speakers who feel, think, and behave like normally speaking individuals when they talk. In essence, the aim is a complete cure. This can be a realistic goal for preschool children. As discussed at length in Chapter 3, most of them experience natural recovery. The many children who receive therapy do well either due to therapy or due to the combination of natural recovery forces and therapy. This goal appears to be similar to Guitar's (2012) therapeutic outcome labeled "spontaneous fluency."

When applied to school-aged children and adults, achieving complete cure in both the fluency and the psychological domains of speaking by means of any of the current therapies has typically been viewed as unrealistic. Clinicians tend to believe in the potential for substantial improvement, but only up to a point (Manning, 2001; Sheehan, 1980). The main reason for being guarded has been the limited long-term success of therapy. Also, such guardedness may have been influenced by organic theories of stuttering that intuitively imply constraints on the power of speech therapy to alter physiological or biochemical structures and processes. There are indications, however, that speech therapy can alter the brain activity of people who stutter (e.g., Boberg, Yeudall, Schopflocher et al., 1983; De Nil et al., 2001). It also remains possible that with the advent of new medical treatments, such as gene therapies, stem cell implants, and so on, full cure may, at some future time, become a realistic goal for the growing number of clients.

Deliberately Fluent Speech

Deliberately fluent speech is produced by the speaker who exercises a conscious mental and/or behavioral monitoring of speech that normally fluent speakers usually do not use. Clearly, this subcategory presents quite a different goal from the first one listed. It is similar to what Guitar (2014) called "controlled fluency" (p. 290) or "superfluency"

(p. 265) as a therapeutic outcome. Most fluency shaping approaches aim for the goal of deliberately fluent speech. Fluency shaping strategies are applied by a client to promote a smooth manner of speaking before stuttering is even anticipated. This goal presents a paradox for some individuals who stutter because one abnormality may have been substituted for another that still makes the person uncomfortable. Also, the required self-monitoring is tremendously difficult, attempting to attend to one's own speech production while simultaneously tracking the development of the intended message. This multitasking demand might even result in triggering some disfluent or stuttered speech, the opposite of the intended outcome.

Managed Stuttering

The goal is to lessen the abnormality of overt stuttering, and, as a by-product, to also decrease its frequency. This objective appears close to what Van Riper (1973) labeled as "fluent stuttering" and to what Guitar (2014) refers to as "acceptable stuttering" (p. 290). Note, however, that what is acceptable, and to whom, is a wide-open question. The goal may also be described as "managed stuttering."

Managed stuttering occurs when the movements involved in the production of discontinuities in the speech stream are managed deliberately by the speaker. This can perhaps be likened to a person with spasmodic extremities attempting to "smooth out" the uncontrollable movement. It is a counterintuitive concept in that most, if not all, of those who stutter seek therapy to get rid of their stuttering, not keep it going. A speaker who applies strategies to smooth out a moment of stuttering, engages in "managed stuttering." A client may choose to work simultaneously on the prior goal of increasing fluency and the goal of decreasing the severity of the remaining stuttering (i.e., manage the stuttering moments).

Improved Cognitive-Emotional Adjustment

The goal is to change emotional and social behavior related to speaking without directly addressing speech itself. Such changes, however, are expected to yield the by-product of diminished stuttering. This broad goal of indirect influence on stuttering may be reached in diverse ways. It may reflect elements of Travis's (1931) concept of mental hygiene, Bryngelson's (1931) ideas of an objective attitude, Sheehan's (1970) role acceptance, and others. In this sense, one could refer to this goal as a form of "attitude control."

General Therapeutic Approaches

What has been done and what can be done to achieve the three optional stuttering treatment objectives presented earlier? The clinical literature reveals numerous therapies, reflecting extremely diverse subjective factors with respect to clinicians' theoretical positions, personal beliefs about stuttering, professional backgrounds, or preferred eclectic strategies. Cultural values and religious beliefs also have had some influence (Leith, 1986; Roberts & Shenker 2007). There are also more objective factors, such as the multidimensional nature of the disorder, that influence the focus and character of the therapy. At times, these factors overlap. It is to be expected that psychologists gear their therapies to the emotional aspect of stuttering, which, in some cases, is a very significant component of the disorder. In a similar vein, speech clinicians tend to focus on the overt speech characteristics, whereas physicians show more interest in body function and medication.

A naive observer of therapy, not knowing for what problem it is provided, may witness that one client soaks his feet in a pail of cold water, a second client is hypnotized, and a third one receives a shot in the rear end. Such an observer will be amused to learn that all three were being treated for stuttering. In fact, it has not been uncommon that a single client received several, if not many, extremely diverse therapies. One of us presented an incomplete list of 16 different therapies, including the three mentioned earlier, that he had received (see Yairi & Ambrose, 2005, p. 402). Also Johnson (1946) listed a good number of therapies that were applied to him.

Unfortunately, not only laypersons are at risk of becoming confused about stuttering therapy. Students and professionals in speech-language pathology, too, are vulnerable. Hence, prior to answering the question of how to accommodate any of the broad treatment aims presented here, the confusion might be lessened by organizing the numerous therapies into a small number of categories based on their commonalities.

There are several reasonable classifications for types of therapy. Examples include:

- Therapies aimed at changing speech directly versus those whose target is to change speech indirectly.
- Aided therapy, such as using delayed auditory feedback (DAF) or electromyography (EMG) instruments, versus unaided therapy, such as stuttering modification or fluency reinforcement.
- Therapies for treating the parents versus therapies in which parents are the agents of treatment.
- Therapies focused on broad permanent change of the disorder, such as psychotherapy, versus therapies focused narrowly on immediate change of the events, such as stuttering modification techniques.

Therapies might also be classified according to how the stuttering problem is conceptualized. Some approaches related to psychotherapy, emotions, and attitudes address stuttering in terms of the "loss of control" definition that Perkins (1990a) defends. Other approaches address stuttering in terms of speech behaviors to be modified by means of operant behavior–based techniques, such as those developed by J. Ingham (1999) or Onslow et al. (2003). Notice the overlap because some therapies can be described within more than one classification system.

Traditionally, stuttering therapies have been informally distinguished according to two categories: antianxiety and anti-stuttering (Williams, 1968). This oversimplified classification fails to consider fundamental differences among approaches, excludes a number of important therapies, and does not accommodate more recent developments. Yairi and Ambrose (2005) offered a more representative nine-category classification of stuttering therapies based on the common theme of the specific techniques that have been employed. In writing this book, the set of possible long-term treatment objectives provides the framework for a scheme that includes 12 general therapeutic approaches for stuttering arranged in three classes:

I. Focus on Improved Cognitive-Emotional Adjustment
1. Resolving psyche and personality disturbances
2. Promoting calmness and relaxation
3. Modifying emotional reactions
4. Modifying cognitive sets
II. Focus on Managed Stuttering
5. Modifying or replacing stutter events
6. Decreasing stutter events
III. Focus on Increased Fluency
A. Achieving Deliberately Fluent Speech
7. Fluency shaping
8. Fluency reinforcement
B. Achieving Naturally Fluent Speech
9. Instrument-based therapies
10. Pharmaceutical treatments
11. Strengthening supporting skills (e.g., oral motor, phonology, language)
12. Environmental management

Having outlined the general therapeutic options, it is important for the student to understand that each represents a number of specific techniques that have been employed to achieve it. For example, personality problems (approach 1) have been dealt with by different types of psychotherapy; relaxation can be realized by practicing certain movements, through meditation, and others. Fluency shaping (approach 7) can be achieved through very slow (stretched) speech or by applying easier voice initiations. Hence, clinicians are faced with the challenge of developing a therapy program by choosing among numerous possibilities. They may opt to pursue one approach by means of a single technique or several techniques, or prefer to pursue therapy through multiple approaches, which, of course, imply also several techniques. As a matter of fact, clinicians have combined and/or integrated stuttering modification with psychologically oriented approaches such as anxiety reduction (Van Riper, 1973), or anxiety reduction with stuttering modification and fluency-generating approaches (Guitar, 2012).

Approaches to stuttering therapies have seen considerable fluctuations in popularity among professionals. Whereas resolving personality problems as the main approach peaked during the first half of the 20th century, at present it is out of favor. The use of various fluency-enhancing techniques, such as slow speech, was employed over a long period of time, lost its popularity during the middle two quarters of the 20th century, and has seen a considerable resurgence since the late 1970s. Finally, some approaches have targeted specific age groups more than others. For example, instrument-based therapies (approach 9) have been applied primarily with adults, whereas environmental management (approach 12) has been applied primarily with preschool children. The major clinical techniques and programs developed within each of these major approaches are described and discussed in subsequent chapters.

Clinical Applications

Developing Appropriate Treatment Objectives

Goal setting with adolescents or adults is best accomplished together with the clients so they are encouraged to feel a sense of ownership of the process. Similarly, the parents of young children should be involved in planning their child's treatment. When developing therapy objectives, clinicians should be clear and completely define all the components according to the following formula:

Treatment objective = who + will do what + to what degree of accuracy + under what conditions

Sometimes even seasoned clinicians overlook the defining conditions and write imprecise or insufficient goals as "John will perform his fluency targets with 95% accuracy." Such a statement may seem sufficient at first, but there is no way of telling when the client has satisfactorily met this objective. It lacks specific information about the nature of the conditions of John's performance (independently? after imitating? given an indirect model?) or the speaking context (on sentences? in spontaneous conversation? during oral reading?) or location (therapy room or classroom?), or even the time frame (in one session? across two consecutive sessions?). Finally, a major problem with the objective stated above is that the measurement basis was not specified. Compare the relative stability of a 95% achievement if the client has performed only 20 utterances as compared to 100 utterances. An example of an objective that specifies the particular task, conditions, and measures needed is "John will independently apply a slow, easy speech initiation strategy on 100 utterances with 95% accuracy during spontaneous conversation with his peers across two consecutive group sessions in the therapy room."

When setting the clinical goals and objectives for persons who stutter, several considerations that are not largely different from those appropriate for individuals with speech sound disorders, are particularly worth noting: Which goals and objectives will make the most impact on the speaker's effectiveness as a communicator? Which steps will the client be most ready and able to undertake? Are there changes that if made in one area will promote change in other areas? Are the conditions and expectations commensurate with the individual's lifestyle and cultural background, communication needs, and/or developmental stage? What will offer the most relief for his or her experiences of communicative stress?

Individual versus Group Therapy Sessions

Therapy can be delivered in a variety of formats, including individual and group. Commensurate with modern technology, recent years have seen a growing trend of therapy via the Internet (Carey & Onslow, 2012). So far, the individual format has dominated stuttering therapy. It is obvious that an individual session in which a client has the therapist's full attention affords the most flexibility for zeroing in on the client's needs. It takes the one-on-one contact for the clinician to have a firsthand understanding of the problem and to get to know the client, consider relative strengths and weaknesses, and together, formulate goals. Initially, many adolescent and even adult clients who stutter are not comfortable sharing feelings, discussing stuttering, or practicing speaking skills in the presence of other clients. Group stuttering therapy in addition to individual therapy, however, can be a particularly valuable component of the overall treatment approach, especially with others at the same age or stage. Advantages of group therapy are discussed in Chapter 11. Sometimes, it may be the only format available. Regardless, the clinician has to make a decision about the format or formats of the program.

Implementing Treatment

Several intervention principles that apply broadly in the practice of speech pathology are appropriate for fluency intervention. For example, a long-term goal should be broken down into a progressive sequence of intermediate, short-term, and session-specific objectives. Unrealistic goals can easily lead to a sense of failure even if considerable improvement has been achieved. We next consider some procedures shared in common across approaches to communication disorders treatment in regard to stuttering and fluency intervention.

Increased Awareness and Self-Monitoring

With any speech target, it is important for a client to have a clear awareness of the nature of that target. In fluency therapy, for example, the target may be self-knowledge of the overt features of the disorder, or of his/her avoidance behavior. Generous amounts of modeling and instructional support are important when teaching new target skills. The modeling and feedback are gradually faded out as the client demonstrates consistent success independently. Clinician feedback is best when it offers specific descriptions of performance (e.g., "you touched your lips together gently that time") and should be applied more often than vague general praise (e.g., "good job"). In motor learning terms, knowledge of performance about what movement pattern occurred is more instructive than knowledge of results about whether outcome was successful or not. Adolescent and adult clients need to develop habits of ongoing self-evaluation and self-monitoring, both of the old and newly learned behaviors, to ensure an enduring result. That is, clients need to be able to serve as their own therapist. For this to happen, the client needs plenty of practice in self-evaluation and self-monitoring in the presence of the clinician with whom impressions can be compared/contrasted. Finn (2003c) has reviewed in detail the value of self-regulation in fluency therapy.

Conditions of Practice

In nearly every learning experience, especially for changing speech processes, some component of practice is needed. Although the old adage asserts that "practice makes perfect," the new wisdom warns that "practice makes permanent." So it is important before encouraging repeated practice to ensure the client is performing the target behavior in the desired way. Because it is relatively easy to achieve fluent speech in the confines of the clinical setting, misleading impressions might be formed that only a minimal amount of practice of new skills should be required. The speaking approach, however, needs to be practiced over and over, multiple times and in multiple conditions.

> Some musicians argue that 10,000 hours of practice distinguish the best experts in the musical world. If deliberate practice and perseverance are essential to becoming a top performer, then it may take a concerted investment of time to develop proficient speech management skills The important implication for clinicians: If many hours of practice will be necessary, then the *client* should spend the largest percentage of time talking during their therapy sessions.

The motor learning literature reveals some conditions of practice to enhance learning. Motor practice is most effective when the conditions are varied rather than consistent. One treatment implication may be that rather than practicing the same set of words every clinical session, words sets should be varied continuously. Similarly, instead of the same tone of voice applied consistently in practice, the speaker needs to practice techniques in conditions of varied intonation patterns and stress emphasis. Finally, if motor learning principles (Schmidt & Lee, 2005) apply to speech fluency learning, then 8 hours of practice in 2 days may not be as beneficial as 2 hours of practice on each of 8 days. Still, recent research has raised some questions concerning the effect of practice on people who stutter, showing that after practice, instead of decreasing reaction times and increasing accuracy like normally fluent speakers, people who stutter continue to demonstrate slower reaction times and decreased accuracy in a color recognition naming task (Smits-Bandstra & De Nil, 2009). Further studies are needed of the nature of these apparent speech learning constraints. Under what conditions do people who stutter make improvements in speech performance? Would greater numbers of practice trials afford speech performance gains? If this finding suggests an underlying area of speech performance deficiency where little gain is possible, then what compensatory or adaptive strategies will contribute to speaker success? For example, can a readjustment of jaw position release a stuttering block, as proposed by Zimmermann (1980c)?

Clinicians should realize, however, that extensive practice in stuttering therapy has some unique perspectives compared with practice in other speech disorders, say correcting articulation of speech sounds. Where speech production is concerned, the person with articulation disorders practices to develop fine motor skills, such as tongue placement. In learning how to modify a stuttering block, clients may learn rather quickly the motor adjustment required to reduce tension and get out of the block. The extensive practice with modifying hundreds and thousands of blocks is necessary not so much for developing fine motor skills but to change the clients' beliefs and confidence in what they can do in spite of the anxiety and tension they experience as they talk. People who stutter often feel they have no control over stuttering. Extensive practice in modifying blocks changes this entrenched psychology. In other aspects of stuttering therapy, practice does not involve any motor skills whatsoever. For example, clients learn to identify various features of their overt stuttering by observing themselves in the mirror or listening to their recorded speech. Again, the aim of extensive practice goes beyond the clients' ability to identify all the features. An equally important objective is to increase clients' realization that some aspects of stuttering are their own doing.

Generalization and Transfer

Generalization across many situations, conditions, and people is an essential component of most procedures in stuttering therapy. Even if a client can apply the target strategies in the clinic session, how well can the client apply the strategies in other circumstances? We just mentioned that speech practice should take place in a variety of conditions for better learning. A certain amount of practice across situations, conditions, and people should be incorporated into therapy to facilitate transfer of learning. Incorporating others—family, teachers, and friends—both for motivational support and for practice in variable conditions is important. Some clinical tools of transfer include use of situation hierarchies, event or daily log notations, employing self-regulating habits, and role play. For example, after achieving adequate skills modifying stuttering blocks in the therapy room, clients can practice their skills speaking to other people brought into the therapy room, then in speaking to other people in the clinic, followed by easy situations out of the clinic, and so on. Finn (2003a) highlights the use of everyday, real-life elements in speech therapy and emphasizes that clients must gain a sense of self-efficacy, that is, the belief that they have capacities and skills to enable them to generalize and maintain achievements.

Skill Maintenance and Prevention of Relapse

With adolescent and adult clients, it is almost certain that some will experience relapse following therapy. Thus, clinicians should prepare clients for this possibility before it occurs and gain confidence in being able to recover from speech fluency failures. Some experts have even suggested not dismissing a client until at least one major relapse has been addressed together (Manning, 2001). Another option may be to simulate or role-play such an experience for practice and adjustment of attitudes. Adoption of realistic expectations is important for the prevention of relapse. When too much of a premium is placed on the experience of relatively continuous fluency, the client is apt to be more at risk for problems later on.

   To cope with relapse Blood (1995) created a game for adolescents to change their cognition about speech as a supplement to changing speech motor skills. In the game, called POWER2, players move their pieces along a game board and draw cards to answer questions about a variety of situations (e.g., not being able to say a word to order your food). Players are sometimes required to respond in a way that is constructive and proactive, and, at other times, in a way that is reactive and less productive. By engaging in these opposite types of responses, players gain a better awareness of their nature and what is preferable. Topics and activities in the game raise issues of (1) permission to stutter or not, (2) ownership (of the speaking difficulty), (3) well-being and social support, (4) self-esteem and self-talk,[1] (5) resilience (bouncing back after stuttering moments), and (6) responsibility (handling life and processes of change). Rather than assuming that attitudes will change if speech improves, the idea is to empower the speaker with attitudes and problem-solving approaches that will help him or her be prepared for the bumps in the road ahead. Many clinicians also follow systematic maintenance programs whereby periodic contact with the client, either in person or via telephone, continues after dismissal from the regular therapy. This is typically done with decreasing frequency.

Other clinicians have employed video self-modeling (VSM) following fluency shaping treatment to improve maintenance of treatment. After the completion of treatment, 89 clients were randomly assigned to either standard maintenance or to standard maintenance plus VSM. Those in the latter group viewed stutter-free videos of themselves each day for 1 month. The addition of VSM did not improve speech outcomes, as measured by percent syllables stuttered, at either 1 or 6 months posttreatment testing. At the latter assessment, however, self-rating of stuttering severity by the VSM group was 10% better than that of the control group, and satisfaction with speech fluency was 20% better; quality of life was also better for the VSM group (Cream et al. 2010).

Evidence-Based Practice

During the past 25 years, the concept of evidence-based practice (EBP) has come to occupy greater centrality in speech-language pathology, including stuttering (Bernstein Ratner, 2005). This is the current trend among other health professions, especially those concerned with behavioral health management. In its strictest meaning, the philosophy of EBP is that therapy must be supported by research findings which provide positive evidence of its effectiveness. Framed more broadly, evidence-based treatment is a clinical decision-making process that integrates (a) the best scientific evidence with (b) an individual clinician's expertise (Sackett, Rosenberg, Gray et al., 1996). Finally, the triangular model of evidence-based practice endorsed by ASHA at their Web site integrates a third element: (c) client/patient/caregiver perspectives. Although clinicians and researchers may debate the question of primacy among the three elements, each of them is essential to a valid clinical decision-making process.

The value of scientific evidence is obvious. It is dangerous for clinicians to trust subjective impressions of what works. Suspicion must be upheld because in too many cases,

---

[1]Self-talk, and its application in therapy, is addressed in Chapter 11.

clinicians' instincts have been completely wrong. The stuttering literature is filled with a host of unfounded clinician advice to parents of preschool children just beginning to stutter, such as "ignore the child's stuttering, be a good listener, use simple language and short sentences, and have the child go to bed early." These suggestions, and other advice, have remained popular, although their clinical merit has rarely ever, if at all, been tested. Furthermore, there have been studies that negated some advice, showing, for example, that calling attention to stuttering in young children may in some cases actually reduce it (Martin et al., 1972; Wingate, 1976). Other scholars concluded that the premise underlying clinicians' admonition for parents to reduce the length and complexity of their utterances when conversing with their children has no experimental support. In fact, caution was raised about potential harmful effects from following this advice on the child's language development (Miles & Bernstein Ratner, 2001).

> There are virtually no data on the effects of being a good listener, style of toilet training, early bedtime, and so on, on children's stuttering. Similarly, although research has revealed that parents of children who stutter tend to be overprotective, the direct effect of increase or decrease in overprotectiveness on stuttering has not yet been demonstrated. Although none of these forms of advice have been shown to work, they are still being disseminated in parent counseling. Ingham and Cordes (1998) stated that a range of popular treatments persists even in the face of evidence showing them to be ineffective. In other words, the sole justification for the therapy is the clinician's "feeling" that it works. We doubt that such practices would be met with much tolerance in medicine.

Although in earlier times there was limited knowledge about how to evaluate treatment effectiveness, progress has been made. There is a current body of information to guide clinicians in how to search for the best available evidence. Students of speech-language pathology learn to differentiate among levels of evidence (ASHA, 2004). Progress in treatment testing has also been reported in several reviews of the clinical research literature (Bothe, Ingham, & Ingham, 2009; Herder, Howard, Nye et al., 2006).

The value of "clinical expertise" to treatment decisions is obvious for several reasons. First, the scientific literature has multiple limitations: (1) available treatment effectiveness data are limited, (2) research has been plagued by various methodological weaknesses, (3) critical measurements have often been overlooked, (4) interpretations of the data vary greatly, and (5) the evidence might not always be particularly meaningful to the individual client. (See Lilienfeld, 2003, for an interesting discussion of these issues.) Second, the clinician's interpretation of the client's needs is paramount to selecting and applying treatment effectively.

Finally, the value of the client/caregiver's perspective is tantamount in clinical decision making. In his article on the topic of self-regulation and stuttering, Finn (2003c) stated that "an evidence based-framework can be described as an empirically-driven, measurement-based, client-sensitive approach for selecting treatments" (p. 209). ASHA's

EBP position statement guides clinicians to "recognize the needs, abilities, values, preferences, and interests of individuals and families to whom they provide clinical services, and integrate those factors along with best current research evidence and their clinical expertise in making clinical decisions" (ASHA, 2005a). This means that clinical decisions require discernment on the part of clinicians who must sometimes work in support of a client's opinions and circumstances, and at other times work to effect change in a client's opinions and circumstances.

> Another important question is to what extent a given evidence-based program allows the clinician any flexibility and creativity? Suppose a hospital or clinical center adopts a specific assessment-treatment protocol for individuals who stutter. Should a clinician only practice the one approved protocol in each case? If the protocol has a defined set of steps, must the clinician follow all the steps in the exact order? If not, how many steps can be omitted or re-sequenced? At what point do the changes amount to a substantial deviation from the approved research-based treatment? And what about tested programs that do not yield meaningful results from the client's perspective, for example, what if the person who stutters cares more about overcoming fears of speaking in social events than about being 100% fluent?

A Case Study to Illustrate the Steps in EBP

The challenges associated with EBP are illustrated with a practical case applying a five-step process outlined by Sackett, Straus, Richardson et al. (2000). A 7-year-old African American boy is referred for stuttering treatment. The first step is to develop a clinical question (e.g., Will advising parents and teachers to speak more slowly to the child provide a supportive environmental factor toward his smooth speech?).

The second step, finding the best relevant information, may uncover several studies pertinent to the clinical question (e.g., Guitar & Marchinkowski, 2001; Zebrowski, Weiss, Savelkoul et al., 1996). This step involves challenging decisions about how many and which search engines to use, what keywords to search on, and when the search has been sufficient.

Step 3 raises the issue of how to engage in critical examination of the studies that are found. This is one important reason for including research methods courses in the university curriculum of speech-language pathology programs. The studies should be examined for their background, rationale, participants, procedures and conditions (controlled factors), measures, reliability, results, and implications. A clinician may note that the articles mainly found that children who stutter benefit from slower speaking rates by their parents. But what if the gender and stuttering symptoms of her client do not match any of the children in the studies under scrutiny? What if there are no studies to be found with children of the same age and culture? Are the results still applicable to her client? Even if generalizing results is a sensible option, is it justified in this case? An adult's model of slow speech may enhance child fluency but not necessarily by slowing the speech of the child (Stephenson-Opsal & Bernstein Ratner, 1988). Perhaps more critical factors may be operating. For example, Bernstein Ratner (2004) explained that longer turn-taking latencies may be the effective outcome of instructing parents to slow their speech, and that the increased latency of adult responses might be the factor that enhances fluency as suggested by Newman and Smit (1989). Based on the set of articles identified in step 2, the clinician may conclude that she needs to advise adults to slow their speech around the child. She would explain that the slow-paced environmental condition is beneficial to fluency even though the child is not apt to mirror this speech rate. However, if the additional review article is found (Bernstein Ratner, 2004), the clinician may conclude that she should advise parents to wait before responding to their child, increasing the latency of conversational turn taking.

With the fourth step, application, the clinician would instruct the adults who speak with the child according to her findings, duplicating the type of instructions given in the research studies. In the fifth step, evaluation, the effect of the procedure on the child's fluency is determined. Finally, if the outcome does not indicate a substantial effect, the clinician will have to determine whether her instructions were insufficient or whether the evidence does not apply for the specific client. In our opinion, this five-step process, although challenging, is nonetheless valuable.

The Client-Clinician Relationship

The roles that the speech clinician will serve during stuttering intervention are diverse: counselor, coach, educational resource, and comrade model. The clinician must shift readily among modes of interaction to meet the client's needs. More important, however, are the personal qualities the clinician brings to the therapeutic relationship. Certain qualities facilitate the rapport, trust, and openness necessary to the therapeutic process. Without sufficient trust, clients may not report attitudes and feelings honestly, resulting in misleading data and progress assessment.

The famous clinical psychologist Carl Rogers (1957) asserted that professionals who intend to practice a person-centered approach to facilitating therapeutic change must display qualities of (1) empathy, (2) self-congruence, and (3) unconditional positive regard. Although there are other desired qualities, we believe these three establish an important foundation for the client-clinician relationship in the context of stuttering intervention. Clinicians, and those preparing themselves to become clinicians, who lack experience with people who stutter may find it particularly challenging to display these qualities and facilitate therapeutic change for their clients. These can be developed in several ways, as discussed next.

Empathy

The word *empathy* derives from two sources: the German word *einfühlung* which means "feeling into" and the Greek word *pathos,* which means emotion, feeling, or pity. Empathy is the experience of understanding another person's condition from their perspective. It is placing oneself in another's shoes to feel what that person is feeling. In the clinical setting, empathy is about the clinician's keen appreciation of the nature of the problem as the client sees it and his/her feelings about it. It has been said that only someone who stutters can understand what a person who stutters experiences. Some people go so far as to assert that unless the clinician is a person who stutters or has stuttered, her or his therapy will not be effective. Although it may be true that clinicians who do not have a stuttering history may never fully comprehend the stuttering experience of their clients, several steps can be taken to improve that empathy:

1. Simulating various forms of stuttering in speaking situations with strangers, friends, in public places, on the telephone, and so on, to experience the range of accompanying feelings and listener responses. Feelings experienced prior to, during, and after stuttering, as well as listeners' responses should be examined. Placing oneself in others' shoes facilitates empathy.

2. Participation in stuttering support groups. This affords the opportunity to encounter a greater number of people who stutter, and so become familiar with their feelings about speaking, stuttering, speech therapy, and clinicians. Among other experiences, it can be an eye-opener to sometimes encounter negative opinions about therapy and the reasons for such animosity. These experiences seed ideas for doing things differently in therapy.

3. Reading books written by people who stutter regarding their life, reading newsletters and other publications of support groups keeps ongoing familiarity with what children and adults who stutter are saying about their speech problem. Examples of sources are listed in Table 10.1.

Similarly, watching video commentaries prepared by people who stutter (e.g., *Transcending Stuttering*, etc.) and participation in online groups (e.g., STUTT-L, visit www.mnsu.edu/comdis/kuster/stuttlfaq.html), provide the experience of dialogue about stuttering. Two very good presentations on this topic can be found in the articles by Manning (2004) and Quesal (2010).

Table 10.1	**Support Groups**		
Group	**National Association of Young People Who Stutter**	**National Stuttering Association**	**The Stuttering Foundation**
Newsletter	*Friends*	*Letting Go* (newsletter for adults)	*The Stuttering Foundation Newsletter*
		Family Voices (newsletter for kids, teens, parents)	
Address	38 S. Oyster Bay Rd.	119 W. 40th St.	PO Box 11749
	Syosset, NY 11791	14th Floor	Memphis, TN 38111-0749
		New York, NY 10018	
Web site	www.friendswhostutter.org	www.westutter.org	www.stutteringhelp.org

The concept of empathy has broader applications to understanding the client's needs, views, and expectations. As discussed earlier, speech-language pathologists must heed the call for evidence-based practice. As Quesal (2010) notes, however, most of the existing treatment evidence has been focused on the surface aspects of the stuttering disorder. Although these are critical components, Quesal posits that other factors, such as the feeling of control or loss of control, may be as relevant to clients. What a client feels is a desired therapy outcome has been recognized as an important parameter to include in clinical outcomes research. Bothe and Richardson (2011) referred to the treatment outcome that has "personal significance." We believe that empathy should help clinicians identify what is personally significant to their clients early in the therapeutic process.

Self-Congruence

Self-congruence is about being authentic and genuine. People with self-congruence do not hide or disguise feelings, but own and admit them. They are less apt to play a role rather than being themselves. Self-congruence by professionals enhances the trust of clients because the clinicians are objective and open to perceiving the real selves of others. It creates an atmosphere in which a client can perceive himself or herself more clearly, the negative as well as positive aspects, without experiencing them as a threat. Clinicians can enhance their self-congruence by adopting an objective awareness of their thoughts and feelings through regularly recording self-observations and selecting an entrenched habit for changing or elimination, studying objectively the difficult process of change over the course of several weeks or months.

Unconditional Positive Regard

Psychological health is encouraged when people sense they are completely accepted as they are. The clinician's warmth and high regard toward a client must not have preconditions. To this end, the clinician should be desensitized to stuttering and be comfortable when it occurs. The client must be fully respected and accepted, with or without stuttering. It is not that stuttering must be seen as desirable, only that whether or not stuttering behaviors are observed, the clinician regards the client with full respect and high regard.

Strategies for developing a desensitized attitude toward stuttering by a clinician are similar to what they might be for a client (e.g., watching a videotape of severe stuttering, remaining comfortable and focused on what the speaker has to say). The following self-questions provide guidance in achieving this: What attitudes make it difficult for me to remain comfortable? Is it difficult for me not to be distracted by stuttering? Was it the stuttering itself or pragmatic behaviors that most interfered with my communication with the client? Is how something was said what really matters, or isn't it more important what the intended message was?

Listener respect for the speaker who stutters should also be given attention. By intentionally studying the behaviors of listeners for how they do and do not show their respect for speakers, clinicians may identify ways to improve their own listening behaviors. Examples include reducing tendencies to hurry the speaker by their own fast speaking behaviors, using appropriate and comfortable eye contact, decreasing interruptions, dominating the speaking time, and so on.

Clinicians may also need to examine their own attitudes toward themselves, especially in regard to things disliked. Being overly self-critical can be addressed through the practice of letting go of severe judgments and becoming gentler toward oneself. The point is that the more gently we respond to our own shortcomings, the more gently we are apt to respond to others. This gentleness should not be confused with permissiveness or a relaxed attitude toward self-discipline. Beginning clinicians should be encouraged to self-evaluate their recordings of therapy sessions and minimize the amount of time they spend talking. How can the client accomplish enough practice if the clinician tends to talk 10 times as often (Costello, 1977) in the therapy session?

The client-clinician relationship is especially important to the process of therapeutic change for people who stutter. The qualities just discussed will serve to enhance this relationship. Several authors have addressed this issue with special reference to stuttering in ways that may further enrich your understanding (e.g., Ezrati-Vinacour & Weinstein, 2011; Manning, 2001; Shapiro, 1999; Van Riper, 1975).

Clinical Research

What kind clinical research has been done to provide the sought-after scientific evidence for stuttering therapy? In this respect, a significant distinction exists between clinical *outcomes* and clinical *efficacy* research. The first addresses only whether significant change occurred posttreatment, whereas the latter is concerned with proving that the specific treatment, not something else, is responsible for the change. Treatment efficacy can be considered in terms of two main components: effects and efficiency. An examination of treatment *effects* (i.e., outcomes) is concerned with whether change has occurred, the extent and nature of that change, and client satisfaction. An examination of treatment *efficiency* considers whether the change was cost-effective, whether all parts of the treatment were necessary, and whether another treatment could have worked faster. *Efficacy* ultimately is concerned with how well the treatment achieves both effects and efficiency (Dowden, Stone-Goldman, & Olswang, 2006; Olswang, 1998).

Clinical efficacy research in stuttering can be directed to answer many questions. Examples for *adults:* Does a particular therapeutic approach (e.g., psychotherapy; noise application) result in a long-term cure or decrease in stuttering? Which therapeutic approach (e.g., stuttering management versus fluency management) yields better and/or faster results? Is therapy oriented toward the emotional aspects of stuttering as effective as therapy oriented to the speech aspect? What is the optimal number and frequency of therapy sessions? Examples for young *children:* Are early predictions of chances to exhibit natural recovery accurate? Does early intervention result in a higher percent of complete cure than natural recovery without clinical intervention? Is indirect intervention (parent counseling) as effective as direct therapy with the child? The implications of some of these clinical questions to understanding the nature of stuttering are quite obvious.

Evaluating Efficacy

Efficacy research requires rigorous design. Typically, studies are conducted in laboratories or other controlled settings and employ randomized trials, careful selection of the clinical population, well-trained clinicians, blind data analysis, and so on. One problem is that frequently there is no clear indication for whether such laboratory conditions and levels of reported success can be transferred to treatment conducted in typical work environments that all too often are impossible to control. For example, clients may have other health problems that influence treatment outcome, and the clinicians may be less experienced than those who run the formal study. This leads to effectiveness-focused research that seeks to explore the extent to which the intervention, when deployed in the field, yields the intended results, and factors that interfere with, or increase, the therapeutic results (Association for Applied Psychophysiology and Biofeedback, 2011; Stuart, Treat, & Wade, 2000). Hence a treatment's efficacy may be different than its effectiveness in real field conditions.

Group Studies

The most common clinical research design employs group comparisons in which a certain treatment is administered to participants, with or without a control group, over a certain period. Pre- and posttreatment measurements are made of the behavior under investigation, as well as single or multiple follow-up measures. The strongest efficacy studies are randomized controlled clinical trials characterized by several features. First, they involve a test treatment (therapy) delivered to one group, another treatment or treatments delivered to other groups, and/or a control group receiving no treatment. Second, the clients are assigned into each group randomly. Third, subjects are selected with careful epidemiological, ethnic/culture, and other factors that might impact the results. Natural recovery is one example of such a factor. Testing the effect of new stuttering therapy with children between ages 2 and 4 is likely to be problematic because the high rate of natural recovery in this age group could easily distort the results. Fourth, data analysis is performed at a different site than the treatment center and by independent investigators who are blind to the purpose of the study.

Efficacy research to examine the effect of treatment on speech fluency may be closely tied to theoretical issues and further our scientific knowledge of the stuttering disorder (Olswang, 1993). Studies comparing preschool-age children receiving therapy soon after stuttering onset with children who do not receive treatment should generate important information about developmental processes of early stuttering as well as etiological factors (if the participants characteristics are well described). Similarly, when modified parental behaviors are the experimental variable in a treatment study, we can test hypotheses regarding the role of environmental factors in precipitating stuttering.

Although recent years have seen a growing number of studies concerned with the evaluation of therapies for stuttering, for the most part, they do not constitute randomized clinical trials. In a study that compared the effectiveness of the ISTAR Comprehensive Stuttering Program as employed in the Netherlands and in Canada, the number of participants was small, 22 and 16 respectively; no control groups were employed in either site, hence no random assignment of subjects was possible (Langevin et al., 2006). In Canada, yearly posttherapy follow-up measures were obtained from 18 clients for 5 consecutive years but no control group was employed for comparison (Langevin, Kully, Teshima et al., 2010). There have been, however, a few exceptions. Among them is the Franken, Kielstra-Van der Schalk, and Boelens (2005) study comparing two therapy programs for children using a randomized design, and the Jones et al. (2005) investigation that included 54 children randomly assigned either to receive the Lidcombe Program of intervention or to a nontreatment control group. Carey, O'Brian, Onslow et al., (2010, 2012) compared telehealth versus face-to-face delivery of the Camperdown Program utilizing randomized controlled trials with multiple blinded outcome assessments. On the whole, however, other procedures essential to unbiased clinical trials in stuttering have not been commonly adopted. Such procedures include careful control of subject selection, for example, history of persistent or recovered stuttering in the family, administration of treatment in several clinics, blind analyses of data, and others.

Single-Subject Studies

As mentioned earlier, a rather popular means for conducting clinical research in various behavioral/emotional disorders, including the area of stuttering, has been single-subject studies. These are used to observe any changes occurring in an individual as a result of a treatment or treatments. Whereas typical studies compare groups of subjects, this type of research compares treatment effects on one or several individuals, each examined alone. The term *single-subject study* simply indicates that each participant serves as her or his own control. This is accomplished by looking at the person's performance while alternating between treatment and nontreatment phases of the study. For example, the first phase includes eight consecutive sessions (4 weeks) of no treatment followed by a second eight-session phase in which punishment is administered upon stuttering, followed by a third phase during which reinforcement is administered upon stuttering, followed by a fourth phase of no treatment once again. Such alternating cycles may repeat several times. Thus, whereas typical studies allow for one or just a few observed sessions in which the target behavior is measured, the single-subject design is advantageous in allowing repeated multiple observations of stuttering. McMillan (2004) points out that this feature also minimizes the effect of normal variations.

Several clinical studies in stuttering have employed a single-subject design. For example, Martin et al. (1972) demonstrated the effect of response contingencies with two preschool-age children: one stuttered severely (37% of syllables) and the other moderately (10% of syllables). During the base rate phase (about 3 to 5 sessions), the children talked with the puppeteer examiner. In the treatment phase (10 to 32 sessions), a 10-second period of time-out immediately followed every moment of stuttering. The time-out consisted of the puppet stage sound and lights being turned off. In the final extinction phase (about 10 sessions), the time-out treatment was no longer administered. In both children, stuttering frequency dropped to below 1% and remained at that level after the time-out treatment had been removed. Follow-up visits approximately 1 year posttreatment revealed continued levels below 1% by each child.

Although single-subject experiments do not supply evidence that is as strong as group experiments with respect to generalization of results, they nonetheless play an important role in demonstrating the specific conditions that may affect clinical outcomes. When characteristics or symptoms of single-case subjects (e.g., age, severity level, disfluent behaviors, etc.) match the client being served, similar stages or considerations in treatment may be applicable. Clinicians can apply principles of single-subject design to test the efficacy of their own treatments. In a school setting there are ample opportunities for small breaks that give clinicians a chance to observe whether treatment has been having a beneficial impact when compared to the "no treatment" periods, or whether treatment effects are maintained and generalized in the post-treatment variable conditions. Clinicians must wrestle with the various questions and decide what criteria are indicative of individual client success with therapy.

Issues Regarding Efficacy Research

Aside from the logistical difficulties in pursuing clinical efficacy research, several fundamental questions are yet to be resolved, such as how the effects of therapy should be evidenced. If change in overt stuttering is the target, what parameters should be reported: frequency, duration, severity, clustering of disfluencies, speech naturalness? What other aspects of the disorder should be investigated: for example, changes in attitudes and social adjustment regardless of overt stuttering? Can they serve as sufficient evidence of therapeutic success (see Thomas & Howell, 2001)? Should clients' self-assessment be taken as evidence or only external observations (see Quesal, Yaruss, & Molt, 2004; Rustin, Boterill, & Kelman, 1996)?

Another question is what level of change should be taken as evidence of successful treatment. When stuttering frequency is the measure, should the absolute or percentage change be regarded as a significant indicator of success? Specifically, is a reduction in three stutter events, say from 10 to 7 per 100 words, sufficient evidence supporting the technique employed? If yes, would a reduction in three stutter events from 20 to 17 per 100 words be viewed as sufficient evidence? Or should a specific percentage change, say 30%, be set as minimally acceptable? In that case, someone initially exhibiting 6 stutter events per 100 words would have to drop by only two events, to settle at four events per 100 words. But is a reduction in two events perceptible enough to be meaningful?

A third relevant issue is the amount of treatment and its distribution. Should we stipulate the number of sessions or the overall duration of the program as standard? And, of course, there is the well-known tendency for relapse in adults who stutter, estimated by several investigators as approximately 70% (e.g., Craig, 1998). For how long should follow-ups continue in order to declare success? More research is needed to address the various efficacy questions to guide clinical decision making.

Ethics

The term *ethics* pertains to a set of moral values: what is considered good and bad. Ethics influence the principles of conduct governing an individual or a group's standards of behavior. In the advanced world, just about every professional organization operates with a set of rules to define virtues of action: a code of ethics. The practice of speech pathology involves various encounters between clinicians and clients that are embedded in a moral context. Students of speech pathology engage in general courses and readings that address the domain of clinical ethics in our field, including the ASHA code of ethics, in a more comprehensive manner. Hence, we include here just a brief reminder. Clinical ethics issues include patient rights, confidentiality, truthfulness, informed consent, disclosure of optional treatment, recommendations for treatment, advice, and more.

Four commonly accepted principles of ethics (Watson, Byrd, & Moore, 2011) include:

- **Respect for autonomy:** Clinicians will honor clients' capacity to make fully voluntary and informed decisions related to the treatments they receive. No one should force a treatment on someone who has decided they do not want that treatment. Thus, persons of sufficient age and cognitive maturity are encouraged to actively participate in decisions related to their treatment.

- **Beneficence:** Clinicians do what is necessary to benefit clients. Sufficient scientific underpinnings are essential in order for clients and clinicians to have a reasonable expectation of benefit from the selected procedure. The commitment to beneficence implies that clinicians hold the value of the client well-being utmost in their concern as they make clinical decisions.

- **Nonmaleficence:** Clinicians will act to remove or prevent conditions of potential harm to clients. Clinicians follow the Hippocratic oath to "do no harm" in clinical intervention. If a particular treatment poses some costs or risks (e.g., a drug might have side effects), then these must be weighed carefully in balance against the projected improvements. Here again, clients must be informed regarding all the potential risks of any evaluation or treatment procedures, prior to making voluntarily consent to these conditions.

- **Justice:** This refers to clinician fairness; professionals should show no favoritism or bias in decisions affecting the distribution or delivery of their services to clients. The same opportunity for treatment should be offered to those with similar needs for them. Extra services or special attentions should not be given to some clients and not to others. Costs should be based on fair and reasonable standards applied consistently across individuals.

ASHA's Code of Ethics covers additional principles beyond these four major types, and it is similarly essential for clinicians to practice honesty and trustworthiness (Kummer & Turner, 2011). It should be the aim of all professionals to uphold all these ethical principles in their consultation and delivery of services with clients. The endeavor can be challenging, however; at times it may not be easy to maintain balance among the valued principles. For example, professionals are well aware of the importance of individualizing remediation because there is no "one size fits all" approach to clinical treatment, but the effort to uphold that value could lead to a situation in which clients with relatively similar needs are treated differently. The practice of individualization must be reexamined in cases where delivery of differential treatment creates unfairness. Clients must be afforded the opportunity to receive a consistent set of practices, procedures, and recommendations, so that some are not offered "better" services than others. A good way to demonstrate the magnitude and seriousness of professional ethics as applied to working with people who stutter is through listing questions that might arise in routine clinical practice as we present below. These are categorized according to whether they tend to arise with treatment of adults versus children.

Questions Concerning Ethics

Questions Concerning Adults

1. Is it sound practice to base diagnosis primarily on the judgment of a person who states that he or she stutters?
2. Should I use only strict evidence-based therapies?
3. Is it ethical to tell a client that the goal for therapy is the achievement of normal speech?
4. Is it ethical to instruct a client to stutter on purpose in the clinic or at home as part of the therapy?
5. Is it ethical to instruct a client to stutter on purpose talking to strangers in the street, store clerks, and so on?
6. Is it ethical to use mild electrical shock to punish stuttering?
7. Is it ethical to stop people in the street and stutter to them on purpose just to practice?
8. Is it ethical to substitute one abnormal speech (stuttering) with another (e.g., rhythmic speech)?
9. Is it ethical to recommend purchase of an expensive fluency-aiding instrument rather than providing speech therapy?

Questions Concerning Children

1. Is it ethical to postpone therapy for a preschool-age child immediately after onset, just because of the high chances for natural recovery?
2. Is it ethical to recommend therapy for a preschool-age child immediately after onset, knowing the high chances for natural recovery?
3. Is it ethical to counsel parents to not correct their child's stuttering? To correct it?
4. Is it ethical to counsel parents of a child who stutters to talk to him or her in a simple language?
5. Is it ethical to tell parents that perhaps their behavior caused the child's stuttering?
6. Is it ethical to tell parents that perhaps some of their behavior aggravates the child's stuttering?
7. Is it ethical to train children to be assertive when others make fun of them?

As scientific advances are being made in genetics, drugs, brain imaging, and other areas, more questions arise. Genetics raises several concerns, especially privacy issues. A genetic analysis could bring uninvited results, significant to the individual, as well as current or future children. What should be done with such information? Sometimes obtaining genetic information requires participation from other family members who may be unwilling to cooperate. Is there a proper ethical principle to persuade their participation? A rather sensitive issue is counseling. Suppose an infant is at high risk for stuttering even before the onset of speech. Should parents be counseled? If so, how and when is counseling offered? Who should provide the counseling? Another thorny issue pertains to the use of pharmaceutical agents. Suppose a pharmacological treatment for stuttering has been developed but with some risk that disfluency will persist. Some parents would want their child to take the drug, even though stuttering is not a life-threatening condition. How do parents weigh the risks versus the benefits, especially for the one who has never stuttered? We will not provide any opinions. Indeed, these are serious questions that clinicians should be prepared to answer as they formulate their own personal code of ethics in conjunction with the professionally accepted principles.

Summary

Prior to an examination of various forms of treatment for stuttering, it is important to consider several broad issues that impact clinical decisions. The following points were raised:

- Clinical intervention is ideally based in a theoretical rationale. The absence of strong comprehensive theories of stuttering poses a substantial challenge to this endeavor. Yet successful eclectic therapy programs should be recognized and considered with all other factors.

- Three major potential aims of stuttering treatment were identified: producing fluent speech, reducing stuttering, and improving social-emotional adjustment.

- Twelve general approaches to stuttering treatment were classified into three areas of focus: improved cognitive-emotional adjustment, managed stuttering, and increased fluency.

- The therapeutic nature of the client-clinician relationship can be enhanced by qualities of empathy, self-congruence, and unconditional positive regard. Activities aimed at promoting such qualities were suggested.

- The pursuit of evidence-based practice has both its merits and its hazards. Whereas the merits of evidence-based treatment are obvious, it may also present considerable rigidity in practical implementation.

- The field must face multiple challenges before we can answer all our questions about clinical efficacy. Unfortunately, the limited number of well-controlled clinical research studies pertaining to the treatment of stuttering conducted to date, whether employing group or single-subject design, has left many common clinical practices untested.

- Clinical practice must be conducted within commonly accepted rules of ethics by the society at large and the profession of speech pathology. Ethical questions of special relevance to stuttering were brought to the forefront.

Study Questions and Discussion Topics

1. What is the reasoning behind the advocacy of a therapy-theory link?
2. Do certain forms of evidence-based rationale provide a sufficient basis for treatment even in the absence of a definitive theory of stuttering? Give examples in support of your opinion.
3. What are the three major long-term therapy objectives for stuttering? Explain/discuss the differences among the goals stated.
4. Although the three major treatment goals—fluent speech, reduced stuttering, and improved adjustment—can each be targeted in isolation, these areas also may interact. In your opinion, could progress in each of the areas influence progress in the other two areas? Why?
5. The chapter presented 12 treatment approaches classified into three classes. What are the classes? Elaborate on the uniqueness of each. Explain the differences.
6. If you were charged to categorize these 12 treatment approaches, what classification system would you develop and why? What features would you base your system on?
7. Make a list of the challenges that clinical efficacy research must address in the field of stuttering. Which challenges pose the most serious threats to our progress with treatment knowledge and why?
8. What is your opinion regarding the significance of each of the clinician qualities suggested in this chapter? Do you think they are important? Suggest at least two additional qualities.
9. What would your answers be to the questions listed in the section on ethics?

Suggested Readings

Ambrose, E., & Yairi, E. (2002). The Tudor study: Data and ethics. *American Journal of Speech-Language Pathology, 11,* 190–203.

American Speech-Language-Hearing Association. (2010). *Code of ethics.* Retrieved November 9, 2013, from http://www.asha.org/policy/ET2010-00309.htm

Bernstein Ratner, N. (2005). Evidence-based practice in stuttering: some questions to consider. *Journal of Fluency Disorders, 30,* 163–188.

Bothe, A., Ingham, R., & Ingham, J. (2009). The roles of evidence and information in stuttering treatment. In B. Guitar & R. McCauley (Eds.), *Stuttering treatments: Conventional and emerging interventions* (pp. 341–352). Philadelphia, PA: Lippincott Williams and Wilkins.

Manning, W. (2004). How can you understand? You don't stutter! *Contemporary Issues in Communication Science and Disorders,31,* 58–68.

Packman, A., & Attanasio, J. (2004). Theories and treatment. In *Theoretical issues in stuttering* (pp. 143–156). New York, NY: Psychology Press.

Quesal, R. (2010). Empathy: Perhaps the most important E in EBP. *Seminars in Speech and Language, 31,* 217–226.

Therapy for Adults: Focus on Emotional Reactions

LEARNER OBJECTIVES

Readers of this chapter will be able to:

- Recognize distinguishing characteristics of adults who stutter and their prognostic outlook.
- Examine the potential role of psychotherapy as a form of stuttering intervention.
- Describe the objectives and rationales for a variety of techniques aimed at decreasing or increasing emotional reactions.
- Understand the benefits of group therapy.
- Evaluate past and present efforts of using drugs to treat stuttering.
- Discuss the results of research related to the treatment approaches covered in this chapter.

Adults Who Stutter

You may wonder why the discussion of therapy for the three age groups covered in this part of the book reverses the chronological order, presenting therapy for adults first. The reason for this reversal is that the discussion of therapy for adults allows for a broader exposition of issues, principles, and methods, some of which are also relevant to treatment of preschool and school-age children. Indeed, for a good many years the clinical literature on stuttering focused on adults rather than children. At the time, this trend mirrored the volume of stuttering research literature in relation to age. We note that many of the techniques were originally developed for adults, then adopted for children. Such an age-reversed order of therapy presentation was also followed by Van Riper (1973).

Prior to discussing adult treatment, a basic definitional question arises: At what age are adult therapy methods appropriate? Or, when do children cross the threshold into adulthood? From a biological perspective, physical growth continues until as late as age 22. From a cultural perspective, where Western civilization is predominant, age 18 is a common milestone. From yet another perspective, puberty has been regarded as the transitional period to maturity. From the standpoint of the developmental course of stuttering, Bloodstein and Bernstein Ratner (2008) noted that its most advanced stage was typically reached during adolescence and into adulthood, although sometimes as young as age 10. Similarly, Conture (2001) suggested that individuals in later years of high school and beyond could qualify as adults who stutter. We propose that adult therapy methods may be appropriate a year or two earlier, at about age 15, provided there were no limitations in cognitive or emotional development.

Another important issue when working with adults is their history of past treatments. Because the number of school speech-language clinicians in the United States has substantially increased over the past several decades, it is safe to assume that the number of children they have served has increased as well. This logical inference was substantiated by a survey of adults who stutter that showed over 94% of respondents had received therapy in the past, with the majority reporting more than one treatment experience (Yaruss et al., 2002). Therapy experiences were especially common between the ages of 6 and 12 but often continued into adulthood, mainly prior to age 35.

The prognosis for adult treatment expressed in the literature appears to be rather guarded. Because adults tend to have long histories of stuttering therapy, often they are expected to be more skeptical about their chances for better results "this time around" or to possess well-entrenched stuttering patterns, attitudes, and beliefs about the disorder. One scholar of stuttering stated, "The habituation that adult people who stutter often exhibit implies that their stuttering and related concerns will be fairly resistant to change" (Conture, 2000, p. 284). Other factors, probably stronger, besides attitudes and habituation, however, should be considered.

The prognosis for adults must take into account the critical role of the epidemiological factors that contributed to their persistent form of stuttering. As discussed in Chapter 3, at least 75% of those who begin to stutter exhibit natural recovery in subsequent years. Adults who stutter therefore represent a small remnant of those who have ever stuttered. Their persistence most likely reflects a more robust disorder. In fact, genetics is an important factor underlying both natural recovery and chronic stuttering (Ambrose et al., 1997). Therefore, adult stuttering may be difficult to treat not mainly because of attitudes and resistance, but because of the tenacious nature of this subtype of the stuttering disorder. Clinicians must keep this information in mind before jumping to the conclusion that difficulties in progress are related to clients' attitudes.

There is also an optimistic side to the prognosis for adults who seek therapy. Adult maturity, compared to adolescence, is more apt to support a satisfying process of change. The tendency for greater emotional and social stability with increased age can lead to more "productive attempts at recovery" (Starkweather & Givens-Ackerman, 1997, p. 54). When an adult who stutters continues to seek help, despite a moderate or long history of therapy, it is a positive sign. It suggests hope, motivation to improve, and persistence in spite of past failures. Clients may be ready to change habits of avoidance and more boldly attempt new speaking experiences. The information about past treatments, their results, the clients' feelings about speech therapy, and their clinicians all can be useful toward setting and attaining realistic goals in the present.

Treatments

In presenting the various treatments for adults who stutter, we focus on psychologically oriented therapies and drug therapies. Motor speech-oriented therapies, as well as instrument-based treatments, are presented in Chapter 12. This order also reflects our clinical orientation to stuttering treatment in adults. Unless otherwise indicated, we prefer to begin with some work pertaining to the client's stuttering-related emotional reactions and attitudes, preparing the ground for what we believe to be more productive and stable results of speech-focused therapy.

Chapter 6 presented theories that portrayed stuttering as caused by deep-seated emotional problems, if not disturbances. Whether this is true, there is no doubt that in many afflicted individuals there are emotional components (various reactions) to their stuttering disorder (see Chapter 4). Clinicians know that in no small number of individuals who stutter, the emotional component is so obvious and so strong as to overshadow the stuttered speech. This is one reason why many laypersons think that "stuttering is psychogenic," and why some clinicians treat it as such, attempting to eliminate the psychogenic cause of the stuttering. Most scholars, however, believe that emotionality is not the cause but the result of stuttering, learned and reinforced through unpleasant experiences (see Chapter 6). Being a part of the problem, reduction of emotionality can, and should be, part of the therapeutic agenda. Clinicians, however, must be careful about making undue generalizations because of the wide range of emotional reactivity associated with stuttering. In our experience, some clients report little speech anxiety or emotionality. To them, stuttering is uncomfortable, an unpleasant irritation, but they do not hesitate to speak. Many others, however, are severely oppressed by the disorder.

Treatments to improve the psychoemotional responses of people who stutter do not neatly separate into subcategories of personal and social adjustment, because these two domains are closely related. Nonetheless, based on their major emphasis, the following therapeutic approaches are organized according to a focus on psychotherapy, relaxation, desensitization, social adjustment, and drug therapies. Following, we discuss a variety of psychological methods that have attempted to address personal adjustment and emotional reactions. Whether or not clinicians practice them, they should be knowledgeable about their field and prepared to respond to clients' questions.

Psychotherapy and Relaxation

Over the past century, the meaning of the term *psychotherapy* has broadened to include procedures designed to (1) relieve emotional stress, anxieties, and their associated symptoms; (2) alleviate more serious emotional disorders such as depression; (3) develop positive self-concept and confidence; and (4) improve social adjustment. It involves an analysis of a client's thoughts, feelings, and behavior. The technique rarely requires the client to experiment actively with direct changes in behavior. More typically, psychotherapy aims at bringing about a new awareness concerning the nature or source of the problem, and this insight is expected to alter the client's experience and habitual responses. Thus the psychological awareness transforms the behavior as the client acts in accordance with new insights. In this light, many, if not most, stuttering therapies include certain elements of psychotherapy.

Purposeful, theory-based psychotherapy began toward the end of the 19th century with Sigmund Freud's (1899) technique of psychoanalysis. Psychotherapies are extremely diverse. Wikipedia (2007) lists approximately 140 different methods, reflecting various theoretical orientations and specific techniques. To illustrate the range, among those listed are psychoanalysis, humanistic psychology, cognitive-behavioral therapy, existential therapy, person-centered therapy, holistic therapy, rational-emotive behavior therapy, reality therapy, and primal therapy. Treatment is provided in different formats, such as individual, couples, family, group, and experiential therapy. As for the mode, most psychotherapies rely on spoken conversation, but some employ artwork, drama, playing a narrative story, dance, and other activities. Although sometimes the terms *psychotherapy* and *counseling* are used interchangeably, generally the first term applies to intervention for a serious mental health problem, whereas the second term implies assistance for coping with everyday problems or various difficulties.

Logically, when stuttering was considered a psychoneurotic disorder, psychotherapy was the method to treat it. Although by current standards there is no, or only weak, evidence to support the neurosis hypothesis, anyone who works with clients who stutter would agree that the disorder can strongly affect the mind and emotions of a person who stutters. Having knowledge about psychotherapeutic methods is, therefore, important for practicing clinicians.

Psychoanalysis

Classical Freudian psychoanalysis is aimed at the root problem, not the symptoms. Its ultimate objective is to elevate the unconscious to the conscious level. The clinician creates a relaxed situation, with the patient lying on a couch, in which she or he is encouraged to let thoughts flow in a completely free manner, and in turn say whatever comes to mind in total honesty. The open verbalization of thoughts as they float from one to the next is referred to as *free association*. Whatever the patient says is accepted without criticism. It is assumed that free association in the presence of a neutral therapist, supplemented with dream interpretation, will cause unconscious emotional conflicts to surface so they can be confronted and resolved. Because these ideas were in ascendance at the end of the 19th century and the early decades of the 20th century, one explanation of the stuttering disorder focused on personality conflict within the individual, referencing Freud. In Chapter 6, we explained that this theory viewed stuttering as an overt symptom of an unconscious, deep-seated neurosis. Such development also left its imprints on stuttering therapy, with therapies that were aimed at curing presumed deep-seated personality neuroses traced back to early childhood.

E. Yairi: "I subjected myself to classical psychoanalysis on a weekly basis for a 2-year period while an undergraduate majoring in psychology. To pay for this expensive program, I took hard labor, literally dirty jobs, cleaning multifloor apartment buildings as they went up. I worked odd hours, e.g., 4–7 AM, so that I could make it to classes. To me, therapy was an interesting process but a rather boring experience after a while. My free associations were dull or I was too inhibited to travel to exciting ones. In any event, although I felt better, psychoanalysis had no effect whatsoever on my stuttering. In short, therapy made me a happier stutterer."

Early on, in 1923, Brill reported that among his 600 patients who stuttered, 69 received psychoanalysis with considerable initial success. An 11-year follow-up, however, indicated that only 5 of the 69 patients (7%) were doing "really well." Conceding the large relapse factor, Brill concluded that some subtypes of stuttering will respond well to psychoanalysis, whereas the majority of "true stutterers" are very difficult to treat with the method. In the years that followed, others applied one of several psychotherapies in either individual or group settings (e.g., Barbara, 1962; Brody & Harrison, 1954; Glauber, 1958; Honig, 1947; Murphy & Fitzsimons, 1960; Sadoff & Siegel, 1965) but produced little quantitative data. In 1971, however, Travis reported on clinical experimentation with 30 adult individuals who stutter, all appearing to have conflicts over unmet early childhood needs. The psychotherapy, extending up to 3 years for some clients, yielded mixed results. Only six were considered cured, and five showed substantial improvement. If this subjective assessment is valid, just 35% of the entire group enjoyed a positive to very positive outcome.

In a more extensive study, Webster (1977) examined the clinical records of 648 people treated specifically for stuttering by a team of six psychotherapists at the Speech and Hearing Institute in New York City between 1969 and 1972. No objective counts of disfluencies were made. Outcome was indicated on the following scale: disorder corrected, moderately improved, slightly improved, and unimproved. The disappointing findings indicated that none of the clients fell in the "corrected" category and that moderate improvement in fluency was limited to only 8% of this large sample. In other words, 92% showed either no or only slight improvement. Webster commented that "while psychotherapy may have had some positive effects on the stutterer's psychological well-being, the same treatment seems to have done little to ameliorate the fluency problems of the vast majority of these individuals" (p. 254). Clinicians in the field with extensive experience treating teenagers and adults who stutter also reported that most of their clients who received psychotherapy for their stuttering evaluated it as noneffective as far as their disfluent speech was concerned (e.g., Dodge, personal communication, 2009).

Overall, the effectiveness of psychoanalytic-oriented therapies in reducing stuttering has been limited, and research support for emotional disturbances underlying stuttering has been inconsistent and relatively weak. During the past 40 years or so, the application of psychotherapy as the sole or main therapeutic approach for stuttering lost much ground for three reasons: (1) the failure of research to provide the necessary level of support for the claim that stuttering is a neurotic disorder, (2) the realization that psychotherapy has had very limited success, and (3) the increased availability of speech therapy and its relative, growing effectiveness. At present, the use of psychotherapies as the sole treatment for stuttering appears to be rare. Nevertheless, in assessing obstacles to therapeutic progress, clinicians should consider the client's overall emotional health and the need to obtain other expert evaluation.

Rational-Emotive Therapy

Rational-emotive therapy (RET), originated by Albert Ellis (1973), represented a significant departure from psychoanalysis because with this method, a patient does not merely note and express thoughts but actively takes charge of them. It is considered to be one of the earliest forms of cognitive-behavioral therapy (Phares, 1979). The supposition of cognitive-behavioral therapy is that when a person's way of thinking changes, his or her behavior changes. To understand behavior, examine the underlying thought processes. Detrimental thoughts lead to detrimental behaviors. Beneficial thoughts lead to beneficial behaviors. So one of the premises of RET is that psychoemotional distress arises from the irrational negative thoughts and beliefs people have about themselves, others, or life itself. These thoughts or beliefs can be particularly important if they become *self-fulfilling prophecies*. A self-fulfilling prophecy is a prediction that influences its own outcome. Negative thoughts can set a person up for failures, whereas positive thoughts help to bring about favorable outcomes.

RET emphasizes a reorganization of the person's cognitive and emotional functions. That is, by reexamining beliefs and redefining problems, more suitable patterns of behavior will result. Hence central to this approach is a focus on positive self-talk. Self-talk is the inner dialogue that a person has with his or her self throughout waking hours. An example of negative self-talk might be "I sure am stupid. I hate myself." An example of positive self-talk might be "I like being human. I am a worthwhile person." One of the assumptions of RET is that changing irrational (negative) self-talk into rational (positive) self-talk strengthens consequent emotions. That is, one's thoughts have a direct influence on one's feelings and also on one's behaviors.

RET may be conducted with individuals or with groups. The program includes five steps: (1) Identify the self-talk that occurred when there was an event that activated a self-statement. Example: After making a mistake, the person tells him- or herself, "That was stupid." (2) Look deeper to examine the underlying assumptions and beliefs behind the self-talk. Example: "I believe I must do things right all the time in order to think of myself as worthwhile." (3) Acknowledge the associated feeling(s). Example: "I feel depressed and discouraged." (4) Challenge the irrational assumption and belief. Example: "It's not reasonable to expect perfection from myself. No one always manages to do the right things." (5) Replace the ineffective self-talk with effective self-talk. Example: "I am a worthwhile person. I have permission to be human, and forgive myself when I make mistakes. It benefits nobody when I put myself down." Table 11.1 illustrates how the steps in rational-emotive therapy might be applied to stuttering.

Table 11.1   Example of the Five Steps in Rational-Emotive Therapy Applied to Stuttering

Focus	Step	Stuttering-Related Example
Activating Event	Identify the negative self-talk	"If I stutter now, it will be horrible."
Belief System	Examine underlying assumptions	"Stuttering makes me inadequate."
Consequent Emotion	Acknowledge the feeling	"I feel ashamed and helpless. Poor me."
Dispute Irrational Thinking	Challenge the belief	"Is stuttering what matters most about who I am? No."
Effective Self-Talk	Replace with positive self-talk	"I am a worthwhile person, stuttering or not."

The approach obviously involves an ongoing practice of self-monitoring and self-questioning one's thoughts and beliefs. The changes in emotions or stuttering itself are the indirect result of these cognitive processes. The client's active participation in rational-emotive therapy is more in line with conventional speech therapy methods and should be given more consideration by speech clinicians treating stuttering. One study found this technique was more effective than systematic desensitization in reducing both speaking anxiety and stuttering events (Moleski & Tosi, 1976).

Relaxation

The previously described therapies emphasized the impact of psychoemotional adjustments on physical responses and behaviors. Relaxation therapies emphasize the reverse process. The reduction of physical tensions and responses can deliver a psychoemotional benefit. Thus the dynamics may work in either direction. The physical affects the emotional as well as the emotional affecting the physical.

As we discussed in Chapter 3 about the development of stuttering, and in Chapter 4 about its advanced symptomatology, excessive muscle tension may appear in association with stuttering events from an early stage of the disorder. It becomes more pronounced as stuttering persists over the years. Physical tension in the speech mechanism and the entire head and neck are the most commonly observed locations. Frequently it spreads to other parts of the body, with tightness in the chest, abdomen, and even the extremities. One person who stutters related that even his toes tightened and curled before and during stuttering. We observed a person who used to crush objects held in his hand (e.g., a soda can) when stuttering severely.

Apprehension in anticipation of stuttering, and the mixture of affective reactions during its occurrence, also add a strong component of emotional tension: anxiety. Anxiety is associated with various neurological-physiological changes (e.g., muscle tone and sweat). The physical and emotional tensions are seemingly impossible to separate as one leads to the other. It is difficult to feel mentally relaxed while physically tense. It is well known that anxiety, phobias (unrealistic fears), or panic attacks are associated with physical tension. People with high anxiety have difficulty learning how to release the tension in their muscles, which, in turn, contributes to their experience of anxiety.

Reducing Muscular Tension

Whatever causes it, tension appears to be one of the final expressions of the abnormality of stuttering, presenting a direct obstacle to the necessary smooth movement for speech production. Excessive muscular tension can trigger or intensify the impression of "getting stuck." Here enters the concept of relaxation, which releases both the anxiety and skeletal muscle tension. The rationale for lessening emotional and physical tension is the assumption that it will (1) reduce the frequency and severity of stuttering, and (2) allow the client to attend to modifying speech in a constructive manner when the therapy reaches that stage.

The advice "just relax" is one of the oldest informal instructions offered by laypersons to those who stutter. Although such advice tends to put someone on edge rather than being helpful, relaxing, if possible, may have value. The stiff and uncomfortable sensations of excessive tension seem incompatible with fluent speech movements. There is limited evidence, however, for the inverse assumption that a program of relaxation alone prevents stuttering. Peter Kupferman described his unfulfilled expectations of relaxation exercises in the video *No Words to Say* (Holzman, 1988), stating, "I was really relaxed, but I was still stuttering." Even when a speaker has reduced tension or anxiety to minimal levels, it is still possible to stutter. Thus stuttering therapy usually must involve more than relaxation or desensitization methods alone.

A relaxation component is found in many formal treatment programs. Reference to relaxation can be found in clinicians' writings from the first half of the 19th century. Van Riper (1973, p. 41) cited Hoffman, who in 1840 stated that "the patient must use no muscular effort in the throat, tongue, or lips. Further, he must avoid working other parts of the body, such as the arms, feet, etc. . . . The greatest relaxation of the body must occur during speech." Some clinicians went as far as to propose that relaxation should be the basis for all stuttering therapy regardless of its format (Boome & Richardson, 1947). A comprehensive review of the relevant literature was published by Gilman and Yaruss (2000). Two formal avenues to achieve relaxation include authoritative suggestion and blending mental and physical techniques. A temporary state of relaxation can also be induced with various drugs (discussed later in this chapter).

Authoritative Suggestion and Hypnosis

Strong suggestion by an influential clinician that the client can be relaxed when entering a speaking situation may convince some to the point of success in achieving this goal. Persuasive literature, encouragement by fellow clients in a group setting, as well as other sources may also exert the power of suggestion (Silverman, 2004). When an authority figure, such as the clinician, influences client behavior through the power of suggestion, the technique is called *authoritative suggestion*. Bloodstein (1995) attributed the potential for almost any form of therapy to have temporary success in reducing stuttering to the power of suggestion. He cautioned that this factor complicates the evaluation of any new treatment that may be introduced. Sometimes clients can convince themselves of their ability to rein in a situation, a phenomenon known as *autosuggestion*. Although a considerable amount of suggestion is applied routinely in clinical contexts, its use specifically to induce relaxation is not too common and its effect in stuttering therapy has not been very well evaluated.

Suggestions for keeping calm and relaxed may also be offered under hypnosis. Posthypnotic commands instruct the client how to behave after waking up from the hypnotic state. Hypnosis in stuttering therapy, however, has been minimal. Several clinicians published descriptions of individual cases (e.g., Nao, 1964). In a rare clinical study with a commendable number of 40 participants, Moore (1946, 1959) reported mixed client responses and improvement that lasted only 2 to 3 days. Van Riper (1973) also reported disappointing experiments with the technique. Although the use of hypnosis in stuttering therapy has not drawn much past attention, clinicians should keep in mind the poor results because some people who stutter always seek quick cures.

Blending Physical Relaxation and Mental Desensitization

Much more popular have been relaxation techniques, such as *progressive relaxation* (Jacobson, 1938), that require more direct, active physical and/or mental client participation. Employing the Jacobson technique, the initial sessions begin with a client sitting comfortably in a chair, eyes closed, hands in lap. In a soft relaxed voice, the clinician instructs the client to tighten the fists for a few seconds and then relax, observing the contrast. Similarly, other muscle groups are targeted. Next, the client moves on intentionally to achieve a relaxed sensation (without first tensing) in one muscle group at a time, starting with the feet, progressing upward to the legs, abdomen, chest, shoulders, neck, face, and mouth, breathing slowly in a relaxed manner. The first round may take approximately 5 minutes, but the sequence is repeated several times, checking each muscle group until all reach complete relaxation. Throughout the sequence, the clinician, in a soothing voice, encourages the client to focus on each muscle group until the client reaches a state of being very relaxed, the muscles feel "heavy," and breathing is slow and easy. At the end of the session (20 to 25 minutes), the eyes are opened and there is a definite sense of calmness.

Following a few sessions, the client learns to quickly achieve relaxation in response to clinician's directions, then becomes capable of inducing self-relaxation by repeating the commands mentally. We have routinely demonstrated the procedure during classes, watching many students thoroughly enjoy the experience. Some clinicians have incorporated relaxation in their complex treatment programs with the idea that clients will thereby be better able to implement the various speech techniques regarded as the center of the therapy. Although the skills of relaxation can be learned, implementation in real-life situations can be difficult.

The practice of progressive relaxation has been used in conjunction with the therapeutic program known as *systematic desensitization*. Tyre, Maisto, and Companik (1973) described procedures for systematic desensitization used successfully with a young adult male with moderate stuttering severity. The client was seen for two 55-minute sessions per week for 8 weeks. The first five sessions were spent with training in Jacobson's (1938) deep muscle relaxation techniques. The client was told to practice these techniques daily from that point on. The remaining sessions focused on a reciprocal inhibition program (Wolpe, 1958). This is a behavior therapy aimed at inhibiting one response by pairing it with the occurrence of an incompatible one. For example, when anxiety-evoking stimuli are paired with relaxation, their power is weakened. This is further discussed in the next section. To communicate while deeply relaxed, the client used finger signaling to answer yes/no questions, and indicate feeling anxiety. He was then advanced through imagery exercises through two situational fear-related hierarchies while concentrating on deep muscle relaxation. The program lasted 16 weeks. The stuttering severity scores were diminished from 50 at pretherapy, to 25 posttherapy, to 17 at 6-month follow-up.

Summary of Psychotherapy and Relaxation

Various ideas that stuttering is caused by deep emotional problems traced back to early childhood spurred some interest in psychotherapy as the choice avenue for its treatment, especially as Freud's psychoanalysis approach gained in popularity. The negative findings of research concerned with personality characteristics and emotional adjustment of people who stutter, and clinical reports suggesting that traditional psychoanalysis has had only limited success in the treatment of stuttering, have considerably diminished enthusiasm for this therapeutic approach. Although the speaker's psychoemotional adjustment, more broadly, may be enhanced by a variety of psychotherapeutic approaches, there has been limited evidence of their impact on overt stuttering. Rational-emotive therapy whereby irrational beliefs and negative self-talk are replaced with rational thinking and positive self-talk, appears to be worth further study in stuttering therapy.

As we discussed in Chapter 4, the fearful expectation of stuttering causes considerable apprehension, distress, and anxiety. Such emotional tension is closely linked with physical tension. Physical tensions can be addressed directly through relaxation techniques or indirectly by autosuggestion and hypnosis. The combined application of physical relaxation techniques and mental desensitization has been successful in reducing stuttering. Desensitization principles have played a major role in stuttering therapy over the years and are covered in greater detail in the following sections.

Desensitization

Considerable evidence supports an interaction between stuttering and anxiety or emotional stress. Recall that the review of the literature in Chapter 6 showed a tendency for people with a stuttering disorder to have greater state and trait anxieties. Although the nature of the interaction between those anxieties and stuttering, and the specific implications for intervention have been controversial, many clinicians devote a substantial portion of therapy to the area of emotional reactions. The reason for this clinical focus is not that emotions are believed to be the root cause of the problem, but that they are an integral part of the disorder that interferes with reduction in the overt stuttering.

Although different emotions are experienced prior, during, and after moments of stuttering, it seems that clients and clinicians alike have been concerned primarily with general anxiety and specific fears about anticipated speech (e.g., Brutten & Shoemaker, 1967; Van Riper, 1973). Hence therapy has focused on lessening psychological difficulties and reducing anxiety and fears to the neglect of increasing positive emotions and behaviors, such as assertiveness, self-confidence, and self-image. To this end, behavioral desensitization or anxiolytic drugs have been used. This section deals with the behavioral management of stuttering related anxiety, namely desensitization. Two approaches are discussed in this context: systematic desensitization and desensitization in vivo.

> Desensitization is the process of disassociating negative emotional responses, especially irrational fears (phobias) from the stimuli that evoke them. It allows the person to master anxiety in small doses (Rothbaum, Hodges, Smith, et al., 2000). This is accomplished by being exposed to anxiety-provoking stimuli in a carefully arranged hierarchy, moving from weaker to stronger stimuli, and from a shorter to longer time of exposure. This can be enhanced using reciprocal inhibition techniques. As clients achieve the goal of remaining minimally affected by each of the weaker anxiety-provoking stimuli, they progress to greater challenges.

Systematic Desensitization

Systematic desensitization was developed by psychiatrist Joseph Wolpe (1958) and adapted for stuttering therapy by Brutten and Shoemaker (1967). It is based on the principle of counterconditioning (or reciprocal inhibition). As explained earlier, it seeks to weaken anxiety-provoking stimuli by pairing them with incompatible relaxed states. The first step is to teach relaxation skills (the incompatible response), especially through the progressive relaxation method described earlier.

Having mastered relaxation skills during the first few sessions, the second component of systematic desensitization is introduced by asking a client, while in a state of deep relaxation, to imagine a stimulus (a person, place, situation, and others) that habitually triggers fear and stuttering. The client quickly realizes that she or he experiences considerably milder anxiety facing the situation while relaxed and imagining it. With sufficient repetition, the situation loses its anxiety-provoking power also in reality.

The client, guided by the clinician, ranks a large set of stuttering-provoking situations from least to most distressing. The program then proceeds in a hierarchy of increasing difficulty both within each level and between levels of difficulty. In an anxiety-producing situation like answering the telephone at home, several steps, such as the ones listed below, are involved. At first, each step is only imagined while the client focuses on remaining relaxed:

1. A telephone ringing from the basement of one's home.
2. A telephone ringing at the far side of the same floor of the house, but another person answers it.
3. A telephone ringing in a nearby room, but another person answers it.
4. A telephone ringing in the client's room, but the ringing stops as the client moves toward it.
5. A telephone ringing, and the client picks up the receiver but the caller says it was a wrong number.
6. A telephone ringing, and the client answers it and carries on a brief conversation.

The entire sequence proceeds in one session. When the client feels more comfortable, real telephone calls are planned in progressive steps. Once the client is capable of handling telephone calls, a situation at a higher level in the hierarchy is targeted. The clinician must ascertain that no anxiety is experienced at each level before progressing to the next. The client remains at each step until a relaxed state is reliably achieved. An important advantage of systematic desensitization is that the client can practice reducing the anxiety in many situations in a short time without actually being there. Additionally, clients learn to self-administer the process and maintain the gains through regular practice. From this standpoint, the technique is very efficient. Several studies have reported its effectiveness in reducing stuttering (Fried, 1972; Lanyon, 1969; Tyre et al., 1973). The main drawback is the client's passive role with no speech included in the exercise. Therefore, we recommend that after a client feels comfortable with the imagined situations (e.g., telephone calls), a sequenced hierarchy of real situations of talking is practiced.

It is not clear why systematic desensitization has had limited acceptance by clinicians for treating stuttering. Perhaps this is due to the perception that the technique belongs in the realm of psychologists. In addition, research studies of systematic desensitization may be difficult to interpret because the relative contributions of its multiple dimensions (i.e., relaxation, situational hierarchy, cognitive confrontation, etc.) are not clear. Some research suggests that anxiety-focused approaches to treatment may successfully reduce a speaker's anxiety but not necessarily the stuttering (e.g., Blomgren, Roy, Callister et al., 2005).

Several means of confronting feared situations are possible. Before the computer era, the exposure occurred either through imagery (e.g., imagining a plane flight) or through real-life, or so-called *in vivo*, encounters with the feared situation (e.g., taking an actual plane flight). More recently, computer-simulated exposure (virtual reality) can be used in lieu of in vivo exposure. Research findings indicate that these methods are effective in resolving various anxieties (Rothbaum et al., 2000). An example of using virtual reality experiences to decrease anxiety is shown in this video titled *virtual reality therapy*: http://www.youtube.com/watch?v=CQgKEp_NhHk

Desensitization in Vivo

This technique is used in behavioral therapy when an individual is exposed, in a hierarchical order, to feared, habitually avoided stimuli in real life. It is applied when avoided fears are not regarded as objectively appropriate. Clients learn to face fears directly, stay in the feared experience while remaining calm, proving to themselves that the "danger" is not as bad as they believe it to be. The aim is to lower anxiety and other "negative" emotions although not completely eliminate them. No one can expect to reduce either emotional or physical tension completely or constantly, and sometimes a speaker must feel the intensity but resolve not to hold back speech. In essence, habitual responses to certain stimuli are substantially modified, if not replaced.

Regardless of the method, desensitization has a double purpose. The first is to decrease the frequency of stuttering on the premise that the less fearful the client, the less stuttering is apt to occur. The second is to facilitate an ability to modify moments of stuttered speech because it is difficult to attend to constructive speech changes when a person is anxious. Van Riper (1973) suggested three more specific objectives when applying the technique in stuttering therapy: (1) open confrontation with the disorder, (2) desensitization to the client's own stuttering core behavior, and (3) desensitization to listeners' reactions. To these, one may add desensitization to time pressure, feared speaking situations, size of audience, people in authority, the opposite sex, and more. Next we elaborate on these objectives and provide a brief practical description of procedures, adapted after those of Van Riper, several other sources, and our own experience.

Being Open about Stuttering

Many adults who stutter do not like to look at, listen to, or talk about their stuttering. We have learned from our clients that most parents did not openly discuss stuttering with them except for suggesting to "slow down," "say it again," and so on. Nor did most stuttering children share with parents or siblings their difficulties and the pain brought about by their speech impediment. In one case, a mother of a kindergarten child who stuttered, watching behind an observation mirror, was shocked to learn how upset her child was with children making fun of his speech. She had no idea. The mutual silence usually continues into adulthood. Typically, adults who stutter do not talk about stuttering with friends, coworkers, or even spouses and children. Rarely do they look at themselves in the mirror when speaking. Although the overt stuttering, sometimes severe, is evident and making listeners uncomfortable, whole conversations may be carried on without someone saying a word about the person's stuttering. This reinforces the early-formed taboo. Therefore, we like to begin therapy with encouraging the client to confront the stuttering head on by breaking the silence. For this purpose we prefer Sheehan's (1970) idea of "bringing stuttering out in the open" so that the uncomfortable role of being a stutterer is better tolerated. This approach is pursued in three steps.

First, clients do ample talking with the clinician about their experiences with stuttering during childhood, school-age years, and as an adult, discussing many memories of specific situations, avoidance behaviors, people's reactions, and social impact. Clients are asked to talk about how children made fun of them in school, or about adults who mocked them, general or specific fears of talking, ordering in restaurants, talking on the telephone, tricks they have used to minimize or hide stuttering, problems with job hunting, and more. We suggest to clients to talk about stuttering as if the listeners have no idea what it is, as if they came from another world. (In truth, this assumption is quite valid for most listeners.) In the second step, friends or relatives are invited to sit in on a therapy session or two as the client shares with them what it means to grow up and live with stuttering. Interestingly, some adults who stutter are initially more uncomfortable sharing with people they know than with strangers.

In the third step, clients are encouraged to talk about stuttering with other people in various situations and opportunities out of the clinic (e.g., the workplace or in front of classes). The more clients talk about their stuttering, the more courage is gained as the habitual avoidance response weakens. We review in advance where and with whom they will talk and ask for reports regarding the experiences. Sheehan also viewed the procedure as a means to reduce guilt feelings that trigger stuttering. In a similar vein, Van Riper (1973) conceptualized the process of making a detailed analysis of the features of the client's stuttered speech (identification) as part of the desensitization process, especially in confronting the problem. In our opinion, however, identification procedures are better placed in the section concerned with stuttering-oriented therapy methods.

Role Play

Another useful procedure for confronting the problem of stuttering is *role play*, which can take place in group therapy sessions or by the clinician and client during individual therapy sessions. In some cases, as it fits in the hierarchy of treatment aims, additional persons such as family members, peers, or others can be invited to individual or group therapy sessions to assist in role-play activities.

Role-play participants adopt and act out the roles of people having backgrounds, points of view, personalities, or motivations that are different from their own. Such exercises have been long incorporated in various educational programs, conflict resolution tasks, as well as in psychotherapeutic interventions, for example, *psychodrama* (Moreno, 1953) and *Fixed Role Therapy* (Kelly, 1963). An important element in a successful role play is the creation of dynamic scenarios that fit the objectives of converting relevant feelings and information into a communication discourse. Participants gain insights about other people's beliefs, attitudes, and values, and how and why others perceive and react to them as they do. Admittedly, employing role play in the context of facing stuttering is a bit unusual because a person who stutters cannot be asked to play the role of a stutterer. Nevertheless, the client can see him or herself, and stuttering in general, through the eyes and perspectives of others when they play the role.

In practical terms, the clinician may assume the role of the person who stutters, simulating the client's stuttering patterns while the client plays various roles, such as a friend, employer, professor, telephone operator, waitress, police officer, and others.

Depending on the client's and clinician's genders, another person of the opposite sex may be recruited to assume parts as needed. While playing various roles, the client has ample opportunities to confront the stuttering as portrayed by the clinician or others. As the client converses with the play partners, he or she is encouraged to verbalize impressions of and feelings about the stuttering observed. The clinician can also contribute by acting and expressing attitudes and beliefs that she or he knows are held by the client.

Desensitization to Stuttered Speech

No matter how long and how frequently a person has stuttered, each experience may trigger multiple unpleasant feelings, ranging from embarrassment to tension, entrapment, loss of control, and anxiety (see Chapter 4). Years of strained experiences form a strong association: stuttering arouses anxiety. Although people who stutter may learn to live with it, all too often the feelings associated with stuttered speech are fresh and acute. After more than 70 years of stuttering history, one of us (EY) can personally testify to this. Again, the desensitization process seeks to break the established association between stuttered speech events and emotional reaction. The client is to change his/her automatic reactions and learn that it is possible to be in the midst of a stutter while maintaining a substantially lower reactivity level. What the client needs to understand is that although the long-term objective is to diminish stuttering, this phase of therapy actually requires plenty of stuttering instances for practice to reach the intermediate goal. Many procedures are available, and several common ones are elaborated here.

Negative Practice

To provide quick appreciation of what is meant by experiencing stuttering with diminished emotionality, a technique known as *negative practice* may be used. Negative practice is when an incorrect or opposite behavior is performed in contrast with a target behavior. It rests on the idea advanced by Dunlap (1932) that purposely practicing an undesirable behavior can actually enhance a person's ability to change and eventually eliminate that behavior. The technique is also supported by Viktor Frankl's (1963) principle of *paradoxical intention,* as well as Wolpe's (1990) *reciprocal inhibition.*

In the field of speech pathology negative practice has been used in treating voice and articulation disorders, such as contrasting minimal word pairs (e.g., wug—rug) to highlight target speech sounds. In stuttering therapy, negative practice may also be described as *voluntary stuttering* or *pseudostuttering.* The technique can be applied in a multiple ways, described in the next section, and with a variety of rationales. Historically, it was recommended by Bryngelson (1931) at a time when the prevailing theory was that abnormal hemispheric dominance caused stuttering, and that the stutterer's emotional reactions exacerbated abnormal brain functioning. Regardless, the rationale for voluntary stuttering was reduction of emotional reactions. Clients were to closely display their real stuttering patterns while remaining "objective."

Gregory (2003) recommended negative practice in a form that he referred to as *two degrees of tension*. First, the client imitates the actual stuttering as closely as possible, monitoring the amount of tension, and then imitates the same stuttering but reducing the tension by 50%. Care should be taken not to ease up on the second imitation too much. Gregory opined that the process of gaining control and establishing change is best served if the speaker retains about half of the initial tension. In one sense, any use of voluntary stuttering is also a type of negative practice.

Voluntary Stuttering

For the same desensitization purposes described earlier, three rather different versions of voluntary stuttering are suggested. These versions are referred to as *easy stuttering, simulated real stuttering,* and *freezing*. Any one, two, or all three may be applied, depending on the phase and particular needs of the client.

Relaxed or *easy stuttering,* as it is often referred to, consists of repetitions and prolongations devoid of tension. Our clients have reported that stuttering voluntarily in this manner lowers their anxiety, especially when the speaking rate is also a bit slower. After presenting the objective, rationale, and basic procedure, the clinician begins by demonstrating easy repetitions embedded in sentences of her or his own speech. For example, asking the client, "Wha-wha-wha-what ta-ta-ta-time is it? Or "Te-te-te-tell me abou-bou-bou-bout your job," and "Do you have a ffffreshly baked whole-wheat bread?" Next is the client's turn to practice the technique in short sentences, copying the clinician's speech patterns and reporting impressions after each one. It is essential to reemphasize and monitor the easiness of the repetitions or prolongation, reminding the client of the rationale for the practice: *to experience stuttered speech without the habitual negative emotionality.* As therapy progresses, the client is to easily repeat and prolong in several locations per sentence. Repetitions may vary in length (e.g., three to six iterations per instance and prolongations from 1 to 3 seconds). After satisfactory results, easy stuttering is practiced in a variety of situations. Assignments begin in the clinic with the client phoning various places to ask brief questions while employing the technique. There is no need to be concerned if the easy stuttering is not perceived as "real." The practice will have its intended impact as well supporting the client's realization that it is possible to change.

The second version of voluntary stuttering for desensitization purposes has common roots to the one just described. We refer to it here as *simulated real stuttering*. The objective is to train the client to consciously remain calm while engaging in his/her typical pattern of stuttering, complete with all the tensions and secondary body movements. The client engages in various speaking tasks and, at each stutter event, is to focus on remaining calm through it. Initially, the clinician facilitates the experience by softly saying "remain calm, remain calm" whenever the client stutters, gradually letting the client perform without any external prompt.

A novice observer may wonder why a clinician's instruction to "remain calm" during *simulated real stuttering* is different from the layperson's naive and ineffective admonition of commenting "relax" when stuttering occurs. There are vital differences. A layperson usually feels uncomfortable and intends the advice to alleviate the stuttering. The clinician, by contrast, feels comfortable and gives the instruction to permit and encourage stuttering. Each stutter event is a positive opportunity to practice a more calm response in the face of its occurrence. The client must, by all means, be prepared for the full extent of nonavoidance and open confrontation of stuttering involved with this technique. Frequent evaluation by the clinician and client of the performance and level of success is warranted.

The third useful technique to introduce here is referred to as *freezing*. The client is instructed to hold on to the stuttering posture, natural or voluntary, for as long as the clinician's hand is raised. During this time, he or she is to focus experiencing an unaffected calmness in the presence of the stuttering behavior. The client can continue talking as soon as the clinician's hand is lowered. Using a hierarchical progression, freezing may be started by holding the stutter for 2 or 3 seconds, working up to 15 seconds or longer. As usual, after the desired skill of remaining calm during stuttering has been achieved in the therapy room, the next step is to practice in real-life situations. One client related to us that after he stopped to talk with someone, he kept stuttering on the one word until the other person just walked away.

Desensitization to Listeners

One of the remarkable facts about stuttering is that it occurs almost always when the person who stutters talks to other people, not when talking to self or to companion animals. More speech difficulties are experienced in speaking to perceived unfriendly listeners or groups. Hence desensitization should also directly address this factor in terms of listeners' reactions and audience size. The goal is for the client to achieve the competing response of a comfortable feeling in the presence of various listeners (i.e., the previously anxiety-provoking stimuli), a goal achieved by employing principles similar to those described in the previous sections.

Desensitization to listeners is characterized by its important contribution to the generalization of the therapeutic success. It proceeds by bringing visitors into the safe environment of the therapy room. They may be instructed intentionally to engage in unreceptive responses to stuttering (e.g., smiling, looking down, appearing impatient, helping him or her say a word). The client is to watch the listener/s carefully for their reactions, remaining calm and unaffected by them. A hierarchy made up of various types of voluntary stuttering can be used to ease the client into observing listeners' reactions. The sequence may begin with accessory disfluency types (e.g., many "um's"), progress to repetitions or brief prolongations, and eventually move to longer and more severe stuttering, all while studying listener responses.

Outside activities can be designed to help the client be successful in remaining calm while watching different types of listeners in situations that gradually increase in difficulty. The listener hierarchy may first involve an older person walking in the street, a young man in hurry, a police officer, and so on. Likewise, a hierarchy of audience size from two to three people to a class size can be arranged. Of course, the clinician should work with the client to design unique hierarchies tailored specifically to the set of potential listeners relevant to the client's life and needs.

> One client described a rather classic therapy assignment that reduced his anxiety about listener responses to stuttering. He stood in a public corridor (i.e., at the student union of a university) with a clipboard in hand and asked people passing by to participate in an opinion poll. The polled opinion, in this case, was what people thought about stuttering and about talking with people who stutter. His feelings were transformed by the realization that the vast majority of the people he met were not harboring negative thoughts about stuttering or people who stutter.

One example of such an intensive exposure (also referred to as *flooding* or *implosion*) might be experienced by students and clinicians engaged in making telephone calls to people's homes in conjunction with a fund-raiser for their university or various charity organizations. After 12 calls during 60 minutes, an individual's feelings can be transformed from hesitancy and embarrassment to comfort and confidence, demonstrating the strong effect of such experiences. It is good to keep in mind, however, that adults with long histories of stuttering may harbor a certain amount of speech anxiety regardless of the intensity of the desensitization process or how fluent they become. The feeling that "it" may come back often remains just below the surface.

Summary of Desensitization

Desensitization reduces the person who stutter's negative emotion associated with stuttering. It is based on the principle that the power of a stimulus, such as the sight of a telephone, to evoke anxiety and its stuttering consequence is weakened when the person experiences the stimulus while in a relaxed state. A hierarchy of anxiety-provoking situations, often including imagined experiences, are employed in the *systematic desensitization* approach. Real-life experiences are used for *desensitization in vivo*, where a client learns to gradually reduce anxiety. Psychoemotional adjustment often improves when the speaker learns to confront stuttering rather than suppressing or concealing it. Techniques for confrontation of stuttering include (1) being open about stuttering, (2) use of role play, (3) negative practice of stuttering, and (4) other uses of voluntary stuttering. Various methods of achieving physical and mental relaxation can help in the desensitization process.

Assertiveness Training and Group Therapy

Assertiveness Training

Whereas the previous discussion focused on the personal experience of emotions, particularly anxiety, and modifications of the speaker's reactions to stuttering and oneself as someone who stutters, how these adjustments translate into social experiences may need some direct attention. Improvements in social adjustment are evident when the speaker conveys self-confidence and assertiveness in social situations. These enhance the speaker's overall effectiveness as a communicator and as a self-advocate.

Most normally speaking people find themselves occasionally in situations in which they feel uncomfortable, mistreated, and upset by what others, unjustifiably, say or do to them or to others. They feel wronged, that their dignity or rights were violated, but they are inhibited from making adequate responses. Consider the person who is watching a movie at the theater where a few spectators are making noise nearby that spoils the enjoyment. The person may want to say something to the inconsiderate neighbors but instead holds in the frustration and suffers for 2 hours. In another situation, customers may be served a "well-done" hamburger, although they ordered it "medium." Some people would be reluctant to be so particular as to send it back. These are examples of lack of assertiveness. People who stutter have more inhibitions with behaving assertively because added to the concern with speaking up is the embarrassment of broken speech. Furthermore, they are also likely to encounter behaviors directly related to the stuttering, such as being mocked, that call for appropriate response. Difficulties with assertiveness also interfere with therapy, especially with outside assignments. Some clients are reluctant to make telephone calls or stop people in the street to practice certain speaking assignments, such as stuttering on purpose, not necessarily because of stuttering-related anxiety but because they do not feel right "bothering" others.

A *fight-or-flight* response to an adverse situation is natural. A person actually has not just two, but three choices: aggression (fight or blame the listener), passiveness (flee or avoid the listener), or the most constructive response—assertiveness (reclaim the right to speak up to the other party on equal ground). Assertiveness is the skill of taking positive action toward resolving one's needs without insulting or violating the rights of others.

Another aspect of assertiveness is the exercise of one's right to express feelings and wants. Unfortunately, stuttering often induces a desire to retreat from communication. People who stutter may need to recognize and reclaim their right to state their feelings and wishes. For example, they may at some time want to say: "I like it when people don't try to finish my words," or "I do best when people just listen patiently." Needs for assertive expressions can be met through training programs in which familiar situations, such as those at a movie theater or at a restaurant, can be initially used in role-play fashion.

The situation is planned in the broad sense to preserve some spontaneity; the client (1) orders a medium-rare hamburger while the clinician acts as the server; (2) takes a bite and realizes it was cooked too much; (3) motions to the server, who initially ignores the client; (4) complains to the server who finally responds; (5) expresses anger after the server first argues that the hamburger is just right; and (6) the server complies, ordering another hamburger. No specific wording is suggested. After the scene is performed, clinician and client analyze the verbal responses, body posture, manner, and so on. Improvements are planned and the situation is replayed. Several rounds may be necessary to obtain satisfactory behavior: assertive yet not aggressive nor submissive. Finally, situations more pertinent to the client are selected.

Manual Smith (1975) refers to some assertiveness techniques such as fogging and negative assertion that are helpful at disarming criticism directed against us: People who stutter are apt to benefit by learning these techniques. The first one, *fogging*, is agreeing with the criticism. When an object is thrown into a fog, it is quickly lost from sight. Similarly, fogging is used to make criticisms fade away. An example of fogging by a client who stutters might be to respond to the listener who chides, "Don't you know your own name?" with replies such as "It sure seems like it, doesn't it?" or "I don't know my name or my serial number." Whereas fogging can deflate invalid criticisms, *negative assertion* is used to deflate valid criticisms. It consists of agreeing with or confessing to the shortcoming. For example, the client who stutters could respond to a listener's startled facial expression with the comment "Maybe you've noticed that I stutter."

Sources concerning assertiveness training are numerous and can be found in the scientific literature as well as lay publications. See, for example, Tom Stevens's Web page (Stevens, 2005). Applications concerned specifically with stuttering were reported by Blood (1995). Gendelman (1977) described an assertiveness/confrontation treatment used with at least 200 adolescents who stutter, examined specifically in 40 of them. The approach was based on the theory that stuttering is a conditioned anxiety response (Brutten & Shoemaker, 1967) and a premise that verbal interactions are the stimuli to which speakers must be deconditioned. No time was spent desensitizing clients to stuttering itself, nor to words or sounds that evoke fear. Instead, clients were desensitized to interview situations in which they confronted their listeners with assertive statements related to their underlying fears. The clinician helped clients plan how to express fears in ways most apt to be received favorably by a listener. For example, "It's hard for me to talk with you because I think you don't like me" (p. 87). The subsequent discussion typically brought about explanations and reassurances that made for a more comfortable relationship. Each positive experience created confidence for the next one. Gendelman reported that more than half (23) of the 40 adolescents were normally fluent at the end of treatment, and another fourth (13) had improved. Several months or years later, 22 were either normally fluent or improved. The report is significantly weakened, however, by lack of details and the absence of more objective data pertaining to stuttering frequency and reliability of judgment.

Group Therapy

Group therapy is sometimes provided in conjunction with individual therapy; at times it is the only available service because of the time and cost factors. Although the focus may alternate between speech practice and psychological support, clinicians should be careful not to narrowly address only one of these aims. *The purpose of group therapy in the context of stuttering intervention is to enhance learning and the process of change.*

Rationale

Group therapy presents several advantages. First, a group of people with similar problems provides comfort and support to its members. Second, it provides opportunities and a safe environment for members to express their feedings openly and honestly and share their experiences with others. Members simultaneously give and receive feedback. The open self-expression, feedback, and interaction among members allow group members to view their personal and social issues in new perspectives. Members can discover new interpretations of their problems and find alternative solutions. Third, it can serve to actually practice new responses in interpersonal and social situations. For people who stutter, group therapy can facilitate transfer of learning, in that it presents opportunities to practice speech patterns and other behaviors acquired in individual therapy. They can also share their recent successes and failures in working to overcome their stuttering.

For clinicians, the group presents opportunities to observe the clients' performance and progress in a social situation. At times, group members may subdivide into smaller subgroups or pairs to accomplish beyond-clinic speaking assignments together, tasks that greatly benefit from mutual on-the-spot support. Manning (2001) put it aptly, stating that "the group setting provides opportunities for enhancing as well as maintaining change in both the surface and intrinsic aspect of the syndrome" (p. 297).

The Group

Therapy groups vary in size but we recommend 8 to 10 members as the ideal. Smaller groups of fewer than 5 limit the sense of having "a group" and pose heavier demands for participation on those who attend. There also tends to be less variety of backgrounds and input. Larger groups of more than 10 will limit the potential participation of members. It is important to avoid situations in which one member dominates the discussion by taking too much talking time. The clinician must announce that a reasonable time distribution of group members' participation is desired. Leadership of the group therapy may be handled with different styles. For example, the clinician may select the theme for the session and be active in directing the interaction (e.g., prompting a quiet member to contribute), or the clinician may take a more passive role, letting members steer the session with minimal intervention.

It has been suggested that group experiences for people who stutter serve the dual purposes of therapy and counseling (Luterman, 1991). Some structure and rules, however, are necessary. St. Louis (2007) proposed four characteristics for a typical group therapy session. It should (1) feature a theme and a "lesson"; (2) include something fun; (3) involve some real experiences for the participants, not just ideas; and must (4) "stand alone" as a onetime experience for the participant who shows up only to that one session, even though themes may be ongoing or sequential. Ham (1990) advised clinicians that each member of the group must be considered as an individual.

Activities

Group therapy for stuttering has been employed and described by a number of clinicians. A rare session-by-session account of group therapy with 14 college students who stuttered that provides a useful sample of a structured program, as well as of topics covered, has been presented by Cypreansen (1948). The author reported several indications of positive outcomes. St. Louis (2007) also provides several detailed illustrations of session content and dynamics. Group therapy has been employed in our own respective clinics. Among favorite discussion topics (in question format) we suggest are: (1) How do you feel and what goes through your mind during a moment of stuttering? (2) What does being a person who stutters mean to you? (3) What have been people's reactions to your stuttering: strangers, friends, family members? (4) What motivated you to seek help at this time? (5) Has therapy been helpful? If yes, how? (6) Where would you like to go in therapy? (7) What leads to relapse and what can be done about it? (8) What are three of your strengths or most positive personal assets? Manning (2001) suggested that group activities may involve relaxation exercises, role playing, and public-speaking activities.

Guitar (2014) describes his own experience as a client in a group of seven where Van Riper served as the clinician. Typically, 5 years after termination of therapy, Van Riper measured the treatment outcome using several criteria, such as being rated below 0.5 on the Iowa Severity Scale, showing no avoidance behavior, near zero word or situation fears, and others. Guitar estimated that his group members would have done well if they had the opportunity to be rated. In Australia, group therapy was reported as the vehicle to teach replacement of stuttering with slow stretched speech, gradually shaping it into near normally sounding speech (Howie & Andrews, 1984). This, however, was not the psychological group therapy as described earlier. Instead, the group setting was used primarily as an efficient method to present and practice the new speaking patterns. It is not known, however, whether the significant reduction in stuttering they reported had anything to do with the group setting. Some ideas for clinicians interested in establishing support groups may be found in Bradberry (1997).

Summary of Assertiveness Training and Group Therapy

The speaker who stutters may benefit from an approach that involves more direct social interactions impacted by the disorder of stuttering. Two therapeutic applications that address social adjustment are assertiveness training and group therapy. Whereas desensitization is aimed at reducing certain emotional reactions, these two approaches aim at increasing certain emotions and behaviors. In assertiveness training, the person learns to manage challenging social situations by expressing needs directly and requesting respectful behavior by others. Group therapy affords a variety of benefits including social support and practice of speech strategies in a social situation. Both group size and session format should be considered during therapy planning.

Antianxiety Drugs

It is difficult to determine the most appropriate site in our book for this topic aside from having a special chapter, an unwarranted option in view of the limited scope of the current presentation. Drugs have multiple influences, including physiological, motoric, emotional, and unknown. Some drugs used in stuttering treatment were intended to relieve physiological symptoms (i.e., tension and disfluent events), but most have aimed mainly to control emotionality associated with stuttering, often for antianxiety purposes. Therefore, we have placed their discussion within this chapter pertaining to the emotionality involved in stuttering. We admit, however, to being somewhat arbitrary in choosing this location.

Why Drugs?

Most stuttering therapy approaches described earlier, as well as those we discuss in the following chapters, involve regular face-to-face contact between the client and clinician over a period of time. In fact, the ASHA Code of Ethics states that treatment shall not be carried out solely through correspondence. As discussed below, however, the reality is that the number of people who need speech remediation is expected to continue to expand, whereas the number of professionals needed to provide services not only is inadequate today but will become increasingly smaller relative to the growing demands. Although telehealth may increase the capacities for service delivery, it has limitations in terms of actual outreach, dealing with individual differences, and rate of success. Considering the large worldwide number of people who stutter, the lack of clinical services for so many of them, and the poor economic status of most of the world population, one hopeful promise is seen in effective drugs if they can be developed and made available at affordable prices.

Most people rarely think about the fact that 240 babies are born every minute somewhere in the world. This figure adds up to approximately 130 million new babies each year. Applying the popular 5% incidence of stuttering, it is easy to calculate that, each year, 7.5 million of these babies, if all would live, will begin stuttering within 2–5 years and their parents would benefit from professional help. The accumulation of stuttering cases within several years is staggering. It is simply impossible to train enough speech clinicians and have them available to handle such a continuously swelling caseload. To illustrate the problem, note that in the United States there are approximately 350 speech clinicians per million people. In South Korea and Taiwan, two technologically advanced countries, the numbers are far smaller: 100 and 40 clinicians per million population, respectively. The estimate for India, which has 20% of the world's population, drops sharply to fewer than 1.5 clinicians per million population.

Potentially, drugs could reach large numbers of people who stutter worldwide and could easily be self-administered. Furthermore, availability of safe drugs would change considerably the treatment of stuttering even in conventional clinical settings. Of course, drug distribution and use is not a simple matter. It is expected that for the short- and medium-term future, drugs for stuttering will require a physician's prescription as well as some monitoring. Unfortunately, many areas in the world are served by but a few physicians or qualified nurses who are very busy combating life-threatening diseases. Also, some patients may exhibit negative reactions to the drug. Others may be inconsistent with its timely consumption. There is also the risk of misuse. Nevertheless, modern technology and services have been transforming medical care, for example, with the use of computers for medical consultations, mail-order drugs, and so on. Thus some of the major issues just mentioned will be gradually resolved. Finally, it is not unrealistic to contemplate that scientific progress will eventually yield vastly improved safer drugs that may be sold over the counter.

For the time being, although experimentation with treating stuttering with drugs during the past 100 years has not produced a satisfactory product, recent research progress in several related scientific domains (e.g., physiology, genetics, and pharmacology) make it reasonable to suggest that some pharmaceutical promises could materialize in the near to intermediate future. Therefore, clinicians should become familiar with information as it comes out and be prepared to discuss pros and cons with inquiring clients. Furthermore, because at least for some time to come, drugs will not provide complete cure, they would probably be most effective when integrated with conventional speech therapy.

Drugs for What?

Some drugs are designed specifically for quick relief of symptoms, for example, acetaminophen for relieving headaches. They do not address the cause of the problem. Other drugs, such as insulin, provide a substance the body is no longer able to produce itself, whereas others, for example, Fosamax, actually help rebuild bone density, preventing osteoporosis. In other words, drugs may directly address a disorder or simply relieve symptoms. A basic question arises concerning the specific purposes of drugs for stuttering: What system of the individual who stutters should a drug be directed to? What are its specific intended effects on the organism? The answer can be expected to reflect either one's theoretical outlook on the etiology of stuttering or one's urgency to deal with its symptoms. If stuttering were to be identified as a motor disorder associated with brief muscle spasms, would muscle-relaxant drugs be a reasonable avenue to pursue? If stuttering were associated with underlying anxiety, then one of several antianxiety drugs might provide relief. If stuttering involved high dopamine levels in the brain's speech control areas, drugs affecting these levels would seem to be a reasonable choice. Or, if we believe in multiple etiologies of stuttering, then perhaps more than one drug should be prescribed (e.g., one which controls emotional reactions and one which regulates motor functions). Also, regardless of other considerations, should we pursue drugs that have the properties of altering speech characteristics, for example, to induce slow speech that is known to facilitate fluency?

A question to consider in developing drugs for stuttering is the general strategy for the drug usage. Is the purpose to achieve a constant, long-term effect in the reduction or elimination of stuttering or to trigger the effect intermittently as needed? Would the drug be taken for a short period to produce permanent changes after the drug is withdrawn or will it continue to be consumed to maintain effectiveness? This is a rather fundamental question that should also involve a patient's choice but has not been adequately discussed in the literature. Of course, this issue has implications for the frequency of drug usage. Treatments of many health problems involve multiple daily doses for either short- or long-term use. Some long-term treatments involve once a day or once a week drug consumption, whereas other treatments involve taking the drug once a month. A related consideration is the time required for a drug to take effect. Some drugs may take 2 to 3 weeks for a gradual buildup, others may take an hour or so, whereas some become effective in 1 or 2 minutes. This has important practical implications for the consumer.

The effects of a short-acting calming medication, for example, taken prior to an oral presentation might wear off before a speaker even begins talking. Many years ago, one of us (EY) took such a drug before a presenting at an ASHA convention. With the particular dosage taken, its full-strength effect lasted about 30 to 40 minutes. Being the fourth presenter in the scientific session, much of the drug's calming effect had evaporated by the time it was his turn to speak, creating a last-minute experience of great distress.

Studies of Pharmaceutical Treatments for Stuttering

Experiments with medical drugs for the treatment of stuttering were reported in Europe as early as the late 1800s. In Germany, Gutzmann (see Hogewind, 1940) prescribed one of several drugs, including a bromium preparation, ergotine preparation (with some hallucinogenic properties), and others, depending on his classification of the client's physical constitution. During the first half of the 20th century, reports of drug use appeared sporadically in the literature, often in a less than reassuring scientific context. For example, in 1940, Hogewind, a Dutch physician, published an article in the *Journal of Speech Disorders*, reporting the administration of Bellergal (a combination of several sedatives) to adults who stutter. Starting with a large daily dosage of 3 to 4 tablets for the first fortnight, it was gradually reduced and sometimes stopped for a while. Hogewind commented that "on the whole, the results were satisfactory, sometimes even very good. The patients became calmer, and during the intervals, several asked on their own accord to be allowed to begin with the tablets again, so that they could speak better" (p. 207).

He felt, however, that speech therapy should also be given and that the drug was especially useful during the early phase of the speech therapy as well as in reducing duration and severity of relapses. The Hogewind report is a revealing example of the unsatisfactory quality of the older literature in that it does not provide information about the number of participants, duration of treatment, or the specific dosage contained in the tablets. Similarly, no mention is made of measures of stuttering, or other relevant parameters, before and after treatment. Moreover, there were no follow-ups and no control groups.

Drug treatment for stuttering continued during the 1950s. The belief that stuttering is caused by anxiety prompted a good number of experiments with anxiolytic drugs, that is, drugs prescribed for the treatment of symptoms of anxiety. Following this reasoning Winkelman (1954) used chlorpromazine. Clinicians used meprobamate which works directly on muscles to induce relaxation, as well as having a sedative effect. Di Carlo, Katz, and Batkin (1959), for example, administered the drug to adults who stutter over a 4-week period, concluding as follows:

> "Ten stutterers who were given 600 mg. of meprobamate per day for the first week, 1,200 mg. per day for the second week, 1,600 mg. per day for the third week, and 2,000 mg. per day for the fourth week, showed a reduction in the mean number of stuttered moments. This reduction, while not achieving statistical significance, did show a definite trend and was significant at the .10 level of confidence for the group that received the meprobamate. Nonparametric statistics revealed a statistically significant amount of progressive success with each trial for this group. Their own subjective evaluation confirmed the findings. On the basis of these results, further study is indicated." (pp. 560–561).

The preceding extract reflects the typical findings in this area. A number of other antianxiety drugs, such as alprazolam, were reported to yield some positive results in a minority of the participants. Those who responded positively, however, showed only a very modest reduction in stuttering (see review by Brady, 1991).

A different approach began in the 1960s, after haloperidol was introduced in 1958. Haloperidol is a highly potent antidopamine drug, used primarily in the treatment of psychotic conditions, delirium, and schizophrenia. Dopamine is a hormone and neurotransmitter (a substance that mediates impulses between nerve endings and muscles) that activates five types of dopamine receptors referred to as D1, D2, D3, D4, and D5. It has important roles in brain functioning, including regulation of behavior, cognition, control of movement, mood, attention, and learning. Dopamine dysfunction in the brain, such as depletion from normal level, has been viewed as associated with Parkinson disease, attention deficits, hyperactivity disorders, autism, or surges above normal level in schizophrenia (Arias-Carrión & Pöppel, 2007). An important driving force behind the interest in haloperidol for treatment of stuttering has been the hypothesis that excessive levels of dopamine result in abnormally low metabolism of the cortical speech areas as well as in the *striatum*, a deeper brain structure. Indeed, the presence of considerably larger than normal quantities (50% to 200%) of dopamine in the brains of people who stutter was reported in 1997 by Wu et al.

Because excess dopamine has been suspected as a causal agent in stuttering, drugs that lower dopamine, such as haloperidol, a dopamine D2 receptor blocker, have been investigated experimentally. Research studies of these older generation dopamine antagonists (previously used mostly as antipsychotic medications for hospitalized patients) were reported to improve stuttering symptoms, mainly severity, but typically only in a minority of the participants who stuttered. Andrews and Dozsa (1977), for example, reported improvement in fewer than 20% of the participants. Additionally, the drugs caused poorly tolerated adverse effects, including involuntary movement, drowsiness, and blurred vision, which limited their usage by outpatients, such as people who stutter. Hence a good number of participants ceased participation in the middle of the experiments (e.g., Andrews & Dozsa; 1977; Quinn & Preachy, 1973; Rantala & Petri-Larmi, 1976). A few years later, Prins, Mendelkorn, and Cerf (1980), in a double-blind study, found that whatever statistically significant effects the drug had on reducing the frequency of disfluency, they were too small to be clinically meaningful. Also, reduction in speech interruption occurred primarily on disfluency types more typical to normal speakers, not on the core behaviors of stuttering. All in all, at the time, it appeared that the limited influence on the amelioration of stuttering combined with an unwarranted level of side effects, made haloperidol an undesirable choice for the treatment of stuttering in adults.

A noticeable development occurred in the late 1990s, when second-generation atypical antidopamine drugs, risperidone and olanzapine, were created. They blocked serotonin 5HT2 receptors as well as dopamine D2 receptors and were associated with fewer Parkinson-like side effects of stiffness and tremor. Experiments with these drugs in treating stuttering indicated some improved fluency (e.g., Maguire, Riley, Franklin et al., 2000; Maguire et al., 2004). Stager et al. (2005) concluded from their data that olanzapine is a promising medication for the treatment of stuttering and further research is warranted. It must be noted, however, that olanzapine, risperidone, and similar medications are often associated with substantial weight gain.

Another group of pharmaceuticals, including paroxetine, and those targeting obsessive-compulsive symptoms as well as generalized anxiety, such as citalopram and clomipramine, collectively referred to as *selective serotonin reuptake inhibitor,* or SSRIs, have been experimented with in the treatment of stuttering. These medications are based on *serotonin,* another neurotransmitter that activates neural receptors known as 5-HT. These are different from the neurotransmitter blocked by haloperidol. Another term that better fits this group of drugs is *potent serotonin reuptake inhibitors* because a low dose of all of them has a strong effect in blocking serotonin reuptake. Serotonin is believed to play an important role in inhibiting anger, aggression, moods, and sexuality. Therefore, low-level serotonin may underlie aggressive and angry behaviors, clinical-level depression, obsessive-compulsive disorders, and anxiety disorders. The primary logic for using them in treating stuttering is the possibility that stuttering may share some underlying factors with obsessive-compulsive disorders, given that both involve intrusive repetitive behavior or thoughts. The few experiments conducted with this group of drugs yielded an unclear picture (Burns, Brady, & Kuruvilla 1978; Stager et al., 2005). The data are too few to reach a conclusion but seem to lack promise.

Finally, for the purpose of this brief review, an interesting concept was offered by Brady and Ali (2000) suggesting that two medications might be necessary, especially in severe cases, to deal with the multiple sources of stuttering. They experimented with a combination of alprazolam to reduce anxiety and citalopram, a serotonin reuptake inhibiting drug, to deal with the core symptoms of stuttering. Marked improvement was reported for three adults who stutter. The authors reported that as clients' anxiety subsided, it was possible to gradually eliminate the alprazolam. To sustain improvement in the level of stuttering, however, it was necessary to continue consumption of the citalopram. Regardless of the wisdom of combining these two drugs, the literature indicates that many patients reported trouble with alprazolam and discontinued it.

Recent Developments

In recent years, there was a set of major clinical trials conducted with pagoclone, a relatively new anxiolytic drug related to the sleeping medication zopiclone. In contrast to zopiclone, pagoclone produces its antianxiety effects with little or no sedative or amnesic actions when taken with low doses. The precise action of the drug is not known but it enhances the activity of the $GABA_A$ receptors, a neurotransmitter receptor in the brain that may be disrupted in people who stutter and is also targeted by meprobamate and alprazolam. The Indevus pharmaceutical company, which held the patent for the drug, conducted controlled clinical trials in cooperation with several U.S. clinical and academic institutions with Dr. Gerald Maguire as the leading investigator. The initial publication in a scientific journal reported the largest pharmacologic trial of stuttering ever completed: In an 8-week, placebo-controlled, double-blind, randomized design, 88 adults who stuttered received the drug and 44 received a placebo treatment. This was followed by a 1-year open-label treatment extension. They reported a 40% reduction in stuttering frequency as measured by the Stuttering Severity Instrument. The drug was well tolerated with only minor side effects of headache and fatigue reported by 12% of those treated. Overall, it was concluded that pagoclone may have potential as a pharmacological treatment for stuttering (Maguire et al., 2010). However, the report was severely evaluated by Ingham (2010), especially on the grounds that speech samples were short and probably unreliable. He also contended that 40% improvement fell short as compared to results obtained by some speech therapy methods. In 2009 the Indevus company merged with Endo Pharmaceuticals. A year later, the company announced that the Phase II clinical trials with pagoclone had not met criteria for success and would be discontinued. To our knowledge, Dr. Maguire, at the University of California-Irvine, began a new set of clinical trials in 2010 on the effects of Saphris (asenapine) on stuttering. One can find an on-going blog that follows the effects of medications on stuttering at *stutteringmedication.com*.

Summary of Antianxiety Drugs

We have proposed that the development of drugs for the treatment for stuttering holds great hope for the majority of worldwide PWS who are unable to receive speech therapy, and that conventional therapy will be enhanced by complementary drugs. Although a substantial number of reports on the use of drugs in the treatment of stuttering have been published, many presented observations on a small number of people who stutter, including single cases, during a short period of several weeks. Also, most group studies were not properly controlled according to acceptable high standards for drug research. In a recent analysis of the scientific quality of past work in this area, Saxon and Ludlow (2007) stated that of 75 reports they covered, the vast majority were uncontrolled studies. None were rated at the highest of four possible levels of research quality.

Our brief review shows that although most of the experiments indicated some positive effects, these usually occurred for a minority of the participants. Even when reports could be considered valid, the level of improvement varied from little to moderate and, quite critically, was associated with side effects that are too difficult to cope with by outpatient users, such as people who stutter, engaged in normal life activities. The specific drug effects on overt characteristics of stuttering are also not sufficiently clear. Thus far, speech symptoms have not uniformly improved with drug treatments. Van Borsel, Beck, and Delanghe (2003) concluded that, under medication, the most consistently affected stuttering symptom was reduction in repetition. Other data reviewed, however, indicated that much of the diminished behaviors could be classified as normal disfluency (e.g., interjections, phrase and word repetitions) and to a lesser degree the core stuttering-like disfluencies. Also not too clear is whether the frequency of stuttering or the severity of blocks is most affected. Our guarded view of the current state of the art is reinforced by another critical review of 35 publications pertaining to the use of drugs in the treatment of stuttering. The authors, Bothe, Davidow, Bramlett et al. (2006), concluded that "none of the pharmacological agents tested for stuttering have been shown in methodologically sound reports to improve stuttering frequency to below 5%, to reduce stuttering by at least half, or to improve relevant social, emotional, or cognitive variables. These findings raise questions about the logic supporting the continued use of current pharmacological agents for stuttering" (p. 342); nevertheless, in our opinion further progress in drug treatment for stuttering can be is expected.

Although limited in success thus far, the effort to develop drugs for the treatment of stuttering should continue. As knowledge about the genetics and brain biochemistry properties of the stuttering population expands, it is likely to positively influence the development of stuttering-specific drug formulations. No less important would be efforts to test drugs using more rigorous scientific regimens. The potential to treat millions of people who stutter all over the world is unmatched by the resources and personnel available to provide speech therapy.

Finally, the literature on the applications of drugs for the treatment of stuttering is quite large. Interested readers will find a wealth of organized information in several sources, especially Bothe et al. (2006), Brady (1991), Maguire, Yu, Franklin et al. (2004), and Saxon and Ludlow (2007).

Summary

Although research evidence suggests that emotional and psychological conditions may serve only a rare or minor role in the cause of stuttering, it is clear that when stuttering persists it causes many strong negative emotional responses. These emotions can have a major impact on personal adjustment, and make it difficult for a speaker to attempt speech change. Research and clinical practice in this area can be summarized as follows:

1. Only a subset of people who stutter may need psychotherapy, probably for reasons other than stuttering.

2. Most clients will benefit from attention to their psychological and social adjustment.

3. For a good number of cases, attention to the psychological adjustment may be no less important than the speech modification and fluency-shaping techniques described in the next chapter.

4. A variety of procedures have been developed to improve the management of emotional responses by people who stutter. Mostly, such techniques as relaxation, desensitization, and voluntary stuttering aim at diminishing the level of negative emotionality.

5. Assertiveness training and rationale-emotive therapy principles can be used to increase positive communication behaviors and self-confidence.

6. Unfortunately, for a long time the field had no research-based data concerning the effectiveness of the various clinical methods discussed above.

7. So far, many attempts to develop drugs for the treatment of stuttering have been generally disappointing although recent findings with pagoclone seem to have yielded better results. An effective drug would have a huge impact on the treatment of stuttering worldwide.

Study Questions and Discussion Topics

1. For discussion or essay: Unlike articulation treatment, the intervention approaches for stuttering target a wide range of dimensions, including emotional, physical, and cognitive aspects. Why do you think that is the case?

2. Explain the rationale for desensitization techniques in stuttering therapy. Why might some clients be resistant to such techniques?

3. List as many applications of voluntary stuttering as you can find. Do these all serve as means of desensitization?

4. Describe a time when you did not exercise assertive behavior. Role-play the situation with a fellow student, and act out how you would have liked to have responded with assertiveness.

5. What are the potential benefits and challenges associated with the use of drug treatments for stuttering?

Suggested Readings

Bothe, A., Davidow, J., Bramlett, R., Franic, D., & Ingham, R. (2006). Stuttering treatment research 1970–2005. II: Systematic review incorporating trial quality assessment of pharmacological approaches. *American Journal of Speech-Language Pathology, 15,* 342–352.

Davis, M., Robbins-Eshelman, E., & McKay, M. (1988). *The relaxation and stress reduction workbook.* Oakland, CA: New Harbinger Publications.

Ellis, A., & Harper, R. (1975). *A new guide to rational living.* North Hollywood, CA: Wilshire.

Stevens, T. (2005). Assertion training. Retrieved May 1, 2008, from www.csulb. edu/~tstevens/assertion_training.htm

Van Riper, C. (1973). Desensitization: The reduction of negative emotion. In *The treatment of stuttering* (pp. 266–300). Englewood Cliffs, NJ: Prentice-Hall.

Chapter 12

Therapy for Adults: Focus on Stuttering and Fluency

LEARNER OBJECTIVES

Readers of this chapter will understand:

- Objectives, rationales, and techniques for managing events of stuttered speech.
- Objectives, rationales, and techniques for managing fluency.
- Interventions that rely on instruments.
- Approaches that integrate stuttering and fluency management.

Introduction

As the chapter's title implies, therapies of this type deal more directly with the apparent main impediment and disability involved in the disorder of stuttering. Although for some people who stutter (PWS) the emotional aspect of the problem assumes dominance, it is prudent to keep in mind that, as we know and define it, there would be no stuttering disorder without stuttered speech. Even covert stutterers sometimes experience stuttered speech. Understandably, many people who stutter view speech-oriented therapies as more relevant for them than desensitization. In our experience, their desire to speak without stuttering is expressed more frequently as the impetus for seeking help than any other motivation. Still, not all PWS value fluency over their freedom to speak even if they stutter, without trying to be fluent. Given the choice of talking fluently or talking freely (whether fluent or not), 216 adults who stuttered split their choice with 54% opting for fluency and a substantial minority of 46% preferring speaking freely (Venkatagiri, 2009).

Among the several major therapy approaches that tackle speech directly is that of *stuttering management*, which enjoyed wide acceptance by speech-language clinicians from the 1940s into the 1970s and is still employed by many. Clearly, this is a symptom-oriented approach to the resolution of the stuttering disorder. Its focal point is stutter events, and therefore the client and clinician need stuttering to occur in order to pursue the therapy objectives.[1] Note, however, that in many clinicians' programs, *stuttering management is a stage that follows desensitization*. In the traditional approach to stuttering treatment described by Van Riper (1973), four stages followed this order: identification, desensitization, modification, and stabilization.

---

[1]Some clinicians, for example Van Riper (1973), have included desensitization as a preliminary phase in a stuttering management program. According to our conceptualization, however, it has been placed within the emotionally oriented therapies.

Although symptom oriented, another important aspect underlying the stuttering management approach is the ability of the clinician to help the person who stutters develop a sense of power: that he or she can overcome well-entrenched, stereotyped panic and struggle responses to old cues that yield fluency breakdown, replacing them with planned, controlled speech movements. Prins (1993) asserted that "concerning treatment, self-efficacy theory[2] states that various approaches succeed because individuals become convinced they can successfully execute (i.e., control) the behavior required for a desired outcome. The emphasis, here, is not upon level of skills but on the conviction about their adequacy" (p. 116). Indeed, the motor skills required are not too complicated and can easily be learned. What is important is to alter a speaker's belief in what she or he can do.

> The objective of the extensive practice, then, is not so much to refine motor skills as to alter clients' entrenched belief that stuttering "just happens" to them and is beyond their control (see Williams, 1957). The aim is to develop a cognition that, indeed, people are the masters of their speech and, as such, are able to change it at will.

Although we began the chapter stating the focus is symptom oriented, our discussion and the preceding citation point out that even these approaches still involve significant psychological elements. Van Riper's (1973) traditional program for stuttering management comprises multiple phases. In contrast, the stuttering management program presented here includes just two parts or phases, *identification* and *modification*. Both, however, are rooted in his ideas.

Identification

The overall goal of various *identification* techniques as applied in speech therapy is to raise clients' level of cognition about their speech errors so they can more efficiently correct them. The objective, of course, is to identify all the features of the stuttered speech, becoming closely familiar with all their small details. In the treatment of stuttering, identification has been known, at times, to have significant merit by itself. We have known several adults who showed a large reduction in the overt stuttering just going through it, without practicing any speech modification techniques. Van Riper, too, reported similar experiences. But we have also seen the opposite reaction, especially with mild cases, when the stuttering increased, or at least seemed to intensify for a while, as the client's awareness and attention to stuttering grew. Perhaps it is wise to advise clients of the possibility that stuttering may appear to intensify, so they do not become alarmed if it does. Identification, though, is particularly important as groundwork for the subsequent

---

[2]Bandura's (1986) work is an important reference in this respect.

direct management of overt stuttering through modification. There are two essential phases to the therapeutic program involved in identification: *awareness* and *analysis*.

Rationale

What is the rationale for identification? How does a clinician explain it to clients? Several important reasons are listed and elaborated here:

1. Familiarity with a problem is required for devising an effective means of resolving it (Van Riper, 1973). Although people who stutter are aware of the occurrence of many stuttering events as they speak, they still miss quite a few, especially mild ones. Some are surprised to hear so much stuttering in their tape-recorded speech. As therapy begins, awareness may be general in the sense that speakers merely know that they stutter rather than the specifics of how. People find it difficult to correct something that is unknown to them. *Identification reveals the behaviors that should be targeted for modification,* and thereby also illuminates specific objectives for therapy.

2. Identification requires clients to take an *active role in therapy* early on (Van Riper, 1973). PWS are often under the impression that something will be done, or given to them, in therapy that will make their stuttering go away, similar to experiences they might have had with medical treatment of physical ailments. It is essential, therefore, to instill the idea that behavioral therapy depends almost solely on clients doing the changing. The identification tasks that involve considerable verbal input from clients describing and analyzing their stuttering contribute significantly to creating the desired mind-set.

3. The descriptive language used in identification enhances the ability to *take responsibility for one's own stuttering.* This is based on Williams's (1957) keen observation that people who stutter often relate to stuttering with animistic views. Such views are apparent when a person refers to "my stuttering" as if it is a living entity located somewhere in the body, acting independently, appearing on its own. Or, the person acts as if there is an outside force that makes him or her stutter. People who stutter often say "words get stuck in my throat" as if words are small objects, not sounds resulting from muscle movement. They need to realize that stuttering occurs only when they act to tense their speech muscles, hold their breath, and so on. This can be achieved by analyzing stuttering using language that describes what they do during each instance of stuttering (e.g., "I tensed my jaw").

4. *Identification contributes to desensitization.* The more stuttering is discussed openly and objectively, the more clients' associated emotional reactions lessen. This concept is easily understood because most people, children as well as adults, have experienced that merely talking to a sympathetic listener about what upsets them makes them feel much better.

Phase I: Awareness

The objective of awareness is to increase a client's accuracy in recognizing the occurrence of stutter events. Van Riper (1973) referred to this process as "detection." After discussing the objectives and rationale, the therapy takes on a hierarchical course, progressing from easier to more difficult tasks. Detection can be indicated by saying "there" or using clickers, pushing a button, working a light switch, or other signals. An example of a reasonable sequence may include the following steps:

Table 12.1	A Sample Sequence of Stuttering Detection	
Steps	**Activity**	**Context**
1	The client points out pseudostuttering instances . . .	in the clinician's connected speech
2	The clinician points out stuttering instances . . .	in the client's connected speech
3	The client points out or tallies stuttering instances (and compares with clinician) . . .	in audio or video recordings of his or her own speech
4	The client points out or tallies stuttering instances (and compares with clinician) . . .	in "live" connected speech
5	The client silently makes mental notes about stuttering instances . . .	in various speaking situations without the clinician (e.g., on the phone while looking in the mirror, in face-to-face meetings with people)

It is self-evident that audiovisual feedback can be very useful. Simple counters also facilitate the task. Typically, 95% accuracy is accepted as the criterion for success at each level in the hierarchy, prior to progressing to the next level. Minor, brief stutter events should also be detected and counted. Although these often go unnoticed by the client, they could be important because tension builds up from mild blocks becoming more severe ones.

Phase II: Analysis

Having successfully met the first goal of awareness training, the client moves on to the second part of identification, that of *analysis*, with the objective of becoming familiar with the details of the stutter events. Typically, the client is instructed to talk, pause after each stutter event, and describe what she or he was doing while stuttering—what were the various undesired and unnecessary component behaviors. In line with the rationale just outlined, emphasis is placed on using descriptive language—the "language of responsibility"—as shown in Figure 12.1.

Figure 12.1   Language of Animism Contrasted with Language of Responsibility

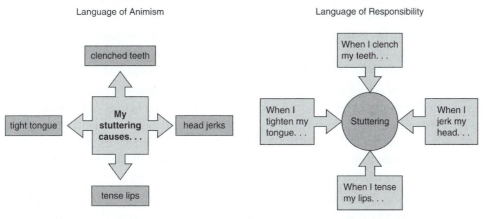

Ask a person who stutters to describe what took place during a stuttering moment, and the individual is apt to say something like "My throat and lips got tight and my breath was cut off," or "My tongue tightened up," a common language used by PWS. By contrast, *language of responsibility* reframes stuttering as an active rather than passive experience. The speaker instead is guided to say, "I tightened my throat. I tensed my lip, and I held my breath" or "I tightened my tongue" to reflect active contribution by describing the event as his or her own doing. The clinician no longer lets the client talk about stuttering as though it is something that happens *to* him or her. This change in language has a great influence on the client's point of view. It minimizes the thinking and feeling that something beyond control makes stuttering happen, and it instills a sense of responsibility for the behavior and a belief that one can change it (Williams, 1957).

Whether stuttering is perceived as something that happens or as something one does may be related to whether clients sense any control over their life more generally. A person's *locus of control* is what one believes about what has an influence over life experiences. An external locus of control is the belief that outside forces have great influence on life events, whereas an internal locus of control is the belief that one's self has a great influence on life events. A few scale measures of locus of control have been developed (J. Riley, G. Riley, & Maguire, 2004). Some research has shown relapse is more likely among those who exhibit an external locus of control (Andrews & Craig, 1988; Craig, Franklin, & Andrews, 1984). In clinical practice, some programs compare pre- and posttreatment measures of locus of control to evaluate progress toward an increased internal locus (Guitar, 2014).

The analysis of stutter events proceeds systematically, including movements directly involved in the speech disfluencies and those involved in the associated secondary characteristics. Here are a few steps:

1. As the client talks, she or he describes and keeps a list of as many behaviors involved in the stuttering as she/he is capable of perceiving without external help

(e.g., "I pressed my lips together on the *p* sound in the word *picture,* then closed the right eye and tilted my head forward"). Because secondary characteristics often are easier to identify, more of these may be analyzed first.

2. The clinician may reintroduce the *freezing technique* by having the client hold on to the stuttering events for several seconds, focusing maximum attention on his or her behaviors, then proceeding with the verbal descriptions.

3. The client continues the analysis task in front of a mirror to facilitate identification of more subtle, or not so subtle, behaviors missed before. The clinician may provide additional refinement by pointing out still additional behaviors missed by the client. Audiovisual forms of feedback (e.g., mirror, recordings, etc.) are particularly helpful for pinpointing the details. Thus all the tense, unnecessary movements that constitute the stutter event are identified.

4. Finally, the client may wish to re-create the stutter event just analyzed, observing again the movements involved, and drawing conclusions as to what should be done to redirect the actions to result in the goal of unimpeded speech, (e.g., start in easy on the vowel, keep the vocal folds open to permit airflow, bring the lips loosely together, etc.). This, in fact, is getting close to the stage of stuttering modification.

Typically, not all steps in either the awareness or the analysis phases are covered in a single session. Time and repeated practice (hundreds of analyses) are needed not only for accurate awareness and analysis but also to impact the client's attitude, understanding, and insight into the problem. It is possible for a person who stutters to demonstrate accurate stuttering analyses early on. Still, *it is extensive practice that brings about change in old beliefs and attitudes*: taking the mystery out of stuttering and developing a strong realization that she or he is indeed doing the actions that constitute stuttering.

Summary of Identification

Exploration, detection, identification, awareness, and analysis of stuttering from an objective, nonemotional perspective has the potential to be the foundation for speech change. Through this process the client and clinician discover what specific stuttering behaviors interfere with speech that should be modified, as well as alter the client's point of view of the nature of his or her problem. Decreased emotionality is a secondary though important outcome. When attention is paid especially to proprioceptive dimensions of speech during exploration, the speaker can start gaining a sense of his or her own controls. Next, those controls are developed through either the modification of stutter events or the production of a whole new manner of fluent speech (i.e., fluency shaping).

Modification

The overall objective of *modification* is to develop the client's skills for changing the habitual stuttering into easier, more relaxed, less abnormal patterns. The changed pattern will be characterized by more continuous, less interrupted speech movements.

The basic tenet is that if a person has to stutter, the stuttering should at least be more acceptable to self and listeners. Such changes are cognitively based and achieved by self-monitoring and redirecting speech movements just after, in the midst of, or in anticipation of stutter events. In short, the aim is more "fluent stuttering."

Prior desensitization training equips the client to respond more calmly and constructively to the stuttering block and change behaviors instead of reacting with a panic that makes the stuttering more severe. Following weeks of extensive analysis as described in the preceding section, the speaker can now quickly identify incorrect positioning, and transform the stuttering-related movements into appropriate speech movements. The theme of *taking responsibility* for stuttering behavior continues to be upheld.

> The learning challenge at this point is how to change speech and, no less importantly, how to be confident in one's ability to take charge of speech. These priorities should be transmitted to the client. Having the will to explore alternatives is also an extremely important therapeutic achievement. The clinician should emphasize the theme of "exploring alternatives" to the client's old rigid struggle responses in anticipation of, or during, moments of stuttering. It is a significant milestone when the client's strong tendency to panic at each moment of stuttering is replaced by a focus on intentional, positive action. It is, as one client summarized "a feeling of power."

The modification phase of stuttering management typically includes three procedural steps, all referenced in time with respect to the stutter event.

Step I: Post-Block Modification

The essence of the first procedure, referred to as *post-block modification* or *cancellation,* is changing the stuttering after it has occurred. In this procedure:

- **The client should complete the stuttered word and then pause.** The clinician ensures that the stuttered speech continues and the client pauses only *after* the stuttered word is completed. Pausing too soon exploits an opportunity to avoid either the stuttering or the word being said. Avoidance of stuttering, however, is not the goal of the technique. Analysis of the stuttering and selecting alternative, more constructive, behaviors are the aim. Based on behavioral theory, the pause is key because the time-out period interrupts the pattern of undesired reinforcement that results each time stuttering is followed by further progress with communication.

- **While pausing, the client quickly (1) identifies and analyzes the stuttering event, (2) reduces tension, and (3) plans necessary changes.** Inasmuch as the client has had ample practice analyzing stuttering during the previous identification phase of the therapy, now he or she can do this quickly. Still, initially the pause may last at least several seconds, or as long as needed, in order to achieve the multiple tasks.

- **Having paused, the client next reproduces the stuttered word but with the appropriate changes,** such as light contact at the lips for the sound /p/ in "picture," easy voice onset on vowels such as *o* in "ocean," and/or a slower progression of movement. The reproduction may be exaggerated to enhance initial learning, by elongating or stretching out the word. Attention is focused on the oral sensation of speech movements and how these may guide adjustments. Sometimes the speaker may pantomime the word before speaking aloud. That is, the client makes a silent mouthing of how the word will be formed prior to speaking it again out loud. Sometimes the stuttered segment can be changed on reproduction using the *bouncing* technique. Bouncing is when a stuttered word or syllable is repeated several times with an easy, very relaxed production on each reiteration, such as in "pi- pi- pi- picture." Because a major goal is to break the client's stereotypic response, emphasizing variations in the new behaviors is important.

Asking the client to restate the rationale for the cancellation technique is important in order to ensure its success. The client may be adequately motivated if the procedure is not found to be more embarrassing than stuttering itself, and if the gratification found by confronting and dealing with stuttering (the feeling of power) exceeds what is felt by avoiding it.

Warning: Clinicians must monitor cancellations carefully because clients could tend to hurry through the procedure, pausing very briefly, with little analysis, slight reduction in tension, and minimal alteration in the movement. All too often the process, especially the pause, seems inconvenient, even embarrassing to a client. It also interferes, although only temporarily, with interpersonal communication. Clients often prefer to bear with their old familiar stuttering than to engage in the pause and awkward new behaviors that deliberately call attention to the act of speaking. This is a time when clinician support is important, as well as the time to review again the rationales for the procedure. Overall it is a means for developing essential management skills as well a realization of being the master of one's own speech. *Clients do not just wait for the word to "come out"; they do something about it.*

Step II: In-Block Modification

Building on skills acquired with the post-block technique, the clinician introduces the second step—*in-block modification,* also referred to as *pullouts.* Assuming the client can now quickly identify and analyze the abnormal movement and tension on the stuttered word, the pause after it is eliminated so that changes are made earlier, as soon as the stuttering occurs.

- As stuttering is detected mid-word, the client identifies and reduces the tension.
- Without pausing or stopping, the client "pulls out" of the block with relaxed, elongated, or easy repeated movements like those described for the post-block modification. For example, an instance of tense repetitions such as "a-a-a-a-ai" is altered "on line" into an easily prolonged "ah→I."

The elimination of the conspicuous pause after the stuttered word greatly improves overall communication and naturally is preferred over the cumbersome post-block procedure. Important: When an in-block attempt fails, the client should immediately switch to a post-block modification as described earlier. Again, intensive practice provides an invaluable boost to a person's feeling of power over his or her speech.

A common problem in stuttering modification therapy is clients' tendency to speak more fluently after becoming comfortable with the clinical environment, hence there may be few opportunities for practicing post-block and in-block modifications. The solution is simple: Instruct the client to stutter on purpose and then use the modification procedure.

Step III: Pre-Block Modification

The third step is the *pre-block* procedure that shifts modification to an even earlier time, prior to the occurrence of the stutter event. As discussed in Chapter 4, people who stutter frequently anticipate upcoming stutter events. Typically, some alterations in speech, including respiration, speaking rate, and tension, build up simultaneously with the anticipation. Van Riper (1971) referred to pre-block preparations as *preparatory sets*.

After spending many hours in therapy analyzing a large number of stutter events, the client can be expected to know much more about what malformed movements will eventually evolve into full-blown stutter events. Having this knowledge and the skill to generate easier speech, the client is now ready to alter those movements:

- As a moment of stuttering is anticipated, but before difficulty ensues, he/she should analyze it and plan a modified approach.
- The client applies various techniques to approach the spoken word(s) differently, using easier, looser movements. For example, the client eases off tension in the jaw and lips, starts in with ease, and elongates the word just in time to mitigate the expected block.

The overall impression might be that of a somewhat more gradual entry into the act of speaking. If the moment passes by too quickly, then either a pull-out (in-block) or a cancellation (post-block) procedure is applied.

The detailed procedural aspects should not create the impression that therapy is, by and large, simply a technical matter. Above all is the importance of being there for the client. The clinician must be a keen observer of the client's feelings and reactions to shift readily from the role of a coach to a counselor. The counselor role requires understanding difficulties as they arise, easing frustrations, and offering encouragement when self-doubt and disappointment about progress are experienced. Also, the clinician-counselor redirects unrealistic expectations for therapy (such as insisting on perfect fluency, or unwillingness to accept gradual progress) and is supportive with other personal issues that may surface.

Summary of Modification

Following intensive identification and analyses of stuttered speech events, therapy proceeds with three modification steps of post-block (cancellation), in-block (pull-out), and pre-block (preparatory set) procedures, each requires changing the stuttering event at a different time in relation to its occurrence: after, during, and prior to. The purpose is to reduce the severity of stuttering rather than to speak fluently. These modification activities aid speakers because they present alternatives to old painful habits and provide them with the sense of an internal locus of control, more specifically, the power to control their speech. Modification also reminds clients that speech is movements, and that oral sensations can guide those movements. These two principles are also central to the fluency-focused therapies described next. Additionally, modification conveys the view that easy stuttering is a better choice than forcing the word out regardless of imperfect speech delivery.

Fluency-Focused Therapies

There has been a long history of attempts to have people who stutter produce fluent speech, often using unusual means. The classic technique of rhythmic speech, paced by metronomic instruments, was practiced in Europe during the early part of the 19th century (see review by Wingate, 1976) or even earlier. Unlike the stuttering management approach that relies on the presence of stutter events to practice modification, a fluency management approach strives to afford people who stutter with completely fluent speech from the start. Rather than change only the stuttering event, the whole manner of speaking is altered. Little or no attention is given to preparing clients for how to handle stuttering should it occur, and usually little emphasis is placed on managing emotional reactions. The assumption is that when the person speaks fluently, negative emotionality, such as anxiety, will dissipate on its own.

Fluency-shaping therapy emerged from three major sources. First was the observation of drastic amelioration of stuttering during externally imposed conditions (e.g., noise, speaking in chorus), suggesting that a common underlying production technique might be the key. A related assumption was that the abnormal motor articulatory, phonatory, and respiratory functions associated with stuttering could be overcome through careful retraining of basic speech gestures. Second, this approach was developed at the time when applications of operant conditioning principles to the treatment of stuttering became popular. These applications emphasized speech modification through reinforcement of behaviors that gradually approximated the target. It was a behavior-shaping approach to speech change. Finally, a third influential factor was the favorable experience of people who stutter with other speaking strategies that provided relief from stuttering, such as slow speech.

Among the obstacles encountered in pursuing this approach are the slow speaking rate, gradual voice onset, articulatory imprecision, and degraded suprasegmentals (e.g., flat intonation) of smoothed speech that are often emphasized and exaggerated at the early stages of programs. Although some forms of deliberate fluency may not sound too abnormal to listeners, it still may be so to the client because it does not sound like his or her own voice. Because typically all speakers sense comfort with the familiar sound of their own voice/speech, success with this form of speech can be challenging. A client must be ready to embrace a new sense of self and keep practicing the new speech pattern despite strange, awkward feelings, knowing that more natural-sounding characteristics will be eventually reinstated as long as fluency is maintained.

In the modern era, several fluency management techniques have incorporated instruments to facilitate, instate, and shape fluency. Other approaches, however, assign considerable responsibility to the clients' active participation and intensive practice. The latter is reviewed here. Therapies that are mostly instrument-dependent are discussed in a separate section.

> The treatment of stuttering via a focus on a fluency-enhancing (or "managing") approach represents both traditional and modern thinking. The main objective is to employ techniques, such as stretched speech, thereby quickly instating fluency in the person who stutters, even if, at least initially, the new speech is often characterized by distorted patterns. These patterns are incompatible with stuttering, however. Once fluency is achieved and stabilized, speech is progressively shaped until it approximates normalcy, with the clinician ensuring that fluency is maintained throughout the various stages. At some point in the shaping process, generalization to the client's everyday environment is initiated.

Fluency-Shaping Basics

Typically, fluency-shaping programs begin by having the person who stutters speak in a novel but totally fluent manner. For example, if the speaker uses a very slow rate, elongating ("stretching") the vowels or the interval between speech segments (e.g., syllables), it induces complete fluency. Because the remarkable change begins with rather abnormal speech patterns, clients may express pessimism or even resentment at being trained to talk in a way that would call as much attention to speech as stuttering itself. Therefore, early counseling is essential to point out that the exaggerated slow speech is temporary. It is only a means to learning correct speech gestures and other fluency skills, and *speech will eventually approximate the normal manner.* Other factors that enhance fluent speech, such as breathing and articulation patterns, as well as vocalization, may be introduced (depending on the particular program), incorporated, and practiced simultaneously with the slow rate. Subsequently, with gradual steps of reinstating normal prosodic parameters, intonation, stress, and rhythm, the slow novel fluent speech pattern is shaped toward increased naturalness.

Ideally, the behavioral skills learned from a fluency-shaping approach should continue to support the smooth flow of speech after treatment. Examples of these skills include slower transitions between syllables, easier vocal initiations, gentle contacts of the articulators, additional airflow to carry the sounds, chunking spoken utterances into shorter phrases, and connecting across words within the phrases. Typical to stuttering therapy for adults, however, transfer of learning is not instantaneous The role of the clinician, therefore, is similar to the music teacher who must help the player (i.e., client) learn to play a new instrument and practice until the skills are ready for public performance (i.e., situations of communicative pressure).

A variety of programs have been developed based on fluency-shaping principles. Clinicians will discover that most commercially available kits will integrate some *fluency shaping* techniques alongside traditional stuttering modification activities, such as identification and voluntary stuttering. The rhythmic speech and stretched speech programs that will be described below are based nearly exclusively on fluency-shaping principles. The behavioral reinforcement approaches that will be described are better classified as *fluency-focused* because they lack the *shaping* component.

Rhythmic Speech

Normal speech is characterized by varying rhythm within and between utterances. As discussed in Chapter 4, when the client adopts a uniform rhythm by keeping equal intervals between syllables, words, or phrases, the resultant fluency promises to be useful for treatment. Under such identical intervals between the spoken units, speech becomes rhythmic and fluency can be maintained across a wide range of speaking rates, whether the intervals between speech units are fast or slow. Slow rhythmic speech has a very different quality from the slow-stretched speech typically induced in fluency-shaping programs described later in the chapter. This is because with stretched speech prosodic variations are possible and even encouraged; but it is not so during rhythmic speech. Even when rhythmic speech is produced at normal speeds, it still sounds robotic.

In an extensive analysis of rhythm and stuttering, Wingate (1976) traced the realization that speaking in rhythm yields fluency to ancient times. After the invention of metronomic devices in the early 1800s, rhythmic speech, with or without metronome pacing, has been employed by clinicians in various countries. Since then, however, the method has been characterized by erratic trends in popularity, but it has never attained widespread implementation by modern era clinicians. A rise in interest, for example, occurred in Europe near the middle of the last century. Dantzig (1940), in the Netherlands, advocated a *syllable tapping* program whereby each syllable was synchronized with a quiet tapping of the client's preferred-hand fingers, progressing from the little finger toward the thumb. The therapy included three stages: (1) practice with deliberate finger tapping per each syllable, (2) minimize the tapping and obscure the view of the fingers, and (3) just imagine finger tapping.

One of us (EY) received rhythmic speech therapy in the 1950s, during his school years in Israel. This was done with and without the aid of metronome pacing. At an advanced stage in therapy, he was asked to swing his thumb from side to side while hiding his hand in the pants pocket. Curiously, a second clinician insisted that swinging the thumb was not a good idea. Instead, he recommended folding the fingers, one at a time, still keeping the hand inside the pocket. In those days, EY was not particularly keen on collecting comparison data.

One rhythmic speech therapy program for stuttering, implemented without the use of the metronome, was referred to as *syllable-timed speech*. It was carried on in the United Kingdom by Andrews, Harris, Garside et al. (1964), who reported its use with 35 clients ranging in age from 11 to 45 years, divided into four age subgroups. The 10-day intensive program consisted of four stages:

1. **Baseline.** Case history and speech samples were recorded. Baseline measures of stuttering were taken.

2. **Teaching Syllable-Timed (S.T.) Speech.** Speech was produced syllable-by-syllable, stressing each syllable evenly, in time to a regular, even rhythm. Practice began with simple sentences composed of one-syllable words. Clients progressed to reading prose and then to conversational speech. If stuttering occurred, the phrase was immediately repeated, paying more attention to timing. By the end of the first 2 hours, most adults and adolescents were speaking fluently but at a slow rate of 80 syllables per minute. To become proficient, considerable practice was necessary, about 50 hours in individual and group therapy over 4 to 5 days.

3. **Generalization.** Over 10 days, every client retained S.T. speech in relaxed group practice sessions that focused on attitudes and concerns regarding stuttering. The group decided when they were ready for practice of S.T. speech outside the clinic, especially in previously difficult situations. Toward the end, clients spent more time accomplishing speaking tasks alone. An important assignment required clients to explain the changes in their speech to family, friends, and people in places of employment. This was done in order to facilitate clients' commitment to speaking fluently upon returning to family or job. By the last day, speech approximated normalcy.

4. **Follow-Up.** For maintenance, a follow-up session for each group was held approximately once a week for 10 weeks. If stuttering occurred, clients were asked to continue talking in S.T. speech for the rest of the day and also practice at home. Next, tape-recorded formal interviews were held every 3 months across 1 year with an unfamiliar staff member. Speech samples were recorded so that speaking rate and stuttering frequency could be compared with respective base rates. Feedback was also obtained from clients' families by means of questionnaires and stuttering severity ratings.

Andrews et al. (1964) presented data showing that all four age subgroups exhibited substantial reduction (20%) in the frequency of stuttering as well as in its rated severity compared to pretreatment measures. The gains remained stable over 1 year after the termination of therapy. Improvement was higher among those who were free of neurotic traits and in groups that also were provided the opportunity to discuss their anxieties and attitudes about speech. Clients with the most severe stuttering showed the least improvement. Similar programs using metronomic instruments are presented later in this chapter. We believe that clinicians should be open to, and familiar with, the technique and apply it within an orderly program, such as the one described above, when they encounter clients who show difficulties with other approaches, or for some reason, prefer this method.

Stretched Speech

Whereas rhythmic or syllable-timed speech did not catch on across wide speech pathology circles, especially in the United States, several programs that emphasized slow, stretched speech were developed from the early 1960s on and gained significant acceptance. We review several of them here.

Conversational Rate Control Therapy

In 1965 Goldiamond reported that when people who stutter read under delayed auditory feedback (DAF), many automatically slowed down and became fluent. Several years later, Curlee and Perkins (1969) were among the first to develop a prototype fluency management therapy program. Motivated by operant conditioning principles, motor speech coordination was facilitated primarily by focusing on speech rate control, often using a DAF device to help the client slow down.

> The delayed auditory feedback (DAF) instrument delivers the sound back to the speaker at a brief delay after speech is uttered. The longer the time delay, the more speech will be produced prior to the speaker's hearing it. This delay induces the speaker to slow down so as not to be ahead of him- or herself. The capability to incrementally increase or decrease the delay is an important element in the Curlee-Perkins conditioning program.

During therapy, the client is prompted to engage in self-formulated conversation while the clinician limits her/his participation as much as possible. Fluency is first established with a 250-millisecond delay, resulting in an extremely slow speaking rate of about 30 words per minute, about 6 times slower than normal. When the client maintains total fluency for two 15-minute talking periods, rate is increased by adjusting the DAF, gradually shifting to faster rates, usually in 50-millisecond increments, as long as the client is able to meet fluency criteria. Also incrementally, both the volume of the DAF and the use of the instrument are diminished until normal speech is achieved without DAF. From the beginning, the client is entrusted with responsibilities for all the program's steps, including criteria for progress and correcting failures. Operant principles are important in the generalization stage.

The initial program in which slow speech was the sole procedure resulted in considerable improvement in the clinical setting as well as in everyday situations. Relapse, however, occurred in more than 50% of the clients (Curlee & Perkins, 1969). Later versions of the therapy regimen (Perkins, 1973a, 1973b) were expanded to include other elements that appeared necessary to shape normal speech, including rate, breath stream management, prosody, and self-confidence. These changes reflected Perkins's position that stuttering is a disorder of timing, characterized by lack of coordination of the various components of the speech system, namely, respiration, phonation, and articulation. Hence therapy should advance compensatory skills that enable stutterers to talk fluently.

In the revised version of the program, fluency-enhancing skills were introduced and added during practice at the exaggerated slow pace. An important skill was continuous airflow throughout the utterance, a behavior typical of normal speakers. While speaking slowly, the client is taught to maintain uninterrupted expiratory airflow on short utterances of three to eight syllables, assuring sufficient air support. Because the slow fluent speech pattern tends to be monotonous, it is further supplemented by practice of normal prosody and emphasis on clear voice quality. Although speech drill is the main aspect of the program, Perkins and Curlee also mention the importance of what they call "psychotherapeutic discussion" that encourages clients to use positive language and discuss success throughout the program. Although these early programs used DAF, it is important to point out that the instrument is not at all essential to pursue them.

> Of course, every procedural step in this and any other approach involves a significant amount of practice in the clinical setting followed by much work to generalize the objective to various environments. To this end, the clinician charts out the therapy goals, teaches the techniques, presents a rationale, supervises the drills, provides feedback, and more. Clients need the clinician's support and encouragement to move behaviors beyond the therapy room to the street, the workplace, and with friends, family, and strangers.

Precision Fluency Shaping

Devised by Webster (1980a, 1980b), precision fluency shaping has probably received more exposure and publicity than any other therapy of its kind. Theoretically, it is based on the assumption that motor abnormalities in articulatory, phonatory, and respiratory functions underlie stuttering, but that these can be overcome through careful retraining of the basic speech gestures. In the past it was presented as an intensive 12-day residential program.

The Webster program begins with immediately instating fluency by having a client speak while stretching the vowels at an extremely slow rate of one syllable per 2 seconds. Thus a two-syllable word would be prolonged over 4 seconds, an even slower rate than what was used in the programs described earlier. Instead of managing rate with DAF, the client is trained to mentally estimate and monitor the different speaking rates. Estimates are aided initially by tracking the seconds on a wristwatch. DAF is reserved for when/if stuttering occurs, and it rarely does.

The objective of the therapy, however, is not just to achieve fluent speech but to have the client attain additional speech gestures that generate fluency. Thus, following extensive practice at an initially slow speaking rate, several articulatory and phonatory behaviors that are even more critical, in Webster's opinion, than the slow rate, are introduced to enhance fluency. These are referred to as *fluency targets*. Perhaps the most notable after slow speech are *gentle voice onset* and *light articulatory contact*.

Continuing with the program, and still using the initial rate of slow-stretched speech:

1. Each vowel is practiced with a gentle voice onset. A computer-controlled bio-feedback loop consisting of a microphone connected to an earpiece provides the speaker with an immediate awareness (audible beeping) concerning the accept-ability of the slope of the gradual voice onset. The instrument serves only as an aid and is not essential to skill learning. The clinician's feedback and guidance can be very effective in helping the client to monitor the softness of the voice initiation.

2. Slow syllables beginning with consonants are practiced in combination with gentle, gradual voice onsets on the initial sound and subsequent vowel. Consonant classes are addressed in the following order:
   a. voiced continuants (e.g., w, l, v, and z) are practiced, such as: W-olf; L-ike; V-ase; Z-oo.
   b. voiceless fricatives (e.g., s, f) are practiced with lower intraoral air pressures in combination with gentle voice onsets, such as: S-un; F-our.
   c. plosive consonants (e.g., b, t, k) are practiced with *light articulatory contacts* in combination with gentle voice onsets, such as: B-owl; T-ime; C-ar.

3. Once these skills are mastered, all are simultaneously implemented in practice on single-syllable words uttered very slowly.

4. Next, the simultaneous fluency targets (slow rate, gentle voice, and light artic-ulation) are incorporated into longer words and then into phrases, all spoken very slowly. Systematic work on respiration, primarily the use of diaphragmatic breathing, is incorporated. For this purpose, another biofeedback device, a dia-phragmatic breathing belt, is used.

5. As might be expected, the next phase in therapy is to gradually increase the speaking rate while maintaining all the fluency targets. Using a stepwise progres-sion, the rate is raised from its initial slow-motion pace of one syllable per 2 sec-onds up to one syllable per second, then up to one word per second (60 words per minute), until finally a slow normal rate of 120 words per minute is reached. Although this pace is more than 10 times faster than the initial rate, it is still slower than the average normal speaking rate of 150 to 180 words per minute.

6. At this point, transfer and generalization begin, including telephone calls, visits to stores, and so on.

In Webster's clinic, participants are reported to spend many hours per day practicing speech. Practice time can be in the context of individual sessions with a clinician, group sessions, or even by them-selves with computer feedback. Although the classic approach involves an intense practice schedule, the basic principles with many similar procedures and steps have been adopted by clinicians in a vari-ety of settings with much lighter schedules, including the typical one or two weekly sessions.

As stated earlier in this chapter, as well as in other chapters of this book, the clinical programs we cite were selected to represent the relevant principles, structure, and techniques for their approaches. Variations on therapy programs, both published and unpublished, have been devised and practiced by clinicians in the field. Other good examples of fluency-enhancing therapies that involve stretched speech, gentle voice, and so on, can be found in Neilsen and Andrews (1992), and Schwartz (1999).

Concerning clinical effectiveness data, in a comprehensive analysis of 42 treatment studies in 1980, Andrews, Guitar, and Howie reported that among several principal treatment approaches, starting with the strongest effectiveness, were prolonged speech, gentle onset, rhythm, and airflow. Other evidence for rate reduction therapies was published two years later by Andrews et al. (1982), who examined responses of three adult men who stutter to various fluency-enhancing conditions. Slowing, syllable-timed speech, and prolonged speech under DAF were found among the strongest of 14 conditions, reducing stuttering by at least 90%. The mean reduction in stuttering frequency, in order from most to least effective conditions, was prolonged speech/DAF (98%), slowing at half one's usual rate (95%), and syllable-timed speech with a metronome at 90 beats per minute (bpm; 91%).

Another study compared the efficiency of fluency-shaping training with 20 adult and adolescent clients who stuttered, half of whom received 16 hours of therapy within 4 days, and the other half, the same amount of therapy over 8 weeks. Both formats produced significant improvement in stuttering and other measures, and both were equivalent on all measures. Generalization of treatment effects was also observed for both groups (James, Ricciardelli, Hunter et al., 1989). Thirteen participants in a PET scan study who received a 3-week intensive modified precision fluency shaping program reduced their stuttering frequency in monologue samples from an average 7% disfluencies (stuttering-like types) pretreatment to 1.6% immediately posttreatment, and 3.46% at a year posttreatment (De Nil et al., 2003). The concern about whether fluency shaping results in posttreatment speech that is still noticeably different was underscored by a study of 32 PWS who took part in a Dutch version of the precision fluency shaping program. Clients were tested immediately posttreatment and again at six months posttreatment. Regardless of whether their speech was perceptibly fluent, listeners still rated their speech as sounding different from the samples of 20 nonstutterers whose speech was also rated (Franken, Boves, Peters et al., 1992).

Behavioral Reinforcement

In Chapter 6, we discussed stuttering within the framework of operant learning theory with an underlying assumption that stuttering is a behavioral response that may be modified by its consequences. Some support to this theory was provided by various experiments showing that stuttering can be diminished through several learning modes, for example, punishment, such as a 5-second time-out period (Martin & Haroldson, 1982), withdrawal of reinforcement (Lanyon & Barocas (1975), and withdrawal of aversive stimuli (Flanagan et al., 1958). Indeed, several therapeutic regimens have been developed contingent on stuttering events.

In the 1970s, early adult treatment studies (Andrews & Ingham, 1972; Ingham, Andrews, & Winkler, 1972) examined whether existing syllable-timed speech programs could be enhanced by application of *token reinforcement* systems. In a token reinforcement system, a client is given some tangible object (i.e., something seen or felt) to reward desired performance. Tokens, the "stimuli" in behavioral terminology, can take any form (e.g., pegs, wooden blocks, etc.) but typically refer to small coinlike pieces resembling poker chips. Clients do not receive tokens when the performance is attempted but not achieved; thus the token reinforcement is contingent on the client's behavioral response. Tokens can be exchanged, like money, for prizes or privileges. The target behavior typically reinforced is fluent speech, but other behaviors may be rewarded too, for example, entering specified speaking situations from a sequential hierarchy (Andrews & Ingham, 1973).

Research has shown that token reinforcement systems can be beneficial both by decreasing the time needed to reach the fluent speech target—greater efficiency—and by the amount of the reduction in stuttering attained—effectiveness (e.g., Andrews & Ingham, 1973;). Some studies, however, have been less supportive, suggesting that token management may be unnecessary if a highly structured intervention system using other forms of reinforcement, such as praise or other verbal feedback, is employed (Howie & Woods, 1982).

> Relevant to this section on fluency-focused therapies, it is worth noting that reinforcement of fluent speech, rather than punishment of stuttering, has been the popular clinical implementation of operant conditioning principles. Generally, such approaches seek to gradually increase the length of fluently produced speech segments as well as the length of time during which fluency can be maintained.

A therapy that integrated the slow-stretched speech technique with operant principles and schedules, referred to as *DAF-prolongation program*, was offered by Ryan (2001b). It contains 12 steps beginning with establishing slow fluent speech at 40 words per minute with or without the aid of a DAF device. Typical of the gradual progress principle, the client begins with reading or saying single sentences fluently.

The contingent reinforcement is "good" or a token. Although the verbal punishment "stop" may be applied if the client stutters, it is used rather infrequently because the stretched speech or the DAF are likely to keep the speech fluent. Ten consecutive fluent responses is the criterion required to advance to the following two steps: The client is to maintain fluent speech for one whole minute, then for 5 minutes at the rate of 40 words per minute (wpm) while reading or talking. Eventually, the speech rate is increased in stepwise progression up to 150 wpm over 5 minutes. Of course, contingencies remain a cardinal feature throughout the program.

Ryan (2001b) stated that he favors the stuttering behavior management program of gradual increase in length and complexity of utterance (GILCU) over prolonged

DAF methods because it is easier to teach and nearly as effective, and has "better generalization, and no negative side effects of abnormal speech" (p. 114). The GILCU program includes two main stages, establishment and identification, combined with home practice. The establishment stage is completed while the client engages in one of three possible activities: reading, monologue, or conversation. The 18-step series is repeated for each of these activity types, as appropriate, for example, a nonreader would not engage in the reading activity. Throughout the progression of steps, both verbal and token reinforcements are administered. The clinician models and instructs the target speech pattern, and evaluates the client's response. Fluent productions are encouraged by the statement "Good" and a token; "Stop; speak fluently" is stated if the client stutters. Ten consecutive fluent responses is the criterion required to advance to the next step. The client is expected to discover his or her own strategies for speaking fluently, which typically involves some form of slowing speech rate. The two stages are outlined as follows:

Stage I. The establishment program takes the client from practicing saying one word at a time ending with talking continuously for 5 minutes.
> Steps 1–6: The client progresses from speaking fluently one word at a time to six consecutive words at a time.
> Steps 7–10: The progression advances from speaking a single sentence fluently to saying four consecutive sentences at a time.
> Steps 11–18: The progression expands from speaking for 30 seconds fluently to 5 minutes fluently.

Stage II. The identification stage is addressed after the first 18 steps are accomplished. That is, after instating fluency with one of the three activities (reading, monologue, or conversation), programs of identification (of stuttering), and home practice are initiated. This backward order of identification (after establishment) appears to serve as the means to develop the client's self-monitoring and self-administration of the program targets. The adolescent or adult client is trained to recognize and count his or her own stuttered words.

Step 1. The three-part identification training sequence begins with a 1-minute speaking activity (i.e., reading, monologue, or conversation) during which the clinician identifies the client's stuttering by stopping the client with the word *there* and then describing and imitating the stuttering while the client observes.

Step 2. The clinician continues saying "there" when the client stutters, and the client overtly counts the moments during another 1-minute speaking activity. To advance between steps, the client's and clinician's counts must agree within one stuttered word.

Step 3. The clinician covertly counts stuttering moments while the client counts covertly. Home practice, during which stuttering is identified and counted, is also included. As previously explained, the establishment stage continues with the other two modes of activities.

Other programs have offered variations on the administration of behavioral reinforcement. For example, James (1981) demonstrated that self-administered response-contingent time-out periods could successfully reduce stuttering in a young adult man. Recall that *time-out* refers to having a speaker stop talking for a short time (several seconds) after she or he stutters. James found that fluency improvement was maintained at 6- and 12-month follow-up assessments after the treatment program. Approximately 15 years later, Hewat, Onslow, Packman et al. (2006) also published a program for training clients in self-administered time-out for stuttering. In this variant, clients learned to make estimations, not only about whether they stuttered, but also about stuttering severity and the passage of time. The improvement among their 22 clients varied, but more than half reduced stuttering by at least 50%. Dr. Betty McMicken, ASHA Fellow, provided the following case study:

12.1 Adult Case Study

Late remediation from stuttering is rather rare. This case study documents the reduction of stuttering in an adult who exhibited long-term persistent stuttering, and the subsequent maintenance of effective speech: fluent, natural sounding, spontaneous, and without external controls.

Client

HL was a 40-year-old male with about a 35-year history of moderate-severe stuttering. Having a long troubled history of drug abuse, as well as various encounters with the law, he lived in a special residential center undergoing a rehabilitation program while also working toward a high school diploma. HL reported that his speech had been a source of emotional pains and also resulted in educational failure, leading him at times to suicidal thoughts. Speech therapies during school were unsuccessful.

Assessment

HL's stuttering baseline was obtained in four modes: conversation, monologue, telephone talk, and reading. On the average, stuttering occurred at a rate of 8–10 stuttered words per minute (SW/M) and was characterized mainly by part-word repetitions, sound prolongations, and facial secondary characteristics. Overall, stuttering was rated as moderate-to-severe. Interjudge reliability in counting stuttering was above 90%. His score on the Erickson S-24 scale was 20 (out of 24), indicating a high level of negative emotions associated with stuttering. Self-rating on a speech naturalness scale (1 = highly natural speech; 9 = highly unnatural speech) was 7–8.

Treatment

Therapy was scheduled for two 50-minute weekly sessions although various schedule conflicts sometimes allowed for only a single session per week. It followed a standard protocol for the Ryan Fluency Program (Ryan, 2001b). During sessions, the main procedure consisted of positive reinforcement with the clinician saying "good" after each of the client's fluent responses. A mild punishment was applied with the clinician saying "stop, speak fluently" if the client's speaking responses were stuttered. At the beginning of the initial interview the client was advised that he may use the *pause time* strategy in anticipation of stuttering, that is, stop for a second and then try to speak fluently. However, except for the first 3 contact hours, this was rarely used. Regardless, *pause times* were counted as stuttered words. Readings were selected from the client's texts; monologue topics focused on text passages of relevance to him. The Conversation mode involved reflections on family and past history. Finally, various communication opportunities with staff and parole committees were used for part of the Transfer activities. HL was encouraged to verbally participate in his required school classes when he felt comfortable with the process.

The criterion for success of the therapy that allowed for progress from one phase to the next was no stuttering during 5 minutes each of reading, conversation, and monologue treatment. A record was kept of the frequency of stuttering for at least once a week. The post-treatment criterion for success was 0.5 SW/M or less in each of the four modes.

Establishment Phase

In this phase, the objective is to achieve the fluency criterion in monologue, conversation, and reading. Total establishment time for the three modalities was 23 hours over 10 weeks. This was considerably longer than the reported mean of 8 hours, perhaps due in part to the inconsistent schedule and other interferences. As suggested in the Ryan program, each of the three modalities: conversation, monologue, and reading was completed prior to initiation of the next. Each task began at the single word level, 10 different word criteria, and progressed through 5 different words and 10 trials. Then the single words were changed to sentences (short to long) and then to a time criteria of 1–5 minutes.

Transfer

The transfer program continued for the next 6 months, with the client being seen 2–3 times a week in a variety of settings. This phase included 61 hours, way above the mean of approximately 12 reported by Ryan (2001b). This extended phase reflects the commitment of the client and the clinician, as well as the many opportunities available in the rehab center. It was also deemed necessary because of the client's past unsuccessful therapy. Practice consisted of 1–2 minute segments of talking time in various settings and activities, such as making telephone calls, giving directions, interviewing different people, talking to policemen, etc. Sessions were held both in and outside of the center, including offices and public parks. Usually there were 3 assignments per session and they consisted of a series of questions: 3 prearranged and 3 spontaneously derived. Immediate unobtrusive hand signals provided positive and negative feedback. When HL joined the center's security team, he had many opportunities to speak with guests as well as over the radio communication system. Occasional stuttering was observed in stressful situations. In clinical sessions, about 5 minutes was spent in the therapy room and the rest on the Center grounds and the street. No more than 1 to 2 SW/M were noted with a transfer session average of 0.5 SW/M.

Maintenance

Maintenance began on a once weekly treatment session with the client also making a 15-minute weekly report over the telephone concerning his speech performance. HL's use of pause time remained at zero during maintenance. The maintenance phase faded gradually. At the time of this report, however, he already had 29 maintenance hours, much more than the average of 11 hours reported by Ryan (2001b). Generally conversations revolved around sensitive topics: family and legal worries, work, and more. The clinician always counted disfluencies during these phone calls.

Final Assessment

Thirteen months after his initial speech assessment, HL spoke extemporaneously about his speech recovery at the graduation ceremony at the Center in front of a large audience. The clinician observed no incidences of stuttering. This was confirmed by several observers who independently related to the clinician that they perceived the speech to be stuttering-free. In two recent conversations, the client again revealed no incidences of stuttering. On the last count of stuttering, there was a total of 1 stuttered word during 50 total minutes of talking time.

The client also showed a very large improvement in rating the naturalness of his speech. Whereas the pre-therapy rating was 7 on a 9-point scale, the posttherapy rating was 1. Finally, whereas his pretherapy score on the Erickson S-24 scale that assesses communication attitudes was a high of 20, the posttherapy score was 6. HL generally spoke at a slower than average rate of 120 to 180 wpm yet in an animated manner. HL stated that he is still getting used to how his new speech feels and sounds, that it requires concentration but that it does feel natural to him, and is much easier to produce under all circumstances. These statements reflect the clinical significance of the treatment, in that "how it feels" is a measurable difference available only to the client. He reported that in certain situations, he tends to become anxious and hurried. Under these circumstances, his speech requires greater focus, but he can handle this.

Summary of Fluency-Focused Therapies

Fluency-focused therapies are not concerned with stutter events but seek to train clients in speech patterns and strategies that are likely to elicit fluency so stuttering does not occur. Most begin with a slowed or rhythmic speech to which other features may be added, such as gentle voicing. Initially, the resultant speech is not normal but fluent. It is practiced, reinforced, and gradually shaped to approximate a more normal rate as well as more typical prosody. Clients progress from basic to more challenging speaking tasks as they acquire the techniques. The focus on speech typically leaves little or no attention to the emotional aspects of the stuttering. Several approaches were described, including rhythmic or syllable-timed speech, conversational rate control, stretched speech, precision fluency shaping, and behavioral reinforcement. Many variations on these approaches exist. Another potential means of generating fluent speech is with the aid of fluency-inducing instruments, such as those discussed next.

Fluency-Inducing Instruments

The discipline of speech pathology has seen a growing number of mechanical instruments employed for both diagnostic and treatment purposes. This trend has also left its marks on clinical management of stuttering as already alluded to in the previous section (e.g., the use of DAF as an aid in fluency-shaping programs). Our experience has shown that most people who stutter indeed wish to discover or obtain a powerful external means to reduce/control their stuttering. The quick, often immediate, and substantive results in achieving fluent speech, the saving in the required therapeutic contact, and the ability to use the instrument either on a permanent basis or when needed most are all attractive features. Although the trend has been growing, the extent of using instruments in stuttering therapy programs has varied from being supplementary to being the main, or even the sole, technique. Whereas in the early conversational speaking rate control of Curlee and Perkins (1969), DAF served as the exclusive means to induce and shape desired rates, it is only one component in the more complex behavioral program outlined by Perkins (1973b). Whereas the voice onset monitor that helps control abruptness of phonation is only one component in a precision fluency shaping program (Webster, 1979), the Edinburgh noise maker serves as the sole technique in the Dewar et al. (1979) treatment program. In some cases the instrument is advertised as if it will be fully sufficient by itself, yet supplemental speech therapy and fluency practice is highly encouraged to enhance user satisfaction.

Instruments employed in stuttering therapy have varied in their background, principles, and purpose. As we discussed in Chapter 4, there are several natural conditions known to induce fluent speech in people who stutter, such as high-level noise, rhythmic speech, singing, and others. Although the reasons for their powerful, yet often temporary, effects remain obscure, investigators and clinicians have been motivated to design instruments, such as miniature noise generators and metronomes, to exploit their potential for practical use. There have been other instruments emerging from laboratory-developed stimuli rather than natural conditions. Examples include DAF, the voice onset monitor (Webster, 1979), and the SpeechEasy (http://speecheasy.com), which provides both delayed and frequency-altered feedback. Instruments employed in stuttering therapy can be classified into four groups according to their principle of operation: (1) speech pacing, (2) auditory masking, (3) physiological feedback, and (4) auditory feedback. Representatives of these categories are briefly reviewed here.

Metronome Pacing of Speech

Although regulated rhythmic speech can be produced without a monitoring instrument, the metronome, often used in music training, has provided a significant boost to the therapeutic application of the technique due to its capability to regulate the length of the desired speech intervals in stuttering therapy. Wingate (1976, p. 154) traces academic records of this technique to the writings of Colombat de l'Isère in 1830, who believed that stuttering was caused by lack of harmony between nervous activity and musculature involved in speech. He discovered that rhythm was the most effective exercise for harmony and then developed a prototype of the metronome, which he called *muthonome*. Although clinicians have employed various metronomic instruments in therapy since the original invention, a fundamental drawback was the impracticality of carrying around the conventional spring-operated desk metronome into everyday situations.

A surge in the use of metronome-paced speech as a major technique in stuttering therapy occurred in the early 1960s when a miniature electric metronome that fit behind the ear (originally one unit behind each ear), like a hearing aid instrument, was first introduced by Meyer and Mair (1963). Based on initial experimentation they found that metronomic beats between 75 and 95 per minute provided the most effective rate. Using improved versions of the instrument, several therapeutic programs were developed, and studies of clinical applications of rhythm were published. In 1968, Brady described a single-unit device, the Pacemaster, in which the rate of the metronomic clicks and their loudness can be adjusted manually. Three years later, Brady (1971) described a systematic therapy program, metronome conditioned speech retraining (MCSR), with accompanied results of the most extensive metronome-paced treatment to date. The program's title reflects Brady's theoretical view that stuttering consists of two components: nonfluencies and anxiety/tension. The MCSR follows five phases and is presented here as a good example of the rhythmic speech method as well as a logically structured, systematic speech therapy program:

Phase I: Obtain nearly 100% fluency using a desk metronome in the clinic. The client determines the most comfortable metronome rate for fluency when reading aloud easy materials. For example, a person with severe stuttering might prefer 40 bpm, whereas a person with moderate stuttering may prefer 80 bpm. The client is to practice speaking with the desk metronome at home for at least 45 minutes a day, first alone, then in the presence of others.

Phase II: Shaping the speech to a more normal rate. Using the desk metronome, the speaking rate is gradually increased by changing the frequency of the metronome beats and by pacing longer speech units per beat, that is, moving from one syllable per beat to words, longer words, and even three to four words per beat. Natural pauses are added. Home practice continues, varying the listeners and their numbers. This phase takes 2 to 3 weeks, ending when the client is able to speak fluently with the metronome at a normal rate of 100 to 160 words per minute and exhibiting no more than 20% of the original disfluency level when speaking without the metronome.

Phase III: The miniature metronome. Because of the excellent mobility of the instrument, the objective is relaxed, fluent speech in virtually all speaking situations. The switch-over to the behind-the-ear metronome, however, may result in a partial setback. In that case, the speaking rate is reduced until fluency is reached again. The client is to construct a hierarchy of speaking situations and practice them in that order. Again, if difficulties occur, the rate is lowered and then gradually increased. Brady sometimes used systematic desensitization techniques to help clients overcome difficulties transferring the metronome-aided fluency to specific situations.

Phase IV: Maintaining fluency without the metronome. The metronome is turned off in less stressful situations and gradually removed from higher stress situations. If stuttering is experienced, the client immediately returns to a strict speech pacing without the metronome. Should difficulties continue, however, the metronome is turned back on.

Phase V: Continuation of training based on responses at Phase IV.

Overall, in spite of several encouraging results of systematic clinical applications of speech pacing, with and without the metronome, the technique met resistance from clinicians in the United States educated within the newly founded profession of speech pathology in the late 1920s. Many regarded it as a "crutch"' rather than a "real" treatment (e.g., Boome & Richardson, 1932). In this respect, it is interesting to note that although Johnson and Rosen (1937) found regulated rhythmic speech to be the most effective of 12 methods they compared, the method aroused little interest in clinical speech pathology circles. Again, we recommend speech clinicians should possess a metronome, have some experience with its application, and consider its use when deemed appropriate, sometimes as a springboard element in the overall therapy program.

In our opinion, speech pacing, like speaking in unison or DAF, should be considered a viable option for clinicians to use as a bridge to fluency. One author (EY) has used the technique with selected adult clients, when needed, in conjunction with other methods, to support the development of fluent speech. A few clients who encountered difficulties with other methods responded so well to rhythmic speech that it became the primary means to improving fluency, even without a portable device. The technique is discussed again later in relation to the treatment of children.

Auditory Masking

The strong effects of white noise on the amelioration of stuttering have been researched extensively and have prompted theoretical implications (see Chapter 4). Although some people who stutter do not improve, as we have seen, or show only limited improvement speaking under noise (Andrews et al., 1982), as auditory-related instrumentation developed, attempts to use masking for clinical management of stuttering also increased. Similar to the metronome case, a critical requirement was that the instrument be small enough to be easily carried by the user out of the laboratory. A first attempt in this direction is seen in a portable noise generator, the Correctophone, constructed in 1939 in the then-Soviet Union by Derazne (1966), who reported good results in treating stuttering. Using an instrument he developed, Van Riper (1973) concluded that whereas continuous masking noise met with clients' objections, turning on the noise only at the beginning of stuttering was more effective. He observed, however, that the fluency obtained exclusively with masking did not generalize, and concluded it was useful only as a supplementary technique to a comprehensive behavioral speech therapy.

A breakthrough occurred in 1963 with the development of a lightweight portable electronic noise generator by Parker and Christopherson (1963) that delivered noise through headphones. Following, other models were developed (e.g., Donovan, 1971; Klein, 1967), including types that delivered white noise and those that delivered pulsating signals, resulting in various clinical applications. For example, Perkins and Curlee

(1969) had three clients use a masker for several days to facilitate transfer of fluency to outside situations.

Perhaps the most systematic, long-term clinical program that relied exclusively on masking noise was reported by Dewar et al. (1979) using a portable masking noise device, the Edinburgh Masker, and its heavier clinical bench model. The device provided an automatically triggered noise. The portable model consisted of a pocket-size noise generator that also housed the on/off switch and volume control. It produced a low-frequency noise but the mean frequency varied, depending on the client's vocal fundamental frequency. The instrument was connected to a throat microphone as well as to a light stethoscope-type headset. Alternatively, it could be connected to individualized ear molds via short plastic tubes arising from behind the neck to minimize visualization. The noise was triggered as soon as the client began talking into the microphone; however, it was also possible to turn the noise on or off manually. The clinical bench model was considerably bigger, and it offered greater frequency and loudness ranges.

The Edinburgh Masker is no longer in production, but because similar devices can be constructed, we provide here some details of the therapy program reported by Dewar et al. (1979). Their group initially included 195 clients (all but two were adults) of whom nearly 75% exhibited severe stuttering. The therapy proceeded as follows:

1. **Baseline.** A speech sample is recorded for future reference assessments and to evaluate stuttering severity.

2. **Client Fitting and Screening.** As the client talks, the bench unit is fitted to provide complete masking of his or her speech. A continuous sound is delivered binaurally. When fluency is achieved, the noise is lowered to a level that just covers normal conversational speech. The device is then switched to the automatic throat microphone. Because of the natural tendency to raise vocal volume when talking in noise (the Lombard effect), the client practices reading until a normal intensity level is reached through instruction or with a sound meter. If a word or a phrase begins with a silent block, the device is activated by the client saying "er" or "mm." Those clients who have problems adjusting to the masker are screened out and excluded beyond this point.

3. **Using the Portable Masker.** Clients are provided with the portable model and instructed to adjust the noise level until speech is fully covered by it. They learn that when the voice rises above the noise level, the effectiveness of the instrument is diminished. Most are able to maintain normal loudness and intonation.

4. **Generalization.** Clients are advised about the ways the masker can be used in everyday situations and are encouraged to experiment with it. The bulk of the therapy activities are concentrated on using the device in various situations. Clients are also encouraged to experiment periodically with turning off the noise while talking, thus testing the carryover effect. In this stage, close clinical monitoring continues.

In contrast to the rich body of laboratory studies on the ameliorating effects of noise on stuttering, nearly all our current knowledge about the application of masking in the clinical setting has come from reports that are not based on adequately controlled studies. The person who began using a noise instrument (the Correctophone) for stuttering therapy in 1939, years later reported good results (Derazne, 1966). According to Van Riper (1973), the instrument was used by many clinicians in eastern Europe but with mixed outcomes. Dr. Trotter, a speech pathologist, described his personal use of masking devices during 50% of the days during a 2.5-year period, about 15 minutes per day. He reported very large reductions of stuttering in many situations with brief, temporary carryover to unaided speech (Trotter & Lesch, 1967).

The largest clinical study of masking noise was published by Dewar et al. (1979) reporting on 195 people who stutter; all but two were adult participants in the program described earlier. Of these, 174 responded well to the masker during the screening phase and proceeded with the program. Follow-up progress was possible in 67 participants who used the device from 6 to 28 months (median = 12 months). Of these, 42% reported the device to be of "great" benefit, 40% as "considerable," and 12% as a "slight" benefit. Interestingly, 67% considered that as a result of using the device, their unaided speech had improved, too. One of the limitations of this study was the reliance on subjective reports rather than speech measures. A much smaller investigation with only three participants found that stuttering reduction varied considerably using noise at the 80-decibel (dB) level over headphones. The two clients whose stuttering was moderate to severe showed the least benefit, 30% and 49% reductions, respectively, compared to the one with mild stuttering, a 77% reduction (Andrews et al., 1982). As is the case with most of these fluency-inducing instruments, individual responses are apt to differ. Nevertheless, the large number of participants who reported a positive outcome in the Dewar et al. (1979) study is impressive. Our own experience with two adults who exhibited moderate-to-severe stuttering was positive with clients reporting considerable satisfaction, especially in conditions of pressure, such as talking in public. Perhaps the unique combination of long-term and intensive daily use (3.3 hours on average) deserves additional research attention.

Students should recall that masking noise is also used in audiological testing to prevent a non-test ear from contributing to a listener's detection of a bone-conducted sound. Considering how much noise is needed to mask the sound of speech for someone listening to oneself talking while wearing headphones, it can be predicted that by adding the volume level of speech (e.g., 55 dB) to the occlusion effect (enhanced bone conduction) from wearing headphones (e.g., 25 db) a level of about 80 dB should be an effective masking noise. Due to the Lombard effect however, the speaker will compensate by spontaneously raising the voice to a louder than expected level, by shouting if necessary, to self-monitor the act of speaking in the presence of such a loud masking noise.

Altered Auditory Feedback

Over several decades clinical researchers have experimented with DAF devices to aid speech fluency (Goldiamond, 1965; Howell, Sackin, & Williams, 1999; Shames & Florence, 1980). Such instruments did not receive much popular attention until the 1990s when they were made small enough to be inconspicuously worn in or around the ear (Kalinowski, Guntupalli, Stuart et al., 2004; Lincoln, Packman, & Onslow, 2006). A set of in-the-ear auditory feedback devices known as the SpeechEasy has been marketed widely and is reviewed here as an example of the general method. Developed by Drs. Joseph Kalinowski, Andrew Stuart, and Michael Rastatter, the patent for the SpeechEasy is owned by the East Carolina University. The SpeechEasy fits into the speaker's ear canal and is indistinguishable visually from a hearing aid. It digitally processes and transforms the speech signal so that there is both a time delay (DAF = delayed auditory feedback) and a pitch shift (FAF = frequency altered feedback). Only the speaker's self-perceptions are altered; others do not hear the sound it delivers to the speaker. Because it is usually applied to only one ear, the speaker's general listening capacities for external sounds are not disrupted.

The SpeechEasy typically is worn monaurally in the speaker's preferred ear, although binaural fittings may also be applied. The time delay is often set to either 50 or 75 milliseconds, with a maximum range up to 220 milliseconds (Antipova, Purdy, Blakeley et al., 2008). The frequency alteration may be shifted up or down at increments of a quarter, half, or one octave above or below the speaker's voice. Mostly, it is shifted either a full octave up or a half octave down. Like hearing aids, the devices are custom-designed to fit each individual's ear(s). Clients are encouraged to wear them constantly, testing the effect in all kinds of speaking situations, returning to the clinic as needed for adjustments and follow-up assessments. At the time of this writing, the cost was several thousand dollars, not including expense of accompanying clinical services.

Frequently, use of the SpeechEasy instrument is supplemented with some speech therapy. Subsequent to the initial fluency assessment and customized fitting, clients may attend several therapy sessions that train them to listen to their altered feedback, adjust their sensorimotor responses, and move past their stuttering blocks. They usually receive literature with exercises and instructions for ongoing practice of fluency skills throughout use of the device. They may be taught to use starters such as "um" or "ah" or to slightly prolong their initial sounds so they can start to hear themselves with the altered feedback (Stuart et al., 2004). Information is lacking, however, about the extent such additional strategies are needed or administered.

The developers explain the effect of the SpeechEasy in terms of its similarity to choral (unison) speech. When a speaker hears both self (via bone conduction and air conduction with the uncovered ear) and altered speech (via the device), the condition may be considered comparable to talking along in unison (or shadowing) with another speaker. Unison or shadowed speech is commonly known to induce fluency in PWS (see Chapter 4). This account offers only a conceptual analogy, however. The theory underlying the effect has not been worked out. The analogy between the SpeechEasy altered auditory feedback effect and choral reading is questionable based on clinical observations. Whereas choral reading never fails, the effect of the device varies from person to person, sometimes within the same individual.

Despite published reports of research related to this form of intervention, reasonable scientific evidence for its effectiveness is still lacking. Unfortunately, independent research did not provide reasonable support. The effect of the SpeechEasy under extra-clinical conditions during a 4-month period was evaluated with 11 stuttering adults. Speech samples were collected every 2 weeks. Qualitative data were also obtained through weekly written logs and an exit questionnaire. Although immediately after fitting of the instrument there was a statistically significant reduction in stuttering, no treatment effect was detected at the end of the 4 months. Individual responses, however, varied greatly with regard to stuttering frequency and subjective satisfaction. The investigators concluded that progress to a more advanced stage of clinical research was not justified (Pollard, Ellis, Finan et al., 2009).

Overall, then, studies have not yet revealed the proportion of individuals who will respond at the "80% to 90%" reduction rates claimed by the developers in the media and at their Web site in 2008. Research has yet to show how long the device can be expected to impact the speaker (weeks, months, or years) who hopes for a lifetime benefit. Many advertisements promise favorable outcomes. Because often the client must apply speech strategies along with the SpeechEasy, it appears likely that the speaker, not the device, still bears the weight of generating an enduring speech change.

> One of us (CS) observed video marketing and local newspaper advertisements regarding the SpeechEasy that carried a strong emotional appeal and demonstration of dramatic speech change. Ads suggest relief from stuttering merely by applying it. CS has known four people who used the device. Two experienced minimal benefit almost from the beginning, despite seeking follow-up adjustments. Two others experienced an initial decrease in stuttering to about half their pre-device level. With time, however, they acclimated to the device and, despite repeated adjustments, did not sustain long-term benefits. One returned to the pre-device level of stuttering, and the other independent of the device went on to develop his own strategies for milder stuttering. The parents of one young man had been so impressed by the device, that they became distributors. Because it was their son who returned to pretreatment stuttering levels, they abandoned their role as distributors after 2 years.

Biofeedback

Biofeedback is the delivery of information about the status or function of one's biological system through an analogous sensory signal. The sensory analog may take the form of tactile, visual, auditory, or combined modes. For example, electromyographic (EMG) biofeedback involves the placement of sensory electrodes on the skin over muscle areas of interest. An electromagnetic gel aids the conductance. When the muscles are contracted, a series of lights are illuminated and a beeping sound increases in volume and speed to reflect the level of that activity.

The effectiveness of EMG feedback for reducing stuttering frequency has been illustrated with a single-subject research design. The research demonstrated that (1) a speaker could be trained to reduce stuttering with the aid of feedback, (2) treatment could be accomplished in just 10 consecutive days, and (3) relatively lasting effects are possible (Guitar, 1975). The investigator examined the use of EMG feedback in stuttering treatment with adult PWS. Surface electrodes were applied to three sites: upper lip, jaw, and neck. Participants were trained to speak with almost resting-level muscle activity. Next, an entire treatment regimen was applied with one participant, a 32-year-old man, who learned to reduce muscle activity just before words that might be stuttered. As treatment progressed, the EMG feedback was removed so the person had to depend on his own perceptions. Stuttering frequency diminished from a mean level of 17% syllables stuttered during baseline to 1% or less with the treatment regimen. This low level was maintained at reassessments both 5 weeks and 9 months posttreatment. Some other clinical EMG studies with PWS also demonstrated relative success with both adolescents and adults (Block, Onslow, Roberts et al., 2004; Lanyon, Barrington, & Newman, 1976).

Summary of Fluency-Inducing Instruments

Several instruments have been developed to take advantage of the effect of fluency-inducing conditions. The portable devices are intended to alleviate stuttering anywhere so the speaker can focus on communication instead of the act of speaking. Nonetheless, a certain amount of attention to speaking is still required. These devices include metronome pacers, auditory maskers, auditory feedback, and biofeedback instruments. Treatments using a mechanical apparatus such as an old-fashioned desk metronome, or electrical systems like DAF or miniature noise generators, usually require some face-to-face contacts between client and clinician, limited as they may be. Devices, even if used independently of clinician contact, present problems in that they can be costly, sensitive to environmental conditions or mishandling, and require ongoing maintenance (e.g., batteries, cleaning) and repair. Individual responses to these instruments vary widely, and not infrequently effects are not sustained over time. Admittedly, we have known a few clients who were pleased by the relief provided by one device or another. Much more long-term research is necessary for each of these instruments.

Integrated Approaches

The sharp contrasts between the stuttering management and fluency-shaping approaches have not prevented clinicians from realizing potential advantages in combining elements of both into eclectic unified therapeutic programs. Both authors of this text have been involved with such endeavors during their professional careers. We have seen satisfying results with both stuttering management and fluency management procedures. Furthermore, based on decades of experience, we hold to the position that a comprehensive approach that also includes early work on facing the stuttering, identification, and attending to the emotional aspects increase the likelihood of success in subsequent speech-oriented stages of therapy involving either stuttering modification or fluency management.

Successful long-term maintenance seems to be supported by attention, in therapy, to reducing the negative emotionality associated with stuttering and increasing the client's positive feelings of self-confidence, assertiveness, and so on. We have worked with clients who formerly underwent only fluency-enhancing therapies who immediately experienced great progress that, unfortunately, proved to be intermittent, if not short lived. Fluency collapsed in situations of relatively mild pressure because they were not skilled in how to calm themselves or take charge of speech-related movements when stuttering occurred. Their well-practiced fluency-enhancing techniques, such as gentle voice onset, could not be executed under stress. We submit, however, that our clinical observations, are not substitute for well-controlled studies.

With respect to integrated therapy, in the early 1970s one of us (EY) devised and implemented selectively such a program (unpublished) that balanced the cognitive-emotional and speech domains of stuttering. It consisted of the following four components:

1. Identification and facing stuttering (bringing it out into the open)
2. Desensitization
3. Fluency-facilitating strategies
4. Stuttering modification

Specific procedures were already described in related sections of Chapter 11 and earlier in this chapter and are not repeated here. Admittedly, we have never quite made up our mind as to the question of order: Which should be introduced first, stuttering management or fluency enhancement procedures? It seems logical to begin with the positive approach of practicing fluent speech, shifting to stuttering managing techniques only when fluency fails. In practicality, however, the order has been changed depending on the client, or else techniques from both approaches have often been introduced simultaneously. Sometimes, instruments have also been used to facilitate work on fluency.

A different concept of integrated therapy was developed by the second author (CS) to merge fluency-shaping and stuttering management techniques. In this approach, fluency-facilitating behaviors (e.g., easy voice onsets, light contacts, etc.) are tailored specifically to the physical locations of tension produced by the client (e.g., easy voice onsets for glottal tension, etc.). These are employed either at the initiation of utterances (where stuttering is most apt to occur) or at the moments when stuttering occurs, as a form of pre-/in-/post-block management of saying the word. The methods are taught concurrently, not as fluency enhancement first and stuttering modification second. The fluency-facilitating behaviors are described as follows:

• Proper breath management—breathe in fully but not beyond; start exhalation just before initiating voice.

- Easy voice onsets—start voice gently with a gradual swell to appropriate loudness during the first vowel.
- Slow rate—initiate the word gradually, stretch the vowel sounds, slide on to the next word.
- Connect between words—continue voice throughout the words within a phrase, saying the phrase like it was one word; focus on moving forward to completion.
- Light articulatory contacts—gently touch the lips, tongue, and other oral structures that come together for sounds; apply minimal pressure, release gradually to glide forward to the next sound.
- Phrasing—group 3–6 syllables into a phrase; pause slightly between phrases; do not succumb to time pressure to start the next phrase right away; remember to connect between words within the phrase.

Others have developed integrated therapies that are similar to those we have described. Schwartz's treatment approach teaches clients to apply speaking skills derived from a fluency-shaping orientation but borrows modification concepts of client responsibility and desensitization counseling to address and reduce emotional reactions. Especially beneficial to student clinicians, Schwartz (1999) offers plenty of examples of exact wording that may be used when teaching clients about topics such as the speech mechanism, slow and smooth speech initiation, connecting across word boundaries, counseling related to stuttering, and more.

Some other well-known examples of integrated therapies include Guitar (2006) and Manning (2001). It is interesting that simultaneously, but independently, the ISTAR Comprehensive Stuttering Program bears a striking similarity to EY's steps. It was first published by Boberg and Kully (1985) and recently updated by Kully, Langevin, and Lomheim (2007). This intensive 3-week program is typically conducted with groups but allows for individual delivery too. The acquisition phase progresses as follows:

1. Clients begin with learning to identify stuttering and reduce tension during stuttering.
2. Fluency skills, such as prolonged vowels, and light articulatory contacts are learned.
3. After all skills are acquired, they are refined and the speech rate is increased from 40 to 60 syllables per minute (spm) to 150 to 190 spm. Skills are practiced at each rate level.
4. Clients learn stuttering modification techniques, such as post-block, in-block, and pre-block.

An important feature of the program is the constant monitoring of progress through self-rating by clients, as well as their rating by peers and clinicians regarding performance and stuttering severity. There is also an effort throughout the program to develop cognitive-behavioral skills aimed at providing knowledge about stuttering, encouraging positive thoughts, understanding feelings, and self-acceptance.

With acquisition accomplished in the first few days of therapy, a very carefully structured maintenance regimen ensures fluent speech is implemented in many situations, with a variety of listeners, as well as in more formal presentations. The program ends with equally intensive preparation for the maintenance phase posttherapy with emphasis on daily warm-up and ongoing practice once the client leaves the clinic. Clinical outcome studies of 42 adolescent and adult participants indicated that after 1 year posttreatment, 10 clients relapsed. Of the remaining 32, 69% maintained a satisfactory level of stuttering frequency (under 3%) and 7% maintained a marginally satisfactory level (3% to 6%) of stuttering (Boberg & Kully, 1994). After 2 years, 80% of the clients reported that they were satisfied with their speech.

Computer and Mass Media-Based Therapy

The past 15 years or so have seen a growing interest in developing and employing multimedia and distance therapy technologies, such as the use of video cameras (via Skype) for client-clinician interaction. One example is the Kassel Stuttering Therapy (KST) program, a computer-assisted German adaptation of fluency shaping. In one study, 400 clients completed the 2- to 3-week inpatient intensive treatment, followed by self-guided speech practice with the aid of computer software. Follow-up disfluency data in four speech situations for 1-year (n = 238), 2-year (n = 69), and 3-year (n = 69) periods remained stable between 3.2% and 3.8% syllables stuttered (Euler, Gudenberg, Jung et al., 2009). Effects were strongest for speech situations with the highest communicative demands. Relapses were mostly temporary and most frequent within the first 6 months after intensive treatment. Speaking rates and speech naturalness increased slightly.

A computer-assisted fluency program known as Modifying Phonation Intervals (MPI) has aided clients in achieving stutter-free and natural-sounding speech. Five PWS were observed to maintain success at least 1 year posttreatment (Ingham, R., Kilgo, Ingham, J., Moglia et al., 2001). The software program receives a transduced signal from a microphone worn around the client's neck that detects phonation. The frequency distribution of the various durations that the voice has been "on" (i.e., the phonation intervals or PIs) are displayed to the client on the computer monitor. Treatment involves four phases:

1. Pretreatment: Obtain baselines of the typical range and distribution of the client's phonation intervals.

2. Establishment: The client establishes stutter-free speech by reducing his or her short-interval target range of PIs by at least 50%, achieved concurrently with target naturalness ratings. Intensive practice takes place for at least a week.

3. Transfer: The client carries over the natural-sounding, stutter-free speech into "real world" assignments for at least five weeks.

4. Maintenance: The client continues to practice additional carry-over assignments separated by longer and longer time periods between tasks; for example, 2 weeks apart, 4 weeks apart, and so on, until success has been demonstrated with a 16-week period between assignments. This phase typically lasts about 9 months.

The MPI program is offered at only a few locations in the United States and Australia, but the sponsors can administer the program completely online through secure Internet access after the client obtains the necessary equipment. During transfer and mainte-nance phases, the clinicians can evaluate progress based on the digital files of recorded conversational speech that clients upload to their shared secure Web site.

Recent publications reflect a growing interest in the telepractice mode of therapy in our field (Cherney & van Vuuren, 2012), including in the area of stuttering (Carey et al. 2012). The American Speech-Language-Hearing Association (2005b) has issued a posi-tion statement on this topic.

Summary

Speech-focused therapies are intended to teach a new way of managing either stuttering events or a style of speaking fluently. In either case, the client is challenged to aban-don previous behaviors and adopt new ones: stutter easier or apply strategies to speak fluently.

Although we cited data supporting some therapy programs, much of the current clinical research has not been particularly strong according to principles discussed in Chapter 8. Research to date has yielded more support for forms of behavioral fluency shaping compared to other approaches. Speech clinicians must apply their indepen-dent professional judgment toward the selection of approaches among those that were described. It is expected that strategies and techniques will be adopted within the larger framework of a holistic process of change tailored to meet unique client needs. The fact remains that no intervention will work with all clients, and individual factors for both the client and the clinician must be incorporated into therapeutic decisions.

Approaches and strategies described in this chapter are summarized as follows:

- Identification or exploration of stuttering-related behaviors in a sequence of two steps: awareness and analysis. The discovery process does not target change itself, but establishes the foundation for eventual change.

- Modification that alters the speaker's response to a stutter event with one of three strategies: post-block modification (cancellation), in-block modification (pull-outs), and pre-block modification (preparatory sets).

- Fluency-focused approaches include fluency shaping, rhythmic speech, stretched speech, rate control therapy, and behavioral reinforcement programs. Some of these programs incorporate fluency inducing instruments such as metronome pacing, auditory masking, altered auditory feedback, and biofeedback.

- The application of instruments appears to create conditions in which speakers may talk fluently without specifically concentrating on the act of speech. Across indi-viduals, the response to such devices varies widely. Even among those who respond initially, it has not been common to see full or lasting relief without supplemental approaches.

- Speech clinicians should proceed with caution as they work with limited research evidence, and must be especially skeptical about successful treatment claims in the broadcast media.
- The era of digital, computer-aided feedback programs creates the possibility of tele-practice that is being used successfully in some locations.

Study Questions and Discussion Topics

1. What are the rationales for the identification and analysis of stutter events?
2. What are the rationales for the pause in the technique of post-block modification?
3. What are the major differences between stuttering management and fluency management approaches to stuttering intervention? Similarities?
4. What are the potential benefits and challenges associated with the use of fluency-inducing instruments for stuttering treatment?
5. What different techniques have been used to establish fluent speech in people who stutter?
6. Why is it not enough to simply establish fluent speech?
7. What different methods have been used to sustain fluent speech after it has been established?
8. What are the advantages and disadvantages of instruments in stuttering therapy?
9. What is your opinion regarding the new telepractice model of service delivery?

Suggested Readings

Guitar, B., & Peters, T. (Eds.). (2004). *Stuttering: An integration of contemporary therapies* (4th ed.). Memphis, TN: Stuttering Foundation of America.

Kully, D., Langevin, M., & Lomheim, H. (2007). Intensive treatment of stuttering in adolescent and adult. In E. Conture & R. Curlee (Eds.), *Stuttering and related disorders of fluency* (3rd ed.). New York, NY: Thieme.

Ryan, B. (2001). *Programmed stuttering therapy program for children and adults* (2nd ed.). Springfield, IL: Charles C. Thomas.

Schwartz, H. D. (1999). *A primer for stuttering therapy.* Boston, MA: Allyn & Bacon.

Van Riper, C. (1973). *The treatment of stuttering.* Englewood Cliffs, NJ: Prentice-Hall.

Chapter 13

Therapy for School-Age Children

LEARNER OBJECTIVES

Readers of this chapter will understand:

- Factors that distinguish school-age children who stutter from speakers at other ages who exhibit stuttering.
- Therapy techniques to manage the emotional and social aspects of stuttering in school-age children.
- Stuttering modification and fluency-enhancing techniques applied to school-age children.
- Methods for incorporating parents in a therapy program for school-age children.
- Current status of clinical research related to stuttering treatment for school-age children.

School-Age Children Who Stutter

Generally, the material discussed in this chapter pertains to children in the first to through sixth grades, typically ages 6 to 12. Although this is a useful frame of reference for organizational and didactic purposes, it is an arbitrary range in that some children at the lower end may be immature for their chronological age, whereas some at the upper end demonstrate advanced maturity for their age. Regardless of the extremes, it is impossible to address many issues discussed in this chapter as equally applied to first/second graders as to fifth/sixth graders. Just imagine a first-grade child and a sixth-grade child, and you will appreciate the differences. Hence you should understand that whatever is addressed here in regard to treatment of school-age children must be adjusted to the level of the individual child. Besides the relatively large age spread, there also is a relatively large spread in the length of stuttering history within the group, depending on the age at onset and the current age. For example, a fifth grader who began stuttering at age 2 presents a 9-year history, whereas a second grader who began stuttering at age 4 has only a 4-year history. Their experience with stuttering and its consequences, therefore, are quite different.

Because school-age children have stuttered for several years, their chances for natural recovery are diminished, although some may still recover (Andrews & Harris, 1964; Yairi & Ambrose, 1999a). By now, these children exhibit chronic stuttering that is more advanced in both its overt and covert manifestations, and more likely to persist for years. Therefore prior to discussing therapy, it would be sensible for clinicians to hone their knowledge of several characteristics of the stuttering disorder in school-age children and consider these factors when preparing to work with this group.

> Those whose stuttering persists constitute a small minority among other children who began stuttering at about the same time as they did, most of whom have recovered. This minority apparently possesses extra genetic components, and perhaps also is influenced by additional environmental factors that result in chronic stuttering. All of these combine to make the disorder more resistant to amelioration, either naturally, or in response to intervention. Hence the ultimate therapy prognoses are guarded and the therapeutic objectives are quite different from those set up for preschool-age children.

Awareness and Emotional Reactions

Being older, with a longer history and more developed cognition than preschoolers, the school-age child who stutters is highly aware of the stuttering (Bloodstein, 1960b) and in many cases has developed self-identification framed as "I am a stutterer." In turn, awareness of one's own stuttering is a major factor underlying the emergence of another important characteristic, a wide range of emotionality associated with the stuttered speech. It begins with feelings of frustration and embarrassment that are soon followed by much stronger reactions, such as shame and anxiety that lead to avoidance of speech. (See Chapter 4 for a more detailed discussion of the developing features of stuttering.) This emotionality also is nurtured by the heightened awareness of stuttering among the child's normally speaking peers, even at early grades as found in an experimental study (Ezrati-Vinacour et al., 2001) and in response to a communication attitude questionnaire (De Nil & Brutten, 1991; Vanryckeghem & Brutten, 1997). Some classmates react overtly by mocking and bullying the stuttering child. It is at this stage that the social impact of the disorder emerges and occupies a substantial portion of the picture. The fear and avoidance of speech, reinforced by peers and other people's reactions, can, and often does, spread to many situations, eventually leading to social withdrawal, the degree of which varies greatly.

One indication of others' attitudes is made evident in research findings showing that even speech-language clinicians working in the schools, the people who may be expected to be most understanding and accepting of children with communication disorders, hold negative stereotypes of school-age children who stutter (Yairi & Williams, 1970). All in all, a general alteration in the nature of the stuttering disorder is seen. Whereas at the very early stages, stuttering was primarily a disorder of speech difficulty, it now has become a disorder with significant emotional, social, and educational components that sometimes overshadow the speech aspect. As children advance to higher grades while they continue to stutter, more of them develop strong emotional reactions associated with stuttering (Rustin, Cook, & Spence, 1995). Furthermore, these children are likely to have little, if any, understanding of the stuttering problem, adding to the complexity of emotions that appear in conjunction with the stuttered speech. Unrealistic explanations and erroneous beliefs take root. As a child, one of us (EY) believed, perhaps correctly, that something wrong in his brain made him stutter and that if struck by lightning, his stutter would be cured. Thus he would walk in the empty streets during nights when particularly severe lightning storms brightened the sky. We worked with a second grader who, while circling his hand around his head, said in an emphatic tone that "something is wrong with my brain." Of course, children vary greatly in the speed and intensity of these new developments, which should be kept in mind as the clinician probes into the problem, planning therapy that deals with its significant variables.

Children may show complex emotional reactions to daily speaking demands at school that interfere with routine classroom tasks. Reading aloud or being called on to answer a question in class can be terrifying for a child who stutters. Fears are heightened regardless of whether the student's turn to read aloud is predictable based on seat row, or whether a "popcorn" method is applied with random student turns. Some children who stutter intentionally drop their pencils as their turns come, thus creating a distraction that "causes" them to lose their place so the teacher will move on to the next child. Others will ask to be excused to the bathroom just as their turns come up.

It is reasonable to conclude that in addition to the overt stuttered speech, treatment may, or should, tackle the negative emotionality associated with (1) moments of stuttering and (2) self-image/self-confidence, as well as (3) social distracters, employing appropriate therapeutic procedures for the child's maturity level. Case Study 13.1 illustrates the emotional and social reactions of one child.

CASE STUDY 13.1   Emotional Reactions of a School-Age Child

"As a school-age child, I (EY) had severe stuttering always hanging over my head. At times it was rather traumatic in its emotional and social impact. Progressing each year to the next grade, having new teachers and a few new children in the class with whom I had to deal (and stutter to), was repeatedly a tense period. I would be dreading the moment when 'they will find out' I stutter, especially those girls whom I happened to like. I avoided speaking in class as long as possible. Moving to another school was a real crisis for the same reasons, just twice magnified due to the larger number of new kids and teachers to meet and expose to my stuttering. When in the lower grades, I would at times cry in class when visitors, such as the principal or a supervisor, came to the classroom and it was my turn to read aloud or answer a question. Throughout school, I used to carefully select my desk location, all in consideration of my stuttering and where I would be less likely to be targeted by the teacher to answer or read, or where I could minimize the impact of the stuttering on peers. A front seat was 'dangerous' because it exposed me directly to the teacher. Also, if I stuttered, the whole class behind me would smile or laugh. A back seat was also undesirable because if I stuttered, the stuttering would thunder over the entire class in front of me. I always ended up selecting a seat in the middle of a side row, by the wall or by the window. It took weeks of constant tension in a new classroom, being anxious that I might be called upon to recite in class, until I finally felt comfortable as the teachers 'learned,' more or less, how to deal with me, and the new kids 'learned' to accept my speech. Some teachers were really good and, in my judgment, contributed significantly to my eventual success."

Overt Stuttering

Another phenomenon or a characteristic of stuttering, mentioned briefly earlier (and in Chapter 4) can be seen as the disorder persists into the school-age years. For a good number of children, there is a significant alteration in the overt stuttering. Whereas repetitions were the most common disfluency type in an earlier period, now the proportion of sound prolongations and complete blocks increases, sometimes becoming dominant. Secondary characteristics, such as facial contortions and respiratory irregularities, increase in variety, frequency, and severity. These developments also contribute to the heightened awareness and emotionality. The implications to the treatment of school-age children are clear: Direct speech therapy should be a central approach. The children are capable of understanding and handling this kind of therapy, although they may be reluctant to apply the techniques outside the clinical space. This is quite different from past controversies regarding the propriety of direct therapy treatment for preschool-age children.

Academic Performance

One possible educational impact of stuttering is in the area of reading. A common practice for assessing the reading abilities of young children is by means of reading fluency measures, such as the Dynamic Indicators of Basic Early Literacy Skills, or DIBELS (Good & Kaminski, 2002). Reading fluency tasks include naming as many letters as possible, reading as many sight words as possible, or making as many rhyming words as possible in a minute. A child's results are compared to norms to determine whether he or she is developing important early literacy skills at a typical rate. For a child who stutters, performance on such tasks may be influenced by stuttering, leading to confusion regarding whether diminished performance is due to challenges with reading or with speaking.

Other possible areas of impact can be noted across a state's public school curriculum benchmarks. Iowa's core curriculum literacy benchmarks expect children in kindergarten to grade 2 to "demonstrate control of oral delivery skills, including using appropriate volume and vocal expression and attending to rate of delivery" (Iowa Department of Education, 2008). The Virginia Department of Education's (2003) English Standards of Learning require fifth-grade students to "maintain eye contact with listeners [English 5.2(a)]," and seventh-grade students to "communicate ideas and information orally in an organized and succinct manner [English 7.1(b)]." Stuttering may interfere with a child's ability to perform according to these benchmarks, potentially limiting his or her ability to make adequate educational progress. Furthermore, children who stutter who habitually say "I don't know," even when they do know an answer because "I don't know" is easier to say, may also risk lower academic grades that do not reflect their actual skills and knowledge. One high school student we know used the "I don't know" response so frequently in her chemistry class, her lack of oral participation points lowered her overall grade in the course to a D.

Keeping an eye on a child's academic achievements, therefore, is warranted because a few studies have reported that children who stutter were several months behind the average control group in either grade placement (Schindler, 1955) or standardized academic skill tests (Williams, Melrose, & Woods, 1969). Among other reasons, it is possible that these findings reflect avoidance of class participation by children who stutter, hence teachers' reluctance to call on them, and a resultant diminished academic effort on the child's part.

The School and Home Factors

As children who stutter progress into the school setting, they are transported from the relatively limited environment of home or day-care center, with a small staff and a small group of similar-age peers, into a significantly expanded world of many children of different ages, larger number of adults, rules, more structured schedules, and so on. Although parents typically maintain centrality in a child's life, teachers and peers assume significant influence. Hence knowing the child's setting and circumstances in the class, including teachers' and peers' attitudes, can help the clinician terminate bad situations (e.g., peers imitating the child's speech). Furthermore, the clinician may be able to alter peers' attitudes in a positive way, recruiting their cooperation in protecting the child from others. As we discuss later, teacher cooperation may be employed as well in facilitating the work done in speech therapy. Therapy also should be oriented to train the child to properly handle adverse situations at school. Consideration must also be given to the setting in which treatment is delivered and its format. A child who attends speech therapy in the public school might receive shorter therapy time per week than in private settings. Not only may therapy time be shorter, public school treatment must often be conducted in groups, not in a one-on-one format. Hence the child may have fewer opportunities to practice new behaviors because treatment time is shared with other children who need opportunities to practice their own new skills.

> When speech-related attitudes are compared between school-age children who stutter and their peers who do not stutter, different trends are observed. Children who stutter tend to show decreased verbal self-confidence as they grow older, while their peers have increased self-confidence in their own verbal abilities (e.g., Vanryckeghem & Brutten, 1997). This evidence highlights the need for intervention with school-age children aimed at enhancing their sense of self-confidence in their own speaking capacities.

Although the child's world has expanded, as mentioned earlier, parents continue to play a central role in the child's life. Therefore, it is wise to consider their participation in the overall therapy program (some, however, may not be suitable for the task). This can be in the form of counseling, as well as active participation in the carryover of the therapy to home (Mallard, 1991). Parents, for example, can remind the child to use the speech strategies practiced in therapy or can conduct brief practice sessions at home (which some programs require). We strongly believe that parental involvement in the therapy, even in small ways, can substantially increase its effectiveness. Unfortunately, in single-parent homes, involvement is much more difficult to achieve. Again, such information is important to obtain and consider.

The Age Factor

Lastly in this list of characteristics, the school-age child who stutters is, in most respects, like others of the same age. For example, because children have not yet developed adult levels of cognition, the clinician's explanations of stuttering, instructions, and rationales given for therapeutic procedures, and so on, should be brief; presented in simple, concrete language; and accompanied by many visible illustrations and demonstrations. Another example is in the level of responsibility assumed in conjunction with therapy. Whereas adult clients are expected to carry out their own home assignments, such as making a set number of telephone calls each day or voluntarily entering conversation with a set number of strangers, second graders should not be expected to perform these kinds of assignments.

Motivation also may be problematic. Whereas adults refer themselves to therapy, young children are referred and brought by parents or identified during school screenings. Although the child who stutters wants to speak better, other attractions (e.g., extracurricular sports activities) compete with attending speech therapy after school. The decisions associated with activity selections often present major dilemmas for parents. Most parents want their child in therapy, hoping to diminish the amount and impact of stuttering before the child gets any older. At the same time, they see the value of their child having a variety of interests and skills and the importance of other activities to their child's self-esteem. In an ideal world, the child does both, but in reality parents sometimes have to choose between the Tuesday-Thursday speech therapy sessions and the Tuesday-Thursday baseball league. There is no one right answer; the best decision will be different for each individual.

Prognosis and Objectives for Therapy

Why Is Stuttering in School-Age Children Difficult to Treat?

The literature on stuttering includes many opinions advocating clinical intervention soon after stuttering onset, typically during the preschool period (e.g., Ingham & Cordes, 1998). The main argument put forward by these scholars and clinicians is that difficulty achieving a cure, or even appreciable progress in stuttering therapy by the time a child enters school, stems from the failure to provide early intervention. They go on to argue that by the time children reach school age, they have bypassed the window of brain plasticity that would have enabled therapy to cause changes in brain processes responsible for speech. Thus stuttering becomes less amenable to treatment. Indeed, clinicians have concluded from experience that it is much more difficult to achieve successful treatment with this age group (also with adults) as compared with reported successes for preschool-age children (e.g., Conture, 2001; Ward, 2006).

If the assertion that school-age children do not respond to stuttering therapy as readily as preschool children is valid, as we believe it is, we hold to a different explanation. In our opinion, the prognosis for school-age children, like that for adults (see Chapter 8), must take into account the critical role of the epidemiological factors that contributed to the persistent form of stuttering. As explained in Chapter 3, school-age children are a small minority (25%, perhaps as small as 15%) of the original population who began stuttering about the same time. This minority failed to exhibit the natural recovery experienced by 75% or more of their stuttering peers. Recent research in genetics (see Chapter 7) has shown that genetics is an important factor underlying natural recovery and chronic stuttering. Hence the difficulties encountered in treating stuttering in school-age children may simply reflect a genetically based, tenacious, more robust, resistant form of stuttering: a different subtype of the disorder. Quite likely, it would have resisted therapy if provided in early years, an assumption supported by the findings that almost all preschool participants in the large Illinois project who persisted did receive therapy (Yairi & Ambrose, 2005). Therefore, the idea that treatment difficulty in school-age children is the fault of negligence to treat them earlier as young children, and that these difficulties should be assigned to lost brain plasticity previously available lacks in any evidence. Furthermore, not only does it fail to recognize the role of genetics, it could have some negative effects as well. First, it places undue pressure to begin treatment as early as possible after onset, when actually it might not be necessary in view of the high rate of natural recovery during that period. Second, if clinicians fail to appreciate that school-age children who stutter present a genetically different subtype of stuttering that is inherently more resistant, it may cause an unjustified sense of failure in clinicians, parents, and clients alike and promote misguided, unrealistically high therapeutic objectives. This also can contribute to clinicians' perceptions that they are "bad" at stuttering therapy, which can lead to negative attitudes toward children who stutter as a group.

Therapy Alternatives and Objectives

Both Van Riper (1973) and Williams (1971) noted that therapy for the school-age child who stutters frequently takes the form of adult therapy with some modifications. We agree that, in general, therapeutic objectives similar to those set out for adults also may be applied to school-age children who stutter. The main difference between therapy for the two groups is not so much in the objectives but in the procedures employed that are adapted to the child's level. As discussed in Chapter 10, there are three major alternatives to consider when setting up long-term therapeutic objectives for stuttering: increased fluency, reduced stuttering, and improved emotional and social adjustment. We are of the opinion that all three should be incorporated, or at least considered, in formulating the objectives for the individual client. For many years, we have practiced comprehensive therapy programs that incorporate these different major approaches.

Under the increased fluency alternative, two subcategories, *naturally fluent* speech and *deliberate fluent* speech, were listed. It has been shown experimentally that it is possible for preschool-age children who stutter to achieve naturally fluent speech that is indistinguishable from that of normally speaking peers (Finn, Ingham, Ambrose et al., 1997). This outcome also entails that the child feels, thinks, and behaves like normally speaking individuals. Unfortunately, close scientific examination of the normalcy of posttherapy speech in school-age children has not been documented. Although achieving naturally fluent speech patterns and all the psychological domains of normal speaking might be possible for school-age children,[1] particularly in lower grades, it is very difficult to erase the self-concept of a "stutterer" and the feeling that stuttering is still there, just waiting to resurface. We feel, therefore, that achieving *deliberately fluent* speech is a more reasonable initial objective. The tenacity of stuttering by this age means that for a fairly long time, fluency will be consciously "controlled" and self-monitored. The child will have to exercise a form of mental and behavioral activity to maintain fluency, which can be daunting at any age.

The idea behind the <u>third alternative</u>, producing more acceptable overt stuttering, is quite different. Here, <u>the client does not strive to be fluent but strives to be able to man-</u><u>age speech movements during stuttering events, movements that yield milder, smooth</u><u>stuttering that is more acceptable to listeners</u> (Van Riper, 1973). Lastly, improved <u>adjustment pertains to changing the broad spectrum of emotional and social behaviors</u> related to speaking. This includes helping the child carefully confront a variety of difficult speaking situations, respond to and cope with potential teasing, and, above all, choose to continue to communicate even when stuttering. Such changes are important in strengthening the client's ability to either work on fluency or on modifying stuttering. Additionally, reducing emotionality also may result in less frequent stuttering as a by-product.

Clinicians should attempt to strike a <u>careful balance</u> between encouraging the goal of <u>easier,</u> <u>smooth speech</u> along with fostering a positive emotional self-acceptance of experiences with <u>stuttering.</u> This balance is important because if a premium is placed on attaining fluency, the child may infer that his or her stuttering is unacceptable and be apt to develop behaviors that merely suppress stuttering. Suppression may be evident, for example, if after a few weeks of therapy, the SLD have significantly decreased, but the Other Disfluencies, such as interjected "ums," have increased. It is best therefore to conduct therapy in the safe environment where stuttering and its modification are acceptable by the clinician at the same time that strategies for fluent speech are explored and practiced.

Speaking partner behavioral adjustments commonly applied during intervention with preschool children are also appropriate with school-age children. Both the clinician and parents can serve as <u>role models of a slower, relaxed approach to talking,</u> of <u>appropriate pausing and phrasing,</u> of frequent easy initiations of speech, and of showing

---

[1]It has been reported that speech therapy can alter the brain waves of people who stutter (e.g., De Nil et al., 2001). The author (EY) believes future advances with medical treatments may yield an increasing number of complete cures.

restraint from interruptions and simultaneous talking.[2] A blend of these environmental support strategies can be combined with the direct instruction offered in treatment sessions. When a school-age child does not have firmly entrenched avoidance habits, objectives designed to prevent or reduce avoidance may be appropriate. The child can be encouraged to go ahead with talking whether stuttering occurs or not, in safe environments created by the clinician and supportive speaking partners, to counteract the natural inclinations to hold back or struggle against the act of speech. Treatment objectives for school-age children otherwise do not differ substantially from those set for adults. For example, objectives may be set for the child to learn about speech and stuttering, to reduce negative emotionality associated with stuttering, to develop assertiveness and self-confidence, to identify and modify stuttering, and/or to facilitate fluency-related skills. The main difference between therapy for adults and school-age children lies in the procedures employed to achieve these objectives and the cognitive and linguistic sophistication of the discussions held between the clinician and child. Of considerable importance, particularly for school-age children, is to promote and encourage appropriate forms of support in the child's home and school environments. Like adults, every child's needs will be different, and so therapy must be individualized.

School-based clinicians may be familiar with the phrase "adversely affects educational performance" (from IDEA: Individuals with Disabilities Education Act, 1997), a key criterion indicating whether children who stutter are eligible to receive speech therapy. Unfortunately, the widely recognized phrase is often misunderstood. Some have interpreted it to mean that stuttering must adversely affect a child's grades in order for the student to be eligible for treatment. This, however, is not the case. The 2004 reauthorization of IDEA actually increased the accessibility of services for children who stutter by emphasizing not only academic performance or speech characteristics but also how stuttering affects other aspects of the child's life. Therefore, school-based clinicians should broaden their focus to consider not only the academic issues but also the academic setting. Under IDEA 2004,[3] the academic setting is defined as encompassing regular education classrooms, other education-related settings, and extracurricular and nonacademic activities. This means that not only should the impact of the child's stuttering on performance in the classroom be considered, but also how it impacts success with communication at recess, on the school bus, at lunchtime, and in interactions with peers during school-sponsored clubs and activities. This broader view of the educational impact of stuttering allows for inclusion of a variety of goals in a child's treatment, such as improving communication attitudes, reducing negative reactions to stuttering, educating people in the child's environment, and minimizing the overall impact of the child's stuttering in many domains.

---

[2]Involving parents as role models has a dual purpose: Parents are less apt to adopt unreasonable expectations of their child's ongoing deliberate fluency control when they have attempted ongoing speech changes of themselves and appreciate how difficult the endeavor actually is.

[3]For more information on IDEA 2004, visit http://idea.ed.gov/explore/home.

Too often, school-based speech-language clinicians have set up goals for a child who stutters aimed at the elimination of the stuttering. Because of the persistent nature of stuttering in this population, defining therapeutic success only in terms of decreasing overt speech characteristics, clinicians run into failure of their own making while also overlooking important areas where they can help the child in meaningful ways, such as developing more helpful attitudes about communication that lessen the social impact of the disorder. With the school-age population, what is the success rate for getting children who stutter to be normally fluent all the time? Likely, it is not very high.

> If we use a broad definition of the disorder, taking into account a child's overall communication experience, therapy can be much more successful. In other words, if the stuttering disorder extends beyond speech, then treatment should be more than just speech-focused. Throughout the therapeutic process, parents and teachers need to understand that progress is not measured only in terms of fluency. As with adults, we hold that clinicians should be open to a child's individual needs and capabilities. Hence, they should consider methods for dealing with emotional aspects, modifying stuttering, and enhancing fluency. Sometimes all three may, or even should, be integrated. Goals that are included on a student's Individualized Education Plan should reflect this view.

Goals designed to lower the intensity of a child's negative attitudes, as well as decreasing the behavioral and cognitive reactions that accompany stuttering, are essential to the creation of a broad-based approach toward stuttering management. For example, goals such as "stuttering easily, strengthen self-confidence, and feel good about self" are, in our opinion, more desirable than just "no stuttering and using easy onsets." School-age children who stutter often are relieved to hear this, although parents and teachers may have more difficulty accepting the projection that the child will continue to stutter. This is another reason why parent counseling and education of school personnel are such important components to school-age stuttering therapy.

Another issue in stating goals is the criteria sought to achieve them. In speech-language pathology, many goals for clients, regardless of the disorder, are stated using a percentage-based metric (e.g., "client will do . . . 80% of the time"). Although this structure is legitimate for use in generating goals for a school-age child who stutters, clinicians also should consider other forms of measurement. One way is to develop a list of achievements a child can pursue along a hierarchy from easier to harder situations. For example, if the child's goal is to be able to educate others about stuttering, it does not make sense to state that the child should be able to do this 80% of the time. Instead, the clinician could document that the child can demonstrate the skill in a variety of settings, such as with a teacher, a peer, or parents. A criterion for this type of activity might be written as an all-or-none achievement, such as "the child will educate three individuals about stuttering." If the child does it, a check mark is made, indicating success; if the child has not done it, then no check. Using this method, both clinician and child can see the level of progress by counting up the number of checks on the goal chart, comparing it to the total number of situations listed in the hierarchy. Another example of an alternative measurement criterion may be used for documenting changes in a child's fear or anxiety about a particular speaking situation. The clinician can ask the child to rate the intensity of his or her fear/anxiety before and after entering the situation using a self-rating system on a 1 to 10 scale. The criterion could then be set to a change in self-rating of 2 or more points.

Home and School Environments

Although the school-age child's world is an ever-expanding experience beyond home and family, parents still constitute a major component of that world and should be included in the therapy if at all possible. The physical conditions, however, present challenges. Because most schoolchildren in need receive speech therapy on the school's premises during regular hours, parents are not the ones bringing them in, nor are they present after the session as is the case with many preschool children. Hence the clinician's opportunities for contact with parents are greatly diminished. Furthermore, mothers of school-age children are more likely to work outside the home than mothers of preschool-age children, a fact that also limits their availability. Recognizing the difficulties, all efforts should be made to have at least one or two meetings with a child's parents early in the program, as well as maintaining at least some periodic contact throughout via brief written or e-mail (if available) notes sent to the home. Because the home environment is explored through parent counseling, attention should be given to three objectives: (1) providing information about stuttering, (2) venting parents' feelings, and (3) reduction of interfering factors.

Counseling Parents

Information about Stuttering

We first probe parents concerning knowledge about stuttering that they may have acquired from various sources, such as the Internet, newspaper articles, relatives, doctors, and others. Misinformation should be dispelled, followed by a brief presentation of the essential state-of-the-art information. One pair of parents suspected that their child stuttered as punishment for *their* misbehavior, an inaccurate tax report. One father was convinced that his child stuttered to annoy him. Responding to the most frequently asked question, "What causes stuttering?" the clinician proceeds by presenting the main theoretical views about stuttering: (a) psychological, (b) learning, (c) organic, and (d) multiple causation, succinctly explaining each one. In this context, it is useful to point out that research has not provided reasonable support to the psychological and learning theories as the cause, although the two factors do play an important role in the further development and maintenance of the disorder. For example, emotional reactions often become an important part of the disorder *after* it has begun. These emotional components are the result of stuttering, not the cause of it as laypeople and some health professionals, such as pediatricians, tend to believe (Yairi & Carrico, 1992). Moreover, recent research findings have implicated intricate neurological and motor components. These data, combined with information about the genetic bases of stuttering, should serve to alleviate possible parental guilt feelings, blaming their behavior as the cause of the stuttering.

Additional information about the variability of stuttering, what may trigger ups and downs in its frequency, and the emotional and social implications of stuttering should be provided. Many parents are aware mostly of the overt stuttering. Because many, if not most, schoolchildren rarely share their concerns about stuttering with parents, and because parents often feel uncomfortable asking, they have a vague, or no, idea of the devastating emotional components of the disorder. They may not know, for example, that their child sits tense during class, dreading being called to answer a question or recite something, that he fears the ringing telephone at home, or that she suffers mockery by a few kids in school. Some parents were utterly shocked to discover situations like these when watching behind a two-way mirror as their child conversed with us.

The fact that environment plays a substantial role in the shaping and maintenance of stuttering should be used to advise parents that they can create more favorable conditions at home that might improve the child's life. Later on, they may be asked to contribute in other ways to the therapy program. Simple suggestions for reducing undue stressful communication demands on the child, avoiding or minimizing other unnecessary pressures at home, stopping parents' and/or siblings' negative responses to stuttering, reviewing and alleviating other stressful family interaction patterns, and concrete suggestions for how to handle the child's moments of stuttering should be offered and discussed. It is also wise to teach and encourage parents to notice when their child is communicating well, such as telling a funny story, finishing a difficult word, being polite, or taking conversational turns. Focusing on desired communication behaviors is as important as focusing exclusively on stuttering, so that the child develops awareness of what he or she needs to do to be a good communicator whether stuttering or not. Because this may be a rare opportunity for having face-to-face communication with one or both parents, a brief and simple presentation of only several key suggestions is recommended.

Attending to Parents' Feelings

Having lived with a child's stuttering for several years, some parents may have toned down the initially strong emotional reactions they had at the time of onset. They may have become accustomed to hearing their child's abnormal speech and try not to call negative attention to it. It does not mean, however, that they are at peace with the handicap—nor does it mean that strong emotions will not resurface. It's not uncommon for parents to become highly anxious or upset when important life events present themselves, such as the child transitioning from elementary to middle school, because communication demands can be quite different. Other life events that may cause parents anxiety include religious rituals such as confirmation or a bar mitzvah, making a speech to earn Eagle Scout status, or trying out for a school play. Being worried about the social consequences of stuttering, parents may have become highly protective. Parents naturally want what is best for their child; they do not want him or her to experience the pain or shame of stuttering. Protectiveness may lead to limiting social interactions for those children who stutter, speaking for them in public places, and making decisions about social arrangements based on the stuttering. They (parents) may develop compensatory habits themselves, stepping in to bridge the gap for the child's difficulty initiating communication. Because public stuttering may bring pain and embarrassment to parents and family as well as the child, their nonverbal behaviors and management of situations may send a strong message that stuttering is a stigma. But the problem is that the message to "avoid stuttering" will thereby suggest "avoid communicating." The child's avoidance of communication is worse than openly stuttering. Neither the family nor the child may realize they are taking this path.

Our clinical experience has shown that many parents of school-age children remain concerned about the stuttering, disappointed in their hopes for recovery, frustrated by their inability to help and/or by unsuccessful treatment, concerned about the child's current suffering as well as his or her future (e.g., career), and sometimes continue to harbor guilt feelings about their possible contribution to the disorder. DiLollo and Manning (2007) noted that parents of children who continue to stutter can exhibit many grieving reactions, such as denial, anger, and depression. Therefore, within the limited opportunities available for interacting with parents, spending a portion of the time to allow them to express their feelings certainly is beneficial. It also provides the clinician with insight into the child's more intricate and intimate home environment and the kind of cooperation that might be possible to gain from parents. A few simple questions are often sufficient to facilitate this avenue. Some of these may have been discussed as part of the initial evaluation if the parents participated. We have found these or similar questions enable most parents to talk at length, for example:

- What happened when stuttering began?
- What did you think caused it?
- How did you react then?
- How do you feel about it now?
- What kind of a child is your son/daughter? Tell me about his/her personality, strengths, and weaknesses.
- Does he/she spend time with friends?

As DiLollo and Manning (2007) suggested, the next goal is to encourage parents to redirect their emotional energy from grieving toward involvement in the treatment and supporting the child. Parental participation in a support group, if one is accessible, can facilitate understanding and support for the child (Manning, 2001). Parents are more apt to listen to the clinician and apply her practical suggestions if the clinician has developed sufficient rapport first, providing supportive listening and ample opportunity for venting of emotions.

Interfering Factors

Another objective to pursue with parents is the identification of factors that might interfere with, or facilitate, progress. This can be achieved by directing a few questions that probe relations among the family members, such as:

- How do your spouse and other children react to the stuttering?
- How do the children get along?
- Do you talk about the stuttering at home?
- Do you and your spouse agree on how to handle the child's stuttering?
- Generally, how are things at home these days?

As is the case with preschoolers, parents of school-aged children can enhance the child's progress by offering a number of practical support strategies at home. Research indicates that communication partners can support fluent speech with several behaviors: slowing the pace of their conversational speech, following rules of conversational turn-taking (i.e., not interrupting), and delaying their conversational responses (Bernstein Ratner, 2004). Perhaps more than anything else, just encouraging their child to go ahead and express what he or she wants to say, even if there is stuttering, is the most important type of support parents can offer. Providing an environment in which the child feels free to talk openly about his or her speech and stuttering is another important way parents can support their child. Parents are often unsure that talking openly about stuttering with their child is a good idea. This is where a clinician can be especially helpful to the family. Schoolteachers as well as parents can be apprised of these strategies.

Teachers and Peers

If you talk with adults who stutter about their experiences in elementary school as children who stutter, you may hear different stories about encounters with schoolteachers. Although some are remembered as being sensitive, understanding, and supportive, others are remembered for responses to stuttering that caused pain. Examples of the latter are anecdotes about teachers who made a child put marbles in his mouth or who stood by passively when peers mocked or laughed. Even when an infraction is minor and the teacher meant well, the pain of embarrassment or unfair treatment can be indelibly etched in a child's memory. These memorable responses by teachers can come from opposite sides of the coin, either circumstances for talking were unusually spotlighted or the child was unfairly deprived of an opportunity to speak. The findings of two studies illustrate some of the potential problems in the school environment. The first one asked school speech-language clinicians to assign adjectives to children who stutter, resulting in a list of rather negative personality descriptors and other unfavorable characteristics (Yairi & Williams, 1970). More than two decades later, a group of investigators used similar methods targeting schoolteachers with similar results: Teachers hold a predominantly unfavorable, stereotypic view of the characteristics of children who stutter (Lass et al., 1992).

To help teachers and children avert these potential unpleasant experiences and painful memories, it is vitally important for clinicians to educate teachers and school personnel about stuttering. Teachers need to know about the need to check in with a child who stutters privately regarding the types of talking opportunities she or he will be comfortable with in school. They need to know that the child often wants and needs to talk even if he or she stutters, but they also need to be sensitive to averting talking circumstances that can be emotionally threatening. Having reached an understanding with the child, possible ways to facilitate class participation initially might be to ask the child questions that require short answers or to have the child demonstrate on the whiteboard step-by-step solutions to math problems that can be done with minimal talking demands. Besides, it is quite likely that if the child talks while writing on the board, there will be no stuttering. They also may reach an understanding that the child will not be asked to read aloud to the whole class, if the child so wishes. Use of simple cues, such as the child raising a closed hand to indicate "I know the answer, but please don't call on me," versus an open hand to indicate "I know the answer and would like to be called on," can be negotiated by the teacher and child so that the child is encouraged to participate to the degree that feels safe. Teachers (or adults, parents, etc.) should *not* make a unilateral decision to exclude a child from a speaking task without checking in with the child. The speech clinician needs to communicate with teachers and parents about the level of participation appropriate to the child's progress with therapy, and facilitate, with all involved, a hierarchy that moves the child toward greater classroom communication at a rate that keeps fear at a minimum.

Teachers need to understand the nature of the potential anxiousness that can build up prior to being called on, before having to say one's name, or when expected to take a turn talking in front of peers. This may be one of the difficult things to achieve because most people simply are unaware of the strong emotional component of stuttering. The teacher needs to appreciate his or her important role to instruct peers not to laugh at or tease or think less of the child who stutters. Teachers should be educated about the general objectives of the therapy program and the general procedure. When therapy is focused on certain behaviors (e.g., pullouts or gentle voice onset), a cooperative teacher is in a position to provide reinforcement, although not in front of the class. Teachers also may be advised that stuttering can be addressed in the class within units on diversity. Everyone has different characteristics, and how one talks is just one such difference, like height, weight, or skin color. A number of available curricular programs for preventing teasing and bullying apply to all students in a classroom, not just the student who stutters.

The speech clinician also needs to ensure that teachers and other school personnel are provided with basic facts about stuttering. They need to know that children can be very intelligent and still stutter and that periods of fluency do not mean the child has an ability to control or stop stuttering from occurring. It is important to dispel the misguided popular folklore that has been passed around, like the belief that stuttering was caused by the parents. School personnel need to have their questions answered, such as: "Can I look directly at the child when he talks, or is that apt to make him stutter more?" Teachers should also feel confident that if they have a question about how to handle a given situation with a specific child, that it's OK to talk with that child about his or her wishes. Here is our brief information sheet that clinicians may hand to teachers (and other school personal) who have a child who stutters in their class.

Children Who Stutter: Basic Information and Advice for Teachers

1. Most children begin stuttering between ages 2 and 4. The school-age child who stutters (CWS) has had several years of unpleasant experiences with the disorder.

2. Stuttering is not a "bad habit." Although the specific cause is not known, it is related to genetics but also is very sensitive to environmental forces, such as pressure and people's reactions to it.

3. The disorder afflicts the child in several ways, with the two most important being (a) the observable speech difficulties, and (b) the strong emotional reactions, often hidden, especially shame and intense fears of talking that lead to avoidance. If asked a question in the class, the CWS may reply, "I do not know" just because he or she is afraid of stuttering in front of the other children. The child's apprehension can rise substantially just anticipating that he or she will be asked to recite orally. An experience of severe stuttering in class may cause devastation for several days.

4. Aside from the overt stuttering and emotions associated with it, research has shown that CWS, as a group, are similar to children who do not stutter in nearly all other respects (e.g., personality and intelligence).

5. Children who stutter may experience serious difficulties when they move to a new school and face a new teacher and new peers who become acquainted with the fact that they stutter. They may feel extremely embarrassed, especially at the beginning of the year when their stuttering is first "exposed." The first 2 to 3 weeks are especially critical for teachers to be understanding and provide support and comfort to the child.

6. The testimonies of many CWS and their parents indicate that the teacher's understanding and cooperation can be critical to emotional experiences in school in ways that the speech-language clinician may be unable to impact. The most important areas where teachers can help are (a) peers' reactions toward the child who stutters, (b) class participation, and (c) cooperation and support (to varying degrees) with the speech therapy.

7. Not infrequently, the CWS is the subject of mockery, sometimes bullying. A single inconsiderate classmate can make life miserable for the child. The teacher should be alert to this possibility. You may observe such peers' behavior or you may learn about it through an open talk with the CWS. The offender should be confronted and counseled individually. Also, you may explain to the whole class about the damage that such behavior might inflict. The class discussion should occur when the CWS is absent from the classroom.

8. In regard to the child's verbal participation in class, it is best to have an open discussion with him or her privately and come to an agreement as to the desired type and frequency of oral recitation. For example, the child may prefer to respond to questions that call for brief answers but not like to read aloud. Alternatively, or additionally, solving math problems on the whiteboard could

be a desired mode of participation, for example. Teachers also may call on the child early before anxiety builds too much or when they know the child has the answer to the question.

9. There are several conditions in which the CWS typically experiences fluent speech. For example, singing, talking in chorus, talking in rhythm, timing some movement with talking, speaking in a different dialect, high or low pitch, whispering, and so on. These can be used to allow participation in plays and other class projects involving verbal performance.

10. Teachers can contribute substantially to the success of speech therapy in ways that require minimal time. As the child practices various ways of changing speaking behaviors in therapy, such as maintaining eye contact, slowing down, or reducing tension during a stuttered word, some feedback in class is important. You can employ two or three agreed-upon nonverbal signals (e.g., one as a reminder to the child to use the technique, one for reinforcement of good performance, etc.). Again, this should be discussed with the child and the speech-language clinician.

Additional information for teachers may be found in several other sources:

Rind, P., & Rind, E. (1988). *The stutterer in the classroom: A guide to the teacher.* New Rochelle, NY: Stuttering Resource Foundation. Found at http://www.isastutter.org/CDRomProject/teacher/stutter_classroom.html
Scott, L. (2008). *The child who stutters at school: Notes to the teacher.* Memphis, TN: Stuttering Foundation of America. Found at http://www.stutteringhelp.org/sites/default/files/Migrate/tips_for_teachers4_08.pdf
Stammering Association. Information for teachers found at http://www.stammering.org/teachers_info.html

Therapy: Explaining Stuttering

As mentioned earlier, what is happening during stuttering is somewhat of a mystery to most people who stutter, certainly to children. Whereas some clinicians prefer a narrow therapeutic path, such as reinforcing fluency (e.g., the GILCU or Lidcombe methods described later in the chapter) we present here a comprehensive approach. An early goal to pursue in therapy is providing the child with a reasonable understanding of the stuttering in the context of speech production in general (Williams, 1971). Some of the ways that this objective can be accomplished are described next.

The Speech System

Using a simple three-dimensional model or a good-sized diagram of the upper body, the clinician explains the sequence of events that result in speech: inhaling air, exhaling it through the two vocal folds ("voice box") that vibrate to produce voice, continuing upward into the throat and mouth. The air forces its way out through a series of moving parts in the mouth, such as the tongue, lips, and jaw, that results in many other speech sounds, depending on the shape and postures of these structures. The emphasis is on the continuous, smooth movement that characterizes normal speech. This can be demonstrated by the clinician as she or he talks, highlighting the ongoing movement of the lips, jaw, and tongue (Guitar, 2014; Williams, 1971). Simple and descriptive terms can be applied, such as the *speech helpers* suggested by Runyan and Runyan (2007).

What Can Go Wrong with the Speech System?

The clinician may count on the probability that many schoolchildren have had opportunities to observe babies as they start learning to talk by uttering many repetitions and stretching sounds and syllables (i.e., babbling), to eventually mastering short words and brief phrases. These disfluencies are normal. Many older children and adults continue to occasionally hesitate when talking or repeat and stretch sounds and syllables. This too is normal. We do not know why, but some children begin repeating and prolonging much more than the usual and also with much more tension. This is different. This kind of speech is made worse when the person becomes concerned about the repetitions and prolongations, gets even more uptight, and tries to force the words out by tensing up the speech muscles in many places (point to them in the diagram). The more one tenses, the more difficult it becomes for the speech system to move smoothly. *This is what stuttering is.* It is the tensing and forcing that causes much of the stuttering and the unpleasant feeling of getting stuck. In other words, an emphasis is placed on the idea that children are making talking harder for themselves. They need to go ahead and let themselves talk instead of investing so much energy fighting the stuttering. This also is an opportunity to point out other activities in which children are engaged that do not go well or even fail when the child gets panicked and uses excessive tension attempting to get out of it (e.g., activities like learning how to ride a bicycle or swim). Tensed, panicked, disorganized movement is what makes swimmers feel they are drowning.

Experimentation

At this point, the child is encouraged to experiment with speaking behaviors that actually make talking difficult or impossible altogether. For example, inhale, then tighten the throat on purpose, then attempt to speak. Nothing comes out, neither air nor speech. Similarly, the child is asked to speak while purposely pressing the lips together, or talk while forcing the tongue against the hard palate. This is what Dean Williams (1971) wisely referred to as *hard speech*. Next, proceeding with additional experimentation, the opposite concept, *easy speech*, is soon brought into play by asking the child to first say a word the hard way and then say it again easily, without physical tension.

The difference between *hard speech* and *easy speech* also can be illustrated with non-speech behaviors, say by asking the child to shake hands "really hard" and then do it again easily, gently, and slowly. Several comparisons of hard and easy speech are practiced. Children thus gain some insight into their own contribution to the stuttering and also may begin realizing that they can do something about it. Overall, such demonstration and experimentation are practical ways to help children comprehend more abstract explanations of the problem of stuttering that the clinician provides. The fact that they can change from hard to easy speech also might help in reducing the upheaval that the child often experiences during stuttering. At this point, limited practice is sufficient. At a later stage in the therapy, when the program is focused on identification and speech modification, much more extensive practice will be resumed.

The process of strengthening a client's learning by contrasting two opposing behaviors is called *negative practice*. In fluency therapy, the experience of flexibly performing the *hard speech* versus the *easy speech* highlights the parameters of the easy speech that the child is endeavoring to learn. The procedure is similar to the negative practice employed in articulation therapy, when a child is required to contrastively produce a target phoneme in both the incorrect and correct ways to enhance learning of the new skill.

Therapy: Focus on Emotional Reactions

School-age children who stutter present a wide range of emotions reacting to, and resulting from, stuttering. Clinicians, however, should exercise caution against undue generalization. Just because a child stutters, does not mean he or she necessarily possesses strong reactions; some children show no hesitation responding to, or initiating, telephone calls, whereas others make themselves disappear as soon as the phone rings. Smith (1999) referred to this as the nonlinearity of the stuttering problem. Making assumptions about a child's emotional reactions based on the severity of the speech behavior should be avoided. We knew one child whose overt stuttering was approximately 4%, typically regarded as very mild in severity. Her speech was smooth and natural and only occasionally disrupted by brief repetitions. This child, however, was terrified to be called on in class and would engage in a number of avoidance strategies, such as asking to go to the bathroom if she anticipated the teacher was going to ask her a question. Another child who presented with severe stuttering, including long blocks and visible facial tension, always volunteered to be the reporter for his small groups during class projects. Hence some prior probing of this domain is warranted. If problems are identified, a comprehensive stuttering treatment program should address them in a direct manner, in addition to whatever other approach(es) are pursued to address speech patterns. This is an example of a therapeutic objective that is similar to that encountered in adult therapy. The question, however, is how this objective can be best accomplished with children.

As suggested earlier, a milder (less aggressive) approach is applied in multiple ways: simple presentation of the problem and the therapy objective(s), use of concrete instead of abstract language, and avoidance of lengthy abstract explanations but use of ample meaningful examples, simplified procedures, and demands that are not too challenging. As with adults, we advocate a two-pronged approach when working on the emotional aspect. One approach is aimed at diminishing negative emotionality by means of desensitization. The second approach is aimed at increasing positive self-perception and assertiveness.

Adapted Desensitization Activities

Applying a milder approach, particularly with children in lower grades for whom desensitization is deemed necessary, procedures should not require a child to enter boldly into unpleasant or challenging situations as is sometimes employed with adults. For example, an 8-year-old should not be asked to go up to a stranger and hold on to a stutter for seconds while attempting to remain calm. Van Riper (1973) has commented that the *systematic desensitization* technique is not particularly useful with schoolchildren. For early steps, exposure to stuttering identification techniques is useful, such as having the child identify *hard speech* events made purposefully by the clinician, or in video or audio speech samples that the clinician recorded of his or her own speech. Van Riper (1973) also recommended that clinicians put stuttering in their own mouth for various purposes. These activities begin with exposure to mild-to-moderate rather than severe stuttering. If the child is ready to describe the feelings, reactions are elicited and discussed. Videos of other children and adults who stutter that are available for purchase as part of various clinical programs also are very useful for this purpose (e.g., *Stuttering: For Kids by Kids,* distributed by the Stuttering Foundation of America). Besides providing greater exposure to stuttering, selecting video samples of gradually more severe stuttering helps make the point that the child is not alone in stuttering. Children also may find comfort from age-appropriate literature containing characters who stutter. An example is the Mary Maroney book series by Suzy Kline in which the main character is a second-grade girl who stutters. Another is found in a story about a squirrel who stutters who learns about self-respect in *Stuttering Stan Takes a Stand* by Artie Knapp. (A list of children's literature that deals with stuttering can be found at http://www.mnsu.edu/comdis/kuster/Bookstore/childrensbooks.html)

Because a sense of isolation is one of the most difficult aspects of stuttering, finding videos of children, even older children who stutter, who talk about their experiences can be helpful. If a group therapy experience is possible, it too can help in this regard. (A range within one or two grades among group members seems to work best.) As the children converse, or as each speaks in turn about a given topic, the rest of the group signals the moments when the speaker stutters but without any expectation that speech should be changed. Typically, this activity is rather entertaining to the children, creating a feeling that should reduce the pain of stuttering. "Playing" with stuttering behaviors, being willing to voluntarily produce some stuttered speech in the accepting clinical environment, with the clinician's participating in the activity, helps create an atmosphere of openness and also is desensitizing in that it makes the children feel more comfortable with stuttering (Healey et al., 2004; Ramig & Bennett, 1997). This type of relaxed handling of stuttering is expected to be partially transformed into more calm reactions during genuine speaking situations when stutter events occur. As a contrasting activity, it has been suggested that children, especially in a group, may be asked to compete in a demonstration of the "most possible stuttering." Because of the artificiality involved, this tends to be an amusing and fun activity that, again, provides the child with experiences of stuttering without pain—the objective of desensitization (Emerick, 1970).

After several sessions, desensitization proceeds into more sensitive materials with the children being asked to share experiences they have had with adults or peers who have made fun of them. This more serious issue could be more difficult for some children and should be handled carefully. As often is the case, however, when a person talks about what hurts, the hard feelings subside. The aim of sharing their experiences is to express and release emotional tensions rather than bottling them up inside. Many other procedures have been suggested, such as telling jokes about stuttering. Another one presents the child with brief descriptions of several situations, accompanied with illustrating drawings, each involving a child who stutters and listeners. For each, the child is to select one of several listed emotional descriptors—shame, disappointment, fear, anger, pride, triumph, and confidence—in order to describe what the person in the situation feels (Guitar & Reville, 1997). This, as well as other sources, provides plenty of reasonable ideas concerning desensitization for children. Some are listed at the end of the chapter. Clinicians, however, should devise their own procedures to suit their clients, incorporating suggestions offered by the child or the group. In doing so, clinicians should keep in mind that the goal is to reduce painful feelings associated with stuttering.

In addition to becoming less reactive to the stuttering itself, children need opportunities to openly express their emotions, just like the parents do. Relevant activities may include drawing pictures of their stuttering, drawing pictures of people who scare them or make fun of them and then tear them up, writing brief essays about their stuttering, or becoming the experts who teach fellow classmates about stuttering (Emerick, 1970). More positive self-perceptions also can be encouraged by having children engage in activities such as making a list of things they like about themselves, things that they are good at, and in developing a talent that they can share with others. Also, having children role-play responses that convey confidence and assertiveness can be beneficial. One of the best sources for activities to help children talk about their feelings is *The School-Age Child Who Stutters: Working Effectively with Attitudes and Emotions* by Chmela and Reardon (2001), published by the Stuttering Foundation of America. The Stuttering Foundation of America has other resources for addressing various topics, such as teasing, bullying, and self-perceptions.

Teasing and Assertiveness

Teasing is a rather frequent problem confronted by schoolchildren who stutter as our clients have reported to us. Among others, it indicates their lower acceptance by peers (Davis, Howell, & Cook, 2002). Teasing is making comments that embarrass and hurt. Often a teaser thinks everyone finds it fun to make light of a matter, and does not understand how feelings have been hurt. At times it is done purposely to hurt. Clinicians should be aware of the risk and probe children in this regard because some children will not bring it up themselves. Here, the teacher's cooperation is of the utmost importance. Teachers should see to it that the teaser understands the seriousness of his or her negative behavior and stops it. The child who stutters also can be helped through assertiveness training. Many schools now have curricula that address teasing and bullying behavior.

Assertiveness and assertiveness training were discussed in Chapter 11 in relation to adults. It was suggested that most people occasionally find themselves in situations where they feel they have been wronged by others or that their dignity or rights were violated. Still, they are inhibited from making adequate responses. We offer the example of a person watching a movie at the theater while a few spectators disrupt the show with loud talk and laughs that spoil the enjoyment. The person badly wants to say something to the inconsiderate people but, instead, keeps silent, holding in frustration and suffers. Assertiveness is the skill of taking action toward resolving one's needs without insulting or violating the rights of others. The child who stutters, however, faces a double challenge: first, the typical anxiety of just speaking in a difficult situation and, second, speaking up assertively (e.g., protecting his or her rights).

Assertive responses can be developed typically through specific, short role-play programs in which familiar situations, such as peers mocking the child's stuttering, are rehearsed and the child's reaction are properly modified. As we explained in Chapter 11, a situation is planned only in general outline to allow for some spontaneity. For example, the child who stutters is playing in the schoolyard during lunch break. Another child, played by the clinician or another child in the group, passes by saying, "Hi, you stu-stu-stutter boy. You talk funny." Several optional responses are provided in advance (e.g., "So what?" "Better watch it, you may catch it," "Sticks and stones may break my bones, but words will never hurt me"; see Van Riper, 1973, p. 435). The situation is replayed several times with feedback, reinforcement, and suggestions for improvements. The clinician emphasizes that the desired behavior is being assertive, not aggressive. The child is then asked to recall other situations, not necessarily involving reactions to stuttering, where more assertiveness would have been desired (e.g., standing in line at McDonald's when an adult is barging in front of him). These are practiced through role play until the desired behavior is achieved (Murphy, Yaruss, & Quesal, 2007b). We have employed this technique for many years and witnessed great enthusiasm and satisfaction expressed by children as they were practicing. The effectiveness of the method with children has been shown experimentally. In one study with normally fluent 8- to 11-year-olds, targeted behaviors included ratio of eye contact to speech duration, loudness of speech, and several new responses. Results indicated an increase in each target behavior, as well as in rating of overall assertiveness by judges not familiar with the study (Bornstein, Bellack, & Hersen, 1977). Several relevant sources are listed at the end of this section.

Bullying

Bullying perhaps can be viewed as a more intense and severe level of hurting people than teasing. It is intentionally harming another person emotionally through frequent verbal harassment, sometimes also through physical assault, or even forcing another person to do something against his or her will. This can be done by one person or a group ganging up on their victim. The bully may have a need to experience a sense of power and superiority over others. Usually, adults need to get involved to establish and enforce rules prohibiting the bullying. Although teasing of children who stutter is quite common, "hard bullying" is not too common. Nevertheless, teachers need to frame stuttering as one type of observable personal difference and instruct children to accept the stuttering without offending comments. Clinicians should be alert as well as inform teachers about the increased risk to the child who stutters. Children who are bullied need comfort, support, and a clear message the problem belongs to the bully, not to themselves. In a recent study, 608 school children participated in an educational program about stuttering and bullying (awareness and prevention). Employing two questionnaire instruments, their data revealed that such educational programs have the potential to effect positive changes in peer attitudes toward children who stutter and toward bullying (Langevin & Prasad, 2012). Additional information regarding assertiveness training and addressing bullying/teasing may be found at the following Web sites:

- http://www.csulb.edu/~tstevens/assert%20req.html
- http://www.stopbullying.gov/

Therapy: Focus on Stuttering and Fluency

Identification and Analysis

Earlier in the chapter, we referred to simple identification of stuttering procedures as one of several useful techniques applied in working on desensitization. For that purpose, activities were mostly in terms of observing others or self and pointing out stuttering events when they occur. For clinicians who feel comfortable with traditional approaches to stuttering therapy, continuing into more extensive, somewhat more detailed, identification activities may be a reasonable option as the program progresses closer toward a focus on speech modification. This time, however, stuttering events are not only identified as they occur, they are also analyzed for their special characteristics. Again, the objectives and rationale are similar to those for adults, but the procedures are adjusted to suit children's level and abilities. At this stage, the clinician explains to the child, in a simple manner, why it is a good idea to get to know his or her own stuttering by taking a closer look at it from different angles. Essentially, the question asked is, "What is going on when you stutter?" but it is preferable to word the question as, "What do *you* do when you stutter that makes speech more difficult?" The parallel procedure with adolescents and adults tends to explore stuttering in great detail. Analysis with school-age children, however, especially at lower grades, should be focused on a limited number, say three to five, of the child's main stuttering characteristics. Getting into too many details could be counterproductive.

Using mirrors and videos taken of him or her, the child is guided to examine the most frequently occurring disfluency types (e.g., repetition and prolongation) as well as the most obvious secondary characteristics and the focal points of tension associated with them. The child's readiness to observe audio and videos of self should be recognized in advance. For some children, seeing themselves stuttering on video may be too emotionally intense. Working in front of a mirror for some time may be a good intermediate step prior to introducing video observation and analysis. Some difficulties can be expected because, as Conture (2001) pointed out, many speech movements and postures involved are not observable. The clinician helps the child describe the behaviors, for example, "I stretched the 'Wh' sound in the word *where* and at the same time I tensed my lips." Or, "I repeated 'I-I-I' and at the same time twisted my head to the side." Of course, the use of the language of responsibility, for example, "I twisted my head to the side," is purposely injected to help the child realize that what he or she does can also be changed. (This concept was discussed in Chapter 12.) Additional help is necessary to provide the child with a better idea of the unseen behaviors, for example, when blocking on the sound /k/, pressing the back of the tongue against the palate. The clinician can demonstrate these movements and postures using one hand as the tongue and the other one as the palate. Models of the speech mechanism are useful for this purpose, as is the videotape *Stuttering and the School-age Child* (by the Stuttering Foundation of America). If extensive practice, that is, the many analyses of the main stuttering features that we pursue in therapy, leads the child to recognize additional characteristics, there is no reason not to permit him or her to expand the behavior repertoire being analyzed.

Another useful aspect of the analysis technique is in guiding the child to differentiate the severity level of stuttering events, for example "light," "middle," and "hard" stuttering. Greater awareness of the variability may drive home the point that, depending on the individual case, much of the problem is not as bad as the few severe stuttering events may lead the child to believe. With children, special terms can help add a more gamelike feeling to the processes of therapy. Clinicians can involve children in making up their own terms. For example, an older child who likes golf might enjoy referring to a cancellation as a "mulligan." Examples of possible terms are shown in Table 13.1 based on analogies to video recordings, football games, show terms, and more.

Table 13.1	**Examples of Terms Used in Therapy with School-Age Children**			
Behavior	**Video Terms**	**Show Terms**	**Football Terms**	**For Young Children**
Talking too quickly	"Fast forward"	"Run through"	"Rushing"	"Rabbit talk"
Repetition	"Rewinds"	"False starts"	"Fumbles"	"Bumpy talk"
Prolongation	"Long plays"	"Delays"	"Holdings"	"Sticky talk"
Stopping talking	"Pause"	"Cut"	"Time-out"	"Red light"
Starting talking	"Play" or "Resume"	"Roll 'em"	"In play"	"Green light"
Cancellation or pullout	"Erase" and "Record over"	"Restart" or "Take 2"	"Instant replay"	"Yellow light"
Talking slowly	"Slow play"	"Slow motion"	"Stretching"	"Turtle talk"

Changing Speech

There is no clear demarcation where work on identification ends and speech modification begins. Often, some practice on modification is incorporated while working on identification. When a child identifies and analyzes a stuttering event, it sometimes is inviting to show him or her how to "correct" it, how to switch from "hard speech" to "easy speech." Nonetheless, when therapy has progressed to the point where speech modification calls for a more prominent focus, several options are available. First, as just described, the clinician may opt to proceed with the traditional Van Riper's (1973) approach aimed at having the client learn to modify the form of stuttering, making it more acceptable to listeners. The second option is to employ operant conditioning techniques to gradually increase the length of fluent speech segments (Ryan, 1979). Third, the clinician may pursue fluency-generating techniques, such as those developed by Webster (1980a, 1980b). All these were described in Chapter 12.

Stuttering Modification

We prefer to begin with at least a brief stuttering modification program following some of Van Riper's (1973) ideas because skills acquired through the procedures provide clients with the feeling that they can do something that directly combats the stuttering, the source of the pain, frustration, and feeling of helplessness. (See Chapter 12 for a more detailed description of the stuttering modification techniques.) Adapted to the child's level, the modification procedures we select are easily demonstrable, well understood, and typically well received. It is worth pointing out that a child who is trained primarily with fluency-shaping techniques will benefit from some practice with stuttering modification because of the likelihood to be in situations when fluency is lost. It is then that the ability to also *manage* stuttering is extremely useful in helping the child get back on the fluency track. Without experiences of managing stuttering, the child may be incapable of regaining a hold on the fluency-generating techniques.

For the sake of simplification, with children in early school grades, the stuttering modification program may be limited to perhaps only the *in-block* procedure, also known as *pullout*. In our experience, young children do better with pullouts, preferring it to the post-block modification (*cancellation*). The pre-block procedure appears to be too abstract and difficult for them altogether. The clinician demonstrates a stuttering block while saying, for example, the word *picture,* with clear tensed lips on the /p/ sound. For demonstration purposes, the tension is reduced in the most obvious manner, as the word is uttered smoothly with some elongation or by easily repeating the syllable /pi/ two or three times. We tell the child, "Let's *pull out* of the stuttering," or "Let's switch from hard speech into easy speech." Visual illustrations, such as a drawing symbolizing the block with spikes that gradually decrease in size, turning into an arrow projected upward and forward in moderate angle, or making a fist for the block, slowly changing into an open hand to illustrate the release, might be useful with some children. The practice begins with releasing many purposeful stuttering blocks and then continues into changing an authentic stuttering event during reading or conversation. The child is encouraged to "feel the change" and recognize it is of his or her own doing. It is important here to note a small, although potentially significant, deviation from Van Riper's (1973) writings. Whereas he advocated "teaching the child to stutter easily" (p. 441) and "to show him how to stutter in a new way" (p. 442), Williams (1971) preferred altering the language used, opining that the child must learn to "talk easily rather than hard." In particular, Williams favored teaching the child to modify a stuttering block into easy repetitions before moving on with the word. Using this language ("talk easily"), he explained, shifts the frame of references from that of a "stutterer" to that of a "speaker." As the child stutters, the clinician may join his stuttering and demonstrate the desired transition.

With a young child, a demonstration is more effective than several explanations. With children at more advanced grades, say fourth to sixth, stuttering modification can be more elaborate, including the post-block procedure that requires the client to stop after stuttering, reduce tension, and say the word again in an easier fashion. The practice of modification with the clinician should progress into a generalization program. *Important: Among the first people who should be included in this process are the child's parents.* Their presence in some sessions can help significantly. Often, children are reluctant to use therapy techniques at home because parents and sibling might think it is odd and react in unpredictable ways. Parent presence in therapy sessions releases much of the pressure and also allows them to encourage the child.

Fluency Facilitating Speaking Skills

Following the traditional therapy approaches outlined here, including desensitization, identification, and modification, we proceed by shifting focus to the more recent fluency-generating approach as discussed in detail in Chapter 12. We have pursued such integration of approaches since the 1970s and have been impressed with the advantages provided by each. Other clinicians, however, may elect to employ only the fluency-generating approach.

The clinician explains the change in the direction of therapy, conveying the general idea that "now, when you have learned a lot about stuttering and have practiced techniques that let you release stuttering blocks without getting panicked, it is time to also learn what can be done to speak more fluently to begin with so that fewer instances of stuttering occur." The clinician states that four ways of talking will be practiced that help produce stutter-free speech:

1. Slow, stretched spoken phrases
2. Gentle voice initiated with airflow
3. Light articulatory contact
4. Continuous articulatory movements

These are the *fluency targets*, as they are often referred to in the literature. Each is explained and demonstrated. A general plan is outlined whereby each of the four speaking patterns will be practiced, then gradually merged into the ongoing speech.

1. Establish slow, stretched speech, about one word per second (with adults the initial rate is much slower, one word per 2 seconds). Start with one-syllable words and then move to two-syllable words. Clinician provides models until the child catches on.

2. Introduce gentle voice onset. Demonstrate by contrasting hard and gentle attempts at voicing. Have the child do the same. Simulate the desired vocal fold movement with the two hands lightly vibrating against each other. Then, practice easy voice initiation, starting with words that begin with vowels, sliding from near whisper to normal loudness. Next, practice words that begin with voiceless consonants.

3. Introduce light articulatory contact. As in the earlier example, demonstrate hard and easy contacts, like in saying the /k/ and the /p/ sounds. Have the child do the same in order to feel the difference and become aware that the hard contact stops the airflow. Provide visual simulations, such as producing the /k/ sound by holding the fist of one hand (representing the tongue) against the second flat hand (representing the palate). The contact can be hard or the fist just slides easily along the hand surface while saying words like *kite, take,* and so on. Contrast hard and easy release of these and other classes of sounds.

4. Integrate gentle voice onset and light contact with slow speech, using one- and two-syllable words, keeping the same rate of one word per second. This complicated task requires more practice than the previous steps.

5. Increase the length of the utterances to three to four words but still keep the same initial slow rate.

6. Introduce continuous speech movement and continuous airflow throughout the phrase. As children practice talking slowly in short phrases, they are being urged to attend to the constant ongoing motion of the jaw, lips, and tongue: how the words blend into each other without stopping in between. This is the essence of normal speech. Most speakers do not stop in the middle of or between words. Again, models, videos, hand motions, and other illustrations should be used to highlight this important characteristic.

7. Proceed to practice longer sentences while also increasing the rate to two words per second. This rate is the low end where some parts of normal speech reach. All along, pay attention to the other basic targets of gentle voice, light contact. The continuous movement target is easier to practice in longer sentences.

8. Proceed to conversational speech, keeping the slow rate. A variety of conversation topics can be incorporated, such as those found at the Conversation Starters Web site (http://www.conversationstarters.com).

9. Transfer to several selected situations, then to a range of life situations.

We again emphasize that considerable flexibility should be exercised in pursuing the program's steps. Some may need to be eliminated or altered; much depends on the child's age and ability to follow. For example, with an 8-year-old, the clinician may begin with a faster rate, although still perceptibly slower than normal, using short phrases rather than single words. We have had noticeable success with variations of this program, working with children ages 8 to 12. For the most part, however, this was done in a clinical setting, not in the schools, and we enjoyed excellent cooperation from parents who participated in the sessions when asked to, and also used slow speech while interacting with the child. Years later, one child who initially exhibited moderate-to-severe stuttering won a state speaking award.

Generalization

A significant number, perhaps most, of a school-age child's communication situations take place in school. Thus the school setting presents a very real and appropriate setting for generalizing treatment goals into real-life settings. It is because school-based clinicians work directly in the school setting that they have a significant advantage over clinicians in other settings in terms of helping children who stutter. If possible, and when children are ready, clinicians should attempt to get them out of the therapy room and immediately begin to facilitate generalization of techniques: for example, walking the school hallways. Then the approach is extended to other settings where children spend time, asking them to complete brief homework activities outside the school environment. More specific examples of strategies for generalization could include using materials from the classroom in all practice activities; bringing in a friend, sibling, or a teacher to the therapy session; teaching other people in the children's environment about stuttering, and so on, and holding parts of therapy sessions on the playground, in the gym, and/or the library. Learning to modify speech while engaged in activities that require divided attention, such as walking, participating in a conversation with multiple listeners, talking in environments with lots of background noise, or using different loudness levels like those in a classroom versus on the playground, are all hierarchies that should be explored and practiced. Another interesting generalization activity, contract cards, is described by Chmela (2006). The child, clinician, and teacher (or other adult, such as a scout master) develop a contract for the child's participation. For the contract, the child agrees to demonstrate participation in a specific way such as using a speech tool to provide an answer in class during social studies. The contract is written on an index card, and following the social studies lesson, the child would take the card to the teacher and they would both sign it to indicate the child had fulfilled the contract. The card would then be returned to the clinician and discussed in the next therapy session. In essence, methods like these bring therapy into the real world.

Other Therapy Programs

The literature presents a number of other therapeutic programs for school-age children that reflect differences in approaches and scope. We next summarize a few of them to demonstrate their range.

Conditioning Fluent Speech

In Chapter 6, stuttering was discussed within the framework of operant learning principles, such as positive reinforcement, punishment, extinction, and negative reinforcement, that were used to portray stuttering as a response modified by its consequences. Applications of these principles can be seen in several early therapy regimens (e.g., Haroldson, Martin, & Starr, 1968; Rickard & Mundy, 1965). Bar (1971) trained parents to reinforce fluent utterances in their child's speech using verbal contingencies. Two programs are presented here.

Gradual Increase in Length and Complexity of Utterance (GILCU)

The *GILCU* program (Ryan & Ryan 1995) was described in Chapter 12 in the context of therapy for adults who stutter. It may be even more suitable for school-age children. The main objective is to gradually increase the client's length of fluent speech by means of immediate positive or negative feedback about the speech behavior. The program includes three parts, oral reading, monologue, and conversation, each composed of a similar progression through 18 steps. In each case, the 18 steps are divided into four levels. Within a speaking context, the client gradually progresses from one-word fluent responses to 5 consecutive minutes of connected speech. The criterion for advancing between steps is 10 consecutive fluent responses. Table 13.2 lists the target responses corresponding to each set of steps. In practice, the client is instructed to speak fluently, and each fluent response is reinforced by the clinician's feedback of "Good" and/or delivery of a token. Stuttered responses are followed by feedback such as, "Stop; speak fluently." After the child has completed the first 18 steps to attain 5 minutes of fluent reading in the clinic, the parents are trained to apply the reinforcement system at home. The fluent reading responses are reviewed each session while the client proceeds through the same 18 steps in monologue and then ultimately in conversation.

The effectiveness of this approach was investigated in a study of 12 school-age children seen for 30-minute sessions twice weekly for an average of about 8 weeks; 9 showed a drop from 6.0 to 0.4 mean stuttered words per minute under the establishment stage administered in public school settings. Follow-up measures taken 14 months after the

---

Table 13.2   Target Responses Corresponding to the Sets of Steps in the GILCU Program

Set of Steps	GILCU Target Responses
Steps 1–6	One word to six words
Steps 7–10	One sentence to four sentences
Steps 11–16	30 seconds to 3 minutes
Steps 17–18	3–5 minutes

maintenance stage revealed a mean 0.6 stuttered words per minute for 6 of these children (Ryan & Ryan, 1995). See Chapter 12 for more information about the GILCU.

The Lidcombe Program

Developed by Australian speech-language clinicians, this program has been directed mostly to preschool-age children. Hence more detailed information is presented in Chapter 14. The Lidcombe Program focuses on reinforcing fluent speech on the one hand and pointing out stuttered events on the other. Although the authors view responses to stuttering as "neutral," their corrective nature also can be characterized as "punishment" in operant conditioning terminology. That is, the stuttering response is followed by verbal stimuli designed to decrease that behavior. The program relies primarily on parents' administration of the procedures at home (Onslow et al., 2003). Although Onslow and colleagues opined that stuttering in children older than 6 years is less responsive to parental contingencies, the program also has been also successfully applied to school-age children between 6 and 12 years of age.

The initial sessions are conducted in the clinical setting as the clinician demonstrates to parents when and how to apply verbal contingencies: positive reinforcement of the child's fluent speech but requesting a reattempt or giving neutral feedback related to stuttered speech. Fluent utterances are rewarded with responses such as, "That was smooth speech" and similar reinforcing praises. Stuttered utterances are met with corrective feedback such as, "That was bumpy speech." In addition to verbal contingencies, the child also may be instructed to correct the stuttering (e.g., "Say it again to smooth it out"). In general, many more reinforcing praises than corrective comments are made. When parents are thought to be proficient with the procedures, the therapy is transferred to the home, starting with a few brief structured practice sessions per day conducted by the trained parent. Shortly thereafter, contingencies are applied in various home situations. Parents monitor progress by daily rating of stuttering severity. Progress also is evaluated by the clinician during periodic visits to the clinic. Two small studies that evaluated the effectiveness of the Lidcombe Program with school-age children demonstrated considerable lower frequency of stuttering at the end of treatment and at a 12-month follow-up (Lincoln, Onslow, Lewis et al., 1996) and between 2 and 41-month (mean = 15) follow-ups (Koushik, Shenker, & Onslow, 2009).

Integrated Programs

Fluency Rules Program   Developed by C. Runyan and S. Runyan (updated in 2007), this program requires a child to adhere to three rule classes totaling seven rules that are basically instructional procedures. They appear simple to present to children and easily understood by them.

Universal Rules: (1) Speak slowly (turtle speech). (2) Say a word only once. (3) Say it short.
Primary Rules: (4) Use speech breathing. (5) Start voice box running smoothly.

Secondary Rules: (6) Touch "speech helpers" together smoothly. (7) Use only "speech helpers" to talk.

As you can see, the therapy emphasizes fluency-enhancing techniques (rules 1, 4, 5, and 6) with additional important elements designed to control stuttering, mainly by limiting its occurrence or duration, that is, learning what not to do (rules 2, 3, and 7) rather than how to modify stuttering according to the traditional Van Riper techniques. For example, rule 7 directs the child to avoid making nonspeech behaviors, or secondary characteristics. The therapy is conducted twice or three times per week in the school environment in a nonstructured manner with the children sitting on the floor and engaged in conversational speech and games. Speech is kept slow although not abnormally slow. An example may be made of the children's TV host, Mister Rogers, who speaks more slowly than most people but remains within the normal range of natural rates. Symbolic therapy materials, such as turtles and snails to characterize slow speech, and rabbits and racehorses to indicate that speech is too fast, are generously employed. Parents also are encouraged to speak at a normal slow rate. Significant attention is given to carryover and transfer to the classroom and home. This requires active cooperation of teachers who are to remind the child to adhere to the rules via agreed-on signals. The authors reported generally positive results for a total of 32 children, mostly in the lower school grades with treatment lasting 9 months on average.

A Comprehensive Stuttering Program for School-Age Children (CSP-SC) This program, which addresses both overt stuttering behaviors and the emotional domain of the disorder, was developed in Canada over a 20-year period, specifically for children ages 7 to 12 years (Kully & Boberg, 1991; Langevin, Kully, & Ross-Harold, 2007). It is designed to be delivered in a 4-week intensive format with groups of six to eight children. However, it has been delivered in other formats in the clinic as well as through interactive mass media, for example, telehealth therapy (Kully, 2002). In several aspects it bears significant similarities to our comprehensive program described earlier in the chapter. These are the CSP-SC's four main components:

1. Speech-related goals achieved through both fluency-enhancing and stuttering management techniques.
2. Attitudinal-emotional goals that include reduction in fears and avoidance as well as an increase in assertiveness, positive attitudes toward communication, and social skills.
3. Self-management goals, such as developing problem-solving and self-monitoring skills, as well as the ability to plan and carry out practice activities.
4. Environmental goals that basically include parent counseling regarding the nature of stuttering and an understanding of and cooperation with the therapy program.

Work on each component proceeds along three stages: acquisition, transfer, and maintenance. Practice on fluency skills during the first two phases is delivered in small groups of two children. Emotional aspects are dealt with in several formats from larger groups to individual sessions. The authors reported therapy outcomes for four school-children. For three of them, stuttering was reduced by 52% to 75% within 6 to 19 months follow-up. Later follow-ups with parents indicated good maintenance of the gains. The fourth child presented a relapse 2 months posttherapy.

Family Stuttering Programs

A unique and less well-known therapeutic approach that differs from the programs described earlier attempts to expand therapy significantly beyond the emphasis on the child to include a circle of people in his or her home and school environments (Mallard, 1991). We believe it contains some ideas that might also be useful to clinicians who prefer other programs. Influenced by the work of Rustin and her colleagues in England (e.g., Rustin & Cook, 1983), Mallard's approach reflects the belief that, inasmuch as communication is a social skill, therapy must take into account the social environment in which the child communicates. His program is "based on the assumption that inter-vention with individuals who influence the communication environment of the stut-tering child is the critical component in the treatment of stuttering children" (Mallard, 1991, p. 22). According to this model, successful therapy can only be achieved when the person who stutters and those in the person's communication environment work together. Hence the entire immediate family, including parents, siblings, grandparents (spouses in adult cases), and the home environment structure, as well as teachers and the classroom structure, and their respective modes of communication, are very rel-evant if carryover of improved speech is to take place. Therapy is focused on two main goals: speech control and the acquisition of social skills that enable the new speech pat-terns to be employed in the child's environments. Changes are expected for the child and in the child's communication environment as well.

Therapy is delivered either in a 2-week intensive group program or a nonintensive format. The program begins with an explanatory meeting in which the entire family is present. Next is a 3-week phase during which each parent must initiate twice a week a 5-minute Talk Time with the child at home. Each parent submits a weekly evalua-tive report about these assignments. An important rationale for the Talk Time is that it establishes a routine for parent-child communication. It also creates the basis for home speech assignments.

Next, weekly therapy sessions are initiated with the family. Various discussion topics are offered by the clinician, beginning with problem-solving procedures, followed by exercises of resolving actual problems. The objective is to get the family to view stutter-ing as a problem that can be solved, not necessarily a disorder that must be treated. Many of the problems raised by the child and family appear to be in regard to coping with the stuttering. For example, a child who has to give an oral report in class may be more concerned about how to handle peers' teasing rather than talking without stuttering.

Options are listed and considered, and a response to the specific problem is selected. Other topics/assignments include social skills training such as turn taking, observation, and listening. These topics also can provide for home assignments as needed. In therapy, parents may be asked to mimic their child's stuttering in order to appreciate what he or she is experiencing all the time. They also could be asked to engage in this activity at home during Talk Times because it provides insight for why the child avoids talking. All sessions begin with an evaluation of the previous week's assignments.

Work on speech begins after a few sessions. The first step is for the child and family to understand normal speech processes and what is happening during stuttering. Next, the participants, with the clinician's guidance, select a few techniques for changing speech, such as maintaining eye contact with conversational partners, stuttering voluntarily (for desensitization purposes), or stuttering in a relaxed manner. All therapy sessions are conducted with the family present (Mallard, 1998). The effects of these speech changes are discussed. The child and parents are to practice all speech modification techniques at home during Talk Time. The speech modification sequence generally begins with keeping eye contact during moments of stuttering and then moves to stuttering easily with control and maintaining eye contact. Emphasis is placed on stuttering without tension or avoidance. Training in social skills, such as turn taking and problem solving, continues.

In a school setting, open discussion ensues to explain the child's stuttering to the teacher, the various nonobservable aspects of it, what is done in therapy, and how the teacher can help, for example, selecting a time for the child to use his or her speech control procedures and agreeing on reinforcement signals. According to Mallard, when following a family-based problem-solving model of treatment, the role of the speech-language pathologist changes from that of the primary service provider to that of a monitor of how the child, parents, and significant others in the child's communication environment are progressing. Clinicians who opt to implement this program should be aware that no formal research data have been published for its evaluation.

Seth, a 7-year-old male, began stuttering at around age 2. Although no family history of stuttering was reported, his younger brother, Abel, exhibited atypical disfluency from an early age as well. Mrs. Eve, Seth's mother, stated the boys were most disfluent when tired or excited or when talking to certain people, such as strangers or their grandmother who was reported to be highly critical. After reviewing past treatment with Mrs. Eve, Seth was identified to need work on two areas: fluent speech strategies and conversational turn taking (i.e., not interrupting) with his brother. Fluent speech strategies were addressed in each session (e.g., light touches of the articulators, easy starts, a slow approach), but of special note was an activity devised for improving turn-taking skills, described next.

Each session followed a routine format that consisted of approximately three activities. First, Seth and the clinician participated in a group play activity with Mrs. Eve, Abel (brother), and Abel's clinician. They engaged in structured game activities in which each participant took turns talking and playing in the game. The second task was a structured storytelling activity with the clinician only. The third and last activity was the least structured and most conversational. Seth and the clinician either conversed while making an art project or engaged in a show-and-tell activity based on items brought from home. During all activities, the clinician indirectly modeled a slow relaxed rate of speech, plenty of pausing, and short utterance lengths.

Turn-taking behaviors were addressed during the group activities. A "speaking block" (wooden block) was used as a visual/tactile cue during all of the group sessions to promote appropriate turn taking (i.e., no interruptions). Seth and Abel were told that only the person holding the speaking block could talk. Good listening skills were demonstrated and described, and the boys were told to sit quietly and listen to the person holding the speaking block. They were also instructed to not interrupt. During each session, the clinician served as a "referee"; she was allowed to talk without the speaking block in order to provide feedback (e.g., "You don't have the speaking block"). Initially the activities were structured so that participants took rotating turns either describing a picture or saying something about a chosen topic. During the last two sessions, the activities were more conversational in manner. A topic was chosen and the participants raised their hands, passed the block, and discussed a topic rather than rotating turns. After each topic change, the referee asked participants to evaluate their own turn-taking behavior, to promote self-monitoring.

During storytelling and description activities, the clinician cued language organization by prompting Seth to apply the terms: *first, then, next,* and *last* to aid sequencing. The clinician also provided visual cues consisting of pictures representing the parts of a story (i.e., people, place, time, event, start and ending). To encourage a slower rate, Seth was instructed to say only one thing at a time that would permit the clinician to transcribe (write down) his statements verbatim to make a book from his story. Seth drew pictures for his story that were attached to each page of the eventual book. Verbal reinforcement (e.g., "I like the way you spoke with a slow, easy start") was provided intermittently. In addition, a hand signal in which the clinician put her hands together and slowly pulled them apart was used to remind Seth to "stretch out his words" as they had practiced when learning this fluent speech strategy.

Group Therapy

Principles and basic methods of group therapy were presented in Chapter 11 in regard to treatment of adults who stutter. Generally, group therapy also is applicable for school-children who stutter, and several examples were presented earlier in this chapter. The school setting is conducive because the children are already under one roof, and clinicians often look for ways to economize their time. Groups typically are small because not too many children who stutter are found in a single school. Groups also are restricted in size because age/grade difference may cause problems. We recommend group members come from a narrow range of no more than two grade levels. Often clinicians group children who stutter with other children of the same age who are working on nonfluency speech goals because of constraints related to their time and availability. If handled well, a mixed group still can provide an effective forum for therapy, but care should be taken with this arrangement to ensure that it is a "safe" and comfortable environment in which to stutter. Leith (1984) advocated what he called a *shaping group* as part of stuttering treatment program in the school environment and listed several advantages of heterogeneous groups: The interaction among members is more natural, opportunities to practice new speech patterns in front of people who do not stutter are more like real-life situations, feedback to expressed feelings tends to be more objective from children who do not stutter, and all benefit from learning that children have other problems. The shaping group format requires all members to actively participate in the discussions, monitor the speech behaviors of the other children, as well as administer reward and penalties. The clinician assumes a less active role.

Clinical Research

In the first edition of this book (2011), we noted that in spite of the appreciable amount of clinically related literature pertaining to school-age children who stutter, it appears that research related to intervention with this age group has been limited. Considerably more research is available for treatment with younger children and adult populations. Very few reasonably controlled clinical efficacy studies were conducted exclusively with school-age children (6 to 12 years of age). This is partly due to the tendency in a good number of studies to use a wider age range of participants. For example, Ryan and Ryan (1995) included children between the ages of 7 and 17. It may also be a reflection of how school-age children who stutter access therapy; many of these children are served within the school setting, where conducting methodologically sound clinical research can be challenging. After a comprehensive review of 162 articles pertaining to stuttering treatment results for preschool-age children through adulthood, only 39 were found to satisfy four of five methodological criteria to be considered as meeting clinical trial quality (Bothe, Davidow, Bramlett et al., 2006). Perusing this list we found only five reported data for children between 6 and 14 years of age. Of these, three reports included only one to three participants. Unfortunately, not much has been changed since then. A similar assessment was expressed by Nippold (2011).

Perhaps an exception is the exemplary investigation conducted in Australia by Craig and a large group of collaborators (1996). They compared effectiveness among three therapy methods: intensive smooth speech, intensive electromyography (EMG) feedback, and home-based smooth speech. Each group was composed of 25 to 27 children. These also were compared with a nontreatment control group of 20 stuttering children. Progress was assessed in terms of percentage of syllables stuttered and speaking rate (number of syllable spoken per minute). A 12-month follow-up was conducted. Comparisons were made in several speaking environments (e.g., clinic, home, and telephone). By the end of therapy, the frequency of stuttering in all treatment groups improved by 85% to 90%, decreasing to under 1% stuttered syllables. By the 1-year follow-up, there was a slight increase in stuttering to the 3% level on average. No change occurred in the control group. The authors concluded that the three approaches were very successful for 70% of the children, with the EMG and home treatment showing the best results. In a follow-up study, Hancock et al. (1998) compared the same children after a mean of 4 years posttreatment. Long-term effects of the therapy continued to be good in that the children in the three treatment groups maintained stuttering frequency similar to what they had demonstrated at the 1-year follow-up in the first study. Effectiveness was not significantly different among the three approaches. Later investigators, however, attempting to replicate the EMG portion of Craig et al.'s study were not as successful (Block et al., 2004). Given the initial finding that all three treatment approaches met with comparable success, it may be that the specific methods employed are less important than the broad aim of an approach to speech management with reduced tension. Similarly, it has been difficult to establish that any particular approach to treatment of phonological disorders is better than another as long as the sound targets have been selected appropriately (Kamhi, 2006).

Other studies have reported various degrees of success, although they fell short of tight methodology. For example, earlier in the chapter we referred to a study that tested the Lidcombe Program administered to school-age children (Lincoln et al., 1996). Eleven children, ages 7 to 12, were treated using this method. The investigators reported that a median of 12 hour-long treatment sessions was required to reach 1.5% stuttered syllables in speech samples recorded within-clinic as well as in three everyday speaking situations out of the clinic. The lower stuttering frequency at the end of the treatment was maintained by all the children at a 12-month follow-up. Parents were either "satisfied" or "very satisfied" with their children's speech posttreatment. A second study of the effectiveness of the Lidcombe Program with 11 school children also reported good results although it suffered from methodological inconsistencies (Koushik et al., 2009).

Another recent interest in treatment research involving school-age children took the form of a case study of a 9-year-old boy who, in addition to stuttering modification and fluency-enhancing therapies, was exposed to several techniques aimed at reducing emotional reactions. Following treatment, the child exhibited improved communication attitudes and reduced frequency and severity of stuttering (Murphy, Yaruss, & Quesal, 2007a). It is difficult, however, to determine whether changes in stuttering resulted from the attitude treatment or if attitude improvement could have resulted from the effect of reduced stuttering. Clearly, if clinicians are to practice data-based therapy, a considerably larger number of investigations looking at various approaches must be conducted employing rigorous scientific methodologies.

Summary

Clinicians who work with school-age children who stutter should be cognizant of the special characteristics of stuttering in this age group, the increased severity of the overt stuttering, the high level of awareness of stuttering, emergence of strong emotional reactions associated with the speaking difficulties, the growing impact of social forces on the disorder, and the persistent nature of the disorder that has set in. This last item has clinical implications to goal setting and expectation of progress. It means that progress

LEARNER OBJECTIVES

Readers of this chapter will understand:

- The historical background of therapy for early stuttering.
- Considerations regarding intervention for preschool children who stutter.
- The range of treatment objectives for this subpopulation.
- Clinical programs representing the current major treatment approaches.
- Research issues concerned with treatment of preschoolers who stutter.

General Considerations

Having reviewed and discussed the treatment of stuttering in adults and school-age children, we now shift attention to general approaches, specific techniques, and programs that have been offered for the treatment of preschool-age children. Chapter 2, which focused on the distribution of the stuttering population, established that the overwhelming majority of people who stutter experience the onset of the disorder (incidence) during the preschool period, ages 2 to 5, mostly before age 3. Additionally, the data show that the prevalence of stuttering (the percentage of people who exhibit active stuttering) is also the largest in this age group.[1]

In spite of these indisputable facts, systematic clinical intervention programs designed specifically for preschool-age children who stutter were relatively late to appear, and for a long time they lacked the breadth of treatment methods offered to adults who stutter. This trend paralleled the one seen in the research domain that, for many years, favored adults who stutter. This scenario reflects several realities. First has been the lingering "hands off the child" attitude toward treatment of early stuttering that was promoted especially in the United States. Second may have been a tendency toward thinking that stuttering in children and adults was all the same. Third, university laboratories and clinics were mainly accessible to college students. Fortunately, the trend has been reversed, and the past three decades have seen a substantial increase both in clinical programs and clinical research pertaining to preschool-age children who stutter. The following brief historical account of past therapies for this age group is intended to provide a broadened perspective on current clinical issues and therapy programs.

---

[1]One study (Craig et al., 2002), however, suggested a peak prevalence in the 6- to 10-year age group.

415

Therapeutic interventions for early childhood stuttering have operated with different philosophies that have alternated over the years, reflecting changes in the dominant thinking of mainstream speech pathology in respect to direct and indirect intervention modes. The distinction between the two in regard to stuttering is not clear. For some clinicians, for example Conture (2001), the criterion is based on the approach to a child's speech. An indirect approach does *not* explicitly, overtly, or directly prompt the child to speak fluently. Rather, the focus is on changing the child's environment, especially parents' behavior or the child's emotionality. Direct approaches involve explicit attempts to modify the child's speech. Our interpretation, by contrast, encompasses a wider context of what is considered direct therapy.

In this context, the term *direct therapy* applies to methods in which the clients themselves are subjected to treatment. In addition to methods in which the child who stutters receives guidance for making speech changes (speech therapy), psychologically oriented therapy and/or physical stimulation of parts of the body (e.g., oral structures) are viewed as direct therapy. For example, play therapy with the child as a participant in a process aimed at altering his or her emotionality and behavior is direct therapy. Although play therapy does not deal with speech modification, it is a method that requires a very direct contact between clinician and child. A therapy that is limited to physical stimulation of oral muscles (not speech therapy) is also viewed as direct.

In view of the constraints placed on early intervention, particularly by the client's age and the nature of the early stuttering, discussed later, it is interesting to note the diversity of treatments that have been applied. In that light, it also is surprising that many share a fair number of objectives with the major therapeutic approaches listed in Chapter 10 for older children and adults. The procedures, however, have been adapted to suit young children.

Direct Treatments

As stated above, direct therapy is when the client is the immediate recipient of the treatment, being speech- or nonspeech-oriented. Toward the end of the 19th century and the first decades of the 20th century, the most frequently advocated types of programs involved direct therapy. They leaned toward what we have referred to as *fluency enhancement*, that is, the elicitation and subsequent practice of talking patterns that produce fluent speech, rather than modification of instances of stuttering. Such philosophy was particularly dominant in Europe. In fact, today's popular approaches were practiced more than 100 years ago.

European Methods

According to Pay and Sirotkina (1955), Russian clinicians devised intensive programs, including all-day clinics, that required children as young as 2 years of age to memorize and repeat sentences, tell picture stories, rehearse questions and answers, and drill rhythmic activities. These activities perhaps reflected a strong view, held in eastern Europe, that stuttering is also a disorder of language. Hence enriching the child's vocabulary and expressive language were important therapeutic objectives (Daskalov, 1962). Others focused on developing speech breathing and easy phonation to facilitate fluency. Music and singing were also favored because they introduced rhythm into the speech pattern, a condition that yields fluency. In one program, the children practiced coordinating speech utterances with body movements and music to facilitate speech rhythm. Although some attention was given to modification of emotional reactions, there was more emphasis on regimented rest and sleep to achieve relaxation, which, in turn, was supposed to facilitate fluency. Even sedation was sometimes used for this purpose (Vlasova, 1962).

By contrast, linguistically oriented therapies were not practiced in western Europe. There, some clinicians employed motorically oriented techniques. These included having children say phrases that were timed with body movements (Pichon & Borel-Maisonny, 1937), teaching them to speak slowly and practice coordination of speech with breathing (Emil-Behnke, 1947), or talking in unison (Kingdon-Ward, 1941). Others devised therapies based on the conception of stuttering as a perceptual disorder that disrupted auditory feedback. Consequently, children were asked to talk while shadowing the clinician's speech so as to not depend on their own feedback (Marland, 1957).

American Methods

A different direct therapy was employed by a few clinicians in the United States who viewed stuttering as a neurological problem affecting muscle coordination. They opted for a nonspeech approach, working with children to manipulate neurological and muscular functions. For example, based on Lee Travis's (1931) theory that stuttering results from lack of cerebral dominance, Johnson (1934) thought it was possible to eliminate early stuttering by retraining the child's handedness, shifting it from left to right. Supposedly, it should have helped the child establish left cerebral dominance. Other clinicians who adhered to the moto-kinesthetic method stimulated the child's speech muscles (e.g., touching the lips or tongue), instructed the correct placement of the speech organs, as well as drilling children in specific speech movement sequences (Young & Hawk, 1955).

A third direct approach reflected psychogenic perspectives of stuttering that relegated the blame for stuttering to the child's neurotic parents. Although some clinicians coming from this orientation directed considerable therapeutic attention to the parents (indirect therapy), the child too was suspected of harboring neurotic reactions that warranted therapy. This gave rise to diverse psychotherapeutic programs, especially play therapy that focused directly on the child (e.g., Harle, 1946). Perhaps the most notable effort was Murphy and Fitzsimons' (1960) extensive play therapy that sought to help children project deep feelings through the highly symbolic medium of play. As we discuss later, the belief was that play serves to bring emotions to a child's awareness, emotions accepted with impunity by the clinician.

Indirect Treatments

Indirect treatments are methods in which those who closely interact with children (i.e., parents, other family members, teachers) are the primary recipients of treatment. The underlying assumption being that improving their emotional well-being and/ or attitudes and behavior will also favorably impact children's speech. An additional assumption is that speech-related behaviors can be influenced by social modeling and environmental conditions.

Indirect approaches were practiced widely in the United States for several decades, especially during the middle of the 20th century, reflecting a popular belief in the parental role in the cause of stuttering. When the trend shifted to direct treatments, few realized it was not such a bold move but merely returning to interventions that had existed for long time, particularly in other countries.

> A 180-degree shift in philosophy occurred in the late 1930s when direct speech and nonspeech therapies were largely abandoned for 30 to 40 years in favor of indirect therapies that focused on parents, leaving children out of the therapeutic contact (hence the expression "indirect"). This has been referred to often as the "hands off the child" philosophy. Typical of the voluminous literature of that period is Schuell's (1949) statement that "it is impossible to escape the need for working with the parents of the young child who stutters" (p. 251). This change occurred for several reasons, mostly because of the combined effects of the diagnosogenic theory and certain aspects of psychogenic theories of stuttering.

Psychotherapy for Parents

As we discussed in Chapter 6, psychogenic theories traced stuttering to parents, mainly mothers, having neurotic personalities. A pathological mother-child relationship, it was postulated, encumbered the child with deep emotional conflicts, eventually expressed as stuttering. Hence the neurotic parent(s) became an important target of intervention, calling for psychotherapies to help them achieve emotional adjustment and insight into their unhealthy relations with the child. Glauber (1958) prescribed traditional psychoanalysis, primarily for the mother, viewed as the main source of conflict and anxiety. Other members of the nuclear family also received therapy as deemed necessary. Glasner (1949) was another clinician to include extensive psychiatric guidance for family members, although not in the form of psychoanalysis. The underlying assumption was that to alleviate a child's neurotic behaviors, parents had to recognize their own problems and redirect their relationships with the child. Psychotherapy for parents of children who stutter, however, was practiced only by a few psychiatrists and psychologists. This form of intervention never became commonplace, probably because the vast majority of parents of children who stutter are, in fact, neither neurotic nor in need of psychotherapy. An additional factor is the complexity and costs of this kind of treatment.

Parent Counseling

In a very different vein, the diagnosogenic theory (Johnson & Associates, 1959), a learning theory, also placed the blame for stuttering on parents, especially their child-rearing practices and overreaction to a child's normal disfluency. This view gained support from several studies that found parents of children who stutter to be more demanding, or to exert more pressure on their children as compared with parents of normally fluent children (see review by Yairi, 1997). These impressions emanated the logic that intervention should target parents, not children, with counseling geared toward changing the pressure behaviors employed in routines of child rearing. Note that this is very different from psychotherapies aimed at correcting a parental personality disorder. Another rationale for keeping children out of active participation in therapy was the strong belief that heightened awareness of disfluent speech would be instrumental in transforming it into full-fledged stuttering (e.g., Bluemel, 1932).

Many speech-language clinicians adopted parent counseling as the preferred form of intervention for early childhood stuttering. Most programs were mounted to instruct parents in what was regarded as "good parenthood," as well as providing them with guidance related to handling stuttering. The typical advice of how to respond and how not to respond to the child's stuttering rendered this counseling with a direct authoritarian character.

Johnson's approach (1948) emphasized parent education about speech development, the normalcy of disfluencies, and his contention that the overreactions of overanxious parents to normal disfluency caused stuttering. Parents were told that they should not feel or show any concern about stuttering, and that they should avoid any negative responses to it, be patient listeners when the child stuttered, and avoid giving suggestions to help the child through moments of stuttering. Clinicians who followed this approach often prescribed specific details of planned parent-child activities. Similar counseling approaches were offered by Schuell (1949) and by Brown (1949).

Winds of Change

After more than 3 decades dominated by the philosophy of indirect treatment for early childhood stuttering, winds of change eventually altered the clinical landscape of the field. An important reason for this was the decline of Johnson's diagnosogenic theory, a central foundation of the therapeutic approach. Among contrary evidence were data showing that, close to the onset of stuttering, the speech of young CWS was substantially different from that of NFC, indicating that stuttering was fundamentally different from normal disfluency rather than an outgrowth of it (Throneburg & Yairi, 1994; Yairi & Lewis, 1984). Additionally, studies inspired by operant conditioning theories demonstrated that stuttering, instead of being increased, could actually be reduced by calling attention to it (Martin et al., 1972; Reed & Godden, 1977), and there was growing evidence for genetic factors underlying stuttering (Kidd, 1977). At the same time, a new, much larger, generation of speech-language clinicians was more willing to recognize of what appeared to be insufficiencies of the limited indirect intervention as reflected in cases of children who persisted in stuttering in spite of all the counseling given to their parents. Hence renewed interest in direct treatment, either speech or more psychologically oriented, emerged by the 1980s. Parental involvement, however, has continued, and, in some programs, remained a prominent feature.

> How do clinicians best educate parents who have no previous experiences with stuttering about the responses they must encourage versus prevent, as well as an understanding about how to view stuttering in light of their child's future and individual potential? One way their perspective can be enhanced is through opportunities to meet adults who stutter, either individually or by attending a local stuttering support group. Adults who stutter can offer insights about what they wished their parents had known and done during their childhood years. As well, books by people who stutter and/or about famous people who stutter can offer valuable education to parents of children who stutter.

Current Issues Concerning Early Intervention

Prior to presenting current approaches to clinical management for preschool children who stutter, it is important to keep in mind a few facts and factors that influence general clinical considerations for this age group. Several of these pertain to the characteristics of stuttering, whereas others pertain to the preschool age itself.

Factors Pertaining to Stuttering

The most notable factor is the strong prospect for *natural recovery*. Inasmuch as stuttering is expected to improve or expire on its own accord, a logical question to be asked is whether intervention should be pursued for every child. Treatment is expensive and presents a burden to the family in several other respects. If the clinician shares our view that not all children who begin stuttering require intervention, the next questions become *who* should receive treatment and *when*? Some answers may be found in the information about chances for natural recovery or risks for chronic stuttering, as well as other considerations (e.g., parents' reactions) presented in Chapters 3 and 13. This issue is further discussed later in this chapter.

Another factor is *awareness* of stuttering. Although some indications of awareness are seen in a good number of children younger than 4, they tend to be unstable, perhaps because the history of the disorder is too short to trigger complex emotional or social reactions. It is uncommon, for example, for a preschool-age child who stutters to be teased by peers. In light of this, we believe a third significant factor should be recognized: In its early stages, stuttering is primarily a disorder of speech. The intensive attention to emotionality by many clinicians treating adults becomes secondary in the treatment of most cases of early childhood stuttering where the focus is on changing the child's speech patterns and environment.

Factors Pertaining to Age

There are three important factors in this category:

1. Preschoolers who stutter, like most of their peers, function with limited cognitive and language skills. They have limited, if any, comprehension of the stuttering problem as understood by adults or of the nature of therapy goals, or similar considerations. Therefore, speech therapy with young children should be conducted with minimal instruction or explanation. Instead, it should be rich with demonstrations, and the clinician should use simple language. Modeling (e.g., slow speech) and simple feedback to reinforce (increase) or punish (decrease) certain behaviors become prominent.

2. Preschoolers who stutter do not ask for therapy but are brought in by worried parents. Hence therapy should also focus in some way on the parents' feelings about, reactions to, and interactions with the child.

3. Home and the immediate family constitute an overwhelming portion of the child's world. Therefore, it would be wise, as well as productive, to have the parents involved in the child's therapy so that they can cooperate and carry on some of the procedures at home (e.g., model slow speech).

Who Should Be Treated? When?

During the period when indirect treatment of early childhood stuttering was popular among speech clinicians, especially in the United States, the prevailing view was that no child should receive therapy. As described, intervention was focused on parents, primarily in the form of standard counseling and sometimes in the form of psychotherapy. As direct therapies were revived and more widely practiced during the past 35 years, an opposing view was voiced: Every child should be treated as soon as possible (e.g., Starkweather et al., 1990). In between these two extremes, a third view also emerged: Therapy should be offered selectively, primarily to those at high risk for developing persistent stuttering (Andrews, 1984; Curlee, 1993; Curlee & Yairi, 1997; Ryan, 2001a; Yairi & Ambrose, 2005). Other children should be monitored during a waiting period. We agree with this view and submit that it is supported by current scientific information, by well-grounded practical concerns, and by ethical considerations.

From objective scientific perspectives, the documented high percentage of natural recovery (see Chapter 3) implies that it is not necessary to provide therapy to all children who begin stuttering because most of them will recover on their own accord. Furthermore, although information necessary to make precise predictions of which children will recover and which will continue to stutter is incomplete, the current research does permit identification of those children with the highest risk for persistent stuttering. Certainly, these children should be recommended for therapy. More detailed considerations of pertinent risk factors were discussed in Chapter 13.

> From a practical perspective, treating a group of children, 75% to 80% of whom will do well on their own, might be a questionable use of professional and budgetary resources, diverting resources from those who need them most. At least one health insurance company, to our knowledge, has questioned paying for therapy for early stuttering in view of natural recovery prospects. Surely there are not enough clinicians in this country, let alone the many countries outside the United States, to do the job if every child who begins stuttering is referred for treatment. Additionally, bringing a child for therapy can be a significant burden on the family, for example, in terms of availability of working parents, cost, time (driving to and from the clinic), lack of insurance participation, impact on the rest of the family, and more. Should the family and the child go through all these inconveniences if they are not needed? Clinicians should exercise their best judgment based on research evidence, and participate in decisions with parents weighing the costs/benefits for individual cases.

Finally, there is the issue of ethics. Some clinicians have posited that delaying therapy is unethical because it places the child at unnecessary risk and because delay reduces the success of therapy at older ages (Ingham & Cordes, 1998). Another surprising argument has been that therapy should be provided to all children because it will not hurt (Bernstein Ratner, 1997b). We, however, agree with Yairi and Ambrose (2005) who countered by suggesting that providing *unnecessary* treatment might be considered unethical. They also argued that therapy should be given on a positive basis: Because it is necessary and helps, not because it would not hurt. Unfortunately, when clinicians counsel parents, they often exaggerate the urgency for immediate therapy, painting a dark, less than objective possible prognosis. So what general clinical strategy for preschool children who just began stuttering should be pursued? The answer is that therapy should be delivered selectively. For most of these children a waiting period is our preferred option. Even proponents of early intervention suggest flexibility in regard to when treatment should begin (Packman & Onslow, 1999). Ingham and Cordes (1998) proposed waiting up to 6 months from the time of onset before initiating intervention. Yairi and Ambrose (2005) suggested that a longer waiting period, 9 to 12 months, to observe a shift toward recovery is justified by data from their longitudinal study. At that point in time, those who will recover become more identifiable. Given that some high-risk children are easily identified for immediate intervention, for example, boys whose fathers also stutter, disagreement among scholars and clinicians about the timing of intervention for those who fail to show signs of early recovery is primarily in regard to the specific length of the waiting, not to the wisdom of the decision to wait.

Concerns that delayed intervention will harm future therapy, if it becomes necessary, should be alleviated in view of findings of no significant relation between the length of the interval (even 1 year) from stuttering onset to the beginning of therapy or with the amount of therapy required for a desired outcome (Jones, Onslow, Harrison et al., 2000; Kingston, Huber, Onslow et al., 2003). Attribution of low therapeutic success rates in school-age children to long delays of treatment in early stages of the disorder does not hold water for another reason. This is because school-age children who stutter constitute a small minority who resisted natural recovery, a tendency shown to be determined, at least in part, by genetic factors (see Chapter 7). They may not respond well to therapy primarily because they have a more resistant type of stuttering. Thus decisions regarding the timing for intervention are based on each child's combination of risk factors, indication of progress or lack of it, and unique circumstances. In short, at the present, there are general guidelines (see Chapter 13) but no definite rules as to when intervention should begin.

Current Therapies

As we pointed out earlier, direct treatments for early childhood stuttering, common during the first few decades of the 20th century, were overtaken by indirect therapies from about the late 1930s. The wheel, however, kept on turning. The years since the mid-1970s have witnessed the reemergence of direct treatment programs in which children's speech is at the center. Parent counseling, though, has remained an integral part of most therapies. Furthermore, there has also been a tendency to have parents participate in the therapy sessions and assume an active role in its administration at home. To help clinicians and students better comprehend the sometimes confusing pool of current therapies for preschool-age children, we have organized them in four classes according to their main procedural focus: therapies that focus on (1) modifying speech motor patterns, (2) reinforcing fluency and punishing stuttering via operant conditioning, (3) altering parent-child interaction, and (4) modifying the emotional domain. We also make reference to another class, integrated therapies, which attempt to incorporate several of these into a single program. Finally, parent counseling, which is included, one way or another, in most therapy programs was already covered in the previous chapter. Here we offer an overview of sample programs for each of the therapy classes.

Focus on Speech/Motor Patterns

Therapies in this class geared toward preschool children reflect some differences in theoretical frame of reference and vary in specific procedures compared to those applied with adolescents or adults. They are similar in principle, however, to the parallel class of adult therapies in that they rely primarily on fluency-generating techniques. Although stuttered speech and emotional aspects may receive some attention, these are secondary and do not constitute a central part of the main therapy. Five programs are presented here as examples.[2]

---

[2]Among other programs are those suggested by Meyers Fosnot and Woodford (1992) and Bøstrup and Møller (1990).

Easy Speaking Voice

The underlying assumption of Shine's (1980) Easy Speaking Voice program, one of the first in this group, is that physiologic and aerodynamic factors, such as laryngeal tension and airflow rate, result in stuttering and should be altered. Its stated objective is to have the child understand and incorporate the concept of an "easy speaking voice." The twice-weekly sessions present a mixture of training in two skills: (1) gentle voice and (2) slow speaking rate. The program begins with drills in saying single-syllable words using a whispered voice and "stretched" speech. Picture stimuli for words the child can speak fluently are used to facilitate practice. An extremely soft voice (whisper is encouraged) is practiced initially and gradually altered into a more normal speaking voice. Activities are highly structured to minimize stuttered conversational speech. From fluently spoken single-syllable words, the child progresses to practice of longer speech segments, up to the conversation level. Some speaking activities other than structured drills on words and sentences are included in each session to facilitate transfer. A storybook and a surprise box afford opportunities to practice different standard phrases, and a language lotto game allows for the practice of asking and answering questions. All speech is executed with a soft voice and slow rate. Generalization activities are incorporated at each intermediate level of speech size segment when the criterion for fluency (0.5 or fewer stuttered words per minute) is reached at that level. When generalization is successful at the conversation level, the therapy shifts into a 1-year maintenance schedule as the frequency of clinical visits is gradually diminished.

Stuttering Intervention Program

A rather similar therapy to that of Shine is seen in Pindzola's (1987) Stuttering Intervention Program (SIP), which is purported to be rooted in the demands and capacities model (see Chapter 6.) Inasmuch as stuttering results from a child's insufficient capacities, which are not specified, to cope with demands placed on the speech system, SIP strives to increase those capacities so that fluent speech can be produced. Children are drilled intensively with three speech patterns (targets) that promote fluency: slow-stretched speech, soft speaking voice, and smooth flow of speech. These motoric strategies are enhanced by control of linguistic content, which at the beginning permits only short, simple utterances (e.g., single-syllable words) and progresses to longer complex utterances. Soft voice, especially on the first syllable of an utterance, and smoothly connected speech are introduced and practiced. The target of smooth flow of speech means blending of syllables and words within a breath group to maintain continuous movement. To facilitate pacing and blending, the child moves the index finger from side to side while talking. Practice takes place in the clinical setting and at home under parental supervision.

The Illinois Programs

In the late 1970s, one of us (EY), at the University of Illinois Stuttering Research Program, independently developed a therapy regimen similar in several fundamentals to the two therapies just described with an emphasis on slow-stretched speech.

It emerged after several years during which we experimented with rhythmic speech therapy. To us, both methods, slow rate and rhythmic speech, were summed up in the theoretical notion espoused by Van Riper (1971) and others that stuttering is a disorder of mistiming of speech movement associated with difficulties in planning upcoming speech sequences. These result in articulatory discoordination.[3] Such difficulties, we hypothesized, are particularly pronounced during the second and third years of life, a period of accelerated speech development and the time most typical for the onset of stuttering. Hence slow, regulated speech should allow the child more time for the planning and execution of the required coordination of movements. Although the therapies focus on speech manipulation, parent counseling has remained an integral aspect of the two programs.

Rhythmic Speech   Our experimentation with direct speech therapy began with metronomic-paced speech that forces the speaker into monotonous rhythm and a highly controlled speaking rate. Van Riper (1973) employed rhythmic speech, such as rhymes and "Indian talk" in his therapeutic regimen for preschoolers. The technique, however, did not attract much interest, and there has been but a single published study of metronome-paced speech applied to this age group (Coppolla & Yairi, 1982). We demonstrated that even 2-year-old children can master the technique and attend to the task. The program contained four steps:

1. Practice of saying bisyllabic words (e.g., *baseball, hotdog*) paced by a desk metronome at 80 beats per minute (bpm). A stimulus picture is presented for each word accompanied with the clinician's voiced model. Gradually progress to 120 bpm.

2. Similarly progress from 80 to 120 bpm with 2- to 3-word utterances, such as "ride school bus." Abundant reinforcement is applied. Also, periodic diversions to other activities if the child becomes tired.

3. After several sessions, the most comfortable metronomic rate for each child, typically 104 to 112 bpm, is determined and used through the rest of the program as the children advanced to practice phrases and sentences as well as during questions, storytelling, and simple brief exchanges.

4. The last few sessions are devoted to practicing rhythmic speech without metronomic pacing. Brief meetings with parents are held throughout the program to assess progress at home and answer questions. Parents reluctant to model rhythmic speech at home are encouraged to slow down their own speech, especially when talking to the child.

---

[3]It is interesting to note here the phenomenon of coarticulation, which involves a "looking ahead" in the execution of speech sequences. For example, research has shown that lip rounding for the vowel "u" in *construe* can already be detected four sounds earlier, during the formation of the "n" (Daniloff & Moll, 1968).

Moderate success in decreasing stuttering and in generalization at home was reported. The children actually appeared to have fun with the robotic-type speech. It was concluded that rhythmic speech practice should be considered an option in conjunction with other techniques, or as the main technique in selected cases.

Slow-Stretched Speech   As our experimentation with treatment of early stuttering progressed, we eventually adopted slow-stretched speech as the preferred technique because it sounds more acceptable to parents who were more willing to model it for their children than rhythmic speech. The three general objectives are to (1) provide children and their parents with intensive exposure to slow speech, (2) provide the child with ample practice of slow speech, and (3) provide parents with practice of slow speech as well as to prepare them to carry on with it at home. The program combines structured and unstructured speech activities in which the clinician always presents the child and parents with extensive modeling of slow speech. Parent counseling sessions were held periodically to deal with their concerns, provide specific advice when called for, and to obtain progress reports.

As you will see below, the clinician begins with modeling slow speech in unstructured play activities. This is followed by drills in structured activities, starting with slow speech in short segments enhanced by visual stimuli and verbal modeling, progressing to speaking slowly without external cues. The complexity and length of the speaking materials are gradually increased along with the speaking rate. To minimize children's loss of interest, short structured drills are alternated with unstructured free play. Parents first observe and later assume more active roles in the sessions, learning to speak slowly and gaining experience of doing so while interacting with the child. To provide a better sense of constructing a therapy program, the 12-session 6-week sequence, 45 to 50 minutes per session, twice per week, is outlined here.

Week 1: Sessions 1–2

The two sessions are dedicated to establishing good clinician-child relationship, introducing slow speech, and assessing the child's reaction to it. Parents do not observe. Each session has three parts.

1. Fifteen minutes of free play and relaxed conversation create a comfortable atmosphere. The clinician serves as an indirect model: (a) engaging the child in unstructured slow-paced play conducive to slow speech (e.g., making forms with plastic clay); (b) bombarding the child with a model of slow speech, about 1 word per second, while interacting (e.g., "are you making a ball?"); and (c) echoing in a slow, easy manner the child's stuttered or fast speech. That is, if the child stutters, or says a sentence fast even if fluently, the clinician repeats (echoes) the word or the phrase in a slow-stretched manner.

2. Fifteen minutes of structured speech practice. The clinician directly models single words containing one or two syllables at 1 word per second while presenting 20 to 30 picture cards, one at a time, saying the word for each picture. For example: *chair, school bus, hotdog.* The clinician instructs the child to "say it like I say it." The child

may be limited and that chances for complete recovery are low. Some key points raised in this chapter include:

- There is a certain degree of similarity among school-age children, adolescents, and adults who stutter in terms of broad therapeutic objectives and approaches.
- Management of the emotional component of the disorder, traditional stuttering modification, and fluency shaping all may be applied.
- For children within the age range of 6 to 12 years, therapy may vary significantly, depending on the age, level of emotional and cognitive maturity, and the potential for family and teachers' cooperation.
- Individual as well as group therapy formats can be pursued successfully. Many activities differ in that skills and strategies often are instructed in the context of imaginative terminology, games, and fun activities.
- To help prevent negative communication experiences at school, the clinician needs to be proactive to educate school personnel about stuttering and support the self-confidence and esteem of children who stutter. Problems of teasing and bullying may need to be addressed.
- Parent involvement in the therapy process, if possible, is extremely desirable.

There seems to be an overall clinical impression that improvement in stuttering in school-age children as the result of therapy is more difficult to achieve and sustain than it is in preschool-age children. We believe that this limitation reflects, in large part, a more resistant form of stuttering. Still, treatment efficacy research with school-age children has been very limited and the impression just mentioned should be viewed with caution. Although further studies are necessary to reach any conclusions, it is possible that specific methods are less important than whether the child learns to initiate and manage speech with reduced tension.

Study Questions and Discussion Topics

1. What are the particular stuttering characteristics of school-age children that should be considered in regard to therapy? In what ways do they differ from those of preschool-age children who stutter?
2. What are the particular emotional and social characteristics of school-age children who stutter that should be considered in regard to therapy? In what ways do they differ from those of preschool-age children and adults who stutter?
3. What are the potential roles of parents in the clinical management of school-age children who stutter?
4. Given the choice between employing the GILCU program or the Lidcombe Program, which one would be your preference, and/or under which conditions? Explain why.
5. Given the choice between employing the fluency-enhancing program or a stuttering modification program, which one will be your preference and/or under which conditions? Explain why.
6. Compare your response to question 5 in relation to treating adults who stutter. Explain why it does or does not differ.

Websites

Family Voices: http://www.westutter.org/what-is-stuttering/newsletters/

Friends—National Association of Young People Who Stutter: http://www
.friendswhostutter.org

Stuttering Foundation of America, For Kids Web site: http://www.stutteringhelp.org/kids

Stuttering home page Just for Kids Web site: http://www.mnsu.edu/comdis/kuster/kids/
kids.html

Suggested Readings

Chmela, K., & Reardon, N. (2001). *The school-age child who stutters: Working effectively with attitudes and emotions.* Memphis, TN: Stuttering Foundation of America.

Guitar, B., & Reville, J. (1997). *Easy talker.* Austin, TX: Pro-Ed.

Langevin, M., Kully, D., & Ross-Harold, B. (2007). A comprehensive stuttering program for school-age children with strategies for managing teasing and bullying. In E. Conture & R. Curlee (Eds.), *Stuttering and related disorders* (3rd ed., pp. 131–150). New York, NY: Thieme.

Ramig, P., & Bennett, E. (1997). Clinical management of children: Direct management strategy. In R. F. Curlee & G. M. Siegel (Eds.), *Nature and treatment of stuttering: New directions* (2nd ed., pp. 292–312). Boston, MA: Allyn & Bacon.

Runyan, C., & Runyan, S. (2007). A fluency rules therapy program for young children in the public schools. In E. Conture & R. Curlee (Eds.), *Stuttering and related disorders* (3rd ed., pp. 101–114). New York, NY: Thieme.

Yaruss, J., Coleman, & Quesal, R. (2012). Stuttering in school-age children: A comprehensive approach to treatment. [Letter to the Editor]. *Language, Speech & Hearing Services in Schools, 43,* 536–548.

Chapter 14

Therapy for Preschool-Age Children

LEARNER OBJECTIVES

Readers of this chapter will understand:

- The historical background of therapy for early stuttering.
- Considerations regarding intervention for preschool children who stutter.
- The range of treatment objectives for this subpopulation.
- Clinical programs representing the current major treatment approaches.
- Research issues concerned with treatment of preschoolers who stutter.

General Considerations

Having reviewed and discussed the treatment of stuttering in adults and school-age children, we now shift attention to general approaches, specific techniques, and programs that have been offered for the treatment of preschool-age children. Chapter 2, which focused on the distribution of the stuttering population, established that the overwhelming majority of people who stutter experience the onset of the disorder (incidence) during the preschool period, ages 2 to 5, mostly before age 3. Additionally, the data show that the prevalence of stuttering (the percentage of people who exhibit active stuttering) is also the largest in this age group.[1]

In spite of these indisputable facts, systematic clinical intervention programs designed specifically for preschool-age children who stutter were relatively late to appear, and for a long time they lacked the breadth of treatment methods offered to adults who stutter. This trend paralleled the one seen in the research domain that, for many years, favored adults who stutter. This scenario reflects several realities. First has been the lingering "hands off the child" attitude toward treatment of early stuttering that was promoted especially in the United States. Second may have been a tendency toward thinking that stuttering in children and adults was all the same. Third, university laboratories and clinics were mainly accessible to college students. Fortunately, the trend has been reversed, and the past three decades have seen a substantial increase both in clinical programs and clinical research pertaining to preschool-age children who stutter. The following brief historical account of past therapies for this age group is intended to provide a broadened perspective on current clinical issues and therapy programs.

---

[1]One study (Craig et al., 2002), however, suggested a peak prevalence in the 6- to 10-year age group.

A Brief Historical Review

Therapeutic interventions for early childhood stuttering have operated with different philosophies that have alternated over the years, reflecting changes in the dominant thinking of mainstream speech pathology in respect to direct and indirect intervention modes. The distinction between the two in regard to stuttering is not clear. For some clinicians, for example Conture (2001), the criterion is based on the approach to a child's speech. An indirect approach does *not* explicitly, overtly, or directly prompt the child to speak fluently. Rather, the focus is on changing the child's environment, especially parents' behavior or the child's emotionality. Direct approaches involve explicit attempts to modify the child's speech. Our interpretation, by contrast, encompasses a wider context of what is considered direct therapy.

> In this context, the term *direct therapy* applies to methods in which the clients themselves are subjected to treatment. In addition to methods in which the child who stutters receives guidance for making speech changes (speech therapy), psychologically oriented therapy and/or physical stimulation of parts of the body (e.g., oral structures) are viewed as direct therapy. For example, play therapy with the child as a participant in a process aimed at altering his or her emotionality and behavior is direct therapy. Although play therapy does not deal with speech modification, it is a method that requires a very direct contact between clinician and child. A therapy that is limited to physical stimulation of oral muscles (not speech therapy) is also viewed as direct.

In view of the constraints placed on early intervention, particularly by the client's age and the nature of the early stuttering, discussed later, it is interesting to note the diversity of treatments that have been applied. In that light, it also is surprising that many share a fair number of objectives with the major therapeutic approaches listed in Chapter 10 for older children and adults. The procedures, however, have been adapted to suit young children.

Direct Treatments

As stated above, direct therapy is when the client is the immediate recipient of the treatment, being speech- or nonspeech-oriented. Toward the end of the 19th century and the first decades of the 20th century, the most frequently advocated types of programs involved direct therapy. They leaned toward what we have referred to as *fluency enhancement*, that is, the elicitation and subsequent practice of talking patterns that produce fluent speech, rather than modification of instances of stuttering. Such philosophy was particularly dominant in Europe. In fact, today's popular approaches were practiced more than 100 years ago.

European Methods

According to Pay and Sirotkina (1955), Russian clinicians devised intensive programs, including all-day clinics, that required children as young as 2 years of age to memorize and repeat sentences, tell picture stories, rehearse questions and answers, and

1. Free-play/conversation time involving parental participation.

2. Structured drill is carried out with a focus on short stories aided by several sequence cards. The clinician uses 4- to 6-word sentences telling the brief story depicted in a picture sequence. Next, the parents repeat, sentence by sentence, after the clinician, pointing to the appropriate picture in the series. Next, the parents ask the child to repeat the same sequence following the modeling. Lastly, the child is to tell the sentence sequence without a model. The clinician intervenes when needed.

3. Structured activity in the form of a simple dialogue. The clinician, using the slow speaking rate, asks the child questions about the sequenced stories used in activity. The child is requested to respond with 4- to 6-word sentences using the slow speech rate practiced earlier. A model is provided at the beginning and as needed as the practice progresses.

4. A few minutes of free-play activities.

Week 6: Sessions 11–12

The changes for the week are (1) a progression to longer speaking tasks, (2) a greater role for the parents, and (3) increased speaking rate to 2 words per second (about 120 words per minute).

1. Beginning with unstructured activities, the clinician introduces the faster speaking rate (still slower than normal). Echoing continues with occasional reminders to use "slow, easy speech" or the feedback "this was slow and easy."

2. Proceeding to a more structured activity, the clinician tells a story that may be somewhat longer than in the card sequence materials. Short sentences, at the new rate, are used. The child is to repeat his or her version of it maintaining slow speech. Parents learn how to practice similar activities at home.

3. Return to free play/conversation. Now, the parent assumes the sole role in modeling, monitoring, and echoing the child's speech.

4. Similar to part #2, practice during storytelling. The parent takes over as the teller and model. The child repeats and practices with the parent.

In our experience, a 6-week therapy is sufficient for the first round. The program may be repeated or continued if necessary after a few weeks off, allowing for assessment of child progress and parental reactions. Data for six children with moderate-to-severe stuttering who were between 13 to 29 months post-onset when therapy commenced, presented changes in SLD, comparing two pretherapy and two posttherapy testing points. Four children demonstrated substantial improvement between the pre- and initial posttherapy testing. Six months later, 3 of the 6 children exhibited substantial improvement, 2 showed modest or minimal improvement, and the remaining child exhibited a substantial increase in stuttering (Yairi & Ambrose, 2005, p. 453). Perhaps differences in the chronic nature or the individual child's stuttering may explain the variable improvement in spite of the intensive treatment. But, as explained, the purpose of presenting the program in a step-by-step fashion is to provide clinicians with concrete ideas about how to plan and execute a systematic, logical therapy program that addresses the child's stuttering and also guides parents in cooperating, thus increasing potential attainment. Clinicians, however, should be flexible, for example, selecting other speaking rates, altering order of progress or time distribution among activities. The point is that if there are good reasons to believe that slow speech is helpful, this could be a reasonable approach to pursue in a systematic manner.

Speech Motor Training

A unique current treatment for early childhood stuttering that belongs in this class of therapies is the Speech Motor Training program (Riley & Riley, 1985, 1999). It was motivated by data interpreted to show that children who stutter exhibit reduced integration of the speech motor system. Hence its goal is to develop, or strengthen, speech motor control by correcting the deficient oral speech movement sequences necessary for normal production of syllables by means of extensive drill. The target is uninterrupted production of multiple iterations of nonsense syllable sequences at the fastest rate possible while maintaining accuracy.

The 14-stage program begins with the child practicing sequences of meaningless syllables, such as "vami" and "nimu." The meaningless content's aim is to minimize cognitive self-monitoring. Also, nonwords may pose less risk of triggering stuttering than real words. Gradually, the number of syllables increases from 1 to 4, the speaking rate from 1 to 3 syllables per second, and the unvoiced consonants from 0 to 2. The complexity is also increased from the CV structure at level 1 to the CVCVCCVVC structure at level 14. The extensive drill in the speech motor skills contributes to successful long-term maintenance of fluency gains because, as the Rileys explain, overlearned motor skills tend to remain stable. Their reported data for six children who underwent 24 therapy sessions indicated that stuttering frequency was diminished by 49% and its severity by 46%. One of us (CS) has had modest experience with this technique and found it supportive toward fluency gains in conjunction with other strategies (e.g., slower easier speech) in the case of a young school-age child who had relatively weak diadochokinetic syllable sequencing skills.

Focus on Operant Conditioning

In Chapter 6, stuttering was discussed within the framework of operant learning theory with an underlying assumption that it is a behavioral response modifiable by its consequences. Research has supported this view, showing that stuttering can be diminished through punishment, withdrawal of reinforcement, and withdrawal of aversive stimuli. A well-known, although small, controlled laboratory study by Martin et al. (1972) demonstrated the power of operant conditioning also on the diminution of stuttering in preschool children. They had two children converse with a lighted puppet. Each time the child stuttered, the puppet stopped talking and the light was turned off for 10 seconds (removal of reinforcement). At the end of the program, stuttering was reduced in the clinic and home. Actually, however, operant-based stuttering therapy for young children was practiced before that study as seen in the clinical programs developed by Bar (1971) and Ryan (1971). Whereas some forms of punishment and withdrawal of reinforcement have been incorporated in therapeutic regimens for children, positive reinforcement of fluent speech rather than punishment of stuttering has received greater emphasis. Bar (1971) applied positive reinforcement, whereas Van Riper (1973) used both. Describing his early clinical experimentations he wrote, "by intermittently and casually showing more attention and appreciation of the child's fluent communication but only ordinary acceptance of his stuttering speech, we have been able to get marked gain in fluency by this simple procedure and without the child's conscious awareness of the contingency" (cf. p. 409). Two current programs that represent the approach applied to preschool children are described below.

Extended Length of Utterance (ELU)

The ELU program was devised by Janis Costello Ingham (Costello, 1983; J. Ingham, 1999) for young CWS and bears similarities to the GILCU program for school-age children described in Chapter 13. Primarily achieved through positive reinforcement of fluent speech, it seeks to gradually increase the length of fluently produced speech segments, as well as the length of time during which fluency can be maintained. With contingent feedback and following a stepwise progression, the child learns to produce the desired speech more frequently. The main speaking contexts of the ELU program (e.g., picture naming) make it particularly suitable for preschool children. The clinician reinforces fluency with verbal feedback, such as "Good talking!" or "Excellent speech!" while the contingent instruction "Stop" is made after moments of stuttering. Token reinforcements may also be administered. The objective is to maintain fluency throughout the elicited speech responses.

The ELU is a highly structured 20-step program in which the target utterances progress through a sequence from monosyllabic words to longer utterances and up to 5 minutes connected speech. Table 14.1 describes the target contexts for fluent speech associated with the 20 steps grouped into four sets.

Table 14.1   Target Responses Corresponding to the Sets of Steps in the ELU Program

Set	ELU Target Responses
Steps 1–6	Monosyllabic to 6-syllable utterances
Steps 7–11	3- to 30-second monologues
Steps 12–16	1- to 5-minute monologues
Steps 17–20	2- to 5-minute conversations

To conduct the therapy, the clinician needs the following stimulus materials: 50 picture cards to elicit monosyllabic words, a list of 50 two-syllable words, a list of 50 two-syllable phrases, and 50 each of 3-, 4-, 5-, 6-syllable words and phrases. Progress is monitored by measuring the percentage of correct (fluent) utterances, numbers of syllables spoken, and numbers of trials to reach criterion. Stage advancement requires a certain number of consecutive fluent trials (e.g., 10 consecutive correct productions for steps 1 through 13). Another feature of the program is that when the simple contingencies are insufficient, other "additives" may be included, such as reduced speaking rate, gentle voice onset, reduced linguistic complexity, and/or modification of attitudes.

The ELU program received support in two very small studies. Riley and Ingham (2000) treated six children and reported 63.5% median reduction in stuttering frequency from pre- to posttherapy. Onslow (1996) reported on one child who produced less than 0.5% syllables stuttered at follow-up assessment. Still unknown is the extent to which all 20 steps are needed and how many children need "additives" and altering for various aspects of the program. Another program of interest in which reinforcement is applied to increasingly longer fluent speech segments is the Stocker Probe Technique (Stocker & Goldfarb, 1995). Its special feature is the heavy emphasis placed on a systematic increase in linguistic complexity of the verbal content practiced at each progressive level of difficulty.

The Lidcombe Program

The application of operant conditioning principles to the treatment of preschool children who stutter through heavy parental participation began with a large project pioneered by Bar (1971). He published a clinical program in which parents of 59 stuttering preschoolers were trained in reinforcing fluent utterances in their child's speech using verbal contingencies such as "I like the way you said this word." Surprisingly, and rather unfortunately, Bar's contribution to the recently popular reliance on parent-administered conditioning therapy is almost never acknowledged. Perhaps it had a substantial influence on the later appearance in Australia of the Lidcombe Program for early stuttering (Onslow et al., 2003) that has gained considerable international popularity. It delivers direct speech therapy for the child and rests heavily on parents' active participation in carrying out the therapy at home. The therapy is tied to operant learning principles: contingent verbal positive reinforcement of the child's fluent speech and contingent verbal mild disapproval ("punishment" in operant conditioning terminology) of stuttered speech. Still, it is not as rigid as the typical operant program in terms of progressive stage, criteria for progress, and tight contingency schedules.

The best age for children to receive this therapy may be from 4 to 6 years. Children ages 2 to 3 took a much longer time to respond and benefit. When a child is older than 6 years, stuttering tends to already be more complicated and less responsive to parental response. To be accepted for standard therapy, a child must exhibit "unambiguous stuttering. For some research studies, however, eligibility criteria also required more than 6% syllables stuttered, be at least 6 months post-onset, and have no other cognitive or linguistic disorders.

The first stage aims at achieving near zero stuttering. Treatment begins with several 1-hour weekly sessions conducted by the clinician with the parents initially passively observing while learning the principles and administration of verbal contingencies to their child's stutter-free as well as stuttered speech. The child is encouraged to speak during play or other activities, and the clinician is keen on providing praise or acknowledgment when the child is fluent by saying, "That was smooth speech" and similar reinforcing praises. But when the child stutters, the clinician responds with mild corrective feedback in the form of acknowledgment of stuttering (e.g., "That was bumpy speech"). A previous overall 5:1 ratio of praises to corrections has been dropped. No particular speaking rate or pattern is targeted.

There are, however, additional important features to the program that expand it outside the parameters of operant procedures, for example, self-evaluation. At times, after either fluent or stuttered speech, the child is requested to evaluate his or her own speech with a question such as "Was that smooth speech?" There are also requests for self-correction. After stuttering had occurred, instead of the usual acknowledgment, the clinician may say, "Can you fix that bump?" or combines an acknowledgment with self-correction: "That was bumpy. Say it again to smooth it out." The program, however, does not include practice in modifying instances of stuttering. The child is left to experiment on his or her own.

Parental involvement is an essential part of the whole program. As mentioned, they attend all early sessions together with their child and are trained to deliver the therapy at home. Parents demonstrate the ability to administer the procedures in the clinic, and the speech-language pathologist (SLP) gives feedback to ensure that the treatment is appropriate. The SLP demonstrates necessary adjustments to be made in the coming week, taking into account how the child is responding to the therapy.

As parents become more proficient, they apply contingencies at home, starting with two designated 10-minute talking sessions per day to increase stutter-free speech at home, first applying positive reinforcement, and then adding corrective feedback for stuttered speech. Gradually, the structured home sessions are reduced and contingencies are applied in unstructured life routines. The contingency schedule is intermittent rather than after every utterance. Parents must not feel uncomfortable or judgmental of stuttering when they apply the contingencies.

The practice sessions in the clinic are gradually reduced after the child has been stutter-free at home for a sufficient time, typically 3 consecutive weeks. Parents use a 10-point stuttering severity rating scale (1 = no stuttering, 2 = extremely mild stuttering, and 10 = extremely severe stuttering) to indicate daily fluctuations. Progress is also monitored by the clinician's measurement of percentage of stuttered syllables (%SS) taken at the start of each visit to the clinic. Past research indicated that the treatment time to complete stage 1 varies around a median of 11 clinic visits, with 90% of children completing stage 1 in 22 clinic visits. The median number has been revised to 16 sessions (Rousseau, Packman, Onslow et al., 2007).

When stuttering frequency reaches the level of absent or very low stuttering, both within and beyond the clinic, and for 3 consecutive weeks, the program continues with the second stage, maintenance. The objective is to maintain the fluency criteria while the parental verbal contingencies are withdrawn and the frequency of clinic visits decreases. Parents and child visit the clinic a few times for monitoring changes in the stuttering and making adjustments in the parents' handling of it. Follow-up continues for a while to ensure long-term gains. As will be presented later in the chapter, the Lidcombe Program has been subjected to considerable clinical effectiveness research with promising published findings. More information can be found on the Internet guide http://sydney .edu.au/health-sciences/asrc/health_professionals/asrc_download.shtml

> The Lidcombe Program has several strengths. It is administered in natural settings so that no generalization targets are necessary. Children enjoy the talking activities that always involve connected speech. The program is not too complicated to implement, and parents and children do not find themselves uncertain about how to respond to stuttering. There are several limitations to the program, however. Some parents are neither careful nor particularly capable of following the home management aspects, and it is not easily altered for children with cognitive or language delays. Minor deviations in the regimen can compromise its effects, and not all parents are prepared to be consistent in carrying it out. The approach does not address disfluency that may be ambiguous with respect to stuttering. Finally research by Bonelli, Dixon, Bernstein Ratner et al. (2000) suggested that children may be responding to the intervention by simplifying their language to stay within fluency capacities and possibly pushing their stuttering under the surface.

Focus on Parent-Child Interaction

Indirect therapies, alluded to earlier in the chapter, were initially driven by theories that parents are the major cause of stuttering. Hence it was quite logical to conclude that parents should be the main target for clinical intervention. Although these ideas have substantially diminished over the years, they have been replaced by strong beliefs that, regardless of whether parents are the cause of stuttering, they exert powerful influences on the characteristics the disorder takes on throughout its developmental course, including the child's emotional adjustment and ways of coping. Thus various degrees of traditional, individual, face-to-face parent counseling aimed at altering behaviors with, and attitudes toward, the child have remained an important component in many current therapy programs for young children. Furthermore, as seen in the Lidcombe program, parents are sometimes recruited to actually deliver speech therapy at home.

Several clinicians, however, have opted to focus on changing the home environment, especially the nature of the parent-child interaction, by engaging parents in ongoing activities, not just providing standard advice in analyzing and altering behaviors. Simultaneously, these programs also involve the child in various ways, such as teaching better interpersonal communication skills. They do not, however, exclude more direct speech therapy. Sometimes it is employed as a secondary procedure. In this section, we review a few programs in which modifying the home environment is either *the* focus or one of a few major foci of therapy.

Interaction Therapy

The main objectives of interaction therapy are to involve both parents, if possible, in an active process of helping them develop and refine constructive behaviors that support the child's fluency through their interaction style. It also aims at dealing with parental anxiety, as well as with the child's self-confidence and behavior.

The Parent Child Interaction program, developed by clinicians in the United Kingdom (Rustin et al., 1996), exemplifies this approach. The therapy is anchored in the assumption that stuttering, as a multifactorial disorder, can be improved through manipulating a child's environment. Nevertheless, direct speech therapy may be implemented as necessary. At an earlier time, the program emphasized teaching parents what *not* to do in order to decrease their child's stuttering. This was done by analyzing videotaped parent-child interactions for potential parental behavior that could undermine fluent speech. In a recent development (Kelman & Nicholas, 2008), the therapy took on a more positive approach, building on parents' intuitive understanding of what their child needs to be more fluent, increasing and reinforcing their ability for helpful interactions in the home environment.

Following a thorough assessment of the child and the home environment, the program proceeds in four phases:

1. **Establishing Talking Time.** Parents should secure at home a brief *talking time* or *special time* when each parent makes a commitment to spend 5 minutes, three to six times per week, playing and talking with the child. It is an opportunity for quality time for the child and parent to spend together, a basic feature of the approach. During these periods, the parents are encouraged to implement their chosen interaction strategies. They are to listen carefully to what is being said, acknowledge the child's speaking difficulty, and maintain an open dialogue with the child about it.

2. **Weekly Clinical Sessions.** Typically, parents learn to master the routine of special times within a few days. These are set up during the initial therapy session, leading to the next phase, which involves six weekly sessions held in the clinic. Sessions begin with feedback concerning the previous weeks' special times. Then, a few minutes of child-parent interaction are video recorded. The parents and clinician review the video together and discuss it. This allows parents to take a step back, consider what they are already doing to help their child's fluency and what should be altered or improved. From such analysis and discussion, a target behavior for the parents to employ in the coming week is agreed on. Examples of typical interaction targets are for the parents to follow the child's lead, slow down their speech rate, listen more attentively, be aware of conversational turn taking, have a balance of questions and comments, extend response time latency (giving the child time to initiate, respond, and finish his/her talking), and employ language that is appropriate to the child's level. Parents are encouraged to think about why that interaction target may be helpful for the

child's fluency. The interaction target is first practiced in the clinic before being applied at home during the special times.

3. **Consolidation Period.** The six weekly clinical sessions are followed by a 6-week consolidation period during which the behaviors targeted for change are implemented at home. The clinician monitors the case weekly through parent-written progress reports.

4. **Follow-up.** The last phase consists of 3-month follow-ups for at least a year. If the child persists in stuttering, further sessions to work on interaction strategies or family strategies may be carried out. If needed, direct therapy is implemented and the child is taught a variety of strategies for managing speech.

To date, research evidence for the effectiveness of the interaction therapy has been minimal. A significant reduction in stuttering after therapy, sustained during the consolidation period, was reported for just one child by Matthews, Williams, and Pring (1997). A more recent single-subject design study that included six preschool-age children, ages 3 years 3 months to 4 years 10 months, indicated that, by the end of the follow-up phase of the program, four exhibited statistically significant reduction in stuttering frequency with both parents and one child improved only with one parent. The sixth child required direct speech therapy in order to improve (Millard, Nicholas, & Cook, 2008).

Parent-Child Groups

The Parent-Child Groups program (Conture & Melnick, 1999) is another example of an intervention in early childhood stuttering that places priority on improving the home environment and interpersonal communication skills rather than on achieving perfect fluency. It has three foci: (1) communication *interaction*, (2) child and parent *attitudes* toward speech, and (3) speech production *behavior*. Delivery is in the form of two small groups: one for children within a limited age range (e.g., 3 to 5 years old) and one for their parents. Both meet once per week over a 12-week period. The procedures bear similarity to those employed by Wyatt and Herzan (1962) and Egolf, Shames, Johnson et al. (1972).

Through modeling and direct instruction, children improve interaction skills with rules such as "listen when another person speaks," "refrain from talking when someone else talks," and "wait patiently for your turn to talk." Direct speech therapy is administered only occasionally, mainly when progress is slow or when the excessive overt stuttering calls for it. In that case, the child is taught through modeling and direct instruction to make the stuttering easy. Parents, in their group, are educated about the possible negative effects on stuttering of frequent interruptions, talking for the child, talking in long complex utterances, talking with excessively rapid rate, and frequent correction of stuttering. Desired behaviors are suggested and/or modeled for the parents. Parents are encouraged to use normally slow speech, as well as short, simple sentences. Also, they either observe part of the child's sessions and/or participate in them. The program is described in greater detail by Guitar (2014, pp. 242–245).

Integrative and Alternative Strategies

In Chapter 12 we discussed attempts to combine several approaches to therapy for adults who stutter into a single program. Integrated methods and those that offer specific alternative or combined treatments also exist for preschool children. The mixture of parent counseling and direct speech therapy is certainly very common. One program that clearly attempts differential treatment based on the developmental status of the stuttering was offered by Gregory and Hill in 1984 (also in Gregory, 1999) and employs three strategies.

The first, *preventive parent counseling,* is the preferred strategy for a child who mostly exhibits disfluencies typical of normally speaking children but whose parents are concerned. Parents receive one or two counseling sessions concerning speech development and styles of communication and interaction that may increase or decrease disfluency. Some follow-up takes place too.

Prescriptive parent counseling, the second, is aimed at children with mild stuttering. In addition to the counseling already described, parents are taught to keep daily charts of the child's stuttering behaviors, awareness, and reactions. This information is used in the counseling. The program also includes four to six therapy sessions with the child, emphasizing modeling of easy, relaxed speech, first by the clinician and then the parent.

Comprehensive therapy program, the third strategy, is for children whose speech contains frequent stuttering events and perhaps also concomitant disorders in speech, language, and/or behavior. It includes the counseling and charting techniques employed in the first two strategies but goes beyond. This is an intensive program in which parents receive weekly counseling and the child is seen two to four times weekly for approximately 6 to 12 months. The child's therapy may include desensitization, modeling of slow, easy fluent speech in increasingly longer and more complicated speech segments, and language structure.

The Helsingborg Hospital Model

The most comprehensive program in this category that also yielded results for a good number of clients was developed in Helsingborg, Sweden.

Cecilia Lundstrom and Marie Garsten (2000, 2012) developed a model of program delivery for preschoolers who stutter that offers flexible intervention options. By virtue of its rich options, it shies away from an all-or-nothing approach of providing immediate intervention on the one hand, or delayed intervention decisions on the other one. The model includes six components:

1. Initial parent counseling (This is the core of the model and is always held first.)
2. Assessment of the child's speech and language
3. Parent support groups combined with a child playgroup
4. Individual follow-up after completion of the group activity
5. Individual or group therapy, followed by contact with the parents
6. Intensive therapy for stuttering children and their parents

Intervention always begins with one or two parent counseling sessions following the Caplan (1970) mental health consultation, a model that has much in common with cognitive therapy. Otherwise, parents may elect any or all components in which the child and they participate. The parents relate information about familial stuttering history, onset of stuttering, and so on. Through active questioning parents are led to explore the stuttering problem and verbalize their observations, thoughts, and feelings. This results in new ideas on how to support the child. The clinician provides information about stuttering that also aims to alleviate guilt feelings. Most parents want to analyze situations at home and try new strategies, then come back for additional counseling.

The child playgroup meets once per week for 5 weeks. It is a nondemanding environment with a nonavoidance emphasis, seeking to encourage the child to communicate regardless of stuttering. Having the CWS play together is viewed as very important for its psychological value. Some direct stuttering modification is done via play, such as using animal toys that talk in different ways, or they observe and make comments about different kinds of stuttering in the clinician's speech. Clinicians talk openly about stuttering, even with the young children. The parent support group, guided by a clinician, meets at the same time. Parents present to each other their children and their stuttering problem and there is an exchange of experiences. Individual follow-up is usually only one visit after group therapy to give parents feedback and discuss further intervention. For individual therapy, parents can choose among three options: integrated stuttering therapy, the Palin Parent Child Interaction program, or the Lidcombe Program. Although preschool in Sweden extends through age 6, all of the procedures and programs described above are employed with 2- to 5-year-old children. Parents also receive counseling and participate in a support group.

Two follow-up studies were conducted in which questionnaires were sent to parents of 110 children of whom 41 were reported to have a familial history of persistent stuttering. Families were contacted 2–5 years after the first visit. Questionnaires were returned by 74 families. Among other results, the survey showed that *counselling only* was selected most by parents. Furthermore, it was usually the only one needed to achieve parent satisfaction. Of the respondents, 41(54%) reported that their child had stopped stuttering. This moderate recovery rate is expected in view of the high percent of persistent familial stuttering. Among the rest, 28 had little stuttering, 3 had considerable stuttering and 2 children had severe stuttering.

Focus on Emotionality

As previously discussed, the past 3 decades or so have seen a strong return trend toward direct therapy in which modification of children's speech has been popular. Still, within the overall trend, there have been a few attempts to include psychologically oriented therapies in which the child is the focus and immediate recipient of the treatment. Hence these are classified as "direct" as well. Their objectives and methods varied widely. Van Riper (1973) had in mind the prevention of future development of negative emotionality (e.g., avoidance of talking). To increase the child's interest in talking and verbal output, he advocated "fun" activities that elicited more speech. Hence speech becomes associated with joyful experiences.

Other methods bear greater similarities to psychotherapy with objectives that vary from resolving the child's emotional conflicts and difficulties in mother-child emotional ties, to increasing the child's self-confidence and interpersonal skills. Although most speech-language clinicians are not trained in this area, we feel it is worthwhile to be informed about the methods and their applications. Some children may benefit from referrals to a trained professional. The two therapies presented here reflect this approach.

Psychotherapeutic Play

Play has long been viewed as an essential component of healthy child development, both emotionally and cognitively. There are many forms and variations of play therapy. It may be directive and structured, even geared toward specific trauma by presenting play materials relevant to the child's stressful experiences, thus facilitating release of the associated emotions. The technique, originally offered by Levy (1938), is known as *release therapy.*

> Psychologists believe that play provides a vehicle to express experiences and feelings in the most natural way available to children and also allows them to work through inner anxieties. Froebel (1903, p. 22) asserted that play alone "is the free expression of what is in the child's soul." Play therapy is built on these assumptions by helping children communicate what they cannot verbalize. The play is seen as having therapeutic value similar to free association for adult psychoanalysis because it leads to the child's unconscious (Klein, 1932, 1955; A. Freud, 1946).

A different technique is nondirective play, which later became known as *client-centered therapy* (Rogers, 1951). Its objective is to provide a secure relationship between the child and an adult—the clinician, and help the child resolve emotional problems. Virginia Axline (1947) expanded on Rogers's work (1942), and her approach to nondirective child play therapy has been among the most widely practiced. These are the main principles:

- The clinician does not direct the child's actions or conversations. The child plays, or behaves otherwise, as he or she wishes. Only minimal limitations are established (e.g., the child cannot hurt self or others).
- The clinician develops a warm relationship with the child, accepting him or her as is. A permissive atmosphere must be created that allows the child complete freedom to express feelings.
- The clinician should be able to recognize those feelings during play and reflects them back so to help the child gain insight into his or her behavior.
- The child should be given ample opportunities to solve problems and make choices and changes.

As the child plays, the clinician reflects on the activity (e.g., "Johnny tore down the block tower. Johnny is angry."). The clinician is careful to state observations without making interpretations. Nonetheless, there may be times when the clinician reflects back in such a manner that she or he becomes directive in interpreting the child's inner world (e.g., is the emotion anger or frustration? Was the tower knocked down partly by accident before it was on purpose?). Hence the concept of *nondirective therapy* should be understood as a relative one.

According to Kenjo (2005, p. 9), "In Japan, the primary treatments with younger children, including those with severe stuttering, have for a long time been play therapy and modification of the environment." Wakaba (1983, 1999), also in Japan, posited that a good number of preschool children who stutter experienced insufficient maternal attachment in infancy and, therefore, she has preferred psychotherapeutic play. Her treatment was strongly influenced by the Axline (1947) approach. In addition to the common focus on accepting and reflecting the child's emotions, thoughts, and aggressive behaviors, special attention is given to the child's stuttering experience and its impact. Of course, the clinician must accept the stuttering. Therapy varies from two or three sessions for a child exhibiting mild stuttering to long-term (several years) for a child with a severe, complicated problem. Small group therapy conducted with the same method of free play is warranted when social interaction emerges as a problem. In weekly parent counseling, the clinician discusses with the mother any changes in the child's stuttering, positive social and aggressive behaviors, or regression to seeking attachment to the mother.

Drama Therapy

Drama therapy is very different in concept and procedures than those based in free play. It employs theater techniques to promote the psychological health of individuals, couples, families, and groups. Drama therapy appears to be an outgrowth of psychodrama (Moreno, 1946) and role play. Rather than being aimed at treating deeply seated emotional conflicts rooted in infancy, the objectives are to reduce fear, increase self-confidence, stimulate positive attitudes toward communication, and explore and resolve unhealthy patterns of personal relations. So far, drama therapy has been practiced at a rather modest level in the treatment of stuttering. Its main advocates have been Professor Tomaiuoli and her team in Rome (Tomaiuoli et al., 2007).

Applied to young children who stutter, the technique uses stories that are played on a stage by a group. Stories are selected in consideration of the characters, the reality problems they present, and suitability to the clients' needs. Children's complex problems and concerns, such as being isolated, clumsy, or mocked, are simplified and projected through the story's characters that the children assume. The children act out the different roles within the same tale. The clinician participates in the play, serving as a verbal and behavioral model for the child and parents. Also family members become involved, taking roles in the play. One example for the method is creating a play based on the story "Skittle the Baby Elephant" who is clumsy in his movements. Negative peer reactions instill in him inferiority feelings and shyness. He resolves the situation by displaying other positive aspects about himself and eventually overcomes the handicap. Through acting the role the child learn to overcome problems similar to real ones but in a less fearful environment. The different tales allow the child to play and interact with different personalities, and through these he or she realizes what the optimal behavior is, including assertiveness, to achieve the objective.

Through acting, the child moves closer to experiencing real-world situations. Because the play, however, is somewhat removed from reality, those situations become less stressful. The play also teaches the child to figure out solutions, adopt optimal behavior, and change habitual responses. Although not dealing directly with speech modification, the play acting does help the child cope better with the stuttering, improve self-confidence, and function well in various educational programs and society. Greater fluency is a by-product.

At the end of a typical 6-month program that entails two weekly sessions, the children put on a show in a real theater for an audience of families and friends. One of us (EY) had several opportunities to attend this theater while visiting the Rome center. Seeing the stuttering children stage an hour-long play and display courage in spite of some stuttering is an uplifting emotional experience.

Tomaiuoli et al. (2007) reported results for 10 preschool children without histories of treatment who completed the entire therapy program. Their data indicated statistically significant reduction in typical and atypical speech disfluency in several speaking situations. Additional data showed improvement in the children's withdrawal behavior and their difficulties with problem solving.

Clinical Research

Past and Current Research

Research concerning the efficacy of therapy for stuttering in preschool-age children has been slow to take place. Research questions are: Does a specific therapy work? If yes, is it better than other therapies? Until the early 1990s, only six relevant studies, with a total of 14 subjects, were identified (Yairi, 1993). With a few exceptions, published therapy programs have not undergone even remotely appropriate controlled research to document either effectiveness or efficacy. For example, seven different therapies published in a compendium edited by Fosnot (1995) were not accompanied with supporting data. Some critics argued that several clinicians advocate techniques that research has actually shown ineffective (Ingham & Cordes, 1999).

In view of scant past research, it is encouraging to note rising clinical research activities since the 1990s that have included more children and encompassed a wide range of therapies. Among other studies, overall success in reducing the frequency of stuttering was reported for a group of 5 children using the ELU method (Riley & Ingham, 1995), 6 children using speech motor training (Riley & Riley, 1999), 19 children using play therapy (Wakaba, 1999), 110 children using mainly parent counseling (Lundstrom & Garsten, 2012), 32 children using child-parent therapy groups (Richels & Conture, 2007), 6 children using slow speech (Yairi & Ambrose, 2005), 10 children using drama therapy (Tomaiuoli et al., 2007), 6 children using parent-child interaction therapy (Millard et al., 2008), and more.

A related research direction has been pursued to study the effect of parents' speaking rate on their child's disfluency, motivated by the fact that a number of therapies and parent counseling programs encourage parents to speak slowly, hoping to influence the child into adopting slower speech that, in turn, should reduce disfluency. Three small studies with a total of 13 mother-child pairs revealed that that when mothers slowed down their speaking rate, the children's fluency improved, although children's speaking rate was not lowered (Guitar et al., 1992; Starkweather & Gottwald, 1984; Stephanson-Opsal & Bernstein Ratner, 1988). Little effect of parents' slowing down their speech on children's speaking rate was also reported for 20 normally speaking children and their mothers (Bernstein Ratner, 1992). The length of the exposure to slow speech, however, was short, and there were individual variations. Similar findings with five parent-child dyads were reported by Zebrowski et al. (1996), although in their study there was a uniform trend toward reduction in the children's speaking rate. Guitar and Marchinkoski (2001) studied six mother-child dyads employing improved procedures that included a substantially reduced (50%) parent speech rate. These investigators were the first to report statistically significantly reduced speaking rate in five children. Clearly, much more research of this critical issue is required, paying attention to the length of exposure and the specific speaking rate required of parents.

A promising, more systematic, clinical research program concerned with young children who stutter has been tested by an Australian team who provided better baseline data, clearer procedures, and follow-up. Starting with a small preliminary study of four children who received a few hours of therapy with the Lidcombe technique described earlier, it was reported that none of them exhibited stuttering 9 months after treatment. Subsequent studies were larger in scope (Onslow, Costa, & Rue, 1990). One study included 47 children who were followed for 2 to 7 years. Speech samples recorded at home by parents indicated that near zero stuttering was maintained (Lincoln & Onslow, 1997). Other studies have been reported on 250 participants (Jones et al., 2000) and 29 participants (Rousseau et al., 2007). They concluded that a median of 11 clinical visits was sufficient to achieve near zero stuttering. Also, allowing a waiting period between stuttering onset and the initiation of therapy did not necessitate increased treatment time. Randomized studies in which children who stuttered were assigned to treatment and no-treatment groups were reported by Jones et al. (2005) for 54 children; Lattermann, Euler, & Neumann (2008), for 46 children; and Lewis, Packman, Onslow et al. (2008) for 18 children. Overall, therapy resulted in a lower level of stuttering compared to no therapy.

Weaknesses and Other Issues in Research

In spite of the welcome progress, the state of the art of clinical research for early childhood stuttering is afflicted by one, or several, experimental flaws that impede their credibility. One such failing has been an absent or vague definition of stuttering. For example, the definition of stuttering employed in several studies of "unambiguous stuttering" (e.g., Harrison et al., 2007) is actually a bit ambiguous. Therefore the clinician/investigator may discount instances of stuttering and thus bias the data in a particular direction. Another problem has been the period of baseline measures prior to treatment. If baseline measures are not collected over a sufficient time (e.g., 6 months), children in the midst of natural recovery will not be identified, and the rest of their progress will be erroneously assigned to the effect of therapy. This is a clear weakness in the Lattermann et al. (2008) study. Insufficient follow-up fails to disclose the long-term impact of therapy. For example, Jones et al. (2005) employed a single follow-up 9 months after the initiation of treatment. Hence, the posttreatment interval was shorter than 9 months. Other issues arise from an uncontrolled time period following the onset of the disorder. If children in a clinical study have stuttered for 3 months or a shorter duration prior to the beginning of treatment, as in the Reed and Godden (1977) study, the likelihood for contaminated data is high because at this early stage of stuttering the chance for natural recovery is 80%, if not higher. It should be noted that selecting children who have stuttered for twice as long, at least 6 months, does not improve the situation much. As stated in Chapter 3, for most children who exhibit natural recovery, the recovery process is gradual and may last from 1 to 3 years. A child seen 2 years after onset still has a 47% chance for natural recovery. A similar problem is presented when control children who did not receive treatment are not included. When such studies report successful therapy, the findings should be suspected for contamination by failing to separate the effect of the treatment from that of natural processes. Also, genetic research has shown that children from families with histories of recovered stuttering also tend to recover on their own (Ambrose et al., 1997). Hence, family history is a significant variable to control in such studies.

Clinical studies in stuttering have suffered from a number of shortcomings. There have been weaknesses related to participant recruitment, such as small numbers of participants, an age range that is too wide or too limited, and inadequate attention to gender distribution. Procedural drawbacks have included (1) too small or unspecified speech sample size, (2) limited types of measures, and (3) insufficient or no treatment follow-up. Finally, there has been an absence of several elements regarded as critical in the general field of human health research:

- Random assignment of participants into various treatment groups
- Administration of the treatment in several sites by different clinicians
- Data analyses in locations and by people not involved in the data collection
- Comparison of different treatments instead of investigation of only one treatment

Fortunately, most recent research has attempted to accommodate at least some of the previously mentioned concerns. A clinical study regarding the effectiveness of the Lidcombe Program carried out in New Zealand was careful to employ a no-treatment control group (Jones et al., 2005). Of the 54 stuttering children, ages 3 to 6, enrolled in the study, 47 remained for the 9-month follow-up. Of these, 27 were randomly assigned to the treatment group and 20 to the nontreatment group. Children had to be at least 6 months post-onset and had received no therapy during the year prior to the start of the study. The results indicated that children in both groups improved substantially by the follow-up, but those receiving therapy made better progress found to be statistically and clinically significant. We note, however, that the seven children who did not complete the study were 9 months older, on average, than the rest of the group. It is important to point out, that the older the child (and 9 months is a big difference at this age), the less they are likely to recover. Had these participants continued with the study, somewhat different findings could have resulted. Another study conducted in the Netherlands by Franken et al. (2005) compared two very different therapies: the Lidcombe Program and a treatment based on the demands and capacities model (Gottwald & Starkweather, 1999). Here, 32 children were randomly assigned to their two treatment groups, and each child received 12 therapy sessions. No statistically significant differences were revealed between the two treatments in the decrease of stuttering frequency, and parents evaluated the two treatments as equal.

In addition to conducting more, larger, and better controlled studies, future research should attempt to separate the multiple aspects of therapy programs to find out which ones do, or do not, contribute to their outcomes. For example, what are the relative contributions of the parents' group versus the children's group in the Parent-Child Group program? Which of the various elements of the Lidcombe and ELU programs are essential versus extraneous?

General Reflections

Earlier in the chapter, a background discussion of therapy for preschool-age children who stutter pointed out two main sources of constraints on treatment for this subpopulation: age and the characteristics of the problem. In spite of these, the review has revealed a broad range of major treatment approaches. As is the case with adults who stutter, no consensus has been reached concerning best practices of treatment with young children who stutter. Most of the general approaches are based on the same, or similar, principles to those used with adults. Clinicians, however, had to sometimes employ or devise procedures that were more suitable to a child's level. Hence, inasmuch as 3-year-olds are not capable of verbalizing complicated emotions in ways that many adult clients can, clinicians electing to focus on the general approach of modifying emotional reactions have employed play therapy as a vehicle for children to vent feelings. If children cannot comprehend or follow direct instructions to change their speaking patterns, clinicians who prefer the general approach of fluency shaping have adapted by applying modeling as an alternative procedure to accommodate the approach. Those clinicians whose general approach involves operant conditioning methods to reinforce fluency or extinguish stuttering have not had to adapt procedures too drastically from those used for adults.

Overall, it appears that the most unique therapeutic approach for preschool children in contrast to adult intervention has been the indirect modification of the environment via various modes, be it psychotherapy for the parents (Glauber, 1958), direct parent counseling (Johnson, 1961a; Sander, 1959), interaction therapy (Kelman & Nicholas, 2008), or others. Another relatively unique therapy for children is the Speech Motor Training program (Riley & Riley, 1999), which has not been practiced widely. This evaluation, however, does not mean that modifying the child's environment has been the most effective among other approaches. Unfortunately, clinical research has been late to arrive on the scene and has mostly been focused on the effectiveness of a single therapy. Comparative clinical treatment has been minimal. Still, it has been encouraging to witness growing clinical research activities concerned with the preschool age who stutter. Future research should strive to follow more careful methodologies in terms of controlling various parameters of subject selection, employing control groups, and using multiple sites and separate data collection and data analysis teams and sites, and analyzing the effect of specific elements and steps in each program. A major question that deserves more discussion, and certainly much more research, is which children require immediate intervention and which ones can be left to recover on their own. As stated earlier in the chapter, declarations of apparent "consensus" in favor of early intervention for all children (e.g., Jones et al., 2005) are less than accurate, demand much stronger scientific basis, and certainly do not consider the reality of the ratio between available services and the population in need.

Summary

During the early part of the 20th century, therapies for preschoolers who stutter focused directly on the children. A shift toward indirect therapy, targeting parents and other significant people in the home environment, occurred early in 1940s, reflecting the rise of the diagnosogenic theory. Another shift reversal—a renewed interest in bringing the child closer to the therapeutic focus—began in the mid-1970s and has grown in popularity among clinicians. Clinical research pertaining to the treatment of this age group was slow to begin but has seen a significant rise during the past two decades. Still, tightly controlled clinical trials on a large scale have not been reported.

Several critical considerations concerning treatment of stuttering in preschool-age children were highlighted:

- Special characteristics of early stuttering
- A child's awareness (or lack of) of the stuttering
- Natural recovery
- Cognitive and emotional limits in young children
- Need to adjust therapeutic technique to children's age

- Great influence of the home environment
- Parent counseling as an integral aspect of various approaches, including those with emphasis on direct speech modification

Current major therapy approaches for preschoolers who stutter can be distinguished according to their focus. Each of these has been pursued through several different programs and techniques, making the overall field quite rich. These areas were briefly described:

- Speech/motor patterns
- Operant conditioning
- Parent-child interaction
- Emotionality
- Integrated therapies

Study Questions and Discussion Topics

1. Compare the general objectives and procedures of direct and indirect therapy approaches for early childhood stuttering. What are the theoretical rationales for the two?
2. What special issues pertaining to age and the disorder characteristics should be considered regarding therapy for preschool-age children who stutter? List and explain.
3. Describe the differences in the nature of parental involvement in the following programs discussed in the chapter: (a) the authors' speech rate therapy, (b) Lidcombe, (c) parent-child interaction, and (d) parent-child groups.
4. What are the principles and procedures employed in psychotherapeutic play methods?
5. What are the principles and procedure employed in the extended length of utterance program?
6. Discuss the methodological issues faced in pursuing clinical efficacy research regarding stuttering therapy in preschool-age children.

Suggested Readings

Axline, V. (1947). *Play therapy.* New York, NY: Ballantine Books.

Harrison, E., Onslow, M., & Rousseau, I. (2007). Lidcombe Program 2007: Clinical tales and clinical trials. In E. Conture & R. Curlee (Eds.), *Stuttering and related disorders* (3rd ed.). New York, NY: Thieme.

Ingham, J. C. (1999). Behavioral treatment of young children who stutter: An extended length of utterance method. In R. F. Curlee (Ed.), *Stuttering and related disorders of fluency* (2nd ed., pp. 80–100). New York, NY: Thieme.

Kelman, E., & Nicholas, A. (2008). *Practical intervention for early childhood stammering: Palin PCI approach.* Milton Keynes, UK: Speechmark.

Riley, G., & Riley, J. (1999). Speech motor training. In M. Onslow & A. Packman (Eds.), *The handbook of early stuttering intervention* (pp. 139–158). San Diego, CA: Singular.

Yairi, E., & Ambrose, N. (2005). *Early childhood stuttering.* Austin, TX: Pro-Ed. See Chapters 3, 12, and 13.

Chapter 15

Other Fluency Disorders; Cultural and Bilingual Issues

LEARNER OBJECTIVES

Readers of this chapter will understand:

- The distinction between stuttering and other fluency disorders.
- Principles of diagnosis, evaluation, and treatment of cluttering.
- Principles of diagnosis, evaluation, and treatment of neurogenic stuttering.
- Principles of diagnosis, evaluation, and treatment of psychogenic stuttering.
- Stuttering and fluency issues for those with multiple languages and cultures.

Introduction

If we accept the definition of stuttering, proposed in Chapter 1, as a speech holding pattern (repetition, prolongation, blocks) in an attempted delivery of articulatory gestures for syllables or elements of syllables, then it follows that when other forms of disfluency disrupt speech, they may represent other fluency disorders. Further, suppose a disorder is characterized by one or all of the stuttering characteristics just listed but also by different features, for example, a sudden acquired onset at adulthood following a head injury. This too may be classified as an "other fluency disorder," even though the speech characteristics may meet criteria for "stuttering." Examples include the child with impairment of language formulation that causes excessive disfluency *not* characterized as stuttering-like (SLD), or the child whose speech fluency is solely affected by an irregular pattern of pauses and breaths mid-utterance. It is important for speech-language clinicians to consider the other fluency disorders that may be encountered because not all disfluent speech is regarded as stuttering.

There are childhood forms and "acquired" adult-onset forms of other fluency disorders. Several of the disfluency types observed in classic developmental stuttering may be seen, but the etiology, symptomatology, and various phenomena surrounding the disordered speech tend to be different. Psychogenic stuttering and neurogenic stuttering are examples of acquired fluency disorders. Table 15.1 outlines the set of other fluency disorders addressed in this chapter.

Table 15.1 Other Disfluency Disorders in Children and Adults	
Age Group	**Fluency Disorder**
Childhood	**Developmental:**
	Unusual breathing patterns
	Word-final disfluency
	Language disorders
	Cluttering
Adulthood	**Acquired:**
	Neurogenic stuttering
	Psychogenic stuttering

Childhood Disorders

The speech-language clinician who engages in a fluency evaluation needs to be aware that sometimes speech is excessively disfluent but not stuttered. The following examples are not meant to be exhaustive but represent typical clinical encounters. They include (1) unusual pausing/breathing patterns, (2) word-final disfluencies, (3) disfluency secondary to language disorders, and (4) cluttering.

Unusual Breathing Patterns

Like stuttering, the cause of other childhood fluency problems is not well understood. Why does a child who previously spoke with no noticeable problem of smoothness suddenly one day adopt an unusual pattern of inhaling in the middle of words? Was it a physical immaturity in respiratory capacity that failed to sustain utterances to completion without interruption? Were there hormonal changes that led to shallow breathing? Did situational pressures and heightened emotions cause muscular tensions and rigid postures leading to insufficient breath support? Or was it merely a compensatory solution to timing turned into a habit, for example, secondary to an attempt to say more words than the airstream would carry?

Published literature suggests that abnormal breathing patterns, both nonspeech and speech, at any age, can be observed secondary to a variety of physical impairments, including but not limited to asthma, dysarthrias, traumatic brain injury (Murdoch, Pitt, Theodoros et al., 1999), deafness (Waltzman & Cohen, 2000), and Tourette's syndrome (Jagger et al., 1982). Usually the abnormal breathing of these populations is accompanied by disruptions to dimensions of vocal quality and intelligibility as well. A pattern of pausing or breathing mid-word without any other physical, speech, or language impairments represents an isolated fluency disorder with an unknown origin. No specific literature on this speech problem was found at the time of this writing. Nonetheless, one of us (CS) has observed three such cases in elementary school–age children, who demonstrated only unusual patterns of pausing/breathing interrupting the flow of speech. The particular patterns of pausing or breathing in these fluency disorders vary with the individual child, just as they do for stuttering, but here is a potential example characterizing this type of problem:

Unusual Breathing: A Sample Case

Description: CS was asked by a second-grade teacher to evaluate a child for a stuttering/ fluency problem. She said that for the past few weeks the child had been talking with an odd pattern that seemed like a kind of stuttering. When assessed, the boy's only disfluent speech behavior was his propensity to breathe in the middle of words. These occurred at the noticeable frequency of every few sentences. The boy exhibited no physical tension or effortful struggle to speak and had never had a history of any other fluency or stuttering problems. He was not aware of the disrupted speech or embarrassed by it. He did not have any unusual speaking rate, articulation, voice features, or hearing problems. Although noticeably distracting, the etiology appeared to be a superficial matter of mismanaged speech production. Because his speech pattern was not a form of stuttering, he readily responded to systematic instruction for breathing in appropriate locations.

Intervention: The intervention for the boy just described did not need to address reduction of any physical tension or emotional reaction during speech because such features were absent. Inasmuch as the problem was determined to be mismanaged speech execution, an approach similar to that used with a traditional articulation disorder was applied. That is, the boy was taught to change his habit of breathing mid-word. Ear training served as the starting point. He learned to identify and contrast the inappropriate breathing behavior with appropriate breathing behavior, listening to these models in the clinician's speech. Next, skills of accurate detection of the inappropriate versus appropriate breathing pattern in audio recordings of his own speech were developed. In the third step, he was taught to plan breath locations appropriately for oral reading and for scripts of conversational speech. These planned speech tasks were then produced for audio recordings. After each segment of several utterances or longer segments, the child was asked to self-evaluate his breathing behavior. The recordings were reviewed together to check on how well he had self-evaluated. When consistent and independent ability to produce speech segments with appropriate breathing patterns was demonstrated in the therapy room, the teacher reported carryover into the classroom speaking activities. Finally, the child had learned where breaths should take place and had developed the ability to self-monitor and use his own judgment to generate appropriate breathing behavior when he talked. The therapy and the remediation process were completed in only a handful of sessions.

Word-Final Disfluency

People who stutter rarely do so on the final syllables of words. The research literature includes just a few accounts of people with disfluency patterns consisting of sound or syllable repetitions occurring at the ends of words (e.g., Cosyns, Mortier, Corthals et al.,

2010; McAllister & Kingston, 2005). Sometimes a language learning deficiency or a brain injury were involved as etiological factors, but others were found to be completely normal. For example, two school-age boys, who were described as having no other known impairments, produced mainly word-final part-word repetitions. It was noted that these disruptions occurred at all positions within the sentence (initial, medial, final) but primarily at sentence-medial locations. An example is *"I don't think—nk we got the whole way through those"* (McAllister & Kingston, 2005, p. 261). No tension, awareness, avoidance or negative reaction, or secondary behaviors were displayed, similar to the breathing/pausing cases described by CS previously. McAllister and Kingston argue that because words affected by this form of disruption have already been spoken prior to the repeated final segment(s), these disfluencies minimally impact listener comprehension and likely raise little concern by anyone. They suggest the possibility that such disfluencies, as the only pattern, should not be viewed as constituting a communicative disorder. When the disruptions are sufficiently frequent, however, they may distract and/or bother both teachers and parents alike, resulting in a referral to a speech-language clinician. Again, CS has encountered two or three such cases.

Cognitive-linguistic processing appears to be the most probable etiology, but it is still uncertain what factors lead to this less typical form of disfluent behavior. Although most speakers mark a delay in an upcoming decision of what words to say next by uttering the neutral syllables of "uh" or "um" or with a silent pause, reiterations of the word ending may serve as the holding pattern to mark where a speaker has left off until ready to complete the rest of the utterance. Of course these questions then arise: Why is the latter method used as the holding pattern rather than the more common methods of interjecting syllables or pausing? And why are speakers so remarkably unaware of such features having occurred? Motoric perseveration, palilalia, and behavioral compulsion have been conjectured as other possible explanations, but these types of repetitive acts tend to have different features[1] and are diagnosed in association with neurogenic or psychogenic causes. Further research is necessary to confirm whether the proposed underlying etiology applies or whether some other conditions are involved. The following case example illustrates a clinical approach to this kind of problem:

Word-Final Disfluency: A Sample Case

Description: Another speech-language clinician referred a 10-year-old who was "stuttering." The child displayed chiefly word-final repetitions; other forms of disfluency were at normal, rarely occurring levels. No tension, awareness, or negative reactions were evident. Language testing revealed within average to above-average range receptive vocabulary and receptive/expressive abilities. The early adolescent temperament questionnaire completed by the boy revealed no remarkable issues. He was reportedly well adjusted psychologically and had an unremarkable

---

[1]In palilalia, the word repetitions become progressively faster and less audible in loudness (Duffy, 1995).

medical history. During both oral reading and conversation, the boy displayed frequent repetitions of sounds or syllables at the ends of words, such as "We left Saturday-ay-ay morning," "There was a hole-ole in the side of it," and "It took a good-ood four hours." The word-final repetitions occurred on 56% (28 of 50) of utterances. Other forms of disfluency occurred at minimal frequencies. There was no apparent emotional reaction to the disfluency, nor other atypical speech, voice, or language behaviors. The boy passed hearing and oral mechanism screenings. His academic performance was reported to be typical for his age.

Intervention: A traditional approach to speech production training was adopted, starting with sensory/perceptual training and progressing to production training following a hierarchy from phrase level, to sentence level, and finally to a conversational context. Enhanced awareness and self-monitoring of speech began with an initial exercise in perceptual awareness in which the child was asked to identify same-different phrase pairs produced by the clinician (e.g., *"Are these two sentences exactly the same or are they said in some way that is different?: It was four months ago. It was four-our months ago."* After a consistent detection of the target behavior was established in the clinician's speech, the child was asked to review and listen to audio-recorded segments of his own speech to detect whether they were said smoothly or with the repeated word ending. When detection and description of his own productions was at least 90% (more than 45 of 50), he was to engage in a kind of "cancellation" in which he repeated the utterance smoothly after the detection of the atypical repetitions. Verbal encouragement and positive reinforcement of accurate detection and smooth reproduction were generously applied. As the child increased his awareness and practice of speech in various activities, occurrences of the behavior progressively decreased both in and out of the clinic.

Language Disorders

Disfluent Speech in Disordered Language

The nature of disfluent speech typical of language disorders has been documented in several scientific sources (e.g., Boscolo, Bernstein Ratner, & Rescorla, 2002). According to Thordardottir and Weismer (2002) children with specific language impairment (SLI) produce a preponderance of maze revisions, phrase repetitions, and circumlocutions compared to children with normal language matched for mean length of utterance (MLU). Surprisingly, interjections are used with lower frequency among children with SLI compared to those with normal language.

It is reasonable to expect that children with language disorders may tend to be more disfluent because when a person struggles with formulating a message, it is often evident in hesitations and disruptions to the flow of talking. An investigation of the speech of children with SLI in story narratives revealed significantly greater levels of both SLD and other disfluencies (Boscolo et al., 2002) than in normally fluent children. The 1% SLD level, however, is still considerably smaller than the low 3% SLD often regarded as the minimal criterion for stuttering.

Several other studies have not found differences in disfluency frequencies between children with SLI and those with normally developing language (e.g., Lees, Anderson, & Martin, 1999; Scott & Windsor, 2000). The absence of differences in these cases could have been because the language difficulty tends to affect phrase-level rather than word-level speech fluency. It has been shown that as language (syntactic) complexity increases, the number of disfluent utterances increases rather than the number of disfluencies altogether (Bernstein Ratner & Sih, 1987).

In addition to observations of phrase-level disfluency, formal and informal language assessment of disfluent children with SLI may reveal weaknesses in word-finding skills, short-term memory, expressive semantic and syntactic abilities, and pragmatic skills (Miller et al., 2005). Thus their disfluencies arise because of delays and difficulties generating the language forms needed to express ideas. Emotionally, they tend to feel frustrated or upset with the communication failure they experience more generally, rather than embarrassed or disturbed by the disfluency specifically.

Stuttering and Concomitant Language Disorders

As we discussed in Chapters 3 and 4, there are children for whom stuttering and language disorders coexist. Research has suggested a higher prevalence of other communication disorders in children who stutter than in the general population, with concomitant language disorders ranking second behind articulation/phonology disorders (Arndt & Healey, 2001; Blood et al., 2003; Hall et al., 2007). As we have previously stated, however, the extent of such coexisting disorders in different age groups is controversial. It is currently not known why there is this tendency for coexisting disorders. Perhaps children who stutter are at higher risk for developing other problems, or alternatively, children with other problems may be at greater risk to develop stuttering. Perhaps stuttering and other communication disorders are both related to a common underlying problem, or perhaps the treatment for communication disorders somehow raises a child's risk for stuttering. J. Riley (1971) actually proposed two subtypes that rest on a language-physiology distinction: children exhibiting only concomitant language deficits, and those exhibiting inferior motor skills. Nippold (2002, 2012a) questioned whether the tendency for co-occurring communication disorders actually exists. Besides procedural weaknesses in past data that she identified, she also argued that children who stutter who have additional disorders are identified for intervention more often than children who exhibit only stuttering. Indeed, a good number of stuttering prevalence studies used data gathered from school clinician caseloads, which perhaps were not representative of the larger population of children who stutter.

The presence of multiple disorders creates a need for additional remediation decisions. The clinician must decide whether to treat the multiple problems sequentially or concurrently. If sequential treatment is selected, then which disorder will be treated first? Will the first target be the stuttering or the other disorder(s)? Several factors may enter into the decision of order, for example, relative severity of each problem, relative ease of expected success remediating each problem, and relative concern or distress experienced related to each problem.

Alternatively, if a concurrent treatment approach is selected (instead of sequential) then other decisions will have to be made about the implementation of the therapeutic approaches. Options include (1) a simultaneous blending of strategies or approaches to the two disorders, (2) cycling or rotating between the treatments of the two disorders within each session, or (3) simultaneous but adapted or altered approaches to the disorders (e.g., no direct corrections, no imitation demands, etc.). Arndt and Healey (2001) surveyed 241 speech clinicians from a variety of U.S. states and found this order of most to least preferred treatment options: simultaneous approach, other approach (e.g., address only language), cycling approach, concurrent approach but without calling attention to language errors, treating fluency fully first. Of course, preferences are not evidence of what constitutes best practice, but these findings do tell us what clinicians may generally be doing.

Other research evidence tends to support a simultaneous but adapted approach. More specifically, an indirect approach to phonological disorders is recommended in children who stutter due to concern that direct speech correction may adversely affect stuttering (Bernstein Ratner, 1995; Conture, Louko, & Edwards, 1993). For example, a fluency-shaping protocol would be combined with focused speech models for phonology without direct feedback on the speech (i.e., giving no attention to errors). Altered approaches to articulation or language targets may involve their practice in simultaneous conditions of speaking slowly, monitored rate/rhythm, smooth transitions between words, reduced interruptions in group situations, longer turn-taking latencies, and use of an easy, relaxed speaking manner (e.g., Byrd et al., 2007). Progressive speaking contexts related to utterance length and complexity should be carefully controlled to ensure success in both areas. If a direct approach to correction is applied, then it is advised that the phonological targets be practiced in a relaxed, unhurried manner, avoiding excessive motoric/linguistic demands.

The dual advantage of treating the two disorders concurrently are (1) progress may be made in both areas without delaying attention to one of the problems, and (2) a broad versus narrow focus on communication effectiveness is more holistic. The disadvantage is that it can be difficult to select an optimal speaking context. For example, the child might benefit most from a conversational context for fluency but need phrase-level practice for the articulation or language problem. Stuttering frequency and severity should be monitored during treatment for other speech/language targets, so that if fluency worsens, appropriate adjustments are made such as easing production accuracy demands, slowing pace of production or activity demands, or reducing linguistic context demands (Conture, 2001).

When children are being treated for multiple communication problems, parents need to be informed that progress may need more time. They need to be counseled in employing support strategies for the fluency (slower pace, longer turn-taking latencies, not correcting errors, etc.) and understand that although these strategies optimize the potential for fluency, they are not directly related to the cause of either stuttering or fluency. Note, however, when parents are asked to provide some sort of home practice for two behaviors at the same time (e.g., stuttering and language), it may be too overwhelming for both the parents and child.

Language and Disfluency: Other Considerations

Several investigators have revealed that disfluent speech may arise secondary to language therapy (Hall, 2011; Merits-Patterson & Reed, 1981). It was proposed that perhaps therapy promotes uncertainty with language formulation that leads to greater disfluency (Hall, 1977). In keeping with the demands-capacities model (Adams, 1990), one may also hypothesize that producing sentences of greater length and complexity may be exceeding the child's fluency capacities. A further possibility that has not received much attention is that greater speech disruptions arise from more frequent attempts to self-monitor ongoing speech (Bernstein Ratner & Healey, 1999). In contrast to precipitating disfluent speech, speech and language therapy can decrease disfluency as was shown in the case of one child following language therapy for narrative organization (Sieff & Hooyman, 2006). Improved fluency may be expected if the disfluency is primarily based on language formulation impairment. Clinicians should remember that if the correct focus in therapy is chosen, then the treatment progresses, but focusing on stuttering when the problem is in language formulation could lead to a lack of progress.

Following is a brief description of a school-age child who presented a fluency problem (not stuttering) associated with a language disorder.

Language Disorders: A Sample Case

Description: An 11-year-old boy was referred for an assessment by his parents, who reported concern about his poor communication abilities. His story explanations were disorganized and disfluent with many revisions and restarts (phrase repetitions). He passed hearing and oral mechanism screenings but scored below age level on formal tests of expressive language. His difficulties with word-finding were evident in his overuse of empty words such as *thing, stuff, like that,* and a below-average score on a formal test of word-finding. He was performing below age/grade level in both reading and writing.

Intervention: The approach in therapy to this fluency issue was indirectly addressed through strengthening the child's language skills. The speech clinician collaborated with the special education specialist and classroom teacher to identify and select a target vocabulary and concepts to incorporate into therapy activities. Word-finding ability was improved by boosting semantic associations through elaboration training and categorical organization tasks (Owens, 2010; Wallach & Butler, 1994), as well as phonological awareness (e.g., rhyming and phoneme segmentation). These involved the targeted classroom-related vocabulary. Concepts were strengthened with description tasks involving use of terminology to compare/contrast characteristics (Owens, 2010). For example, for geography concepts, he was prompted to compare/contrast vocabulary pairs such as *plain* versus *plateau, cape* versus *peninsula,* and more. With each pair, he was prompted with questions of "How are they alike? How are they different?" Language organization and sequencing was improved through activities involving narrative schemes. For example, the child had to develop scripts for a variety of his daily routines, practice with sequenced pictures, and drill with story grammars (e.g., telling and retelling the stories of his vacation trips, field trips, holiday events, etc.). Although some difficulties persisted, his fluency improved as he developed more consistent strategies for telling about objects and events.

Cluttering

Cluttering is a disorder expressed as rapid, imprecise, disrhythmic, and disorganized production of speech. The nature of cluttering has been controversial. Whereas it was previously described as an impairment of central language processes (Weiss, 1967), more recently it has been depicted more as a problem involving central speech planning processes. St. Louis has spearheaded a "lowest common denominator" definition of cluttering: a disorder characterized by perceived abnormally rapid, irregular speech rate (St. Louis, Myers, Bakker et al., 2007; St. Louis & Schulte, 2011). The rate aberrances are in turn associated with excessive disfluencies (mainly of normal types), pauses that do not conform to syntactic and semantic rules, and excessive coarticulation across sounds resulting in reduced speech intelligibility. Understandably, speaking at a rate above a person's given capacity reduces the time available for executing precise articulatory gestures, as well as for proper inflections that influence meaning. Myers (2013) posits that cluttering is more broadly based, often involving higher-level language formulation and organization difficulties when expressing large speech quantities such as narratives in informal and unguarded speaking situations. What aspect of the encoding process is disturbed, however, is not known. Alm (2004b) suggested neurological bases for cluttering implicating hyperactivation and disregulation of the medial frontal cortex that may be secondary to disinhibited basal ganglia circuits resulting from a hyperactive dopamine system.

Data on the incidence and prevalence of cluttering are sparse. One study conducted among German school children reported 1.5% (Becker & Grundmann, 1971). This figure is suspiciously high in our opinion. Confusion regarding definitions has made it difficult for clinicians and investigators to identify the disorder in either an isolated form or in conjunction with other speech/language problems. Daly (1996) reported that, based on his own caseload, those who purely clutter constituted only 5% of his cluttering caseload. What is emerging, is that cluttering co-occurs with stuttering more often than most speech-language clinicians seem to be aware of. Approximately 30% of cases of PWS also exhibit cluttering according to Preus (1981) while Daly (1996) puts the figure at 40%. In our experience, however, this figure is also an overestimate. Daly's estimates may hint that a number of past research studies of stuttering could have been conducted with participants who also cluttered. Some inconsistent findings among studies may have resulted from an imprecise identification of participants.

It has been opined that cluttering begins during childhood, but, unlike stuttering, the problem does not cause sufficient concern to bring it to the attention of the clinician for differential diagnosis (Daly & Burnett, 1999; St. Louis et al., 2007). The tendency for its later identification as compared with developmental stuttering could be related to (1) the typical lack of awareness or concern by the speaker, and/or (2) the tendency for other accompanying impairments to overshadow the problem of disfluent speech. It also stands to reason that inasmuch as cluttering manifests itself best in running speech, it will be detected in school-age children and adults more often than preschool children who speak in shorter segments. Perhaps this is why school-age children and adults are those who are seen for therapy.

In our opinion, there is no evidence for an observable "cluttering onset," that is, that a child's speech was initially normal, then, either gradually or suddenly, cluttering appeared. Perhaps, like some cases of language delay, the difficulties that are present even from the beginning do not resolve when expected with maturation. Thus it takes more time to raise parents' and other people's concern. As Myers (2013) points out, an important distinction from stuttering is that cluttering cannot be quantified in terms of the number of occurrences of discrete cluttered events. The whole speech output is involved. This is especially so because more than one dimension of communication contributes to the perception of cluttering. For example, an individual may exhibit a fast and/or irregular rate, inefficient linguistic encoding reflected in poor topic maintenance, as well as numerous interfering linguistic formulation behaviors, such as fillers, incomplete phrases, and revisions. There is also poor speech intelligibility due to vowel neutralizations and the deletion of sounds and syllables in multisyllabic words. The lack or reduced degree of self-awareness of speech difficulty appears to be particularly distinctive between stuttering and cluttering because individuals who stutter are usually keenly aware they have a speech problem, presenting with embarrassment and fear about speaking.

Children who clutter present a wide variety of characteristics and ability sets. The following list provides examples of characteristics that may be observed in children who clutter (Daly, 1996; St. Louis et al., 2007):

- Excessive repetitions of all kinds (part-word, whole-word, phrase)
- Incomplete words and phrases, revisions that reduce the predictability of the message (by contrast, in stuttering the message is predicted and listeners just wait for the person to get it out)
- Fast bursts of speech; choppy rhythm
- Imprecise, slurred articulation; sound transpositions
- Short attention span and poor concentration
- Little or no awareness of cluttering behaviors and the impact of these behaviors on the listener
- Deficits in self-monitoring of speech/language behaviors in general
- Deficits in expressive language, reading, writing skills

There is considerable controversy over the features that should comprise the obligatory symptoms of cluttering. Some scholars include excessively fast speaking rate as essential (St. Louis et al., 2007); others argue that excessively fast speech rate should not be a key feature (Daly & Burnett, 1999). For example, cluttering has been characterized as primarily consisting of excessive repetitions (Daly, 1996). Interestingly, research has shown that the speaking rate and amount of disfluency of people who clutter (PWC) are not necessarily greater than that of control peers (Bakker, Myers, Raphael et al., 2011; Myers, Bakker, St. Louis et al., 2012). At least from a clinical perspective, Myers (2013) advocates the idea that PWC speak faster than their capacity to encode a message coherently and cohesively.

Research is needed to reveal the nature of factors leading to an impression of faster than normal speech rate for those who clutter. It is possible that they do not pause appropriately at clause or sentence boundaries, whereas those who stutter, even if their overall rates may prove similar, may pause more appropriately. Also, excessive rate may be perceived when a speaker does not observe the temporal relationships typically associated with word and syllable composition. For example, a speaker may collapse and combine the gestures for a three-word (and three-syllable) utterance: "Did you eat?" into an utterance that sounds like one syllable: "Jeet?" or the two-syllable remark "Let's go!" may be shortened to "Sko!" Bretherton-Furness and Ward (2012) compared performance of 8 clutterers (including 3 stutterer-clutterers) and 6 normally fluent controls on language tasks. Participants were selected using a rate-based definition of cluttering proposed by St. Louis and Schulte (2011). There were mixed findings on performance tasks, such as naming members of semantic categories, leading the investigators to propose further studies of the lexical processing by this population.

The characteristics that distinguish the disfluencies of cluttering from those of language learning disabilities are ambiguous. The disfluencies of cluttering appear to be almost exclusively an excess of "other" or "normal" disfluencies rather than SLD types that would be characteristic of stuttering (Conture & Curlee, 2007). An analysis of clutterers' speech samples by Myers et al., (2012) found that the most to least prevalent disfluency types were interjections, revisions, word repetitions, unfinished utterances, and phrase repetitions. The 18 clutterers and 20 normally fluent speakers exhibited similar proportions of typical disfluencies in their speech, 97% for the clutterers and 98% for the normally fluent controls. Comparable frequency data between groups supports the idea that disfluency excess is not the principal symptom of cluttering.

Assessment of Cluttering

The assessment of cluttering involves the standard components of obtaining case history and background information, a description of the client's speech characteristics, and observing the conditions and variables affecting the client's speech (e.g., imitation, rote or automatic speech tasks, oral reading, utterance length, and linguistic complexity). It is important to obtain extended speech samples to capture a client's narrative skills as well as cluttering severity. The client is more likely to clutter when speaking in informal, unguarded situations in which there is less monitoring, such as chatting with friends. Beyond the usual disfluency frequency and type analysis obtained from the speech sample, measures of speech rate and temporal features (e.g., pause locations and timing) will be informative. Consideration of personal factors related to the client's home, school, social and/or work environment and the impact of the communication disorder on the individual's life should be included.

It is important to thoroughly assess speech and language abilities, including articulation in both word and connected speech contexts, language skills (i.e., receptive and expressive vocabulary, semantics, syntax, pragmatics), and academic reading and writing abilities. The clinician should be sure to note the client's speech-language error awareness and self-monitoring skills. How frequently are self-corrections attempted? In this respect, clinicians should observe the client's self-awareness of various dimensions associated with cluttering, such as speaking rate, intelligibility, and so forth. Some PWC can become aware of the problem during short stretches of talk.

Methods of cluttering assessment include formal norm-referenced tests, informal tests, or checklists of characteristics (Table 15.2), such as the one here based on information provided in both Daly (1996) and St. Louis et al. (2007):

Table 15.2

Cluttering Characteristics Checklist	Other Common Characteristics
• Excessive nonstuttering disfluencies	• Atypical grammatical errors
• Excessive repetitions (all types)	• Atypical speech sound errors
• Excessive speech rate	• Poor auditory awareness
• Poor use of pauses during speech	• Reading problems
• Articulatory imprecision	• Writing problems
• Short attention span and poor concentration	• Unregulated vocal quality
• Poorly organized thinking and narratives	• Impulsive, forceful personality
• Lack of awareness of cluttering problem	

While formal standardized tests may be given, they are not sufficient for assessing the language problems of clutterers. The main reason standardized language tests do not capture their linguistic formulation problems is that they tend to be older and have more fully developed language abilities. Clinicians should probe the narrative skills of PWC. As indicated above, the more informal, spontaneous, extemporaneous, and offhand the talk, the more likely one can tap the severity of a client's cluttering.

To capture the multifaceted and perceptual nature of cluttering, Bakker and Myers (2011) developed the Cluttering Severity Instrument (CSI). This assessment tool (freely downloadable at http://associations.missouristate.edu/ICA), allows clinicians to rate the perceived severity of cluttering based on the following communication dimensions: overall intelligibility, rate and rate regularity, prosody, typical disfluency, precision of articulation, language organization, and discourse management. The CSI also permits documenting the percent of the sample perceived as cluttered.

Treatment

Considering the most obvious characteristic of cluttering, accelerated speaking rate, it is quite understandable why rate control seems to have been the main approach to treatment. The rationale for a reduced speech rate is so that motoric and linguistic encoding demands do not exceed client abilities. Various techniques mentioned in previous chapters in regard to the treatment of stuttering, including delayed auditory feedback (DAF), may be applied. Typically, PWC are not fully aware that others have difficulty understanding them. Hence these clients need to develop skills to monitor the integrity of verbal output, awareness of the listener's verbal and nonverbal reactions, and appropriateness of subsequent responses to the listener.

Literature is lacking however, regarding evidence-based treatment of cluttering. A single case study was reported by Daly and Burnett (1996) including only broad treatment goals and description of the implementation in schools. Emphasis was placed on description of evaluation methods. Using two case studies, St. Louis et al. (1996) reported on the efficacy of delayed auditory feedback for the treatment of cluttering. While both PWC made progress during treatment, the clients showed varying degrees of ability to transfer the gains. More recently, Myers (2011) proposed a cognitive-behavioral approach for the treatment of cluttering centered on rate control that incorporates three objectives. These are listed below with a few examples of procedures.

1. Develop awareness and understanding of the nature of cluttering and associated behaviors.
   - With children, this can be accomplished through the use of age-appropriate analogies, such as listening to radio commercials that use fast speech; imagining a fast-going train is derailed and getting all jumbled-up; a driver that brakes erratically; difficulties in finding things in a cluttered, disorganized closet.
   - Use of language references to cluttered speech as "mumble jumble," and "nice and crisp" for precise articulation, can be helpful.
   - Include discussions of the impact of the client's cluttered speech on many aspects of life, such as making friends and class participation.

2. Develop skills in slower rate of verbal output.
   - Specific instructions are given for pausing between phrases, punctuation marks, breath groups, and so on. To increase awareness of spoken rhythm, finger tapping or arm motions coincide with syllables.
   - Apply delayed auditory feedback to slow the client down.
   - Have the client shadow the clinician's speech; use negative practice to contrast excessively fast versus slow speech.
   - Train client to recognize inner states associated with compulsive behaviors that trigger hurried speech. Clients need to learn how to moderate and diminish their rate.

3. Develop skills for monitoring, moderating, and modulating behaviors.
   - Have the client listen to their own recorded speech samples to identify problems.

- Clients can attend to the sensation while experimenting with variations in their own speaking rates, comparing fast and slow. Similarly, experimenting with the sensation of tempo variations during other physical activities such as raising/lowering one's arm.

- Clients should take notice when listeners do not understand what was said. Watching and analyzing video samples of other speakers can help with this skill.

- Clients can role-play various characters as in a skit to experience different speaking patterns.

- Monitor and modulate articulation and intelligibility, language organization, and prosody. To these ends, the client practices exaggerated articulatory gestures to highlight sensory feedback associated with precise and firm posturing. Attend to word endings and unstressed syllables, and consonant clusters. Stressed syllables are emphasized through longer durations and prosodic variations.

- Clients should become acquainted in advance with the essential or important parts of the message they are trying to convey, especially if it is long. That is, clients should attend to organizing thoughts before speaking. To this end, visuals are used, such as cards as reminders of the proper order of presentation. For practice, clinicians can present a story that is disorganized in terms of context and grammar and have clients identify the reason why the narrative lacks coherence, then improve its order.

- Clients should develop awareness of their own discourse patterns; count interruptions and breakdowns during conversation. Clinicians simulate the clients' discourse behaviors and the clients reflect on self-observation of the behavior.

- Role play is used to act out interruptions and conversational breakdowns.

Interested clinicians can find numerous suggestions for specific procedures in the chapter by Myers (2011). Also, a list of resources related to cluttering can be found at the Stuttering Home Page (http://www.mnsu.edu/comdis/kuster/cluttering.html).

Cluttering: A Sample Case

Description: A 9-year-old boy was referred by parents for a fluency evaluation. He previously received speech therapy for several years through a birth-to-3 program due to late speech and language development. His mother reported he had frequent ear infections until the age of 7 years. He had begun to stutter at approximately age 4 when he was putting longer sentences together. Formal tests of his language revealed average receptive vocabulary and language skills, but expressive language skills placed him near the 15th percentile for his age. Stuttering severity was mild, with 3% of syllables characterized by SLD, primarily part-word and whole-word repetitions. His frequency of other disfluencies was 7% and consisted mainly of interjections ("um, uh") and revisions. Speech imprecision was noted in the form of sound transpositions (e.g., "aminal" for *animal*) and syllable elisions (e.g., "pop-lar" for *popular* and "cuppla" for *couple of*). An oral motor assessment of diadochokinesis (DDK) revealed that he reached typical speeds of repetitive syllables but produced irregular rhythms and inaccurate targets, mainly sound transpositions ("pakata" for "pataka"). The clinician had a subjective impression of a fast rate of speech, with frequent rushing into his utterances. Both the parent and clinician observed that the child did not appear concerned or aware of speech disfluencies.

Intervention: A three-pronged treatment approach to improve temporal aspects (slower rate and phrasing), increased self-monitoring, and phonological awareness was pursued. To modify speed of talking, the clinician modeled a slow-natural rate while continuously sliding her finger across the table to cue the start and end points of the spoken utterance. The child was to imitate both the finger sliding and the slow manner of speaking while repeating the utterance. The hierarchy of speaking tasks progressed from short multisyllable words and phrases to longer sentences, and finally to conversation. The modeling hierarchy progressed from imitation to indirect model (clinician models the manner of speaking but not using the same words), and eventually to no model. On the longer sentences, the clinician modeled pauses and phrasing, along with appropriate breath support. Pausing and phrasing were addressed in both spontaneous speech and oral reading. To prepare for oral reading, the child and clinician searched the passage for the commas and sentences to mark them in big red circles as a sign of where to stop. At first the clinician modeled how to read and follow the stop signs; later the child engaged in locating as well as observing the stop signs. Because the perception of fast rate was often due to insufficient pauses, during talking activities the clinician would instruct, "Tell me one thing and stop." "Now tell me one more thing and stop." To address self-monitoring, the child and clinician observed a videotape of the child talking and together engaged in finding segments when the child's speech was hard to follow either due to disfluencies, imprecise articulation, or irregular rate and rhythm. The clinician and child came up with three terms to label the targets of concern: *smooth, clear,* and *restful.* Thus, on an almost utterance-by- utterance basis, they would evaluate "How smooth (connected)?" "How clear (articulated)?" and/or "How restful (not rushed)?" In early stages, the clinician would attempt to exactly imitate the child's utterance with the manner of talking, and then offer a contrasting production of the same sentence improved on one of the target parameters, and ask, "Which sentence sounded clearer?" (or smoother, or more restful, depending on the parameter targeted). Later on, after many examples had been reviewed, the child was asked to produce the contrasting productions, such as "Say that sentence for me in a way that is more restful." Clarity was also addressed by activities to improve phonological awareness by, together, analyzing the multisyllabic words the child produced. For example, the clinician might say "stadium." Let's listen to its parts: "sta- dee- um." How many parts are there?" Or sometimes, "Say each part one at a time with me" (or in imitation, or independently, depending on the readiness of the child). "What sound does each part start with?" "What sound does 'sta' start with?" "What does 'dee' start with?" "Now I will make each part longer and connect them to say: staaaay-deeee-uuuumm (no breaks between syllables); now you say it that way." Eventually, it continued with, "Now I will put that word in a sentence (said at a slow-natural rate). The stadium was crowded." "Say that sentence the way I did." "Is there another sentence you could make with that word?"

Acquired Stuttering

Neurogenic Stuttering

Adults, and less frequently children, who suffered one or several of a wide range of brain injuries or other neurological diseases occasionally exhibit, among other problems, disfluent speech that shares similarities with stuttering. Usually there is a history of normal speech prior to the injury or disease. Those more commonly affected are in the geriatric subpopulation, although stroke-related stuttering has been documented in a 2-year-old (Nass, Sclireler, & Heier, 2008). It is remarkable that lesions of many different areas of the brain are associated with an increase in disfluent or stuttered speech: left hemisphere, right hemisphere, frontal, parietal, and temporal cortical regions, corpus callosum, basal ganglia, brainstem, and cerebellum (Van Borsel, Van Lierde, Van Cauweberge et al., 1998). That is, pyramidal, extrapyramidal, and corticobulbar motor systems have been implicated separately.

A neurogenic disorder of any type by definition results from an impairment of the nervous system. Thus the term *neurogenic stuttering* is applied when there is clear evidence that the speaker's disfluent speech was acquired in connection with a neurological lesion (Duffy, 1995; Helm-Estabrooks, 1999). The term, however, should be applied with caution because much of the disfluent speech of brain-damaged people cannot be regarded as stuttering, and most brain-damaged people do not exhibit neurogenic stuttering. In a study comparing the disfluent speech of 15 individuals with Broca's aphasia and right hemiplegia, 15 nonaphasics with left hemiplegia, and 15 normally speaking people, the frequency of disfluency in the aphasic group was 3 times greater than that of either control group. Most of the disfluencies uttered by those with aphasia, however, were of the type commonly found in the speech of normal speakers (Yairi et al., 1981). Although many challenges are related to the issue of what to refer to as "neurogenic stuttering" (Helm-Estabrooks, 1999), there are times when the speech disruptions observed in neurogenic stuttering are indistinguishable from characteristics of developmental stuttering (Van Borsel & Tailleau, 2001). In some cases disfluent speech becomes chronic; in other cases it is transient (Jokel, De Nil, & Sharpe, 2007).

Another type of neurogenically based disfluent speech pattern is *palilalia,* in which the same word or phrase is repeated over and over. A delayed pattern of repetitive, stereotypical spoken utterances or echolalia is most commonly seen in children with autism or other severe developmental communication disorders. Palilalia must also be differentiated from stuttering. Although often palilalia has been characterized as diminishing in loudness and increasing in rate with successive iterations, this may not always be the case (Kent & Lapointe, 1982). Research has shown that the intervention known as *tact correction* aids in the reduction of palilalia while simultaneously increasing appropriate vocalizations (Karmali, Greer, Nuzzolo-Gomez et al., 2005; Guzinski, Cihon, & Eshleman, 2012). The reasons for palilalia and for the success of this form of intervention are not well understood.

Another potential source of repetitive speech behavior is Tourette's syndrome (TS). TS is an inherited neurological disorder named for the French neurologist Gilles de la Tourette, who in 1885 first described this condition primarily characterized by motor tics. In some cases, stuttering and TS may co-occur, but there is also evidence to suggest that the disfluencies of TS are distinctive from those of stuttering, cluttering, and palilalia (Van Borsel, Goethals, & Vanryckeghem, 2004). It is interesting to note that behavioral intervention for tics is similar to some stuttering intervention techniques. For example, when *habit reversal training* is applied, the client is taught to self-monitor for the early indications that a tic is going to occur. The client learns to apply a competing response intended to disrupt (not suppress) the escalation of the impending tic (Piacentini et al., 2010).

Characteristics and Differential Diagnosis

As in developmental stuttering, there is great diversity in the symptoms and characteristics of acquired neurogenic stuttering. A variety of core and accessory disfluency types have been described: sound prolongations, part-word repetitions, tonic blocks, hesitation pauses, interjections, and word prolongations. In many cases, stuttering-like disfluencies are the main speech characteristic (e.g., Ackermann, Hertrich, Ziegler et al., 1996; Helm-Estabrooks & Hotz, 1998). Tonic blocks on word-initial locations were predominant in the speech of five patients with basal ganglia injuries (Tani & Sakai, 2011). These speech disruptions can occur in the absence of any symptoms of aphasia or cognitive disability (Hamano et al., 2005). More commonly, however, the fluency disruptions are accompanied by other neurologically based speech problems, such as slurred articulation resulting from dysarthria, halted speech resulting from apraxia, as well as voice disorders, cognitive disturbances impairing memory, and language disorders such as aphasia (Ardila & Lopez, 1986). Some patients also exhibit emotional tension, depression, or anxiety (Roth, Aronson, & Davis, 1989), whereas others have relatively little concomitant affective reactions (Market, Montague, Buffalo et al., 1990). In five patients with stuttering following basal ganglia lesions, only one, who had the most frequent stuttering, complained of anxiety about disfluencies (Tani & Sakai, 2011). Interestingly, two of the five patients displayed concomitant behaviors consisting of facial grimaces.

As stated, only a few brain-damaged individuals exhibit what can be diagnosed as neurogenic stuttering, and they too reveal several important differences from the much more common developmental stuttering. The following list offers several examples of features that may contrast neurogenic stuttering from developmental stuttering (Helm-Estabrooks, 1999):

- The onset is acquired, usually in adulthood
- A neurological impairment has been confirmed
- Speech disfluency is less variable across situations
- Stuttering occurs across all the words of an utterance, not mainly on initial words

- Content and function words are stuttered equally
- The person may be frustrated but not usually embarrassed by stuttering
- Secondary behaviors are less likely
- An adaptation effect is less likely
- Stuttering also occurs on highly automatic speech tasks

There are mixed reports concerning the absence of an adaptation effect listed above (e.g., Ardila & Lopez, 1986; Nowack & Stone, 1987), although it was present for others (Hamano et al., 2005; Tani & Sakai, 2011). No reports have been found pertaining to the consistency effect in neurogenic stuttering. Also, note in the preceding list that the distribution of stuttered events in the speech stream is wider than it is in developmental stuttering. Given this reduced predictability regarding locations, it is tempting to hypothesize that the consistency effect as well may be smaller than the 69% reported by Johnson and Leutenegger (1955, p. 211). A low consistency effect supports the impression that neurogenic stuttering represents a separate form of fluency disorder. For further explanations of the adaptation and consistency effects, see Chapter 4.

A survey of speech clinicians regarding 58 Dutch-speaking individuals with neurogenic stuttering revealed some interesting results. Theys, Van Wieringen, and De Nil (2008) observed that more than a quarter (27%) of the 164 clinicians who were serving populations with neurological disorders had worked with one or more patients with neurogenic stuttering. These results suggested that it is a more common problem than previously thought. In addition, patient characteristics contrasted with previously listed criteria in a few ways. A larger proportion than expected, 39% of patients, displayed an adaptation effect. Secondary characteristics, also supposedly rare, were noted among 40%. A remarkable majority (64%) of patients were reported to have emotional reactions to their stuttering, but data upheld the impression that irritation rather than anxiety is a more common response.

Assessment and Treatment of Neurogenic Stuttering

The assessment of neurogenic stuttering includes areas very similar to those of cluttering, but the expected findings differ. In addition to the standard components, such as case history, description of speech characteristics, speaking rate and other temporal features, emotional and social impact, it is important to assess other dimensions of speech and language that may have been affected by the neurological disorder. In this case, however, the types of problems with articulation, language, cognition and memory, and capacities to self-correct errors will all be evaluated relative to the client's premorbid abilities. The potential for spontaneous recovery following the injury and the medical prognosis will also be important.

Treatments of neurogenic stuttering have included a variety of approaches: traditional therapies of stuttering modification and/or fluency shaping, biofeedback, speech rate changes, pacing, delayed auditory feedback, cognitive therapy, voice therapy techniques, respiration training, relaxation exercises, and similar techniques toward an easier approach to speech movements. Medical interventions have included surgery, thalamic stimulation, subcutaneous nerve stimulation, and prescription drugs.

Neurogenic Stuttering: A Sample Case

Description: A 55-year-old woman was referred for a speech-language evaluation secondary to a brain hemorrhage. Medical scans revealed diffuse injury to the right temporal lobe. Speech characteristics included sound/syllable repetitions and postural fixations in all positions of words and utterances. Content and function words were stuttered with proportionately the same frequency. Stuttering occurred during both conversational and oral reading speech samples. No adaptation effect was observed. Although she was also disfluent on automatic speech tasks (e.g., counting, swearing, saying the alphabet), her language skills, both receptive and expressive, were normal. Only mild signs of frustration with speech disruptions were observed.

Intervention: Therapeutic probes revealed improved fluency when speaking each syllable while tapping the beat and when slowing the initiation and connectedness across words in sentences. A pacing board (see Figure 15.1) was introduced to facilitate the client's self-monitoring of rhythm and slow speaking rate. The clinician demonstrated the use of the board by pointing to a space for each syllable as she talked, and the client then imitated. Independent use of the board was targeted in a hierarchy of speaking tasks progressing from short phrases to longer sentences. A drawing of a simple pacing board is seen in Figure 15.1. When the client was consistently successful with the pacing board, she was instructed to look up from the board and make eye contact with the clinician while talking, maintaining a similar rate/rhythm. After consistently fluent speech was maintained in the therapy room, transfer of fluency in multiple outside settings was accomplished after developing an individualized situation hierarchy, starting with easier settings and progressing to more difficult.

Figure 15.1   Pacing Board

Psychogenic Stuttering

Psychogenic stuttering occurs when there is a sudden onset of chronic abnormal disfluency following a psychoemotional trauma, and the speech disorder is not found to be associated with an organic etiology (Baumgartner, 1999). It is a rare condition and should not be confused with cases of adults with previously existing developmental stuttering who experience a new episode of stuttering triggered by psychoemotional factors. The term *psychogenic disorder* is also sometimes used interchangeably with "functional disorder" and "somatic disorder." The original cause of this form of stuttering is emotional breakdown or psychological trauma, such as firsthand views of the tragedies of war. Its core symptomatology includes the essential disfluency features included in our definition of stuttering (see Chapter 1).

A variety of disfluency types have been observed among individuals with psychogenic stuttering, although repetitions are frequently cited (Mahr & Leith, 1992). The dynamics of psychogenic stuttering are similar to that of other psychogenic speech disorders, such as functional aphonia and functional dysphonia. Instead of a loss of voice or hoarseness secondary to an emotional trauma, however, disfluent speech is a symptom of what the psychopathological literature refers to as a *conversion reaction* (Breuer & Freud, 1936). As we discussed in Chapter 6, a conversion reaction occurs when there is an impairment of physical action or sensation that cannot be explained by organic disease or a medical condition, and it arises following deep unconscious conflict. More than one psychosomatic illness sometimes arises in the same individual, but a person who has had another form of conversion reaction is not necessarily inclined to develop psychogenic stuttering. In one person a conversion reaction results in a paralyzed limb; in another it causes loss of speech. Why the symptoms vary across individuals remains unknown. Possible reasons for the variation, however, include the potential of secondary gains from the particular symptom (e.g., being excused from responsibility for a communication role) or a symbolic expression of the psychological conflict (e.g., being blocked from expressing one's opinions). People typically have no awareness of the nature of the problem or the secondary gain that it may have. In contrast to developmental stuttering, they often are emotionally apathetic toward the stuttering, a response that has been termed *la belle indifférence* (Roth, Aronson, & Davis, 1989).

In a retrospective examination of 184 cases of sudden onset adult stuttering, Roth et al. (1989) found that 100 had suspected psychogenic components. Diagnoses included neurogenic stuttering, psychogenic stuttering, a mixed diagnosis (psychogenic + neurogenic), or undetermined origin. Among the 100 with psychogenic stuttering, 12 met criteria for closer scrutiny. Six men and six women, ages 21 to 79 years, with no childhood history of stuttering and for whom neurological diagnoses had been ruled out, all underwent psychiatric, medical, and speech pathology examinations. The characteristics of their psychogenic stuttering cases were in turn described. Their stuttering problem had lasted from 1.5 to 4 years. Speech characteristics included repetitions, prolongations, and blocks that ranged in severity from mild to severe. Nine had some episodes of normal speech. Eleven were classified as "conversion reaction." Psychologically, six experienced acute stress, four chronic stress, and one undetermined stress. All had associated somatic complaints as well, such as headache, backache, leg pain, chest pain, numbness or tingling of an extremity, staring spells, fatigue, fainting, panic attacks, choking sensation, hyperventilation, memory loss, or ringing in the ears. Muscle contractions or twitches occurred among six of them. Eleven experienced a recovery of some fluent speech: five from individual speech therapy, one from group therapy, one from the evaluation processes, and four from spontaneous recovery.

Depression appears to be a common diagnosis among individuals with psychogenic stuttering (Roth et al., 1989). Other potential psychological conditions that may be present include schizophrenia, neurosis, and psychosis. Assessment and diagnosis by a licensed psychiatric or psychotherapy professional is warranted. It is important that health-care professionals maintain a respectful stance toward the client because it is vital to the process of healing. When a client believes his or her symptoms represent a physical ailment, recovery is not aided by being told that the symptoms are psychological. Instead, improvement is based in the client's acquisition of skills and strategies. Similar to conventional stuttering treatment, as the speaker gains self-confidence in his or her own capacities to manage the speech symptoms with new behavioral responses, the problem weakens and progressively recedes.

The onset of psychogenic stuttering typically occurs in adulthood and is sudden and rare. It is different from developmental stuttering because the disfluencies usually persist even in typically fluency-inducing conditions such as singing, unison, and delayed auditory feedback (Mahr & Leith, 1992). Also unlike developmental stuttering, the stuttering symptoms have the potential to go into remission rapidly, especially when the period of acute psychological stress has passed and the individual had no issues premorbidly. Concurrent psychological counseling can aid holistic recovery. Caring support and skilled intervention by multiple professionals can be instrumental in facilitating progress. Although the following case description depicts the potential outcome of an improvement, published reports suggest psychogenic stuttering may continue for months or years (Roth, Aronson, & Davis, 1989) and in some cases does not resolve (Mahr & Leith, 1992).

Psychogenic Stuttering: A Sample Case

Description: The speech-language pathologist (SLP) was contacted by a woman looking for help for her husband, age 38, who suddenly began stuttering for no apparent reason. His speech was characterized by frequent stereotypic repetitions of initial syllables: "Whi-whi-which one do you want? "I-I-I like that one." "Let-let-let's get it." He looked people in the eyes, did not avoid speaking situations, and was not particularly bothered by the speech pattern. He had never stuttered before. He was unmotivated to seek help, but his wife encouraged him to do just that. The client also had some unexplained episodes of neck and back pain, for which several medical professionals had been consulted, who found no physical problems. The client had been in good physical health throughout most of his life. The couple's physician suggested they contact the SLP for a consultation. Further discussion revealed the client was seriously depressed and dealing with some stressful interpersonal conflicts within the family. He had recently begun sessions of psychological therapy.

> **Intervention:** The speech clinician began by educating the client about the vocal tract struc-
> tures and their function for speech production. Then strategies for slow, easy initiation of speech
> were taught via modeling and instruction. The client achieved targeted objectives of describing
> his speech movements accurately and modifying moments of simulated stuttering (particularly
> syllable repetitions). Skills were practiced in multiple speaking tasks and situational contexts. The
> client simultaneously gained cognitive-emotional coping skills through the psychological therapy,
> and one day the client came to therapy reporting that his stuttering had disappeared and that his
> attitudes and adjustment with life more generally had improved.

Malingering

On occasion, a family member or professional may wonder whether the symptoms of
stuttering are faked behavior. Malingering, or faking the presence of a disorder, is a remote
possibility when a speaker has something to gain from the diagnosis, especially for financial, legal, or vocational gains (Seery, 2005). Although parents sometimes suspect a child
is stuttering to annoy or gain attention, these are not typical of malingering. Especially if
other characteristics of the developmental disorder fit diagnostic criteria, such as early
stuttering onset, SLD, progression, emotional responses, and fluency-inducing situations,
these should outweigh the suspicions of underlying motives. A child who shows signs that
she or he does *not* want to be stuttering should not be suspected of malingering.

A person who malingers, however, is more apt to show signs that it is favorable to be
acknowledged for stuttering and would be motivated to want to be identified as someone who stutters. Typically, there is an underlying gainful motivation. For example, on
the basis of stuttered speech, criminal identification could be ruled out, a release from
military service granted, and so on. Faked stuttering is apt to lack variability and take
on a stereotypical form. The diagnosis of malingering is aided by the tendency for the
faker's profile and characteristics to be consistent only with what the individual knows
about stuttering. The areas where a malingerer's knowledge is weak, or incompatible
with what we know about stuttering, are apt to give away the charade. Differential diagnosis in the case of a man suspected of a crime who partially malingered stuttering is
described by Seery (2005).

Stuttering in Bilingual and Multicultural Populations

Large waves of immigrants across continents and countries, as well as the ease of trans-
portation for various purposes, have led to societies with far greater numbers of bilingual/
multilingual speakers than ever before. There are millions of multilingual people worldwide, including in the United States (Tucker, 1998; Van Borsel, Maes, & Foulon, 2005)).
It is therefore likely that speech-language clinicians will examine and deliver clinical services to people who stutter who speak more than one language or stutter in more than
one language.

The impacts of culture, religion, social, and demographic factors on attitudes toward
stuttering and on approaches to its treatment is nicely discussed by Ezrati-Vinacour and

Weinstein (2011). Bilingualism may be viewed as one aspect of a speaker's culture, but it is not evaluated based on a singular characteristic. Coalson, Pena, and Byrd (2013) recommend eight necessary variables to describe the language profile of a multilingual speaker (i.e., proficiency, history, function, mode, stability, accent, affect, and covert speech). With regard to history, there can be differences among individuals based on the timing of their acquisition of the second language. Some children are exposed to two languages essentially from birth on. Others may have been exposed to just one language in the home until they started attending a preschool, day-care, or school program where they were exposed to the second language from that point on. In the latter situation, there may be many varied schedules of exposure to the second language (e.g., daily versus two mornings per week, etc.) that contribute to differences among children in the developmental progress of their second-language learning. Yet another situation arises when there are two languages spoken in a home since birth, and a third or additional languages are introduced through other settings. Such diversity should be kept in mind in evaluating current scientific information, which has often been gathered without due consideration of such differences in the sample of participants.

Three main questions should be addressed relative to stuttering among those with diverse cultural and multilingual backgrounds:

1. Incidence: Are those who speak more than one language or come from different cultures apt to be more disfluent?

2. Diagnosis: Are there distinctive stuttering speech characteristics among those who speak more than one language?

3. Treatment: Does cultural background affect beliefs and attitudes about the disorder and should it be considered in the therapeutic approach?

Incidence

In discussing the incidence and prevalence of stuttering (Chapter 2), we pointed out that stuttering has been identified in most parts of the world and in many societies and cultures. Although for certain societies a link was proposed between high incidence and excessive pressure on children's achievements and ability to speak well, and between low incidence and society's tolerant attitudes in these matters, we concluded that, generally, incidence in various parts of the world seems to be similar. Even if exceptionally high or low incidence/prevalence data are valid, which we doubt, research data to support the causative relations are weak. Also, one should keep in mind that either high or low incidence might reflect genetic factors, especially in societies that were not open to outside bloodlines. Current incidence/prevalence data for bilingualism are scant but do not seem to support appreciative deviation from that of the population at large.

Diagnosis

Clinicians should be aware that encounters with different cultural groups and bilingual clients raise the possibility of misinterpretation of data, resulting in possible misdiagnosis of speech and/or language disorders (e.g., Finn & Cordes, 1997). This is reflected in the opinion of several scholars who expressed that examiners' lack of familiarity with African American English (AAE), a dialect spoken by a large number of African Americans, might have led to an erroneous overestimate of stuttering prevalence among African Americans. They claimed that because normal disfluencies, such as revisions, repetitions, filled pauses, and prosodic features, denote various meanings in AAE, the presence of some or all of these linguistic features in a speaker may be mistaken for stuttering by individuals unfamiliar with AAE (Proctor et al., 2008).

Similarly, differential diagnosis of stuttering from normal disfluency in young non-English-speaking children should be approached with caution due to the limited available cross-linguistic research on typical frequencies and types of disfluencies. In this regard, some pilot data suggested that more than 75% of young nonstuttering Spanish-English bilingual children ages 5–6 years produced more than 3 SLDs per 100 words in their Spanish speech samples. This was significantly higher than the proportion of SLD in their English samples (Logan, Byrd, & Gillam, 2012). The fact that none of these children were considered to be stuttering by their caregivers highlights the importance of applying multiple diagnostic criteria. The opinion of caregivers within the child's speaking community is one factor to consider in the process of identifying those who are at risk for fluency disorders.

Another question is whether the listener's familiarity with the client's language influences identification of stuttering. There is no clear answer yet. One study investigated whether bilingual English-Spanish-speaking judges are better at making disfluency judgments in Spanish than monolingual English-speaking judges. No meaningful differences between the two groups of listeners were found (Humphrey, 2004). Other investigators, however, reported that language familiarity does influence stuttering identification. In a series of listener judgment experiments, native speakers of Brazilian Portuguese rated stuttering in Dutch speakers and in Portuguese speakers while native speakers of Dutch rated stuttering in Brazilian Portuguese speakers and in Dutch speakers. Both panels found identification of stuttering more difficult in the foreign language than in the native language (Van Borsel & Britto Pereira, 2005). The investigators suggested that their results might have been different if the judgment had involved languages that are less remote from each other. To test the hypothesis that closeness to the listener's native language is a determining factor when identifying stuttering in an unfamiliar language, three panels judged stuttering in the speech of Dutch speakers. The Dutch- and the English-speaking panels (both Germanic languages) performed better in identifying Dutch PWS and NFS than a panel speaking Brazilian Portuguese, a Romance language (Van Borsel, Leahy, & Brito Pereira, 2008).

One of the primary concerns in the assessment of bilingual speakers who stutter is the examiner's capacity to recognize the occurrence, location, and nature of disfluent behaviors in another language (Finn & Cordes, 1997). A recent study by Einarsdottir and Ingham (2009) showed that experienced speech clinicians were fairly reliable at identifying stuttered intervals in video-recorded samples of preschool children speaking in an unfamiliar language. It is, however, appropriate for clinicians to be cautious about their identification of stuttering and disfluency in bilingual speakers. It can be difficult even when listening to young monolingual children to distinguish a doubling pattern (e.g., "car-car," "bye-bye") from a whole-word repetition. When a young child is speaking in an unfamiliar language with different patterns of prosody, the clinician would do well to make sure that the listeners who are familiar with the child's language would similarly detect speech disruptions. The clinician may need to include a translator, a parent, or another person proficient in the language for assistance and confirmation. A recent review of the literature on stuttering and bilingualism can be found in Roberts and Shenker (2007).

Disfluencies in the speech of those who are learning to speak a second language are a potential distraction for listeners (Corley, MacGregor, & Donaldson, 2007). Distracting behaviors can include unfilled pauses, self-repetitions, inappropriate rate, and fillers/interjections (Rossiter, 2009). Their speech, however, is usually not stuttered, as suggested by the observation that there has been no concern found in published literature about the frequency of SLD being greater than that of other normally fluent speakers. This inference is preliminary, however, and research should be conducted to test whether SLD might be more frequent among second-language learners. Investigations have reported that second-language learners (i.e., those who have only been learning to speak a language for a few years) produce a preponderance of various forms of hesitation (e.g., silent and filled pauses, self-repairs, etc.) that typify language formulation and working memory overload compared to native speakers. The frequency of these behaviors significantly exceeds those produced by monolingual speakers (Temple, 2000). More research is needed to reveal whether the various phenomena of stuttering, such as typical locations, patterns of occurrence, adaptation, fluency-inducing conditions, and so on are equally evident cross-linguistically among speakers who stutter. For example, one study that analyzed speech samples of Spanish-speaking school-age CWS revealed significantly more stuttering on utterances that are longer (i.e., more syllables) and more complex syntactically (Watson, Byrd, & Carlo, 2011).

Treatment

Experimental data regarding the treatment of stuttering in bilingual individuals is quite limited. Reports have been mostly confined to single case studies with no comparison of bilinguals/monolinguals receiving the same treatment. Furthermore, there have been no published studies of treatment outcomes with bilingual children. The basic question of whether fluency treated in one language transfers to the second language has not been answered satisfactorily although some hints that this is the case have been published. In several case studies, the Lidcombe Program was employed with bilingual children (e.g., Bakhtiar & Packman, 2009). In other instances, treatment was provided in two languages simultaneously, or first in one language and then in the other. Overall, the outcomes of all these cases show that fluency increased in both languages spoken by the child, and that treatment outcome was not affected by whether the languages were input simultaneously or sequentially (Shenker, 2011). Nevertheless, when parents of young children who stutter become involved, it is possible to provide treatment in all languages spoken by the child. Also unanswered is the question of whether the child's learning of a second language has any effect on preventing stuttering onset.

So, are there special therapy methods for bilingual people who stutter? Currently the answer is no. Still, relevant considerations for clinicians are the effects of cultural beliefs about the cause of the disorder, attitudes toward the person who stutters, attitudes toward treatment in general, acceptability of specific therapeutic approaches, reactions to specific techniques, and who should be the treatment provider. For example, peoples from some cultures may not react well to certain advice typically given in the United States in parent counseling, or they may not be open to requests that parents participate in the therapy sessions, especially not both parents. In some cultures, adults may not be willing to openly express deep feelings or emotional problems in group therapy. Clinical assignments, such as stuttering on purpose to strangers, may be unacceptable; so is maintaining eye contact with listeners older in age or superior in status; care must be taken regarding gender-based and age-based roles in interactions and more (see Roberts and Shenker, 2007, for other interesting examples).

Keep in mind that cultural influences include many factors. For example, religious beliefs and social class are relevant in addition to ethnicity, race, and geographic locale. One of us has encountered some people who stutter who believed they were afflicted by God and that a minister should provide the counseling. Differences in overt stuttering patterns between African Americans and whites were tied to cultural background, according to Leith and Mims (1975). They concluded that forces within African American culture actually negate certain common clinical approaches. Still, Roberts and Shenker (2007) have cautioned against stereotypes based on cultural background, explaining that a middle-age lawyer from Hong Kong would have more in common with an Anglo architect from the United States than with a young adult street vendor from his own city of Hong Kong. Robinson and Crowe (1998) offer a model of service delivery to be followed when offering services to multicultural populations. They also offer examples of etiological and remediation myths that clinicians may encounter in their work with African American populations.

Several suggestions may help improve services provided to culturally and linguistically diverse populations (Santos & Reese, 1999):

1. Clinicians should understand and learn about the aspects of their cultural practices that may differ from other's ethnic backgrounds.

2. Clinicians should educate themselves about the cultures of the people they serve. What kinds of accomplishments are respected? What do they believe children should be learning and doing? How do they view the roles of family members (parents, grandparents, aunts/uncles, siblings)? What elements of their culture are treated as public versus private? What is their history with educational, health-care, and social services, and does that history affect their outlook regarding these services?

3. Is the literature provided to the client/family appropriate, or might there be implicit or explicit assumptions, beliefs, or values that could be potentially

problematic, disrespectful, or confusing? What mode of presentation (oral, visual, auditory) is best to facilitate understanding of information? Is the literacy level appropriate and technical jargon kept to a minimum or explained sufficiently? If material is translated, is it appropriate given their particular dialect and community? Clinicians may want to find someone to review material beforehand to prevent potential misunderstandings.

4. Does the program of services assume that family members will take an active role in treatment that is not customary in their culture? Professionals must be careful not to presume that parents or family members who do not take an "active" role don't care, when in fact they do but show concern in other ways. Family participation should be adapted to the culture.

Summary

Although classic developmental stuttering is clearly the largest in incidence and most known within the group of fluency disorders, clinicians must be aware of, and familiar with, other fluency disorders in this group, both in regard to differential diagnosis and treatment. There has been minimal research published to reveal how individuals with other fluency disorders are best served. Case samples and potential considerations were discussed that may be useful in clinical decision making. Several points were highlighted in this chapter:

- Fluency disorders with childhood onset include patterns such as unusual breath locations, word-final disfluencies, language-based disfluency, and cluttering.
- Other fluency disorders with adult onset include neurogenic stuttering and psychogenic stuttering.
- Potential overlap in symptomatology can be confusing, masking very different etiologies and the need for different counseling and treatment regimens. Clinicians must carefully evaluate differential diagnostic criteria as they consider neurogenic, psychogenic, or malingering as possible sources of stuttering and disfluent behaviors.
- It is still unclear if bilingualism influences the incidence of stuttering and whether characteristics of stuttering vary across languages spoken by the same individual.
- Research indicates that the frequency and types of normal disfluencies across sociocultural populations varies.
- Cultural values must be considered when therapy is provided to clients of diverse backgrounds.

Study Questions and Discussion Topics

1. What characteristics of neurogenic stuttering differ from those of developmental stuttering?
2. How is treatment of neurogenic stuttering similar to and/or different from that of developmental stuttering?

3. What would lead you to suspect that a client presents psychogenic stuttering?
4. What would be your approaches to treatment of psychogenic stuttering, and why?
5. What characteristics aid the identification of cluttering? What are some reasons why differential diagnosis of cluttering from stuttering may be beneficial?
6. What special considerations need to be made in the treatment of speakers who clutter?
7. What can you do to help ensure your services are culturally appropriate for your clients?

Websites

Brochures on the following topics are available for download in the Resources section of the Stuttering Foundation of America's Web site: http://www.stutteringhelp.org

- Neurogenic stuttering
- Cluttering
- Tourette's syndrome
- Bilingual child

Suggested Readings

Boscolo, B., Bernstein Ratner, N., & Rescorla, L. (2002). Fluency of school-aged children with a history of specific expressive language impairment: An exploratory study. *American Journal of Speech-Language Pathology, 11,* 41–49.

De Nil, L., Jokel, R., & Rochon, E. (2007). Etiology, symptomatology, and treatment of neurogenic stuttering. In E. Conture & R. Curlee (Eds.), *Stuttering and related disorders of fluency* (3rd ed., pp. 326–343). New York, NY: Thieme.

Ezrati-Vinacour, R., & Weinstein, N. (2011). A dialogue among various cultures and its manifestationin stuttering therapy. *Journal of Fluency Disorders, 36,* 174-185.

Roberts, P., & Shenker, R. (2007). Assessment and treatment of stuttering in bilingual speakers. In E. Conture & R. Curlee (Eds.), *Stuttering and related disorders of fluency* (3rd ed., pp. 183–206). New York, NY: Thieme.

Van Borsel, J., Maes, E., & Foulon, K. (2001). Stuttering and bilingualism: A review. *Journal of Fluency Disorders, 26,* 179–205.

References

Ackermann, H., Hertrich, I., Ziegler, W., Bitzer, M., & Bien, S. (1996). Acquired dysfluencies following infarction of left mesiofrontal cortex. *Aphasiology, 10,* 409–417.

Adams, M. (1987). Voice onsets and segment durations of normal speakers and beginning stutterers. *Journal of Fluency Disorders, 12,* 133–139.

Adams, M. (1990). The demands and capacities model: I. Theoretical elaborations. *Journal of Fluency Disorders, 15,* 135–141.

Agnello, J., & Wingate, M. (1972). Some acoustic aspects of stuttered speech. *Journal of Acoustical Society of America, 52,* 159.

Alfonso, P. (1991). Subject definition and selection criteria for stuttering research in adult subjects. *Haskins Laboratories Status Report on Speech Research,* SR-105/106, 231–242.

Alm, P. (2004a). Stuttering, emotions, and heart rate during anticipatory anxiety: A critical review. *Journal of Fluency Disorders, 29,* 123–133.

Alm, P. (2004b). Stuttering and basal ganglia circuits: A critical review of possible relations. *Journal of Communication Disorders, 37,* 325–369.

Ambrose, N., & Yairi, E. (1994). The development of awareness of stuttering in preschool children. *Journal of Fluency Disorders, 19,* 229–245.

Ambrose, N., & Yairi, E. (1995). The role of repetition units in the differential diagnosis of early childhood incipient stuttering. *American Journal of Speech-Language Pathology, 4*(3), 82–88.

Ambrose, N., & Yairi, E. (1999). Normative disfluency data for early childhood stuttering. *Journal of Speech, Language, and Hearing Research, 42,* 895–909.

Ambrose, N., & Yairi, E. (2002). The Tudor study: Data and ethics. *American Journal of Speech-Language Pathology, 11,* 190–203.

Ambrose, N., Cox, N., & Yairi, E. (1997). The genetic basis of persistence and recovery in stuttering. *Journal of Speech, Language, and Hearing Research, 40*(3), 567–580.

Ambrose, N., Yairi, E., & Cox, N. (1993). Genetic aspects of early childhood stuttering. *Journal of Speech and Hearing Research, 36,* 701–706.

American Speech-Language-Hearing Association Special Interest Division 4: Fluency and Fluency Disorders. (1999, March). Terminology pertaining to fluency and fluency disorders: Guidelines. *ASHA, 41*(Suppl. 19), 29–36.

Anderson, J., Pellowski, M., Conture, E., & Kelly, E. (2003). Temperamental characteristics of young children who stutter. *Journal of Speech, Language, and Hearing Research, 46,* 1221–1233.

Anderson, J., & Conture, E. (2000). Language abilities of children who stutter: A preliminary study. *Journal of Fluency Disorders, 25,* 283–304.

Anderson, J., & Conture, E. (2004). Sentence structure priming in young children who do and do not stutter. *Journal of Speech, Language, and Hearing Research, 47,* 552–571.

Anderson, J., Pellowski, M., & Conture, E. (2005). Childhood stuttering and dissociations across linguistic domains. *Journal of Fluency Disorders, 30,* 219–253.

Anderson, J., Wagovich, S., & Hall, N. (2006). Nonword repetition skills in young children who do and do not stutter. *Journal of Fluency Disorders, 31,* 177–199.

Andrews, C., O'Brian, S., Harrison, E., Onslow, M., Packman, A., & Menzies, R. (2012). Syllable-timed speech treatment for school-age children who stutter: A phase 1 trial. *Language, Speech, and Hearing Sciences in Schools, 43,* 359–369.

Andrews, G. (1984). The epidemiology of stuttering. In R. F. Curlee & W. H. Perkins (Eds.), *Nature and treatment of stuttering: New Directions* (pp. 1–12). San Diego, CA: College-Hill.

Andrews, G., & Craig, A. (1988). Prediction of outcome after treatment for stuttering. *British Journal of Psychiatry, 153,* 236–240.

Andrews, G., & Cutler, J. (1974). Stuttering therapy: The relation between changes in symptom level and attitudes. *Journal of Speech and Hearing Disorders, 39,* 312–319.

Andrews, G., & Dozsa, M. (1977). Haloperidol and the treatment of stuttering. *Journal of Fluency Disorders, 2,* 217–224.

Andrews, G., & Harris, M. (1964). *The syndrome of stuttering*: Clinics in developmental medicine, No. 17. London, England: Spastics Society Medical Education and Information Unit in association with Heinemann Medical Books.

Andrews, G., & Ingham, R. (1972). Stuttering: An evaluation of follow-up procedures for syllable-timed speech/token system therapy. *Journal of Communication Disorders, 5*(4), 307–319.

Andrews, G., & Ingham, R. (1973). An analysis of a token economy in stuttering therapy. *Journal of Applied Behavior Analysis, 6*(2), 219–229.

Andrews, G., Craig, A., Feyer, A., Hoddinott, S., Howie, P., & Neilson, M. (1983). Stuttering: A review of research findings and theories circa 1982. *Journal of Speech and Hearing Disorders, 48,* 226–246.

Andrews, G., Guitar, B., & Howie, P. (1980). Meta-analysis of the effects of stuttering treatment. *Journal of Speech and Hearing Disorders, 45,* 287–307.

Andrews, G., Harris, M., Garside, R., & Kay, D. (1964). The inhibition of stuttering by syllable-timed speech.

The syndrome of stuttering. The Spastic Society Medical and Educational Unit. London, England: Heineman.

Andrews, G., Howie, P., Dozsa, M., & Guitar, B. (1982). Stuttering: Speech pattern characteristics under fluency-inducing conditions. *Journal of Speech and Hearing Research, 25,* 208–216.

Andrews, G., Morris-Yates, A., Howie, P., & Martin, N. G. (1991). Genetic factors in stuttering confirmed. *Archives of General Psychiatry, 48,* 1034–1035.

Antipova, E., Purdy, S., Blakeley, M., & Williams, S. (2008). Effects of altered auditory feedback (AAF) on stuttering frequency during monologue speech production. *Journal of Fluency Disorders, 33,* 274–290.

Archibald, L., & De Nil, L. (1999). The relationship between stuttering severity and kinesthetic acuity for jaw movements in adults who stutter. *Journal of Fluency Disorders, 24,* 25–42.

Ardila, A., & Lopez, M. (1986). Severe stuttering associated with right hemisphere lesion. *Brain & Language, 27,* 239–246.

Ardila, A., Bateman, J., & Niño, C. (1994). An epidemiologic study of stuttering. *Journal of Communication Disorders, 27*(1), 37–48.

Arias-Carrión, O., & Pöppel, E. (2007). Dopamine, learning and reward-seeking behavior. *Acta Neurobiological Experimental, 67,* 481–488.

Arndt, J., & Healey, E. C. (2001). Concomitant disorders in school-age children who stutter. *Language, Speech, and Hearing Services in Schools, 32,* 68–78.

Arnott, N. (1928). *Elements of physics* London, England.

Aron, M. (1962). The nature and incidence of stuttering among a Bantu group of school-going children. *Journal of Speech and Hearing Disorders, 27*(2), 116–128.

Aron, M. (1967). The relationships between measurements of stuttering behavior. *Journal of the South African Logopedic Society, 14,* 15–34.

ASHA. (1997–2007). Incidence and prevalence of communication disorders and hearing loss in Children—2008 edition. Retrieved from http://www.asha.org/members/research/ reports/children.htm

ASHA. (2004). Evidence-based practice in communication disorders: An introduction [Technical report]. Retrieved from http://www.asha.org/policy.

ASHA. (2005a). *Evidence-based practice in communication disorders* [Position statement]. Available from http://www.asha.org/policy.

ASHA. (2005b). Speech-language pathologists providing clinical services via telepractice [Position statement]. Retrieved from www.asha.org/policy.

ASHA. (2008). *Speech and language disorders and diseases.* Retrieved from http://www.asha.org/public/speech/disorders/ default.htm

Au-Yeung, J., Gomez, I., & Howell, P. (2003). Exchange of disfluency with age from function words to content words in Spanish speakers who stutter. *Journal of Speech, Language, and Hearing Research, 46,* 754–765.

Au-Yeung, J., Howell, P., Davis, S., Charles, N., & Sackin, S. (2001). UCL survey on bilingualism and stuttering. In H.-G. Bosshardt, J. S. Yaruss, & H. F. M. Peters (Eds.), *Proceedings of the Third World Congress on Fluency Disorders* (pp. 129–132). Nijmegen, Netherlands: Nijmegen University Press.

Avari, D., & Bloodstein, O. (1974). Adjacency and prediction in school-age stutterers. *Journal of Speech and Hearing Research, 17,* 33–40.

Axline, V. (1947). *Play therapy.* London, England: Methuen.

Backus, O. (1938). Incidence of stuttering among the deaf. *Annals of Otology, Rhinology, and Laryngology, 47,* 632–635.

Bakhtiar, M., & Packman, A. (2009). Intervention with the Lidcombe Program for a Bilingual School-Age Child Who Stutters in Iran. *Folia Phoniatrica et Logopaedica, 61,* 300–304.

Bakker, K, Myers, F., Raphael, L., & St. Louis, K. (2011). A preliminary comparison of speech rate, self-evaluation, and disfluency of people who speak exceptionally fast, clutter, or speak normally. In D. Ward & K. Scale Scott (Eds.), *Cluttering: A handbook of research, intervention and education* (pp. 45–65). East Sussex, UK: Psychology Press.

Bakker, K., & Myers, F. (2011). *Cluttering Severity Instrument.* [Computer software and manual]. Retrieved from http://associations.missouristate.edu/ ICA

Bandura, A. (1986). *Social foundations of thought and action: A social cognitive theory.* Englewood Cliffs, NJ: Prentice-Hall.

Bansevicius, D., Westgaard, R., & Jensen, C. (1997). Mental stress of long duration: EMG activity, perceived tension, fatigue, and pain development in pain-free subjects. *Headache, 37,* 499–510.

Bar, A. (1971). The shaping of fluency not the modification of stuttering. *Journal of Communication Disorders, 4,* 1–8.

Barasch, C., Guitar, B., McCauley, R., & Absher, R. (2000). Time perception and disfluency. *Journal of Speech, Language, and Hearing Research, 43,* 1429–1439.

Barbara, D. (1954). *Stuttering: A psychodynamic approach to its understanding and treatment.* New York, NY: Julian Press.

Barbara, D. (1962). *The psychotherapy of stuttering.* Springfield, IL: Charles C. Thomas.

Barlow, D., Hayes, S., & Nelson, R. (1984). *The scientist practitioner: Research and accountability in clinical and educational settings.* New York, NY: Pergamon.

Barr, H. (1940). A quantitative study of specific phenomena observed in stuttering. *Journal of Speech Disorders, 5,* 277–280.

Bauer, J., Hubbard Seery, C., LaBonte, R., & Ruhnke, L. (2008). Voice F0 responses elicited by perturbations in pitch of auditory feedback in individuals that stutter and controls. *Proceedings of Meetings on Acoustics: The 153rd Meeting of the Acoustical Society of America,* Vol. 1 (p. 060004). doi: http://dx.doi.org/10.1121/1.2959144

Bauerly, K., & De Nil L. (2011). Speech sequence skill learning in adults who stutter. *Journal of Fluency Disorders 36,* 349–60.

Baumgartner, J. (1999). Acquired psychogenic stuttering. In R. F. Curlee (Ed.), *Stuttering and related disorders of fluency* (2nd ed.). New York, NY: Thieme.

Beal, D., Gracco, V., Brettschneider, J., Kroll, R., & De Nil, L. (2012). A voxel-based morphometry (VBM) analysis of regional grey and white matter volume abnormalities within the speech production network of children who stutter. *Cortex, 49*(8), 2151–2161. doi:10.1016/j.cortex.2012.08.013

Beal, D., Gracco, V., Lafaille, S., & De Nil, L. (2007). Voxel-based morphometry of auditory and speech-related cortex in stutterers. *Neuroreport, 18*(12), 1257–1260.

Becker, K., & Grundmann, K. (1971). Investigation on incidence and symptomatology of cluttering, *Folia Phoniatrica, 22,* 261–271.

Beijsterveldt, V., Felsenfeld, S., & Boomsma, D. (2010). Bivariate genetic analyses of stuttering and nonfluency in a large sample of 5-year old twins. Journal of Speech, Language, and Hearing Research, 53, 609–619.

Berlin, A. (1954). *An exploratory attempt to isolate types of stuttering* (Unpublished doctoral dissertation). Northwestern University, Evanston, IL.

Bernstein Ratner, N. (1992). Measurable outcomes in instructions to modify normal parent-child verbal interactions: Implications for indirect stuttering therapy. *Journal of Speech and Hearing Research, 35,* 14–20.

Bernstein Ratner, N. (1995). Treating the child who stutters with concomitant language or phonological impairment. *Language, Speech, and Hearing Services in Schools, 26,* 180–186.

Bernstein Ratner, N. (1997a). Stuttering: A psycholinguistic perspective. In R. F. Curlee & G. M. Siegel (Eds.), *Nature and treatment of stuttering: New directions* (2nd ed., pp. 99–127). Boston, MA: Allyn & Bacon.

Bernstein Ratner, N. (1997b). Leaving Las Vegas: Clinical odds and individual outcomes *American Journal of Speech-Language Pathology, 6,* 29–33.

Bernstein Ratner, N. (2004). Caregiver-child interactions and their impact on children's fluency: Implications for treatment. *Language, Speech, and Hearing Services in Schools, 35,* 46–56.

Bernstein Ratner, N. (2005). Evidence-based practice in stuttering: Some questions to consider. *Journal of Fluency Disorders, 30,* 163–188.

Bernstein Ratner, N., & Healey, E. C. (1999). *Stuttering research and practice.* Mahwah, NJ: Erlbaum.

Bernstein Ratner, N., & Sih, C. (1987). The effects of gradual increases in sentence length and complexity on children's dysfluency. *Journal of Speech and Hearing Disorders, 52,* 278–287.

Bernstein Ratner, N., & Silverman, S. (2000). Parental perceptions of children's communicative development at stuttering onset. *Journal of Speech, Language, and Hearing Research, 43,* 1252–1263.

Blanton, S. (1916). A survey of speech defects. *Journal of Educational Psychology, 7*(10), 581–592.

Block, S., Onslow, M., Roberts, R., & White S. (2004). Control of stuttering with EMG feedback. *Advances in Speech-Language Pathology, 6,* 100–106.

Blomgren, M., Roy, N., Callister, T., & Merrill, R. (2005). Intensive stuttering modification therapy: A multidimensional assessment of treatment outcomes. *Journal of Speech, Language, and Hearing Research, 48*(3), 509–523.

Blood, G. (1995). Power: Relapse management with adolescents who stutter. *Language, Speech, and Hearing Services in Schools, 26,* 169–179.).

Blood, G., & Seider, R. (1981). The concomitant problems of young stutterers. *Journal of Speech and Hearing Disorders, 46,* 31–33.

Blood, G., Ridenour, V., Qualls, C., & Scheffner Hammer (2003). Co-occurring disorders in children who stutter. *Journal of Communication Disorders, 36,* 427–448.

Blood, I., Wertz, H., Blood, G., Bennett, S., & Simpson, K. (1997). The effects of life stressors and daily stressors on stuttering. *Journal of Speech, Language, and Hearing Research, 40,* 134–143.

Bloodstein, O. (1944). Studies in the psychology of stuttering: XIX. The relationship between oral reading rate and severity of stuttering. *Journal of Speech Disorders, 9,* 161–173.

Bloodstein, O. (1950). A rating scale study of conditions under which stuttering is reduced or absent. *Journal of Speech and Hearing Disorders, 15,* 29–36.

Bloodstein, O. (1960a). The development of stuttering: I. Changes in nine basic features. *Journal of Speech and Hearing Disorders, 25,* 219–237.

Bloodstein, O. (1960b). The development of stuttering: II. Developmental phases. *Journal of Speech and Hearing Disorders, 25,* 366–376.

Bloodstein, O. (1970). Stuttering and normal disfluency: A continuity hypothesis. *British Journal of Disorders of Communication, 5,* 30–39.

Bloodstein, O. (1981). *A handbook on stuttering.* Chicago, IL: National Easter Seal Society.

Bloodstein, O. (1990). On pluttering, skivering, and floggering: A commentary. *Journal of Speech and Hearing Disorders, 55,* 392–393.

Bloodstein, O. (1995). *A handbook on stuttering* (5th ed.). San Diego, CA: Singular.

Bloodstein, O. (1997). Stuttering as an anticipatory struggle reaction. In R. Curlee and W. Perkins (Eds.),

Nature and treatment of stuttering: New directions (2nd ed.). Boston, MA: Allyn & Bacon.

Bloodstein, O., & Grossman, M. (1981). Early stutterings: Some aspects of their form and distribution. *Journal of Speech and Hearing Research, 24,* 298–302.

Bluemel, C. (1913). *Stammering and cognate defects of speech* (Vol. 1). New York, NY: Stechert.

Bluemel, C. (1932). Primary and secondary stammering. *Quarterly Journal of Speech, 18,* 187–200.

Boberg, E., & Kully, D. (1985). *Comprehensive stuttering program.* San Diego, CA: College-Hill Press.

Boberg, E., & Kully, D. (1994). Long-term results of an intensive treatment program for adults and adolescents who stutter. *Journal of Speech and Hearing Research, 37,* 1050–1059.

Boberg, E., Ewart, B., Mason, G., Lindsay, K., & Wynn, S. (1978). Stuttering in the retarded: II. Prevalence of stuttering in EMR and TMR children. *Mental Retardation Bulletin, 6*(2), 67–76.

Boberg, E., Yeudall, L., Schopflocher, D., & Bo-Lassen, P. (1983). The effect of an intensive behavioral program on the distribution of EEG alpha power in stutterers during the processing of verbal visuospatial information. *Journal of Fluency Disorders, 8,* 245–263.

Boey , R., Van de Heyning, P., Wuyts, F., Heylen, L., Stoop, R., & De Bodt, M. (2009). Awareness and reactions of young stuttering children aged 2–7 years old towards their speech disfluency , Journal of Communication Disorders, 42, 334–346.

Bohme, E. (1977). *Das stotter-syndrome: Aetiologi, dignose, und therapie.* Bern, Switzerland: Verlag Hans Ruber.

Boldon, A. (1955). *The co-existence of, and certain relationship between diabetes and stuttering* (Master's thesis). University of Wisconsin.

Bonelli, P., Dixon, M., Bernstein Ratner, N., & Onslow, M. (2000). Child and parent speech and language following the Lidcombe Programme of early stuttering intervention. *Clinical Linguistics and Phonetics, 14,* 427–446.

Boome, E., & Richardson, M. (1932). *The nature and treatment of stuttering.* New York, NY: Dutton.

Boome, E., & Richardson, M. (1947). *The nature and treatment of stammering* (2nd ed.). London, England: Methuen.

Borden, G., Kim, D., & Spiegler, K. (1987). Acoustics of stop consonants–vowel relationships during fluent and stuttered utterances. *Journal of Fluency Disorders, 12,* 175–184.

Bornstein, M., Bellack, A., & Hersen, M. (1977). Social skill training for unassertive children: A multiple baseline analysis. *Journal of Applied Behavior Analysis, 10,* 183–195.

Boscolo, B., Bernstein Ratner, N., & Rescorla, L. (2002). Fluency of school-aged children with a history of specific expressive language impairment: An exploratory study. *American Journal of Speech-Language Pathology, 11,* 41–49.

Bosshardt, H. (1999). Effects of concurrent mental calculation on stuttering, inhalation, and speech timing. *Journal of Fluency Disorders, 24,* 43–72.

Bosshardt, HG. (2002). Effects of concurrent cognitive processing on the fluency of word repetition: Comparison between persons who do and do not stutter. *Journal of Fluency Disorders, 27,* 93–114.

Bosshardt, HG, Sappok, C, Knipschild, M, & Hölscher, C.(1997). Spontaneous imitation of fundamental frequency and speech rate by nonstutterers and stutterers. Journal of Psycholinguist Research, 26,425–248.

Bøstrup, B., & Møller, B. (1990). Småbørnsstammegrupper (Therapy groups for preschool children who stammer). *Dansk Audiologopædi, 1,* 21–25.

Bothe, A., & Richardson, J. (2011). Statistical, practical, clinical, and personal significance: Definitions and applications in speech-language pathology.

Bothe, A., Davidow, J., Bramlett, R., Franic, D., & Ingham, R. (2006). Stuttering treatment research 1970–2005: II. Systematic review incorporating trial quality assessment of pharmacological approaches. *American Journal of Speech-Language Pathology, 15,* 342–352.

Bothe, A., Ingham, R., & Ingham, J. (2009). The roles of evidence and information in stuttering treatment. In B. Guitar & R. McCauley (Eds.), *Stuttering treatments: Conventional and emerging interventions* (pp. 341–352). Philadelphia, PA: Lippincott Williams and Wilkins.

Boyle, C., Boulet, S., Schieve, L., Cohen, R., Blumberg, S., Yeargin-Allsopp, M., Visser, S., & Kogan, M. (2011). Trends in the Prevalence of Developmental Disabilities in US Children, 1997–2008. *Pediatrics, 34,*: 385–95.

Bradberry, A. (1997). The role of support group in stuttering therapy. *Seminars in Speech and Language, 18,* 391–399.

Brady, G. (1971). Metronome-conditioned speech training for stuttering. *Behavior Therapy, 2,* 129–150.

Brady, J. (1991). The pharmacology of stuttering: A critical review. *American Journal of Psychiatry, 1448,* 1309–1316.

Brady, J., & Ali, Z. (2000). Alprazolam, citalopram and clomipramine for stuttering. *Journal of Clinical Psychopharmacology, 20,* 287.

Brady, P. (1968). A behavioral approach to the treatment of stuttering. *American Journal of Psychiatry, 125,* 843–848.

Brady, W., & Hall, D. (1976). The prevalence of stuttering among school-age children. *Language, Speech, and Hearing Services in Schools, 7*(2), 75–81.

Branscom, M. (1942). The construction and statistical evaluation of a speech fluency test for young children (Master's thesis). University of Iowa.

Branscom, M., Hughes, J., & Oxtoby, E., (1955). Studies of non-fluency in the speech of preschool children.

In W. Johnson & R. Leutenegger (Eds.), *Stuttering in Children and Adults* (pp. 157–180). Minneapolis: University of Minnesota Press.

Bray, M., Kehle, T., Lawless, K., & Theodore, L. (2003). The relationship between self-efficacy and depression to stuttering. *American Journal of Speech-Language Pathology, 12,* 425–431.

Bretherton-Furness, J., & Ward, D. (2012). Lexical access, story re-telling and sequencing skills in adults who clutter and those who do not. *Journal of Fluency Disorders, 37,* 214–224.

Breuer, J., & Freud, S. (1936). Studies in hysteria. *Nervous and Mental Disease* [Monograph Series, No. 61]. New York, NY: Nervous and Mental Disease Publishing.

Brill, A. (1923). Speech disturbances in nervous mental diseases. *Quarterly Journal of Speech, 9,* 129–135.

Brocklehurst, P. (2013). Stuttering prevalence, incidence and recovery rates depend on how we define it: Comment on Yairi & Ambrose's article Epidemiology of stuttering: 21st century advances. *Journal of Fluency Disorders, 38*(3), 290–293.

Brody, M., & Harrison, S. (1954). Group psychotherapy with male stutterers. *International Journal of Group Psychotherapy, 14,* 154–162.

Broomfield, J., & Dodd, B. (2004). Children with speech and language disability: Caseload characteristics. *International Journal of Language & Communication Disorders, 39*(3), 303–324.

Brosch, S., & Pirsig, W. (2001). Stuttering in history and culture. *International Journal of Pediatric Otorhinolaryngology, 59*(2), 81–87.

Brown, R. (1973). *A first language: The early stages.* Cambridge, MA: Harvard College.

Brown, S. (1945). The locus of stuttering in the speech sequence. *Journal of Speech Disorders, 10,* 181–192.

Brown, S. (1949). Advising parents of early stutterers. *Pediatrics, 4,* 170–175.

Brown, S., Ingham, R., Ingham, J., Laird, A., & Fox, P. (2005). Stuttered and fluent speech production: An Ale meta-analysis of functional neuroimaging studies. *Human Brain Mapping, 25,* 105–117.

Bruce, M., & Adams, M. (1978). Effects of two types of motor practice on stuttering adaptation. *Journal of Speech and Hearing Research, 21,* 421–428.

Brutten, E., & Shoemaker, D. (1967). *The modification of stuttering.* Englewood Cliffs, NJ: Prentice-Hall.

Brutten, G. (1985). *Communication Attitude Test Form A.* Rev. 1997. San Diego, CA: Plural Publishing.

Brutten, G., & Dunham, S. (1989). The communication attitude test. A normative study of grade school children. *Journal of Fluency Disorders, 14,* 371–377.

Bryngelson, B. (1931). Treatment of stuttering. *Journal of Expression, 5,* 19–26.

Bryngelson, B. (1932). A photo-phonographic analysis of the vocal disturbances in stuttering. *Psychological Monograph, 43,* 1–30.

Bryngelson, B. (1938). Prognosis of stuttering. *Journal of Speech Disorders, 3,* 121–123.

Bryngelson, B., & Rutherford, B. (1937). A comparative study of laterality of stutterers and non-stutterers. *Journal of Speech Disorders, 2,* 15–16.

Buchel, C., Raedler, T., Sommer, M., Sach, M., Weiller, C., Koch, M. A. (2004). White matter asymmetry in the human brain: A diffusion tensor MRI study. *Cerebral Cortex, 14,* 945–951.

Buck, S., Lees, R., & Cook, F. (2002). The influence of family history of stuttering on the onset of stuttering in young children. *Folia Phoniatrica et Logopaedica, 54,* 117–124.

Burdin, G. (1940). The surgical treatment of stuttering, 1840–1842. *Journal of Speech Disorders, 5,* 43–64.

Burns, D., Brady, J. P., & Kuruvilla, K. (1978). The acute effect of haloperidol and apomorphine on the severity of stuttering. *Biological Psychiatry, 13,* 255–264.

Byrd, C., Wolk, L., & Lockett Davis, B. (2007). Role of phonology in childhood stuttering and its treatment. In E. Conture & R. Curlee (Eds.), *Stuttering and related disorders* (3rd ed., pp. 168–182). New York, NY: Thieme.

Byrd, C., Conture, E., & Ohde, R. (2007). Phonological priming in young children who stutter: Holistic versus incremental processing. *American Journal of Speech-Language Pathology, 16,* 43–53.

Campbell, J., & Hill, D. (1987). *Systematic disfluency analysis.* Unpublished manuscript. Evanston, IL: Northwestern University.

Caplan, G. (1970). *The theory and practice of mental health consultation.* New York, NY: Basic Books.

Caprara, G., & Cervone, D. (2000). *Personality: Determinants, dynamics and potentials.* Cambridge, UK: University Press.

Carey, B., & Onslow, M. (2012). The promise of web-based stuttering treatment. *The ASHA Leader, 17,* 18.

Carey, B., O'Brian, S., Onslow, M., Block, S., Jones, M., & Packman, A. (2010). Randomised controlled non-inferiority trial of a telehealth treatment for chronic stuttering: The Camperdown Program. *International Journal of Language and Communication Disorders, 45,* 108–120.

Carey, B., O'Brian, S., Onslow, M., Packman, A., & Menzies, R. (2012). Webcam delivery of the Camperdown Program for adolescents who stutter: A phase I trial. *Language, Speech, and Hearing Services in Schools, 43,* 370–380.

Carson, C., & Kanter, C. E. (1945). Incidence of stuttering among white and colored school children. *Southern Speech Journal, 10,* 57–59.

Chang, S., Erickson, K., Ambrose, N., Hasegawa-Johnson, M., & Ludlow, C. (2008). Brain anatomy differences in childhood stuttering. *Neuroimage, 39,* 1333–1344.

Chapman, A., & Cooper, E. (1973). Nature of stuttering in a mentally retarded population. *American Journal of Mental Deficiency, 78*(2), 153–157.

Cherney, L., & van Vuuren, S. (2012). Telerehabilitation, virtual therapists, and acquired neurological speech and language disorders. *Seminars in Speech and Language, 33,* 243–257.

Cherry, C., & Sayers, B. (1956). Experiments upon the total inhibition of stammering by external control and some clinical results. *Journal of Psychosomatic Research, 1,* 233–246.

Cherry, C., Sayers, B., & Marland, P. (1955). Experiments on the complete suppression of stammering. *Nature, 176,* 874–875.

Chmela, K. (2006). *The fluency tool kit.* Greenville, SC: Super Duper Publications.

Chmela, K., & Reardon, N. (2001). *The school-age child who stutters: Working effectively with attitudes and emotions.* Memphis, TN: Stuttering Foundation of America.

Choi, D., Conture, E., Walden, T., Lambert, E., & Tumanova, V. (2013). Behavioral inhibition and childhood stuttering. *Journal of Fluency Disorders, 38,* 171–183.

Chon, H., Kraft, S. J., Ambrose, N., & Loucks, T. (2013). Individual variability in delayed auditory feedback (DAF) effects on speech fluency. *Journal of Speech, Language, and Hearing Research, 56,* 489–504.

Choo, A., Loucks, T. M., Chang, S., Ambrose, N., & Zengin, H. (2012). Corpus callosum morphology in children who stutter. *Journal of Communication Disorders, 45*(4), 279–289.

Choo, A., Kraft, S., Olivaro, W., Ambrose, N., Sharma, H., Olivero, W., Chang, S., & Loucks, T. (2011). Corpus callosum differences associated with persistent stuttering in adults. *Journal of Communication Disorders, 44*(4), 470–477.

Civier, O., Tasko, S., & Guenther, F. (2010). Overreliance on auditory feedback may lead to sound/syllable repetitions: Simulations of stuttering and fluency-inducing conditions with a neural model of speech production. *Journal of Fluency Disorders, 35,* 246–279.

Clark, R., & Snyder, M. (1955). Group therapy for parents of preadolescent stutterers. *Group Psychology, 8,* 226–232.

Coalson, G., Pena, E., & Byrd, C. (2013). Description of multilingual participants who stutter. *Journal of Fluency Disorders, 38,* 141–156.

Conelea, C., Rice, K., & Woods, D. (2006). Regulated breathing as a treatment of stuttering. *Journal of Speech and Language Pathology and Applied Behavioral Analysis, 1,* 94–102.

Connally, E., Ward, D., Howell, P., & Watkins, K. (2013). Disrupted white matter in language and motor tracts in developmental stuttering. *Brain & Language.* http://dx.doi.org/10.1016/j.bandl.2013.05.013

Conradi, E. (1904). Psychology and pathology of speech development in the child. *Pedagogical Seminary, 11,* 328–380.

Conture, E. (2000). Dreams of our theoretical nights meet the realities of our empirical days: Stuttering theory and research. In HG. Bosshardt, J. S. Yaruss, & H. F. M. Peters (Eds.), *Fluency disorders: Theory, research, treatment and self-help. Proceedings of the Third World Congress of Fluency Disorders in Nyborg, Denmark* (pp. 3–29). Nijmegen, Netherlands: Nijmegen University Press.

Conture, E. (2001). *Stuttering: Its nature, diagnosis, and treatment.* Boston, MA: Allyn & Bacon.

Conture, E., & Melnick, K. (1999). Parent-child group approach to stuttering in preschool and school-age children. In M. Onslow & A. Packman (Eds.), *Early stuttering: A handbook of intervention strategies* (pp. 17–51). San Diego, CA: Singular.

Conture, E., McCall, G., & Brewer, D. (1977). Laryngeal behavior during stuttering. *Journal of Speech and Hearing Research, 20,* 661–668.

Conture, E. Schwartz, H., & Brewer, D. (1985). Laryngeal behavior during stuttering: A further study. *Journal of Speech and Hearing Research, 28,* 233–240.

Conture, E., & Brayton, E. (1975). The influence of noise on stutterers' different disfluency types. *Journal of Speech and Hearing Research, 18,* 381–384.

Conture, E., & Curlee, R. (2007). *Stuttering and related disorders of fluency* (3rd ed.). New York, NY: Thieme.

Conture, E., & Kelly, E. M. (1991). Young stutterers' non-speech behaviors during stuttering. *Journal of Speech and Hearing Research, 34,* 1041–1056.

Conture, E., Louko, L., & Edwards, M. (1993). Simultaneously treating stuttering and disordered phonology in children: Experimental therapy, preliminary findings. *American Journal of Speech-Language Pathology, 2,* 72–81.

Cooper, E., & Cooper, C. S. (1998). Multicultural considerations in the assessment and treatment of stuttering. In D. Battle (Ed.), *Communication disorders in multicultural populations* (2nd ed., pp. 247–274). Boston, MA: Butterworth-Heinemann.

Cooper, E., & Cooper, C. (1985). *Cooper personalized fluency control therapy* (Rev. ed.). Allen, TX: DLM Teaching Resources.

Coppola, V., & Yairi, E. (1982). Rhythmic speech training with preschool stuttering children: An experimental study. *Journal of Fluency Disorders, 7,* 447–457.

Cordes, A., & Ingham, R. (1994). Time-interval measurement of stuttering: Effects of interval duration. *Journal of Speech and Hearing Research, 37,* 779–788.

Cordes, A., & Ingham, R. (1999). Effects of time-interval judgment training on real-time measurement of stuttering. *Journal of Speech, Language, and Hearing Research, 42,* 862–879.

Coriat, I. (1928). Stammering. A psychoanalytic interpretation. *Nervous Mental Disorder Monographs, Ser. No. 47,* 1–68.

Coriat, I. (1943a). Theory. In E. F. Hahn (Ed.), *Stuttering: Significant theories and therapies* (pp. 28–30). Stanford, CA: Stanford University Press.

Coriat, I. (1943b). The psychoanalytic conception of stammering. *Nervous Child, 2,* 167–171.

Corley, M., MacGregor, L., & Donaldson, D. (2007). It's the way that you, er, say it: Hesitations in speech affect language comprehension. *Cognition, 105,* 658–668.

Costello, J. (1977). Programmed instruction. *Journal of Speech and Hearing Disorders, 42,* 3–28.

Costello, J. (1980). Operant conditioning and the treatment of stuttering. In W. H. Perkins (Ed.), Strategies in Stuttering Therapy. In J. L. Northern (Series Ed.), *Seminars in Speech, Language and Hearing.* New York, NY: Thieme-Stratton.

Costello, J. (1983). Current behavioral treatments for children. In D. Prins & R. Ingham (Eds.), *Treatment of stuttering in early childhood* (pp. 69–112). San Diego, CA: College-Hill.

Costello, J., & Ingham, R. (1984). Assessment strategies for stuttering. In R. Curlee & W. Perkins (Eds.), *Nature and treatment of stuttering: New directions.* Boston, MA: College-Hill.

Cosyns, M., Mortier, G., Corthals, P. Janssens, S., & Van Borsel, J. (2010). Word-final prolongations in an adult male with neurofibromatosis type 1. *Journal of Fluency Disorders, 35,* 235–245.

Cox, N., Kramer, P., & Kidd, K. (1984). Segregation analyses of stuttering. *Genetic Epidemiology, 1,* 245–253.

Craig, A. (1990). An investigation into the relationship between anxiety and stuttering. *Journal of Speech and Hearing Disorders, 55,* 290–294.

Craig, A. (1998). Relapse following treatment of stuttering: A critical review and correlative data. *Journal of Fluency Disorders, 23,* 1–30.

Craig, A., & Tran, Y. (2005). The epidemiology of stuttering: The need for reliable estimates of prevalence and anxiety levels over the lifespan. *Advances in Speech Language Pathology, 7*(1), 41–46.

Craig, A., Franklin, J., & Andrews, G. (1984). A scale to measure locus of control of behaviour. *British Journal of Medical Psychology, 57,* 173–180.

Craig, A., Hancock K., Chang, E., McCready, C., Shepley, A., McCaul, A., et al. (1996). A controlled clinical trial for stuttering in persons aged 9 to 14 years. *Journal of Speech and Hearing Research, 39,* 808–826.

Craig, A., Hancock, K., Tran, Y., & Craig, M. (2003). Anxiety levels in people who stutter: A randomized population study. *Journal of Speech, Language, and Hearing Research, 46,* 1197–1206.

Craig, A., Hancock, K., Tran, Y., Craig, M., & Peters, K. (2002). Epidemiology of stuttering in the community across the entire life span. *Journal of Speech, Language, and Hearing Research, 45,* 1097–1105.

Cream, A., O'Brian, S., Jones, M., Block, S., Harrison, E., Lincoln, M., Hewat, S., & Onslow, M. (2010). Randomized controlled trial of video self-modeling following speech restructuring treatment for stuttering. Journal of Speech, Language, and Hearing Research, 53, 887–897.

Cross, H. (1936). The motor capacities of stutterers. *Archives of Speech, 7,* 112–132.

Curlee, R. (1980). A case selection strategy for young disfluent children. *Seminars in Speech, Language, and Hearing, 1*(4), 277–287.

Curlee, R. (1999). *Stuttering and related disorders of fluency* (2nd ed.). New York, NY: Thieme.

Curlee, R.(1993). Identification and management of beginning stuttering. In R. F. Curlee (Ed.), *Stuttering and related disorders of fluency* (pp. 1–22). New York, NY: Thieme.

Curlee, R., & Perkins, W. (1969). Conversational rate control therapy for stuttering. *Journal of Speech and hearing Disorders, 34,* 245–250.

Curlee, R., & Perkins, W. (1973). Effectiveness of a DAF conditioning program for adolescent and adult stutterers. *Behaviour Research and Therapy, 11*(4), 395–401.

Curlee, R., & Yairi, E. (1997). Early intervention with early childhood stuttering: A critical examination of the data. *American Journal of Speech-Language Pathology, 6,* 8–18.

Cypreansen, L. (1948). Group therapy for adult stutterers. *Journal of Speech and Hearing Disorders, 13,* 313–319.

Dalston, R., Martinkosky, S., & Hinton, V. (1987). Stuttering prevalence among patients at risk for velopharyngeal inadequacy: A preliminary investigation. *Cleft Palate Journal, 24,* 233–239.

Daly, D. (1996). *The source for stuttering and cluttering.* East Moline, IL: Linguisystems.

Daly, D., & Burnett, M. (1996). Cluttering: Assessment, treatment planning and case study illustration. *Journal of Fluency Disorders, 21,* 239–248.

Daly, D., & Burnett, M. (1999). Cluttering: Traditional views and new perspectives. In R. Curlee (Ed.), *Stuttering and related disorders of fluency* (2nd ed.). New York, NY: Thieme.

Daniels, E. (1940). An analysis of the relation between handedness and stuttering with special reference to the Orton-Travis theory of cerebral dominance. *Journal of Speech Disorders, 5,* 309–326.

Daniloff, R., & Moll, K. (1968). Coarticulation of lip rounding. *Journal of Speech and Hearing Research, 11,* 707–721.

Darley, F. (1955). The relationship of parental attitudes and adjustment to the development of stuttering. In W. Johnson & R. R. Leutenegger (Eds.), *Stuttering in children and adults: Thirty years of research at the University of Iowa* (pp. 74–156). Minneapolis: University of Minnesota.

Darley, F., & Spriestersbach, D. (1978). *Diagnostic methods in speech pathology* (2nd ed.). New York, NY: Harper & Row.

Daskalov, D. (1962). Kvoprosu ob osnovnikh printsipakh I metodakh preduprezhdenia lechenia zaikania (Commentary about the basic principles of stuttering prevention and treatment. *Journal of neuropathology and psychiatry). Zhurnal Nevropatologii Psikhiatrii, 62,* 1047–1052.

Davis, D. (1939). The relation of repetitions in the speech of young children to certain measures of language maturity and situational factors: Part I. *Journal of Speech Disorders, 4,* 303–318.

Davis, S., Howell, P., & Cook, F. (2002). Sociodynamic relationships between children who stutter and their non-stuttering classmates. *Journal of Child Psychology and Psychiatry, 43,* 939–947.

Dembowski, J., & Watson, B. (1991). Preparation time and response complexity effects and stutterers' and nonstutterers' acoustic LRT. *Journal of Speech and Hearing Research, 34,* 49–59.

De Nil, L., & Brutten, G. (1991). Speech-associated attitudes of stuttering and normally fluent children. *Journal of Speech and Hearing Research, 34,* 60–66.

De Nil, L., Jokel, R., & Rochon, E. (2007). Etiology, symptomatology, and treatment of neurogenic stuttering. In E. Conture & R. Curlee (Eds.), *Stuttering and related disorders of fluency* (3rd ed., pp. 326–343). New York, NY: Thieme.

De Nil, L., Kroll, R., & Houle, S. (2001). Functional neuroimaging of cerebellar activation during single word reading and verb generation in stuttering and nonstuttering adults. *Neuroscience Letters, 302*(2–3), 77–80.

De Nil, L., Kroll, R., Kapur, S., & Houle, S. (2000). A positron emission tomography study of silent oral single word reading in stuttering and nonstuttering adults. *Journal of Speech, Language, Hearing Research, 43,* 1038–1053.

De Nil, L., Kroll, R., Lafaille, S., & Houle, S. (2003). A positron emission tomography study of short- and long-term treatment effects on functional brain activation in adults who stutter. *Journal of Fluency Disorders, 28,* 357–380.

De Oliveira Martins, V., & Furquim de Andrade, C. (2008). Speech fluency developmental profile in Brazilian Portuguese speakers. *Pró-Fono Revista de Atualização Científica, 20,* 7–13.

Denny, M. & Smith, A. (1992). Gradation in a neuromuscular pattern associated with stuttering. Journal of Speech and Hearing Research, 35, 1216–1229

Denny, M., & Smith, A. (2000). Respiratory control in stuttering speakers: Evidence from respiratory high-frequency oscillations. *Journal of Speech, Language, and Hearing Research, 43,* 1024–1037.

Derazne, J. (1966). Speech pathology in the U.S.S.R. In R.W. Rieber & R. S. Brubaker, (Eds.), *Speech Pathology.* Amsterdam, Netherlands: North Holland.

Dewar, A., Dewar, A., Austin, W., & Brash, H. (1979). The long term use of an automatically triggered auditory feedback masking device in the treatment of stammering. *British Journal of Disorders of Communication, 14,* 219–229.

Di Carlo, L., Katz, J., & Batkin, S. (1959). An exploratory investigation of the effect of meprobamate on stuttering behavior. *Journal of Nervous and Mental Disorders, 128,* 558–561.

Dickson, S. (1971). Incipient stuttering and spontaneous remission of stuttered speech. *Journal of Communication Disorders, 4*(2), 99–110.

DiLollo, A., & Manning, W. (2007). Counseling children who stutter and their parents. In E. Conture & R. Curlee (Eds.), *Stuttering and related disorders* (3rd ed., pp. 115–130). New York, NY: Thieme.

Donaher, J., & Richels, C. (2012). Traits of attention deficit/hyperactivity disorder in school-age children who stutter. *Journal of Fluency Disorders, 37,* 242–252.

Donovan, G. (1971). A new device for the treatment of stuttering. *British Journal of Disorders of Communication, 6,* 86–88.

Dowden, P., Stone-Goldman, J., & Olswang, L. (2006). *Course glossary, SPHSC 500 fall quarter 2006.* Retrieved from University of Washington, http://faculty.washington.edu/lolswang/html/500/glossary2006.pdf

Duchin, S., & Mysak, E. (1987). Disfluency and rate characteristics of young adult, middle-aged, and older males. *Journal of Communication Disorders, 20,* 245–257.

Duffy, J. (1995). *Motor speech disorders.* St. Louis, MO: Mosby.

Dunlap, K. (1932). *Habits: Their making and unmaking.* New York, NY: Liveright.

Dworzynski, K., Remington, A., Rijsdijk, F., Howell, P., & Plomin, R. (2007). Genetic etiology in cases of recovered and persistent stuttering in an unselected longitudinal sample of young twins. *American Journal of Speech and Language Pathology, 16,* 169–178.

Eggers K., De Nil L., & Van den Bergh B. (2010). The efficiency of attentional networks in children who stutter. *Journal of Speech, Language, and Hearing Research, 55,* 946–959.

Eggers, K., De Nil, L., & Van den Bergh, B. (2013). Inhibitory control in childhood stuttering. *Journal of Fluency Disorders, 38,* 1–13.

Egolf, D., Shames, G., Johnson, P., & Kasprisin-Burelli, A. (1972). The use of parent-child interaction patterns in therapy for young stutterers. *Journal of Speech and Hearing Disorders, 37,* 222–232.

Einarsdottir, J., & Ingham, R. (2009). Does language influence the accuracy of judgments of stuttering in children? *Journal of Speech, Language, and Hearing Research, 52,* 766–779.

Eisenson, J. (1958). A perseverative theory of stuttering. In J. Eisenson (Ed.), *Stuttering: A symposium* (pp. 223–271). New York, NY: Harper & Row.

Ellis, A. (1973). *Humanistic psychotherapy: The rational-emotive approach.* New York, NY: McGraw-Hill.

Embrechts, M., Ebben, H., Franke, P., & vandePoel, C. (2000). Temperament: A comparison between children who stutter and children who do not stutter. In H. Bosshardt, J. S. Yaruss, & H. F. M. Peters, (Eds.), *Proceedings of the Third World Congress on Fluency Disorders: Theory, research, treatment and self-help* (pp. 557–562). Nijmegen, Netherlands: University of Nijmegen Press.

Emerick, L. (1970). *Therapy for young stutterers.* Danville, IL: Interstate.

Emil-Behnke, K. (1947). *Stammering: Its nature, causes, and treatment.* London, England: Williams & Norgate.

Erickson, R. (1969). Assessing communication attitudes among stutterers. *Journal of Speech and Hearing Research, 12,* 711–724.

Euler, A, Gudenberg, A., Jung, K., & Neumann, K. (2009). Computergestützte Therapie bei Redeflussstörungen: Die langfristige Wirksamkeit der Kasseler Stottertherapie (Computer assisted therapy for speech flow disturbances: the long term efficacy of the Kassel Stutter Therapy). *Sprache Stimme Gehör, 33,* 193–197.

Ezrati-Vinacour, R., & Levin, I. (2004). The relationship between anxiety and stuttering: A multidimensional approach. *Journal of Fluency Disorders, 29,* 135–148.

Ezrati-Vinacour, R., Platzky, R., & Yairi, E. (2001). The young child's awareness of stuttering-like disfluency. *Journal of Speech, Language, and Hearing Research, 44,* 368–380.

Ezrati-Vinacour, R. & Weinstein, N. (2011). HYPERLINK "http://www.sciencedirect.com/science/article/pii/S0094730X1100009X" A dialogue among various cultures and its manifestation in stuttering therapy. *Journal of fluency disorders, 36* 36:174–85.

Fagan, J. (1984). The relationship of novelty preferences during infancy to later intelligence and later recognition memory. *Intelligence, 8,* 339–346.

Fagan, L. (1931). The relation of dextral training to the onset of stuttering. *Quarterly Journal of Speech, 17,* 73–76.

Fairbanks, G. (1937). Some correlates of sound difficulty in stuttering. *Quarterly Journal of Speech, 23,* 67–69.

Fairbanks, G. (1960). *Voice and articulation drillbook* (2nd ed.). New York, NY: Harper & Row.

Fein, L. (1970). Stuttering as a cue related to the precipitation of moments of stuttering [Abstract]. *ASHA, 12,* 456.

Feinberg, A., Griffen, B., & Levey, M. (2000). Psychological aspects of chronic tonic and clonic stuttering: Suggested therapeutic approaches. *American Journal of Orthopsychiatry, 70*(4), 465–473.

Felsenfeld, S., Kirk, M., Zhu, G., Statham, D., Neale, M., & Martin, N. (2000). A study of the genetic and environmental etiology of stuttering in a selected twin sample. *Behavioral Genetics, 30,* 359–366.

Fenichel, O. (1945). *The psychoanalytic theory of neurosis.* New York, NY: Norton.

Fibiger, S. (1971). Stuttering explained as a physiological tremor. *Speech Transmission Lab Quarterly Progress and Status Report, 2–3,* 1–24.

Finn, P. (2003a). Addressing generalization and maintenance of stuttering treatment in the schools: A critical look. *Journal of Communication Disorders, 36,* 153–164.

Finn, P. (2003b). Evidence-based treatment of stuttering: II. Clinical significance of behavioral stuttering treatments. *Journal of Fluency Disorders, 28,* 209–218.

Finn, P. (2003c). Self-regulation and the management of stuttering. *Seminars in Speech and Language, 24,* 27–32.

Finn, P., & Cordes, A. K. (1997). Multicultural identification and treatment of stuttering: A continuing need for research. *Journal of Fluency Disorders, 22,* 219–236.

Finn, P., Ingham, R., Ambrose, N., & Yairi, E. (1997). Children recovered from stuttering without formal treatment: Perceptual assessment of speech normalcy. *Journal of Speech, Language, and Hearing Research, 40,* 867–876.

Fisher, M. (1970). Stuttering: a psychoanalytic view. *Journal of Contemporary Psychotherapy, 2,* 124–127.

Fitzgerald, H., Djurdjic, S., & Maguin, E. (1992). Assessment of sensitivity to interpersonal stress in stutterers. *Journal of Communication Disorders, 25,* 31–42.

Fivush, R., Gray, J., & Fromhoff, F. (1987). Two-year-olds talk about the past. *Cognitive Development, 2,* 393–409.

Flanagan, B., Goldiamond, I., & Azrin, N. (1958). Operant stuttering: The control of stuttering behavior through response-contingent consequences. *Journal of the Experimental Analysis of Behavior, 1,* 173–177.

Fletcher, J. (1914). An experimental study of stuttering. *American Journal of Psychology, 25,* 201–255.

Fletcher, J. (1928). *The problem of stuttering.* New York, NY: Longmans, Green.

Forster, D. & Webster W. (2001). Speech motor control and interhemispheric relations in recovered and persistent stuttering. *Developmental Neuropsychology, 19,* 125–145.

Fosnot, S. (1995). Some contemporary approaches in treating fluency disorders in preschool-age, and adolescent children. *Language, Speech, and Hearing Services in Schools, 26,* 115–116.

Fossler, H. (1930). Disturbances in breathing during stuttering. *Psychological Monographs, 40,* 1–32.

Foundas, A., Bollich A., Corey, D., Hurley, M., & Heilman, K. (2001). Anomalous anatomy of speech-language areas in adults with persistent developmental stuttering. *Neurology, 57,* 207–215.

Foundas, A., Bollich, A., Feldman, J., Corey, D., Hurley, M., Lemen, L., & Heilman, K. (2004). Aberrant auditory processing and atypical planum temporale in developmental stuttering. *Neurology, 63,* 1640–1646.

Fox, P., Ingham, R., Ingham, J., Hirsch, T., unter Downs, J., Martin, C., Jerabek, P., Glass, P., & Lancaster, J. (1996). A PET study of the neural systems of stuttering. *Nature, 382,* 158–162.

Fox, P., Ingham, R., Ingham, J., Zamarripa, F., Xiong, J., & Lancaster, J. (2000). Brain correlates of stuttering and syllable production: A PET performance-correlation analysis. *Brain, 123,* 1985–2004.

Fraiser, J. (1955). An exploration of stutterers' theories of their own stuttering. In W. Johnson & R. Leutenegger (Eds.), *Stuttering in children and adults* (pp. 317–324). Minneapolis: University of Minnesota Press.

Franic, D., & Bothe, A. (2008). Psychometric evaluation of condition-specific instruments used to assess health-related quality of life, attitudes and related constructs in stuttering. *American Journal of Speech-Language Pathology, 17,* 60–80.

Frankel, V. (1963). *Man's search for meaning.* Boston, MA: Beacon Press.

Franken, M., Boves, L., Peters, H. F. M., Webster, R. (1992). Perceptual evaluation of the speech before and after fluency shaping stuttering therapy. Journal of Fluency Disorders, 17, 223–241.

Franken, M., Kielstra-Van der Schalk, C., & Boelens, H. (2005). Experimental treatment of early stuttering: A preliminary study. *Journal of Fluency Disorders, 30,* 189–199.

Freeman, F., & Ushijima, T. (1978). Laryngeal muscle activity during stuttering. *Journal of Speech and Hearing Research, 21,* 538–562.

Freud, A. (1946). *The psycho-analytic treatment of children.* London, England: Imago.

Freud, S. (1899). *Die Traumdeutung* [*The interpretation of dreams*]. Franz Deuticke: Leipzig & Vienna

Freud, S. (1901). *Psychopathology of everyday life* (translated by A. A. Brill), London, England: T. Fisher Unwin.

Freund, H. (1955). Psychosis and stuttering. *Journal of Nervous and Mental Diseases, 122,* 161–172.

Fried, C. (1972). Behavior therapy and psychoanalysis in the treatment of a severe chronic stutterer. *Journal of Speech and Hearing Disorders, 37,* 347–372.

Fritzell, B. (1976). The prognosis of stuttering in school-children: A 10-year longitudinal study. In *Proceedings of the XVI Congress of the International society of Logopedics and Phoniatrics* (pp. 186–187). Basel, Switzerland: Karger.

Froebel, F. (1903). The education of man. In G. L. Landreth (Ed.), *Play therapy: The art of the relationship.* Muncie, IN: Accelerated Development.

Froeschels, E. (1921). Beitrage zur symptomatologie des stotterns. *Monatsschrift fur Ohren-heilkunde, 55,* 1109–1112.

Froeschels, E. (1943). Pathology and therapy of stuttering. *Nervous Child, 2,* 148–161.

Froeschels, E., & Rieber, R. (1963). The problem of auditory and visual imperceptivity in stutterers. *Folia Phoniatrica, 15,* 13–20.

Furquim de Andrade, C., & De Oliveira Martins, V. (2007). Fluency variation in adolescents. *Clinical Linguistics & Phonetics, 21,* 771–782.

Gendelman, E. (1977). Confrontation in the treatment of stuttering. *Journal of Speech and Hearing Disorders, 42,* 85–89.

Gens, G. (1951). The speech pathologist looks at the mentally deficient child. *Training School Bulletin, 48,* 19–27.

Gillespie, S., & Cooper, E. (1973). Prevalence of speech problems in junior and senior high schools. *Journal of Speech and Hearing Research, 16,* 739–743.

Gilman, M., & Yaruss, J. S. (2000). Stuttering and relaxation: Applications for somatic education in stuttering treatment. *Journal of Fluency Disorders, 25,* 59–76.

Giraud, A., Neumann, K., Bachoud-Levi, A. C., von Gudenberg, A. W., Euler, H. A., Lanfermann, H., & Preibisch, C. (2008). Severity of dysfluency correlates with basal ganglia activity in persistent developmental stuttering. *Brain and Language, 104,* 190–199.

Glasner, P. (1949). Personality characteristics and emotional problems in stutterers under the age of five. *Journal of Speech and Hearing Disorders, 14,* 135–138.

Glasner, P., & Rosenthal, D. (1957). Parental diagnosis of stuttering in young children. *Journal of Speech and Hearing Disorders, 22,* 288–295.

Glauber, P. (1958). Stuttering and personality dynamics. In J. Eisenson (Ed.), *Stuttering: A symposium* (pp. 71–120). New York, NY: Harper & Row.

Glogowski, K. (1976). Is stuttering inherited? *Folia Phoniatrica, 28,* 235–236.

Godai, U., Tatarelli, R., & Bonanni, G. (1976). Stuttering and tics in twins. *Acta Geneticae Medicae et Gemellologiae, 25,* 369–375.

Goldiamond, I. (1965). Stuttering and fluency as manipulatable operant response classes. In L. Krasner and L. Ullman (Eds.), *Research in behavior modification.* New York, NY: Holt, Rinehart and Winston.

Goldman, R., & Fristoe, M. (1986). *Goldman-Fristoe Test of Articulation* (GFTA). Circle Pines, MN: American Guidance Service.

Goldman-Eisler, F. (1961). The significance of changes in the rate of articulation. *Language and Speech, 4,* 171–174.

Good, C., Johnsrude, I., Ashburner, J., Henson, R., Friston, K., & Frackowiak, R. White 2001). Cerebral asymmetry and the effects of sex and handedness on brain structure: A voxel-based morphometric analysis of 465 normal adult human brains. *Neuroimage, 14,* 685–700.

Good, R., & Kaminski, R. A. (Eds.). (2002). *Dynamic indicators of basic early literacy skills, DIBELS* (6th ed.). Eugene, OR: Institute for the Development of Educational Achievement.

Goodstein, L. (1958). Functional speech disorders and personality: A survey of the research. *Journal of Speech and Hearing Research, 1*(4), 359–376.

Gottsleben, R. (1955). The incident of stuttering in a group of mongoloid. *Training School Bulletin, 51,* 209–218.

Gottwald, S., & Starkweather, C. (1999). Stuttering prevention and early intervention: A multiprocess approach. In M. Onslow & A. Packman (Eds.), *The handbook of early stuttering intervention.* San Diego, CA: Singular.

Gray, B. (1965). Theoretical approximations of stuttering adaptation. *Behavior Research and Therapy, 3,* 171–185.

Gray, B., & England, G. (1972). Some effects of anxiety deconditioning upon stuttering frequency. *Journal of Speech and Hearing Research, 15,* 114–122.

Gregg, B., & Yairi E. (2012). Disfluency patterns and phonological skills near stuttering onset. *Journal of Communication Disorders, 45,* 426–438.

Gregg, B., & Yairi, E. (2006). Phonological skills and disfluency levels in preschool children who stutter. *Journal of Communication Disorders, 40,* 97–115.

Gregg, B., & Yairi, E. (2007). Phonological skills and disfluency levels in preschool children who stutter. *Journal of Communication Disorders, 40,* 97–115.

Gregory, H. (1999). Developmental intervention: Differential strategies. In M. Onslow & A. Packman (Eds.), *The handbook of early stuttering intervention* (pp. 83–102). San Diego, CA: Singular.

Gregory, H. (2003). *Stuttering therapy: Rationale and procedures.* Boston, MA: Allyn & Bacon.

Gregory, H., & Hill, D. (1984). Stuttering therapy for children. In W. H. Perkins (Ed.), *Stuttering disorders* (pp. 351–364). New York, NY: Thieme-Stratton.

Gregory, H., & Hill, D. (1999). Differential evaluation—differential therapy for stuttering children. In R. Curlee (Ed.), *Stuttering and related disorders of fluency* (2nd ed.). New York, NY: Thieme.

Greiner, J., Fitzgerald, H., Cooke, P., & Djurdjic, S. (1985). Assessment of sensitivity to interpersonal stress in stutterers and nonstutterers. *Journal of Communication Disorders, 18,* 215–225.

Guenther, F. (1995). Speech sound acquisition, coarticulation, and rate effects in a neural network model of speech production. *Psychological Review, 102,* 594–621.

Guenther, F. (2006). Cortical interactions underlying the production of speech sounds. *Journal of Communication Disorders, 39,* 350–365.

Guitar, B. (1975). Reduction of stuttering frequency using analog electromyographic feedback. *Journal of Speech and Hearing Research, 18,* 672–685.

Guitar, B. (1998). *Stuttering: An integrated approach to its nature and treatment* (2nd ed.). Baltimore, MD: Williams & Wilkins.

Guitar, B. (2006). *Stuttering: An integrated approach to its nature and treatment* (3rd ed.). Baltimore, MD: Lippincott Williams & Wilkins.

Guitar, B. (2014). *Stuttering: An integrated approach to its nature and treatment* (4th ed.). Baltimore, MD: Lippincott Williams & Wilkins.

Guitar, B., & Marchinkoski, L. (2001). Influence of mothers' slower speech on their children's speech rate. *Journal of Speech, Language, and Hearing Research, 44,* 853–861.

Guitar, B., & Reville, J. (1997). *Easy talker.* Austin, TX: Pro-Ed.

Guitar, B., Guitar, C., Neilson, P., O'Dwyer, N., & Andrews, G. (1988). Onset sequencing of selected lip muscles in stutterers and nonstutterers. *Journal of Speech and Hearing Research, 31,* 28–35.

Guitar, B., Schaefer, H., Donahue-Kilburg, G., & Bond, L. (1992). Parent verbal interactions and speech rate: A case study in stuttering. *Journal of Speech and Hearing Research, 35,* 742–754.

Gutzmann, H. (1912). *Sprachheilkunde. Das stottern und seine grundliche beseitigung (*Speech Health Science. Stuttering and it's fundamental elimination). Berlin, Germany: Weber.

Guzinski, E., Cihon, T., & Eshleman, J. (2012). The effects of tact training on stereotypic vocalizations in children with autism. *The Analysis of Verbal Behavior, 28,* 101–110.

Häge, A. (2001). Können kognitive und linguistische Fähigkeiten zur Verlaufsprognose kindlichen Stotterns beitragen? [Cognitive and linguistic abilities in young children: Are they able to predict the further development of stuttering?]. *Sprache Stimme Gehör, 25,* 20–24.

Hahn, E. (1956). *Stuttering: Significant theories and therapies* (2nd ed.). Stanford, CA: Stanford University Press.

Hall, F., Mielke, P., Willeford, J., & Timmons, R. (1976). *National speech & hearing survey.* [Final report, project No. 50978, grant No. OE-32-15-0050-5010 (607)]

Hall, K., & Yairi, E. (1992). Fundamental frequency, jitter, and shimmer in preschoolers who stutter. *Journal of Speech and Hearing Research, 35,* 1002–1008.

Hall, K., Amir, O., & Yairi, E. (1999). A longitudinal investigation of speaking rate in preschool children who stutter. *Journal of Speech, Language, and Hearing Research, 42,* 1367–1377.

Hall, N. (2011). Emergence of stuttering in children with language impairment during the course of language therapy. *Perspectives on School-Based Issues, 12,* 18–25.

Hall, N., Wagovitch, S., & Bernstein Ratner, N. (2007). Language considerations in childhood stuttering. In E. Conture & R. Curlee (Eds.), *Stuttering and related disorders* (3rd ed., pp. 153–167). New York, NY: Thieme.

Hall, P. (1977). The occurrence of disfluencies in language-disordered school-age children. *Journal of Speech and Hearing Disorders, 42,* 364–370.

Ham, R. (1990). *Therapy of stuttering: Preschool through adolescence.* Englewood Cliffs, NJ: Prentice-Hall.

Hamano, T., Hirajcj, S., Kawamura, Y., Hirayama, M., Mutoh, T., & Kuriyama, M. (2005). Acquired stuttering secondary to callosal infarction. *Neurology, 64,* 1092–1093.

Hancock, K., Craig, A., McCready, C., McCaul, A., Costello, D., Campbell, K., et al. (1998). Two- to six-year controlled-trial stuttering outcomes for children and adolescents. *Journal of Speech, Language, and Hearing Research, 41,* 1242–1252.

Hanson, B., Gronhovd, K., & Rice, P. (1981). A shortened version of the Southern Illinois University Speech Situation Checklist for the identification of speech-related anxiety. *Journal of Fluency Disorders, 6,* 351–360.

Harasty, J., & Reed, V. (1994). The prevalence of speech and language impairment in two Sydney metropolitan schools. *Australian Journal of Human Communication Disorders, 22*(1), 1–23.

Harle, M. (1946). Dynamic interpretation and treatment of acute stuttering in a young child. *American Journal of Orthopsychiatry, 16,* 156–162.

Harms, M., & Malone, J. (1939). The relationship of hearing acuity to stammering. *Journal of Speech and Hearing Disorder, 4,* 363–370.

Haroldson, S., Martin, R., & Starr, C. (1968). Time-out as a punishment for stuttering. *Journal of Speech and Hearing Research, 11,* 560–566.

Harrington, J. (1988). Stuttering, delayed auditory feedback and linguistic rhythm. *Journal of Speech and Hearing Research, 31,* 36–47.

Harrison, E., Onslow, M., & Rousseau, I. (2007). Lidcombe Program 2007: Clinical tales and clinical trials. In E. Conture & R. Curlee (Eds.), *Stuttering and related disorders* (3rd ed.). New York, NY: Thieme.

Hartwell, E. (1895). Application of the laws of physical training for the prevention and cure of stuttering. *Proceedings of the International Congress of Education* (2nd ed.). New York, NY: J. J. Little.

Hauner, K., Shriberg, L., Kwiatkowski, J., & Allen, C. (2005). A subtype of speech delay associated with developmental psychosocial involvement. *Journal of Speech, Language, and Hearing Research, 48,* 635–650.

Healey, C., & Gutkin, B. (1984). Analysis of stutterers' voice onset times and fundamental frequency contours during fluency. *Journal of Speech and Hearing Research, 27,* 219–255.

Healey, E. C., & Bernstein B. (1991). Acoustic analysis of young stutterers' and nonstutterers' disfluencies. In H. Peters, W. Hulstijn, & C.W. Starkweather (Eds.). *Speech motor control and stuttering* (pp. 401–407). New York, NY: Elsevier Science.

Healey, E. C., Scott Trautman, L., & Susca, M. (2004). Clinical application of a multidimensional approach to the assessment and treatment of stuttering. *Contemporary Issues in Communication Science and Disorders, 31,* 40–48.

Hearne, A., Packman, A., Onslow, M., & Quine, S. (2008). Stuttering and its treatment in adolescence: The perceptions of people who stutter. *Journal of Fluency Disorders, 33,* 81–98.

Heitmann R., Asbjørnsen A., & Helland T. (2004). Attentional functions in speech fluency disorders. *Logopedics Phoniatrics Vocology, 29,* 119–127.

Helm-Estabrooks, N. (1999). Stuttering associated with acquired neurological disorders. In R. Curlee (Ed.), *Stuttering and related disorders of fluency* (2nd ed.). New York, NY: Thieme.

Helm-Estabrooks, N., & Hotz, G. (1998). Sudden onset of "stuttering" in an adult: Neurogenic or psychogenic? *Seminars in Speech and Language, 19,* 23–29.

Herder, C., Howard, C., Nye, C., et al. (2006). Effectiveness of behavioral stuttering treatment: A systematic review and meta-analysis. *Contemporary Issues in Communication Science and Disorders, 33,* 61–73.

Hewat, S., Onslow, M., Packman, A., & O'Brian, S. (2006). A Phase II clinical trial of self-imposed time-out treatment for stuttering in adults and adolescents. *Disability and Rehabilitation, 28*(1), 33–42.

Hinkle, W. (1971). *A study of subgroups within the stuttering population* (Unpublished doctoral dissertation). Purdue University.

Hogewind, F. (1940). Medical treatment of stuttering. *Journal of Speech Disorders, 5,* 203–208.

Holzman, A. (Co-Producer & Director), & Amick, R. (Co-Producer). (1988). *No words to say* [VHS video]. Available from Amick/Holzman Company, 10061 Riverside Drive, Toluca Lake, CA 91602–2560.

Honig, P. (1947). The stutterer acts it out. *Journal of Speech Disorders, 12,* 105–109.

Howell, P. (2002). The EXPLAN theory of fluency control applied to the treatment of stuttering by altered feedback and operant procedures. In E. Fava (Ed.), *Current Issues in Linguistic Theory series: Pathology and Therapy of Speech Disorders* (pp. 95–118). Amsterdam, Netherlands: John Benjamins.

Howell, P. (2009). Predicting stuttering onset/[E-letter]. Pediatrics,. http://www.pediatrics.aappublications.org/ cgi/eletters/123/1/270 (17.01.09)

Howell, P., & Au-Yeung, J. (1995). The association between stuttering, brown factors, and phonological categories in child stuttering ranging in aged between 2 and 12 years. *Journal of Fluency Disorders, 20,* 331–344.

Howell, P., & Davis, S. (2011). Predicting persistence of and recovery from stuttering by the teenage years based on information gathered at age 8 years. *Journal of Developmental Behavior Pediatrics, 32,* 196–205

Howell, P., & van Borsel, J. (2011). *Multilingual Aspects of Fluency Disorders.* Bristol, England: Multilingual Matters.

Howell, P., Davis, S., & Williams, R. (2008). Late childhood stuttering. *Journal of Speech, Language, and Hearing Research, 51,* 669–684.

Howell, P., Davis, S., & Williams, R. (2009). The effects of bilingualism on stuttering during late childhood. *Archives of Disease in Childhood, 94,* 42–46.

Howell, P., Davis, S., & Williams, S. (2006). Auditory abilities of stuttered speech. *Journal of Speech, Language, and Hearing Research, 52,* 1092–4388.

Howell, P., Davis, S., Patel, H., Cuniffe, P., Downing-Wilson, D., Au-Yeung, J., & Williams, R. (2004). Fluency development and temperament in fluent children and children who stutter. In A. Packman, A. Meltzer, H. F. M. Peters (Eds.), *Theory, research and therapy in fluency disorders. Proceedings of the Fourth World Congress on Fluency Disorders,* IFA Montreal, 250–256.

Howell, P., Sackin, S., & Williams, R. (1999). Differential effects of frequency shifted feedback between child and adult stutterers. *Journal of Fluency Disorders, 24,* 127–136.

Howie, P. (1981). Concordance for stuttering in monozygotic and dizygotic twin pairs. *Journal of Speech and Hearing Research, 24,* 317–321.

Howie, P., & Andrews, G. (1984). Treatment of adult stutterers: Managing fluency. In R. Curlee & W. Perkins (Eds.), *Nature and treatment of stuttering: New directions* (pp. 245–445). San Diego, CA: College-Hill Press.

Howie, P., & Woods, C. (1982). Token reinforcement during the instatement and shaping of fluency in the treatment of stuttering. *Journal of Applied Behavior Analysis, 15,* 55–64.

Hubbard, C., & Prins, D. (1994). Word familiarity, syllabic stress pattern, and stuttering. *Journal of Speech and Hearing Research, 37,* 564–571.

Hubbard, C., & Yairi, E. (1988). Clustering of disfluencies in the speech of stuttering and nonstuttering preschool children. *Journal of Speech and Hearing Research, 31,* 228–233.

Hubbard, C. (1998). Stuttering, stressed syllables, and word onsets. *Journal of Speech, Language, and Hearing Research, 41,* 802–808.

Hull, C. (1943). *Principles of behavior.* New York, NY: Appleton-Century.

Humphrey, B. (2004). Judgments of disfluency in a familiar vs. an unfamiliar language. In A. Packman, A. Meltzer, & H. F. M. Peters (Eds.), *Theory, research and therapy. Proceedings of the Fourth World Congress on Fluency Disorders* (pp. 423–427). Nijmegen, Netherlands: Nijmegen University Press.

IDEA (1997). Individuals with Disabilities Education Act (IDEA 1997). Retrieved from http://www.ed.gov/offices/OSERS/Policy/IDEA/index.html

IDEA (2004). Individuals with Disabilities Education Act (IDEA 2004). Retrieved from http://www2.ed.gov/policy/speced/guid/idea/idea2004.html

Indevus. (2006). http://www.indevus.com/site/index.php?Intemid= 45& id=31&option=comcontent&task=view

Ingham , J. (1976). Onset, prevalence, and recovery from stuttering: A reassessment of findings from the Andrews and Harris study. *Journal of Speech and Hearing Disorders, 41,* 280–281.

Ingham, J. (1999). Behavioral treatment for young children who stutter: An extended length of utterance method. In R. F. Curlee (Ed.), *Stuttering and related disorders of fluency* (2nd ed., pp. 80–109). New York, NY: Thieme.

Ingham, J., & Riley, G. (1998). Guidelines for documentation of treatment efficacy for young children who stutter. *Journal of Speech, Language, and Hearing Research, 41,* 753–770.

Ingham, R. (1990). Commentary on Perkins (1990) and Moore and Perkins (1990): On the valid role of reliability in identifying "What is stuttering?" *Journal of Speech and Hearing Disorders, 55,* 394–397.

Ingham, R. (1999). Performance contingent management of stuttering in adolescents and adults. In R. Curlee (Ed.), *Stuttering and related disorders of fluency* (2nd ed., pp. 200–221). New York, NY: Thieme.

Ingham, R. (2010). Comments on article by Maguire et al: Pagoclone trial: Questionable findings for stuttering treatment. *Journal of Clinical Psychopharmacology, 30,* 649–650.

Ingham, R., & Cordes, A. (1998). Treatment decisions for young children who stutter: Further concerns and complexities. *American Journal of Speech-Language Pathology, 7*(3), 10–19.

Ingham, R., & Cordes, A. (1999). On watching a discipline shoot itself in the foot: Some observations on current trends in stuttering treatment research. In N. Bernstein Ratner & E. C. Healey (Eds.), *Stuttering research and treatment: Bridging the gap* (pp. 211–230). Mahwah, NJ: Erlbaum.

Ingham, R., Andrews, G., & Winkler, R. (1972). Stuttering: A comparative evaluation of the short-term effectiveness of four treatment techniques. *Journal of Communication Disorders, 5*(1), 91–117.

Ingham, R., Fox, P., Ingham, J., & Zamarripa, F. (2000). Is overt speech a prerequisite for the neural activations associated with chronic developmental stuttering? *Brain and Language, 75,* 163–194.

Ingham, R., Fox, P., Ingham, J., Xiong, J., Zamarripa, F., Hardies, L., & Lancaster, J. (2004). Brain correlates of stuttering and syllable production: Gender comparison and replication. *Journal of Speech, Language, and Hearing Research, 47*(2), 321–341.

Ingham, R., Ingham, J., Onslow, M., & Finn, P. (1989). Stutterers' self-ratings of speech naturalness: Assessing effects and reliability. *Journal of Speech, Language, and Hearing Research, 32,* 419–431.

Ingham, R., Kilgo, M., Ingham, J., Moglia R., Belknap. H., & Sanchez, T. (2001). Evaluation of a stuttering treatment based on reduction of short phonation intervals. *Journal of Speech, Language, and Hearing Research, 44,* 1229–1244.

Ingham, R., Warner, A., Byrd, A., & Cotton, J. (2006). Speech effort measurement and stuttering: Investigating the chorus reading effect. *Journal of Speech, Language, and Hearing Research, 49,* 660–670.

Iowa Department of Education. (2008). *Iowa core curriculum.*

Jacobson, E. (1938). *Progressive relaxation.* Chicago, IL: University of Chicago Press.

Jagger, J., Prusoff, B., Cohen, D., Kidd, K., Carbonari, C., & John, K. (1982). The epidemiology of Tourette's syndrome: A pilot study. *Schizophrenia Bulletin, 8,* 257–278.

James, J. (1981). Behavioral self-control of stuttering using time-out from speaking. *Journal of Applied Behavior Analysis, 14*(1), 25–37.

James, J., Ricciardelli, L., Hunter, C., & Rogers, P. (1989). Relative efficacy of intensive and spaced behavioral treatment of stuttering. *Behavior Modification, 13*(3), 376–395.

Jäncke L., Bauer A., Kaiser P., & Kalveram K. (1997). Timing and stiffness in the speech motor control of stuttering and nonstuttering adults. *Journal of Fluency Disorders, 22,* 309–321.

Jäncke, L. (1994). Variability and duration of voice onset time in stuttering and nonstuttering adults. *Journal of Fluency Disorders, 19,* 21–37.

Jäncke, L., Hanggi, J., Steinmetz, H. (2004). Morphological brain differences between adult stutterers and nonstutterers. *BMC Neurology, 4,* 23.

Jayaram, M. (1984). Distribution of stuttering in sentences: Relationship to sentence length and clause position. *Journal of Speech and Hearing Research, 27,* 338–341.

Jewell, E., & Abate, F. (Eds.). (2001). *The new Oxford American dictionary.* New York, NY: Oxford University Press.

Jiang J., Lu C., Peng D., Zhu C., & Howell P. (2012). Classification of types of stuttering symptoms based on brain activity. PLOS ONE, 7(6), - . doi:10.1371/journal.pone.0039747

Johannsen, H. (2001). Der Einfluss von Alter, Geschlecht, symptomatologie, heredität und händigkeit auf den verlauf des stotterns im kindesalter (The influence of age, gender, symptomatology, heredity and hand dominance preference on the course of stuttering during childhood). *Sprache Stimme Gehor, 25,* 14–19.

Johnson, W. (1934). *Stuttering in the preschool child* (Child Welfare Pamphlets No. 37). Iowa City: University of Iowa.

Johnson, W. (1942). A study of the onset and development of stuttering. *Journal of Speech Disorders, 7,* 251–257.

Johnson, W. (1944). The Indians have no word for it: Stuttering in children. *Quarterly Journal of Speech, 30,* 330–337.

Johnson, W. (1946). *People in quandaries: The semantics of personal adjustment.* New York, NY: Harper and Bros.

Johnson, W. (1948). Stuttering. In W. Johnson, S. Brown, J. Curtis, C. Edney, & J. Keaster (Eds.), *Speech handicapped school children.* New York, NY: Harper & Row.

Johnson, W. (1955a). The time, the place, and the problem. In W. Johnson & R. Leutenegger (Eds.), *Stuttering in children and adults.* Minneapolis: University of Minnesota Press.

Johnson, W. (1955b). A study of the onset and development of stuttering. In W. Johnson and R. Leutenegger (Eds.), *Stuttering in children and adults.* Minneapolis: University of Minnesota Press.

Johnson, W. (1958). Introduction: The six men and the stuttering. In J. Eisenson (Ed.), *Stuttering: A symposium* (pp. 123–166). New York, NY: Harper & Row.

Johnson, W. (1961a). Measurements of oral reading and speaking rate and disfluency of adult male and female stutterers and nonstutterers. *Journal of Speech and Hearing Disorders, Monograph Supplement 7,* 1–20.

Johnson, W. (1961b). *Stuttering and what you can do about it.* Minneapolis: University of Minnesota.

Johnson, W., & Associates. (1959). *The onset of stuttering: Research findings and implications.* Minneapolis: University of Minnesota.

Johnson, W., & Brown, S. (1935). Stuttering in relation to various speech sounds. *Quarterly Journal of Speech, 21,* 481–496.

Johnson, W., & Colley, W. H. (1945). The relationship between frequency and duration of moments of stuttering. *Journal of Speech Disorders, 10,* 35–38.

Johnson, W., & Knott, J. (1937). Studies in the psychology of stuttering: I. The distribution of moments of stuttering in successive readings of the same material. *Journal of Speech Disorders, 2,* 17–19.

Johnson, W., & Leutenegger, R. (1955). *Stuttering in children and adults.* Minneapolis: University of Minnesota Press.

Johnson, W., & Millsapps, L. (1937). Studies in the psychology of stuttering: VI. The role of cues representative of stuttering moments during oral reading. *Journal of Speech Disorders, 2,* 101–104.

Johnson, W., & Rosen, L. (1937). Studies in the psychology of stuttering.VII. Effect of certain changes in speech pattern upon frequency of stuttering. *Journal of Speech Disorders, 2,* 195–209.

Johnston, S., Watkin, L., & Macklem, P. (1993). Lung volume changes during relatively fluent speech in stutterers. *Journal of Applied Physiology, 75,* 696–703.

Jokel, R., De Nil, L., & Sharpe, A. (2007). Speech disfluencies in adults with neurogenic stuttering associated with stroke and traumatic brain injury. *Journal of Medical Speech-Language Pathology, 15*(3), 243–261.

Jones, J., & Striemer, D. (2007). Speech disruption during delayed auditory feedback with simultaneous visual feedback. *Journal of the Acoustical Society of America, 122,* EL135–EL141.

Jones, M., Onslow, M., Harrison, E., & Packman, A. (2000). Treating stuttering in young children: Predicting treatment time in the Lidcombe program. *Journal of Speech, Language, and Hearing Research, 43,* 1440–1450.

Jones, M., Onslow, M., Packman, A., Williams, S., Ormond, T., Schwartz, I., et al. (2005). Randomized controlled trial of the Lidcombe programme of early stuttering intervention. *British Medical Journal, 331,* 659–661.

Kalinowski, J., Guntupalli, V., Stuart, A., & Saltuklaroglu, T. (2004). Self-reported efficacy of an ear-level prosthetic device that delivers altered auditory feedback for the management of stuttering. *International Journal of Rehabilitation Research, 27,* 167–170.

Kamhi, A. (2006). Treatment decisions for children with speech–sound disorders. *Language, Speech, and Hearing Services in Schools, 37,* 271–279.

Kamhi, A., & McOsker, T. (1982). Attention and stuttering: Do stutterers think too much about speech? *Journal of Fluency Disorders, 7,* 309–321.

Kang, C, Riazuddin, S., Mundorff, J., Krasnewich, D., Friedman, P., Mullikin, J., & Drayna, D. (2010). Mutations in the lysosomal enzyme–targeting pathway and persistent stuttering. *New England Journal of Medicine, 362,* 677–685.

Karass, J., Walden, T., Conture, E., Graham, C., Arnold, H., Hartfield, K., et al. (2006). Relation of emotional reactivity and regulation to childhood stuttering. *Journal of Communication Disorders, 39,* 402–423.

Karmali, I., Greer, D., Nuzzolo-Gomez, R., Ross, D., & Rivera-Valdes, C. (2005). Reducing palialia by presenting tact corrections to young children with autism. *The Analysis of Verbal Behavior, 21,* 145–153.

Katsovaskaia, I. (1962). The problems of children stuttering. *Deafness, Speech, and Hearing Abstracts, 2,* 296.

Kawai, N., Healey, E. C., & Carrell, T. (2007). Listeners' identification and discrimination of digitally manipulated sounds as prolongations. *Journal of the Acoustical Society of America, 122,* 1102–1110.

Kay, D. (1964). The genetics of stuttering. In G. Andrews & M. Harris (Eds.), *The syndrome of stuttering* (pp. 132–143). London, England: Spastics Society Medical Education and Information Unit.

Kell, C., Neumann, K., vonKriegstein, K., Posenenske, C., vonGudenberg, A, Euler, H., & Giraud, A., (2009). How the brain repairs stuttering. *Brain, 132,* 2747–2760.

Kelly, E., Smith, A., & Goffman, L. (1995). Orofacial muscle activity of children who stutter: A preliminary study. *Journal of Speech and Hearing Research, 38,* 1025–1036.

Kelly, G. (1963). *A theory of personality: The psychology of personal constructs.* New York, NY: Norton.

Kelman, E., & Nicholas, A. (2008). *Practical intervention for early childhood stammering: Palin PCI approach.* Milton Keynes, UK: Speechmark.

Kenjo, M. (2005). Stuttering research and treatment around the world: Japan. *The ASHA Leader, 36,* 9.

Kent, R. (2000). Research on speech motor control and its disorders: A review and prospective. *Journal of Communication Disorders, 33*(5), 391–428.

Kerlinger, F (1986). *Foundation of behavioral research.* 3rd edition. New York: Holt, Rinehart and Winston.

Kidd, K. (1977). A genetic perspective on stuttering. *Journal of Fluency Disorders, 2,* 259–269.

Kidd, K., Kidd, J. R., & Records, M. A. (1978). The possible causes of the sex ratio in stuttering and its implications. *Journal of Fluency Disorders, 3,* 13–23.

Kidd, K., Heimbuch R., & Records M. (1981).Vertical transmission of susceptibility to stuttering with sex-modified expression. *Proceedings of the National Academy of Science USA, 78,* 606–610.

Kingdon-Ward, W. (1941). *Stammering.* London, England: Hamilton.

Kingston, M., Huber, A., Onslow, M., Jones, M., & Packman, A. (2003). Predicting treatment time with the Lidcombe program: Replication and meta-analysis. *International Journal of Language and Communication Disorders, 38,* 165–177.

Klein, J., & Hood, S. (2004). The impact the stuttering on employment opportunities and job performance. *Journal of Fluency Disorders, 29,* 255–273.

Klein, M. (1932). *The psycho-analysis of children.* London, England: Hogarth Press.

Klein, M. (1955). The psychoanalytic play technique. *American Journal of Orthopsychiatry, 25,* 223–237.

Klein, M. (1967). *U.S. Patent No. 3,349,179.* Washington, DC: U.S. Patent and Trademark Office.

Kleinow, J., & Smith, A. (2000). Influences of length and syntactic complexity on the speech motor stability of the fluent speech of adults who stutter. *Journal of Speech, Language, and Hearing Research, 43,* 548–559.

Klingbell, G. (1939). The historical background of the modern speech clinic. *Journal of Speech Disorders, 4,* 115–132.

Kloth, S., Janssen, P., Kraaimaat, F., & Brutten, G. (1995). Speech-motor and linguistic skills of young stutterers prior to onset. *Journal of Fluency Disorders, 20,* 157–170.

Koenisberger, R. (Ed.). (1989). *Churchill's illustrated medical dictionary.* New York, NY: Churchill Livingstone.

Koushik, S., Shenker, R., & Onslow, M. (2009). Follow up of 6-10 year old stuttering children after Lidcombe Program treatment: A Phase I trial. *Journal of Fluency Disorders, 34,* 279–290.

Kraaimaat, F., Vanryckeghem, M., & Van Dam-Baggen, R. (2002). Stuttering and social anxiety. *Journal of Fluency Disorders, 27,* 319–331.

Kraft, SJ. (2010). *Genome-wide association study of persistent developmental stuttering* (Unpublished doctoral dissertation). University of Illinois at Urbana-Champaign.

Kraft, SJ., Cox, N., Evans, P., Ambrose, N., & Yairi, E. (2012). *A novel approach to the identification of stuttering genes.* Presented at the Seventh World Congress of Fluency Disorders, Tours, France.

Kraft, SJ., & Yairi, E. (2012). Genetic bases of stuttering: The state of the art, 2011. *Folia Phoniatrica and Logopaedica, 64,* 34–47.

Kroll, R., & Hood, S. (1976). The influence of task presentation and information load on the adaptation effect in stutterers and normal speakers, *Journal of Communication Disorders, 9,* 95–110.

Kully, D. (2002). Venturing into telehealth: Applying interactive technologies to stuttering treatment. *The ASHA Leader, 7*(1), 6–7, 15.

Kully, D., & Boberg, E. (1988). An investigation of inter-clinic agreement in the identification of fluent and stuttered syllables. *Journal of Fluency Disorders, 13,* 309–318.

Kully, D., & Boberg, E. (1991). Therapy for school aged-children. In W. Perkins (Ed.), *Seminars in speech and language, 12* (pp. 291–300). New York, NY: Thieme.

Kully, D., Langevin, M., & Lomheim, H. (2007). Intensive treatment of stuttering in adolescent and adult. In E. Conture & R. Curlee (Eds.), *Stuttering and related disorders of fluency* (3rd ed.). New York, NY: Thieme.

Kummer, A & Turner, J. (2011). Ethics in the practice of speech-language pathology in health care settings. *Seminars in Speech and Language, 32*(4), 330–337.

Lan, J., Song, M., Pan, C., Zhuang, G., Wang, Y., Ma, W., Chu, Q., Lai, Q., Xu, F., & Li, Y. (2009). Association between dopaminergic genes (SLC6A3 and DRD2) and stuttering among Han Chinese. *Journal of Human Genetics, 54,* 457–460.

Langevin, M., & Prasad, N. (2012). A stuttering education and bullying awareness and prevention resource: A feasibility study. *Language, Speech, and Hearing Services in Schools, 43,* 344–358.

Langevin, M., Huinck, W. J., Kully, D., Peters, H. F. M., Lomheim, H., & Tellers, M. (2006). A cross-cultural, long-term outcome evaluation of the ISTAR comprehensive stuttering program across Dutch and Canadian adults who stutter. *Journal of Fluency Disorders, 31*(4), 229–256.

Langevin, M., Kully, D., & Ross-Harold, B. (2007). A comprehensive stuttering program for school age children with strategies for managing teasing and bullying. In E. Conture & R. Curlee (Eds.), *Stuttering and related disorders* (3rd ed., pp. 131–150). New York, NY: Thieme.

Langevin, M., Kully, D., Teshima, S., Hagler, P., & Narasima N. (2010). Five-year longitudinal treatment outcomes of the ISTAR comprehension stuttering program. *Journal of Fluency Disorders, 35,* 123–140.

Lanyon, R. (1965). The relationship of adaptation and consistency to improvement in stuttering therapy. *Journal of Speech and Hearing Research, 8,* 263–269.

Lanyon, R. (1969). Behavior change in stuttering through systematic desensitization. *Journal of Speech and Hearing Research, 34,* 253–260.

Lanyon, R., & Barocas, V. (1975). Effects of contingent events on stuttering and fluency. *Journal of Consulting and Clinical Psychology, 43,* 786–793.

Lanyon, R., & Duprez, D. (1970). Nonfluency, information, and word length. *Journal of Abnormal Psychology, 76,* 93–97.

Lanyon, R., Barrington, C., & Newman, A. (1976). Modification of stuttering through EMG biofeedback: A preliminary study. *Behavioral Therapy, 7,* 96–103.

LaSalle, L., & Conture, E. (1995). Disfluency clusters of children who stutter: Relation of stutterings to self-repairs. *Journal of Speech and Hearing Research, 38,* 965–977.

Lass, N., Ruscello, D., Schmitt, J., Pannbacker, M., Orlando M., Dean, K., & Ruziska, J. (1992). Teachers' perception of stutterers. *Language, Speech, and Hearing Services in Schools, 23,* 78–81.

Lattermann, C., Euler, H., & Neumann K. (2008). A randomized control trial to investigate the impact of the Lidcombe Program on early stuttering in German-speaking preschoolers. *Journal of Fluency Disorders, 33,* 52–65.

Law, J., Boyle, J., & Harris, F. (2000). Prevalence and natural history of primary speech and language delay: Findings from a systematic review of the literature. *International Journal of Language & Communication Disorders, 35,* 165–188.

Leadholm, B., & Miller, J. (1992). *Language sample analysis: The Wisconsin guide* (Bulletin No. 92424). Madison: Wisconsin Department of Public Instruction.

Leath, W. (1984). *Handbook of stuttering therapy for the school clinician.* San Diego, CA: College-Hill Press.

Leavitt, R. (1974). *The Puerto Ricans: Culture change and language deviance.* Oxford, UK: University of Arizona Press.

Lees, R., Anderson, H., & Martin, P. (1999). The influence of language disorder on fluency: A pilot study. *Journal of Fluency Disorders, 24,* 227–238.

Lehiste, I. (1972). The timing of utterances and linguistic boundaries. *Journal of the Acoustical Society of America, 51,* 2018–2024.

Leith, W. (1984). *Handbook of stuttering therapy for the school clinician.* San Diego, CA: College-Hill Press.

Leith, W. (1986). Treating the stutterer with atypical cultural influences. In K. O. St. Louis, (Ed.), *The atypical stutterer.* San Diego, CA: Academic Press.

Leith, W., & Mims, H. (1975). Cultural influences in the development and treatment of stuttering: A preliminary report on the Black stutterer. *Journal of Speech and Hearing Disorders, 40,* 459–466.

Lemert, E. (1953). Some Indians who stutter. *Journal of Speech and Hearing Disorders, 18,* 168–174.

Lemert, E. (1962). Stuttering and social structure in two pacific societies. *Journal of Speech and Hearing Disorders, 27,* 3–10.

Leutenegger, R. (1957). Adaptation and recovery in the oral reading of stutterers. *Journal of Speech and Hearing Disorders, 22,* 276–287.

Levelt, W. (1989). *Speaking: From intention to articulation.* Cambridge, MA: MIT Press.

Levelt, W., Roelofs, A., & Meyer, A. (1999). A theory of lexical access in speech production. *Behavioral and Brain Sciences, 22,* 1–75.

Levy, D. (1938). Release therapy in young children. In G. L. Landreth (Ed.), *Play therapy: The art of the relationship.* Muncie, IN: Accelerated Development.

Lewis, C., Packman, A., Onslow, M., Simpson, J. & Jones, M. (2008). A phase 1 trial of telehealth delivery of the Lidcombe Program of Early Stuttering Intervention. *American Journal of Speech-Language Pathology, 17,* 139–149.

Lewis, K. (1991). The structure of disfluency behaviors in the speech of stutterers. *Journal of Speech and Hearing Research, 34*(3), 492–500.

Lilienfeld, S. (Ed.). (2003). *Science and pseudoscience in clinical psychology.* New York, NY: Guilford.

Lincoln, M., & Onslow, M. (1997). Long-term outcome of early intervention for stuttering. *American Journal of Speech-Language Pathology, 6,* 51–58.

Lincoln, M., Onslow, M., Lewis, C., & Wilson, L. (1996). A clinical trial of operant treatment for school-age children who stutter. *American Journal of Speech-Language Pathology, 5,* 73–85.

Lincoln, M., Packman, A., & Onslow, M. (2006). Altered auditory feedback and the treatment of stuttering. *Journal of Fluency Disorders, 31,* 71–89.

Lindberg, K. (1900). Zur Haufigkeit des Stotterns bei Schulkindern. *Medizinisch-padagogische Monatsschrift fur die gesamte Sprachheilkunde, 281–286.*

Lingwall, J., & Bergstrand, G. (1979, November). *Perceptual boundaries for judgment of "normal," "abnormal," and "stuttered" prolongations.* Paper presented at the convention of the American Speech-Language-Hearing Association, Atlanta, GA.

Logan, K., & Conture, E. (1997). Selected temporal, grammatical and phonological characteristics of conversational utterances produced by children who stutter. *Journal of Speech and Hearing Research, 40,* 107–120.

Logan, K., & Haj Tas, M. (2007). Effect of sample size on the measurement of stutter-like disfluencies. *Perspectives on Fluency and Fluency Disorders, 17*(3), 3–6.

Logan, K., Byrd, C., & Gillam, R. (2012). *Toward a comprehensive fluency assessment framework: Challenges & solutions.* Paper presented at the Annual Meeting of the American Speech-Language-Hearing Association, Atlanta, GA.

Logan, K., Byrd, C., Mazzocchi, E., & Gillam, R. (2011). Speaking rate characteristics of elementary-school-aged children who do and do not stutter. *Journal of Communication Disorders, 44,* 130–147

Logan, K., Roberts, R., Pretto, A., & Morey, M. (2002). Speaking slowly: Effects of four self-guided training approaches on adults' speech rate and naturalness. *American Journal of Speech Language Pathology, 11,* 163–174.

Long, N., & Dalston, R. (1983). Comprehension abilities of one-year-old infants with cleft lip and palate. *Cleft Palate Journal, 20,* 300.

Loucks, T., Chon, H., & Han, W. (2012). Auditory-vocal integration in adults who stutter. *International Journal of Language and Communication Disorders, 47,* 451–456.

Loucks, T., De Nil, L., & Sasisekaran,, J. (2007). Jaw-phonatory coordination in chronic developmental stuttering. *Journal of Communication Disorders, 40,* 257–272.

Louko, L., Edwards, C., & Conture, E. (1990). Phonological characteristics of young stutterers and their normally fluent peers: Preliminary observations. *Journal of Fluency Disorders, 15,* 191–210.

Louttit, C. M., & Halls, E. (1936). Surveys of speech defects among public school children of Indiana. *Journal of Speech Disorders, 1,* 73–80.

Lowinger, L. (1952). The psychodynamics of stuttering: An evaluation of the factors of aggression and guilt feelings in a group of institutionalized children. *Dissertation Abstracts, 12,* 725.

Lu, C., Chen, C. , Ning, N., Ding, G., Guo, T., Peng, D., Yang, Y., Li, K. & Lin, C. (2011). The neural substrates for atypical planning and execution of word production in stuttering. *Experimental Neurology, 221,* 146–156.

Ludlow, C. (2000). Stuttering: Dysfunction in a complex and dynamic system. *Brain, 123,* 1983–1984.

Ludlow, C., & Loucks, T. (2003). Stuttering: A dynamic motor control disorder. *Journal of Fluency Disorders, 28,* 273–295.

Lundstrom, C., & Garsten, M. (2000). A model for intervention with childhood stuttering. In *Proceedings of the Third World Congress of Fluency Disorders* (pp. 335–340). Nijmigen, Netherlands: Nijmigen University.

Lundström, C., & Garsten, M., (2012). *A model intervention in stuttering in preschool children.* Proceedings of the International Conference on Stuttering, Rome, Italy.

Luterman, D. (1991). *Counseling the communicatively disordered and their families* (2nd ed.). Austin, TX: Pro-Ed.

MacCulloch, M., Eaton, R., & Long, E. (1970). The long-term effect of auditory masking on young stutterers. *British Journal of Disorders of Communication, 5,* 165–173.

MacKay, D. (1970). Spoonerisms: The structure of errors in the serial order of speech. *Neuropsychologia, 8,* 323–350.

MacPherson, M., & Smith, A. (2013). Influences of sentence length and syntactic complexity on the speech motor control of children who stutter. *Journal of Speech, Langauge, and Hearing Research, 56,* 89–102.

Madding, C. (1995). *The stuttering syndrome: Feelings and attitudes of stutterers and non-stutterers among four cultural groups* (Unpublished doctoral dissertation). Claremont Graduate School.

Maguire, G., Franklin, D., Vatakis, N., Morgenshtern, E., Denko, T., Yaruss, J., Spotts C., Davis L., Davis A., Fox P., Soni P., Blomgren M., Silverman A., & Riley G. (2010). Exploratory randomized clinical study of pagoclone in persistent development suttering: the Examining pagaclone for persistent developmental stuttering study. *Journal of Clinical Psychopharmacology, 30,* 48–56.

Maguire, G., Riley, G., Franklin, D., & Gottschalk, L. (2000). Risperidone for the treatment of stuttering. *Journal of Clinical Psychopharmacology, 20,* 479–482.

Maguire, G., Riley, G., Franklin, D., Maguire, M., Nguyen, C., & Brojeni, P. (2004). Olanzapine in the treatment of developmental stuttering: A double-blind, placebo-controlled trial. *Annals of Clinical Psychiatry, 16,* 63–67.

Maguire, G., Yu, B., Franklin, D., & Riley, G. (2004). Alleviating stuttering with pharmacological intervention. *Expert Opinion on Pharmacotherapy, 5,* 1565–1571.

Mahr, G. C., & Torosian, T. (1999). Anxiety and social phobia in stuttering. *Journal of Fluency Disorders 24,* 119–126.

Mahr, G., & Leith, W. (1992). Psychogenic stuttering of adult onset. *Journal of Speech and Hearing Research, 35,* 283–286.

Makuen, G. (1941). Psychology of stuttering. *Journal of Nervous and Mental Disorders, 43,* 68–72.

Mallard, A. (1998). Using problem solving procedures in family management of stuttering. *Journal of Fluency Disorders, 23,* 127–135.

Mallard, A. (1991). Using families to help the school-age stutterer: A case study. In L. Rustin (Ed.), *Parents, families, and the stuttering child* (pp. 72–87). San Diego, CA: Singular.

Manning W., & Beck, G. (2013). Personality dysfunction in adults who stutter: Another look. *Journal of Fluency Disorders, 38*(2), 184–192.

Manning, W. (2001). *Clinical decision making in fluency disorders* (2nd ed.). San Diego, CA: Singular.

Manning, W. (2004). How can you understand? You don't stutter! *Contemporary Issues in Communication Science and Disorders, 31,* 58–68.

Månsson, H. (2000). Childhood stuttering: Incidence and development. *Journal of Fluency Disorders, 25,* 47–57.

Månsson, H. (2005). Stammens kompleksitet og diversitet (Therapy groups for preschool children who stammer). *Dansk Audiologopædi, 41,* 13–33.

Market, K., Montague, J. C., Buffalo, M. D., & Drummond, S. S. (1990). Acquired stuttering: Descriptive data and treatment outcome. *Journal of Fluency Disorders, 15,* 21–33.

Marland, P. (1957). Shadowing: A contribution to the treatment of stuttering. *Folia Phoniatrica, 9,* 242–245.

Martin, R. R., Kuhl, P., & Haroldson, S. (1972). An experimental treatment with two preschool stuttering children. *Journal of Speech and Hearing Research, 15,* 743–752.

Martin, R., & Haroldson, S. (1981). Stuttering identification: Standard definition and moment of stuttering. *Journal of Speech and Hearing Research, 24*(1), 59–63.

Martin, R., & Haroldson, S. (1982). Contingent self-stimulation for stuttering. *Journal of Speech and Hearing Disorders, 47,* 407–413.

Martin, R., & Siegel, G. (1966). The effects of simultaneously punishing stuttering and rewarding fluency. *Journal of Speech and Hearing Research, 9,* 466–475.

Martin, R., Haroldson, S., & Triden, K. (1984). Stuttering and speech naturalness. *Journal of Speech and Hearing Disorders, 49,* 53–58.

Matthews, S., Williams, R., & Pring, T. (1997). Parent-child interaction therapy and dysfluency: A single case study. *European Journal of Disorders of Communication 32,* 1244–1259.

Max, L., & Caruso, A. (1998). Adaptation of stuttering frequency during repeated readings. *Journal of Speech, Language, and Hearing Research, 41,* 1265–1281.

Max, L., & Gracco. V., (2005). Coordination of oral and laryngeal movements in the perceptually fluent speech of adults who stutter. *Journal of Speech, Language, and Hearing Research, 48,* 524–542.

Max, L., Caruso, A., & Gracco, V. (2003). Kinematic analyses of speech, orofacial nonspeech, and finger movements in stuttering and nonstuttering adults. *Journal of Speech, Language, and Hearing Research, 46,* 215–232.

Max, L., Guenther, F., Gracco, V., Ghosh, S., & Wallace, M. (2004). Unstable or insufficiently activated internal models and feedback-biased motor control as sources of dysfluency: A theoretical model of stuttering. *Contemporary Issues in Communication Science and Disorders, 31,* 105–122.

McAllister, J., & Kingston, M. (2005). Final part-word repetitions in school-age children: Two case studies. *Journal of Fluency Disorders, 30,* 255–267.

McClean, M., Goldsmith, H. & Cerf, A. (1984). Lower-lip EMG and displacement during bilabial disfluencies in adult stutterers. *Journal of Speech, Language and Hearing Research, 27,* 342–349.

McClean, M., Kroll, R. & Loftus, N. (1990). Kinematic analysis of lip closure in stutterers' fluent speech. *Journal of Speech, Language, and Hearing Research, 33,* 755–760.

McDearmon, J. (1968). Primary stuttering at the onset of stuttering: A reexamination of data. *Journal of Speech and Hearing Research, 11,* 631–637.

McDevitt, S., & Carey, W. (1978). The measurement of temperament in 3–7 year-old children. *Journal of Child Psychology and Psychiatry and Allied Disciplines, 19,* 245–253.

McKinnon, D., McLeod, S., & Reilly, S. (2007). The prevalence of stuttering, voice, and speech-sound disorders in primary school students in Australia. *Language, Speech, and Hearing Services in Schools, 38,* 5–15.

McLeod, S. & Harrison, L. (2009). Epidemiology of speech and language impairment in a nationally representative sample of 4- to 5-year-old children. *Journal of Speech, Language, and Hearing Research, 52,* 113–129.

McLeod, S., & McKinnon, D. (2007). The prevalence of communication disorders compared with other learning needs in 14,500 primary and secondary school students. *International Journal of Language and Communication Disorders, 42,* 37–59.

McMillan, J. (2004). *Educational research: Fundamentals for the consumer* (4th ed., pp. 227–228). Boston, MA: Allyn & Bacon.

Meltzer, H. (1935). Talkativeness in stuttering and non-stuttering children. *Journal of Genetic Psychology, 46,* 371–390.

Meltzoff, A. (1995). What infant memory tells us about amnesia: Long-term recall and deferred imitation. *Journal of Experimental Child Psychology, 59,* 497–515.

Menzies, R., O'Brian, S., Onslow, M., Packman, A., St Clare, T., Block, S. (2008). An experimental clinical trial of a cognitive-behavior therapy package for chronic stuttering. *Journal of Speech, Language, and Hearing Research, 51,* 1451–1464.

Merits-Patterson, R., & Reed, C. (1981). Disfluencies in the speech of language-delayed children. *Journal of Speech and Hearing Research, 46,* 55–58.

Meyer, V., & Mair, J. (1963). A new technique to control stammering: A preliminary report. *Behavioral Research and Therapy, 1,* 251–254.

Meyers Fosnot, S., & Woodford, L. (1992). *The fluency development system for young children*. Buffalo, NY: United Educational Services.

Meyers, S., & Freeman, F. (1985). Mother and child speech rates as a variable in stuttering and disfluency. *Journal of Speech and Hearing Research, 28,* 436–444.

Miles, S., & Bernstein Ratner, N. (2001). Parental language input to children at stuttering onset. *Journal of Speech, Language, and Hearing Research, 44,* 1116–1130.

Milisen, R., & Johnson, W. (1936). A comparative study of stutterers, former stutterers, and normal speakers whose handedness has been changed. *Archives of Speech, 1,* 61–86.

Millard, S., Nicholas, A., & Cook, F. (2008). Is parent-child interaction therapy effective in reducing stuttering? *Journal of Speech, Language, and Hearing Research, 51,* 636–650.

Miller, J., Long, S., McKinley, N., Thormann, S., Jones, M., & Nockerts, A. (2005). *Language Sample Analysis II: The Wisconsin guide*. Madison: Wisconsin Department of Public Instruction.

Mills, A. W., & Streit, H. (1942). Report of a speech survey, Holyoke, Massachusetts. *Journal of Speech Disorders, 7,* 161–167.

Moleski, R., & Tosi, D. (1976). Comparative psychotherapy: Rational-emotive therapy versus systematic desensitization in the treatment of stuttering. *Journal of Consulting and Clinical Psychology, 44*(2), 309–311.

Montgomery, B., & Fitch, J. (1988). The prevalence of stuttering in the hearing-impaired school age population. *Journal of Speech & Hearing Disorders, 53,* 131–135.

Moore, W. (1946). Hypnosis in a system of therapies for stutterers. *Journal of Speech Disorders, 11,* 117–122.

Moore, W. (1959). A study of the blood chemistry of stutterers under two hypnotic conditions. *Speech Monographs, 26,* 64–68.

Moore, W., Jr., Flowers, P., & Cunko, C. (1981). Some relationships between adaptation and electromyographic activity at laryngeal and masseter sites in stutterers. *Journal of Fluency Disorders, 4,* 149–161.

Moreno, J. (1946). *Psychodrama*. Beacon, NY: Beacon House.

Moreno, J. (1953). *Who shall survive? Foundations of sociometry, group psychotherapy and psychodrama* (2nd ed.). Beacon, NY: Beacon House.

Morgenstern, J. (1956). Socio-economic factors in stuttering. *Journal of Speech and Hearing Disorders, 21,* 25–33.

Morley, M. (1957). *The development and disorders of speech in childhood*. Edinburgh, UK: Livingstone.

Moskowitz, H. (1941). Psychiatric factors in speech correction. *Quarterly Journal of Speech, 27,* 537–541.

Mowrer, D. (1998). Analysis of the sudden onset and disappearance of disfluencies in the speech of a 2½-year-old boy. *Journal of Fluency Disorders, 23,* 103–118.

Murdoch, B., Pitt, G., Theodoros, D., & Ward, E. (1999). Real-time continuous visual biofeedback in the treatment of speech breathing disorders following childhood traumatic brain injury: Report of one case. *Developmental Neurorehabilitation, 3,* 5–20.

Murphy, A., & Fitzsimons, R. (1960). *Stuttering and personality dynamics: Play therapy, projective therapy, and counseling*. New York, NY: Ronald.

Murphy, W., Yaruss, J. S., & Quesal, R. (2007a). Enhancing treatment for school-age children who stutter: I. Reducing negative reactions through desensitization and cognitive restructuring. *Journal of Fluency Disorders, 32,* 121–138.

Murphy, W., Yaruss, J. S., & Quesal, R. (2007b). Enhancing treatment for school-age children who stutter: II. Reducing bullying through role-playing and self-disclosure. *Journal of Fluency Disorders, 32,* 139–162.

Myers, F. (2011). Treatment of cluttering: A cognitive-behavioral approach centered on rate control. In D. Ward & K. Scaler Scott (Eds.), *Cluttering: A handbook of research, intervention and education* (pp. 152–174). East Sussex, UK: Psychology Press.

Myers, F., Bakker, K., St. Louis, K., & Raphael, L. (2012). Disfluencies in cluttered speech. *Journal of Fluency Disorders, 37,* 9–19.

Nao, C. (1964). The results of hypnosis as stuttering therapy. *Mental and Physical Medicine* (Japan), 4, 176–177.

Nass, R., Sclireler, B., & Heier, L. (2008). Acquired stuttering after a second stroke in a two year old. *Developmental Medicine & Child Neurology, 36,* 73–78.

National Institutes of Health. (1997). NIH Publication 97–4232. *Stuttering* Available at http://www.nidcd.nih.gov/health/voice/pages/stutter.aspx

Natke, U., Sandrieser, P., van Ark, M., Pietrowsky, R., & Kalveram, K. (2004). Linguistic stress within-word position, and grammatical class in relation to early childhood stuttering. *Journal of Fluency Disorders, 29,* 109–122.

Neef, N., Sommer, M., Neef, W., vonGudenberg, A., Jung, K., & Wustenberg, T. (2012). Reduced speech perceptual acuity for stop consonants in individuals who stutter. *Journal of Speech, Language, and Hearing Research, 55,* 276–289.

Neely, M. (1960). *An investigation of the incidence of stuttering among elementary school children in the parochial schools of Orleans Parish* (Unpublished master's thesis). Tulane University New Orleans, LA.

Neilson, M., & Andrews, G. (1992). Intensive fluency training of chronic stutterers. In R. Curlee (Ed.), *Stuttering and related disorders of fluency* (pp. 139–165). New York, NY: Thieme.

Neumann, K., Euler, H., Wolff von Gudenberg, A., Giraud, A., Lanfermann, H., Gall, V., et al. (2003). The nature and treatment of stuttering as revealed by fMRI. A within- and between-group comparison. *Journal of Fluency Disorders, 28,* 381–410.

Neumann, K., Preibisch, C., Euler, H., von Gudenberg, A.W., Lanfermann, H., Gall, V., & Giraud, A. L. (2005). Cortical plasticity associated with stuttering therapy. *Journal of Fluency Disorders, 30*(1), 23–39.

Newman, L., & Smit, A. (1989). Some effects of variations in response time latency on speech rate, interruptions, and fluency in children's speech. *Journal of Speech and Hearing Research, 32,* 635–644.

Newman, P. (1963). Adaptation performances of individual stutterers: Implications for research. *Journal of Speech and Hearing Research, 6,* 293–294.

NIH. (2010). (Publication No. 10-4232). Washington, DC: Author

Nilsen, K., Westgaard, R. , Stovner, L., Helde, G., Rø, M., & Sand, T. (2006). Pain induced by low-grade stress in patients with fibromyalgia and chronic shoulder/neck pain, relation to surface electromyography. *European Journal of Pain, 10,* 615–627.

Nippold, M. (2002). Stuttering and phonology: Is there an interaction? *American Journal of Speech-Language Pathology, 11,* 99–110.

Nippold, M. (2004). Phonological and language disorders in children who stutter: Impact on treatment recommendations. *Clinical Linguistics & Phonetics, 18,* 145–159.

Nippold, M. (2011). Stuttering in school-age children: A call for treatment research. *Language, Speech, and Hearing Services in Schools, 42,* 99–101.

Nippold, M. (2012a). Stuttering and language ability in children: Questioning the connection. *American Journal of Speech-Language Pathology, 21,* 183–196.

Nippold, M. (2012b). When a school-age child stutters, let's focus on the primary problem. *Language, Speech, and Hearing Services in Schools, 43,* 549–551.

Nowack, W., & Stone, R. E. (1987). Acquired stuttering and bilateral cerebral disease. *Journal of Fluency Disorders, 12,* 141–146.

Ntourou, K., Conture, E., & Lipsey, M. (2011). Language abilities of children who stutter: A meta-analytical review. *American Journal of Speech-Language Pathology, 20,* 163–179.

Ojemann, R. (1931). Studies in handedness: III. Relation of handedness to speech. *Journal of Educational Psychology, 22,* 120–126.

Okalidou, A., & Kampanaros, M. (2001).Teacher perceptions of communication impairment at screening stage in preschool children living in Patras, Greece. *International Journal of Language and Communication Disorders, 36*(4), 489–502.

Okasha, A., Bishry, Z., Kamel, M., & Hassan, A. H. (1974). Psychosocial study of stammering in Egyptian children. *British Journal of Psychiatry, 124,* 531–533.

Olander, L., Smith, A., & Zelaznik, H. (2010). Evidence that a motor timing deficit is a factor in the development of stuttering. *Journal of Speech, Language, and Hearing Research, 53,* 876–886.

Olswang, L. (1993). Treatment efficacy research: A paradigm for investigating clinical practice and theory. *Journal of Fluency Disorders, 18,* 125–131.

Olswang, L. (1998). Treatment efficacy research. In C. Frattali (Ed.), *Measuring outcomes in speech-language pathology* (pp. 134–150). New York, NY: Thieme.

Onslow, M. (1996). *Behavioral management of stuttering.* San Diego, CA: Singular.

Onslow, M., & Ingham, R. (1987). Speech quality measurement and the management of stuttering. *Journal of Speech and Hearing Disorders, 52,* 2–17.

Onslow, M., Andrews, C., & Lincoln, M. (1994). A control/ experimental trial of an operant treatment for early stuttering. *Journal of Speech and Hearing Research, 37,* 1244–1259.

Onslow, M., Costa, L., Andrews, C., Harrison, E., & Packman, A. (1996). Speech outcomes of a prolonged-speech treatment for stuttering. *Journal of Speech and Hearing Research, 39,* 734–749.

Onslow, M., Packman, A., & Harrison, E. (Eds.). (2003). *The Lidcombe Program of early stuttering intervention: A clinician's guide.* Austin, TX: Pro-Ed.

Onslow, M., van Doorn, J., & Newman, D. (1992). Variability of acoustic segment durations after prolonged-speech treatment for stuttering. *Journal of Speech and Hearing Research, 35,* 529–536.

Ooki, S.(2005). Genetic and environmental influences on stuttering and tics in Japanese twin children. *Twin Research and Human Genetics,, 8,* 69–75.

Ornstein, A., & Manning, W. (1985). Self-efficacy scaling by adult stutterers. *Journal of Communication Disorders, 18,* 313–320.

Otto, F., & Yairi, E. (1976). A disfluency analysis of Down's syndrome and normal subjects. *Journal of Fluency Disorders, 1,* 26–32.

Owens, R. (2010). *Language disorders: A functional approach to assessment and intervention.* Boston, MA: Allyn & Bacon.

Oyler, M. (1996). Vulnerability in stuttering children. *Dissertation Abstracts International Section A: Humanities & Social Sciences, 56*(9-A), 3374.

Ozawa, Y. (1960). Studies of misarticulation in Wakayama district. *Journal of Medicine: University of Osaka, 5,* 319.

Packman, A., & Onslow, M. (1999). Issues in the treatment of early stuttering. In M. Onslow & A. Packman (Eds.), *The handbook of early stuttering intervention* (pp.1–16). San Diego, CA: Singular.

Packman, A., Code, C., & Onslow, M. (2007). On the cause of stuttering: Integrating theory with brain and behavioral research. *Journal of Neurolinguistics, 20,* 353–362.

Paden, E. (2005). Development of phonological abilities. In E. Yairi & N. Ambrose (Eds.), *Early childhood stuttering* (pp. 197–235). Austin, TX: Pro-Ed.

Paden, E., Yairi, E., & Ambrose, N. G. (1999). Early childhood stuttering: II. Initial status of phonological abilities. *Journal of Speech, Language, and Hearing Research, 42,* 1113–1124.

Paden, E., & Yairi, E. (1996). Phonological characteristics of young children with persistent and recovering stuttering. *Journal of Speech and Hearing Research, 39,* 981–990.

Paden, E., Ambrose N., & Yairi, E. (2002). Phonological progress during the first two years of stuttering. *Journal of Speech, Language, and Hearing Research, 44,* 256–267.

Panelli, A., McFarlane, S., & Shipley, K. (1978). Implications of evaluating and intervening with incipient stutterers. *Journal of Fluency Disorders, 3,* 41–50.

Parker, C., & Christopherson, F. (1963). Electronic aid in the treatment of stammer. *Medical Electronics and Biological Engineering, 1,* 121–125.

Patel, R., & Brayton, J. (2009). Identifying prosodic contrasts in utterances produced by 4-, 7-, and 11-year-old children. *Journal of Speech, Language, Hearing Research, 52,* 790–801.

Pavlov, I. (1927). *Conditioned reflexes: An investigation of the physiological activity of the cerebral cortex* (Trans. G. V. Anrep). London, England: Oxford University Press.

Pay, A., & Sirotkina, M. (1955). *My experience in logoped work.* Moscow, Russia: Academy of Education, Institute of Defectology.

Perkins, W. (1969). *Stuttering and discriminative awareness* (SRS Research Grant RD-2275-S, Final Report). Washington, DC: Div. of Res. and Demonstration Grants, Social and Rehabilitation Services, Dept. of Health, Education, and Welfare.

Perkins, W. (1973a). Replacement of stuttering with fluent speech: I. Rationale. *Journal of Speech and Hearing Disorders, 38,* 283–294.

Perkins, W. (1973b). Replacement of stuttering with normal speech: II. Clinical procedures. *Journal of Speech and Hearing Disorders, 38,* 295–303.

Perkins, W. (1990a). What is stuttering? *Journal of Speech and Hearing Disorders, 55,* 370–382.

Perkins, W. (1990b). Gratitude, good intentions, and red herrings: A response to commentaries. *Journal of Speech and Hearing Disorders, 55,* 402–404.

Perkins, W. (1992). *Stuttering prevented.* San Diego, CA: Singular.

Perkins, W., Kent, R., & Curlee, R. F. (1991). A theory of neurolinguistic function in stuttering. *Journal of Speech and Hearing Research, 34*(4), 734–752.

Peters, H. F. M. & Boves, L. (1988). Coordination of aerodynamic and phonatory processes in fluent speech of stutterers. *Journal of Speech, Language, and Hearing Research, 31,* 352–361.

Phares, E. (1979). *Clinical psychology: Concepts, methods, and profession.* Georgetown, Ontario, Canada: Dorsey Press.

Piacentini, J., Woods, D., Scahill, L., Wilheml, S., Peterson, A., Chang, S., Ginsburg, G., Deckersback, T., Dziura, J., Levi-Pearl, S., & Walkup, J. (2010). Behavior therapy for children with Tourette disorder: A randomized controlled trial. *American Medical Association, 303,* 1929–1937.

Pichon, E., & Borel-Maisonny, S. (1937). *Le Bégaiement, sa nature, et son traitement* (Stuttering, its nature and treatment). Paris, France: Masson.

Pindzola, R. (1987). *Stuttering intervention program: Age 3 to grade 3.* Austin, TX: Pro-Ed.

Pindzola, R. H., Jenkins, M. M., & Lokken, K. J. (1989). Speaking rates of young children. *Language, Speech, and Hearing Services in Schools, 20,* 133–138.

Pollard, R., Ellis, J., Finan, D., & Ramig, P. (2009). Effects of the Speech Easy on objective and perceived aspects of stuttering: A 6-month, Phase I clinical trial in naturalistic environments. Journal of Speech, Language, and Hearing Research, 52, 516–533.

Postma, A., & Kolk, H. (1992). Error monitoring in people who stutter: Evidence against auditory feedback deficit theories. *Journal of Speech and Hearing Research, 35,* 1024–1032.

Postma, A., & Kolk, H. (1993). The covert repair hypothesis: Prearticulatory repair processes in normal and stuttered disfluencies. *Journal of Speech and Hearing Research, 36,* 472–487.

Postma, A., Kolk, H., & Povel, D. J. (1991). Disfluencies as resulting from covert self-repairs applied to internal speech errors. In H. F. M. Peters, W. Hulstijn, & C. W. Starkweather (Eds.). Speech motor control and stuttering. Amsterdam, Netherlands: Elsevier Science Publishers.

Poulos, M., & Webster, W. (1991). Family history as a basis for subgrouping people who stutter. *Journal of Speech and Hearing Research, 34,* 5–10.

Preibisch, C., Neumann, K., Raab, P., Euler, H., von Gudenberg, A., Lanfermann, H., et al. (2003). Evidence for compensation for stuttering by the right frontal operculum. *Neuroimage, 20,* 1356–1364.

Preus, A. (1973). Stuttering in Down's syndrome. In Y. LeBrun & R. Hoops (Eds.), *Neurolinguistic approaches to stuttering* (pp. 90–100). The Hague, Netherlands: Mouton.

Preus, A. (1981). *Identifying subgroups of stutterers.* Oslo, Norway: University of Oslo.

Preus, A. (1990). Treatment of mentally retarded stutterers. *Journal of Fluency Disorders, 15,* 223–234.

Prins, D. (1993). Management of stuttering: Treatment of adolescents and adults. In R. Curlee (Ed.), *Stuttering and related disorders of fluency.* New York, NY: Thieme.

Prins, D., & Hubbard, C. (1988). Response contingent stimuli and stuttering: Issues and implications. *Journal of Speech and Hearing Research, 31,* 696–709.

Prins, D., & Hubbard, C. (1990). Acoustical durations of speech segments during stuttering adaptation. *Journal of Speech and Hearing Research, 33,* 494–504.

Prins, D., & Lohr, F. (1972). Behavioral dimensions of stuttered speech. *Journal of Speech and Hearing Research, 15*(1), 61–71.

Prins, D., Hubbard, C., & Krause, M. (1991). Syllabic stress and the occurrence of stuttering. *Journal of Speech and Hearing Research, 34,* 1011–1016.

Prins, D., Mandelkorn, T., & Cerf, A. (1980). Principal and differential effects of Haloperidol and placebo treatments upon speech disfluencies in stutterers.

Journal of Speech, Language, and Hearing Research, 23, 614–629.

Proctor, A., Yairi, E., Duff, M., & Zhang, J. (2008). Prevalence of stuttering in African American preschool children. *Journal of Speech, Language, and Hearing Research, 50,* 1465–1474.

Quarrington, B. (1965). Stuttering as a function of the information value and sentence position of words. *Journal of Abnormal Psychology, 70,* 221–224.

Quesal, R. (2010). Empathy: Perhaps the most important *E* in EBP. *Seminars in Speech and Language, 31,* 217–226.

Quesal, R., Yaruss, J. S., & Molt, L. (2004). Many types of data: Stuttering treatment outcomes beyond fluency. In A. Packman, A. Meltzer, & H. Peters (Eds.), *Theory research and therapy in fluency disorders. Proceedings of the Fourth World Congress on Fluency Disorders* (pp. 218–224). Nijmegen, Netherlands: Nijmegen University Press.

Quinn, P., & Preachy, E. (1973). Haloperidol in the treatment of stutterers. *British Journal of Psychiatry, 123,* 247–248.

Raczek, B., & Adamczyk, B. (2004). Concentration of carbon dioxide in exhaled air in fluent and non-fluent speech. *Folia Phoniatrica Logopedia, 56,* 75–82.

Ramig, P., & Bennett, E. (1997). Clinical management of children: Direct management strategy. In R. F. Curlee & G. M. Siegel (Eds.), *Nature and treatment of stuttering: New directions* (2nd ed., pp. 292–312). Boston, MA: Allyn & Bacon.

Rantala, S., & Petri-Larmi, M. (1976). Haloperidol (serenase) in the treatment of stuttering. *Folia Phoniatrica, 28,* 354–361.

Reed, C., & Godden, A. L. (1977). An experimental treatment using verbal punishment with two preschool stutterers. *Journal of Fluency Disorders, 2,* 225–233.

Reilly, S., Onslow, M., Packman, A., Wake, M., Bavin, E., Prior, M., et al. (2009). Predicting stuttering onset by age of 3: A prospective, community cohort study. *Pediatrics, 123,* 270–277.

Reilly, S., Onslow, M., Packman, Cini,, E. Conway, L., Ukoumunne, O., Bavin, E., Prior, M., Eadie, P., Block, B., & Wake, M. (2013). Natural History of Stuttering to 4 Years of Age: A Prospective Community-Based Study. *Pediatrics, 36,* 460–467.

Retherford, K. (2000). *Guide to analysis of language transcripts* (3rd ed.). Eau Claire, WI: Thinking Publications.

Rheinberger, M., Karlin, I., & Berman, A. (1943). Electroencephalographic and laterality studies of stuttering and non-stuttering children. *Nervous Child, 2,* 117–133.

Riaz, N., Steinberg, S., Ahmad, J., Pluzhnikov, A., Riazuddin, S., Cox, N. J., et al. (2005). Genomewide significant linkage to stuttering on chromosome 12. *American Journal of Human Genetics, 76,* 647–651.

Richels, C., & Conture, E. (2007). An indirect treatment approach for early intervention for childhood stuttering. In E. Conture & R. Curlee (Eds.), *Stuttering and related disorders,* (3rd ed.). New York, NY: Thieme.

Rickard, H., & Mundy, M. (1965). Direct manipulation of stuttering behavior in experimental-clinical approach. In L. Ulman & L. Krasner (Eds.), *Case studies in behavioral modification* (pp. 268–272). New York, NY: Holt, Rinehart and Winston.

Riley, G. (1981). *Stuttering prediction instrument for young children.* Austin, TX: Pro-Ed.

Riley, G. (1994). *Stuttering severity instrument for children and adults* (3rd ed.). Austin, TX: Pro-Ed.

Riley, G. (2009). *SSI-4: Stuttering Severity Instrument* (4th ed.). Austin, TX: Pro-Ed.

Riley, G., & Ingham, J. C. (1995). Vocal response time changes associated with two types of treatment. In C. W. Starkweather & H. M. F. Peters (Eds.), *Stuttering: Proceedings of the First World Congress in Fluency Disorders* (pp. 470–474). New York, NY: Elsevier.

Riley, G., & Ingham, J. C. (2000). Acoustic duration changes associated with two types of treatment for children who stutter. *Journal of Speech, Language, and Hearing Research, 43,* 965–978.

Riley, G., & Riley, J. (1980). Motoric and linguistic variables among children who stutter: A factor analysis. *Journal of Speech and Hearing Disorders, 45*(4), 504–513.

Riley, G., & Riley, J. (1985). *Oral motor assessment and treatment: Improving syllable production.* Austin, TX: Pro-Ed.

Riley, G., & Riley, J. (1999). Speech motor training. In M. Onslow & A. Packman (Eds.), *The handbook of early stuttering intervention* (pp. 139–158). San Diego, CA: Singular.

Riley, G., & Riley, J. (2000). A revised component model for diagnosing and treating children who stutter. *Contemporary Issues in Communication Sciences and Disorders, 27,* 188–199.

Riley, J. (1971). *Language profiles of thirty-nine children who stutter grouped by performance on a motor problems inventory* (Master's thesis). California State University, Fullerton.

Riley, J., Riley, G., & Maguire, G. (2004). Subjective screening of stuttering severity, locus of control and avoidance: Research edition. *Journal of Fluency Disorders, 29,* 51–62.

Rind, E., and Rind, P. (1988). The stutterer in the classroom: A guide for the teacher. Retrieved from http://www.isastutter.org/CDRomProject/teacher/stutter_classroom.html

Robb, M., & Blomgren, M. (1997). Analysis of F2 transition in the speech of stutterers and nonstutterers. *Journal of Fluency Disorders, 22,* 1–16.

Robb, M., Sargent, A. & O'Beirne, G. (2009) Characteristics of disfluency clusters in adults who stutter. *Logopedics Phoniatrics Vocology, 34,* 36–42.

Roberts, P., & Shenker, R. (2007). Assessment and treatment of stuttering in bilingual speakers. In

E. Conture & R. Curlee (Eds.), *Stuttering and related disorders* (3rd ed., pp. 183–206). New York, NY: Thieme.

Roberts, P., Meltzer, A., Wilding, J. (2009). Disfluencies in non-stuttering adults across sample lengths and topics. *Journal of Communication Disorders, 42,* 414–427.

Robinson, F. (1964). *Introduction to stuttering.* Englewood Cliffs, NJ: Prentice-Hall.

Robinson, T., & Crowe, T. (1998). Culture-based considerations in programming for stuttering intervention with African-American clients and their families. *Language, Speech, and Hearing Services in School, 29,* 172–179.

Rogers, C. (1942). *Counseling and psychotherapy.* Boston, MA: Houghton Mifflin.

Rogers, C. (1951). *Client-centered therapy: Its current practice, implications, and theory.* Boston, MA: Houghton Mifflin.

Rogers, C. (1957). The necessary and sufficient conditions of therapeutic personality change. *Journal of Consulting Psychology, 21,* 95–103.

Rommel, D., Hage, A., Kalehne, P., & Johannsen, H. (1999). Developmental, maintenance, and recovery of childhood stuttering: Prospective longitudinal data 3 years after first contact. In K. Baker, L. Rustin, & K. Baker (Eds.), *Proceedings of the Fifth Oxford Disfluency Conference* (pp. 168–182). Chappell Gardner, UK: Windsor, Berkshire.

Rossiter, M. (2009). Perceptions of L2 fluency by native and non-native speakers of English. *Canadian Modern Language Review, 65,* 395–412.

Roth, C., Aronson, A., & Davis, L. (1989). Clinical studies in psychogenic stuttering of adult onset. *Journal of Speech and Hearing Disorders, 54,* 634–646.

Rothbart, K., & Bates, J. (1998). Temperament. In W. Damon (Series Ed.) & N. Eisenberg (Vol. Ed.), *Handbook of child psychology: Vol. 3. Social, emotional and personality development* (5th ed., pp. 105–176). New York: Wiley.

Rothbart, M. & Bates, J. (1998). Temperament. In W. Damon (Series Ed.) & N. Eisenberg (Vol. Ed.), *Handbook of child psychology: Vol. 3. Social, emotional and personality development* (5th ed., pp. 105–176). New York: Wiley. Temperament-Part 1 (pgs. 105–139) & Temperament-Part 2 (pgs. 140–176).

Rothbaum, B., Hodges, L., Smith, S., Lee, J., & Price, L. (2000). A controlled study of virtual reality exposure therapy for the fear of flying. *Journal of Consulting and Clinical Psychology, 68,* 1020–1026.

Rothbart, M., Ahadi, S., Hershey, K., & Fisher, P. (2001). Investigations of temperament at three to seven years: The Children's Behavior Questionnaire. *Child Development, 72,* 1394–1408.

Rousseau, I., Packman, A., Onslow, M., Harrison, E., & Jones, M. (2007). An investigation of language and phonological development and the responsiveness of preschool age children to the Lidcombe program. *Journal of Communication Disorders, 40,* 382–397.

Rubin, D., Wetzler, S., & Nebes, R. (1986). Autobiographical memory across the adult lifespan. In D. Rubin (Ed.), *Autobiographical memory* (pp. 202–221). Cambridge, MA: Cambridge University Press.

Runyan, C., & Runyan, S. (1993). Therapy for school-aged stutterers: An update on the fluency rules program. In R. Curlee (Ed.), *Stuttering and related disorders of fluency* (pp. 101–123). New York: Thieme.

Runyan, C., & Runyan, S. (2007). A fluency rules therapy program for young children in the public schools. In E. Conture & R. Curlee (Eds.), *Stuttering and related disorders* (3rd ed.). New York, NY: Thieme.

Rustin, L., & Cook, F. (1983). Intervention procedures for the disfluent child. In P. Dalton (Ed.), *Approaches to the treatment of stuttering.* London, England: Croom Helm.

Rustin, L., Botterill, W., & Kelman, E. (1996). *Assessment and therapy for young disfluent children: Family interaction.* London, England: Whurr.

Rustin, L., Cook, F., & Spence, R. (1995). *The management of stuttering in adolescence: A communication skills approach.* London, England: Whurr.

Ryan, B. (1971). Operant procedures applied to stuttering therapy for children. *Journal of Speech and Hearing Disorders, 36,* 264–280.

Ryan, B. (1979). Stuttering therapy in a framework of operant conditioning and programmed learning. In H. Gregory (Ed.), *Controversies about Stuttering Therapy* (pp. 129–173). Baltimore, MD: University Park Press.

Ryan, B. (1992). Articulation, language, rate, and fluency characteristics of stuttering and nonstuttering preschool children. *Journal of Speech and Hearing Research, 35,* 333–342.

Ryan, B. (1997). A reanalysis of the stuttering and syllable: Counting data in Kully and Boberg (1988). *Journal of Fluency Disorders, 22,* 331–338.

Ryan, B. (2001a). A longitudinal study of articulation, language, rate, and fluency of 22 preschool children who stutter. *Journal of Fluency Disorders, 26,* 107–127.

Ryan, B. (2001b). *Programmed therapy for stuttering in children and adults* (2nd ed.). Springfield, IL: Charles C. Thomas.

Ryan, B., & Ryan, B. V. (1995). Programmed stuttering treatment for children: Comparison of two establishment programs through transfer, maintenance, and follow-up. *Journal of Speech and Hearing Research, 38,* 61–75.

Sackett, D., Rosenberg, W., Gray, J. A. M., Haynes, R., & Richardson, W. (1996). Evidence based medicine: What it is and what it isn't. *British Medical Journal, 312,* 71–72.

Sackett, D., Straus, S., Richardson, W., Rosenberg, W., & Haynes, R. (2000). *Evidence-based medicine: How to practice and teach EBM.* Edinburgh, Scotland: Churchill Livingstone.

Sadoff, R., & Siegel, R. (1965). Group psychotherapy for stutterers. *International Journal of Group Psychotherapy, 15,* 72–80.

Sander, E. (1959). Counseling parents of stuttering children. *Journal of Speech and Hearing Disorders, 24,* 262–271.

Sander, E. (1961). Reliability of the Iowa Speech Disfluency Test. *Journal of Speech and Hearing Disorders, Monograph Supplement 7,* 21–30.

Sander, E. (1963). Frequency of syllable repetition and "stutter" judgments. *Journal of Speech and Hearing Disorders, 28,* 19–30.

Sander, E. (1968). Interrelations among the responses of mothers to a child's disfluencies. *Speech Monographs, 35,* 187–195.

Sandow, L. (1898). *Mechanik des Stotterns* (The mechanics of stuttering). Nordhausen, Germany: Edler.

Santos, R., & Reese, D. (1999, June). Selecting culturally and linguistically appropriate materials: Suggestions for service providers. *ERIC Digest,* University of Illinois.

Sawyer, J., & Yairi, E. (2006). The effect of sample size on the assessment of stuttering severity. *American Journal of Speech-Language Pathology, 15,* 36–44.

Sawyer, J., & Yairi, E. (2010). Characteristics of disfluency clusters over time in preschool children who stutter. *Journal of Speech, Language, and Hearing Research, 53,* 1191–1205.

Saxon, K., & Ludlow, C. (2007). A critical review of the effect of drug on stuttering. In E. Conture & R. Curlee (Eds.), *Stuttering and other fluency* disorders (3rd ed., pp. 277–294). New York, NY: Thieme.

Scarbrough, H. (1943). A quantitative and qualitative of the electro electroencephalograms of stutterers and non-stutterers. *Journal of Experimental Psychology, 32,* 156–167.

Schaeffer, M., & Shearer, W. (1968). A survey of mentally retarded stutterers. *Mental. Retardation., 6,* 44–45.

Schindler, M. (1955). A study of educational adjustment of stuttering and nonstuttering children. In W. Johnson, & R. R. Leutenegger (Eds.), *Stuttering in children and adults.* Minneapolis: University of Minnesota Press.

Schlanger, B. (1953). Speech examination of a group of institutionalized mentally handicapped children. *Journal of Speech and Hearing Disorders, 18,* 339–349.

Schlanger, B., & Gottsleben, R. (1957). Analysis of speech defects among the institutionalized mentally retarded. *Journal of Speech and Hearing Disorders, 22,* 98–103.

Schmidt, R., & Lee, T. (2005). *Motor control and learning: A behavioral emphasis* (4th ed.). Champaign, IL: Human Kinetics.

Schubert, O. (1966). *The incidence rate of stuttering in a matched group of institutionalized mentally retarded.* Convention address at the American Association of Mental Deficiency, Chicago, IL.

Schuell, H. (1946). Sex differences in relation to stuttering. *Journal of Speech Disorders, 11,* 277–295.

Schuell, H. (1949). Working with parents of stuttering children. *Journal of Speech and Hearing Disorders, 14,* 251–254.

Schwartz, H. (1999). *A primer for stuttering therapy.* Boston, MA: Allyn & Bacon.

Schwartz, H., & Conture E. (1988). Subgrouping young stutterers. *Journal of Speech and Hearing Research, 31,* 62–71.

Schwartz, H., Zebrowski, P., & Conture, E. G. (1990). Behaviors at the onset of stuttering. *Journal of Fluency Disorders, 15,* 77–86.

Schwartz, M. (1976). *Stuttering solved.* Philadelphia, PA: Lippincott.

Schwenk, K., Conture, E., & Walden, T. (2007). Reaction to background stimulation of preschool children who do and do not stutter. *Journal of Communication Disorders, 40,* 129–141.

Scott, C., Trautman, L., & Cairns, D. (2003). *Time pressure and disfluency: An empirical report.* Paper presented at the Fourth World Congress on Fluency Disorders, Montreal, Canada.

Scott, C., & Windsor, J. (2000). General language performance measures in spoken and written narrative and expository discourse of school-age children with language learning disabilities. *Journal of Speech, Language, and Hearing Research, 43,* 324–339.

Seery, C. (2005). Differential diagnosis of stuttering for forensic purposes. *American Journal of Speech-Language Pathology, 14,* 284–297.

Seery, C., Watkins, R., Ambrose, N., & Throneburg, R. (2006). *Non-word repetition by school age children who stutter.* Paper presented at the Annual Convention of the American Speech-Language-Hearing Association, Miami, FL.

Seery, C., Watkins, R., Mangelsdorf, S., & Shigeto, A. (2007). Subtyping stuttering II: Contributions from language and temperament. *Journal of Fluency Disorders, 32,* 197–217.

Sermas, C., & Cox, M. (1982). The stutterer and stuttering: Personality correlates. *Journal of Fluency Disorders, 7,* 141–158.

Shames, G., & Florence, C. (1980). *Stutter free speech: A goal for therapy.* Columbus, OH: Charles E. Merrill.

Shames, G., & Sherrick, C. (1963). A discussion of nonfluency and stuttering as operant behavior. *Journal of Speech and Hearing Disorders, 28,* 3–18.

Shane, M. (1955). Effect on stuttering of alteration in auditory feedback. In W. Johnson & R. Leutenegger (Eds.), *Stuttering in children and adults.* Minneapolis: University of Minnesota Press.

Shapiro, A. (1980). An electromyographic analysis of the fluent and disfluent utterances of several types of stutterers. *Journal of Fluency Disorders, 5,* 203–231.

Shapiro, D. (1999). *Stuttering intervention: A collaborative journey to fluency freedom.* Austin, TX: Pro-Ed.

Sheehan, J. (1953). Theory and treatment of stuttering as an approach-avoidance conflict. *Journal of Psychology, 36,* 27–49.

Sheehan, J. (1958). Conflict theory of stuttering. In J. Eisenson (Ed.), *Stuttering: A symposium* (pp. 123–166). New York, NY: Harper & Row.

Sheehan, J. (1970). *Stuttering: Research and therapy.* New York, NY: Harper & Row.

Sheehan, J. (1980). Problems in the evaluation of progress and outcome. In W. H. Perkins (Ed.), *Seminars in speech, language, and hearing* (pp. 389–401). New York, NY: Thieme.

Sheehan, J., & Martyn, M. (1966). Spontaneous recovery from stuttering. *Journal of Speech and Hearing Research, 9,* 121–135.

Sheehan, J., & Martyn, M. (1970). Stuttering and its disappearance. *Journal of Speech and Hearing Research, 13,* 279–289.

Shenker, R. (2011). Multilingual children who stutter: clinical issues. *Journal of Fluency Disorders, 36,* 186–93.

Shenker, R. C., & Roberts, P. (2006). Long-term outcome of the Lidcombe Program in bilingual children. In J. Au-Yeung, & M. M. Leahy (Eds.), *Proceedings of the International Fluency Association Fifth World Congress* (pp. 431–436). Dublin, Ireland: International Fluency Association.

Sherman, D. (1952). Clinical and experimental use of the Iowa Scale of Severity of Stuttering. *Journal of Speech and Hearing Disorders, 17,* 316–320.

Shine, R. (1980). Direct management of the beginning stutterer. In W. Perkins (Ed.), *Strategies in stuttering therapy* (pp. 339–350). An issue of *Seminars in Speech, Language, and Hearing.* New York, NY: Thieme.

Shugart, Y., Mundorff, J., Kilshaw, J., Doheny, K., Doan, B., Wanyee, J., et al. (2004). Results of a genome-wide linkage scan for stuttering. *American Journal of Medical Genetics, 124,* 133–135.

Sieff, S., & Hooyman, B. (2006). *Language-based disfluency: A child case study.* Paper presented at the convention of the American Speech-Language-Hearing Association, Miami Beach, FL.

Siegel, G. (1998). Stuttering: Theory, research, and therapy. In A. Cordes and R. J. Ingham (Eds.), *Treatment efficacy for stuttering: A search for empirical bases.* San Diego, CA: Singular.

Silverman, E., & Zimmer, C. (1979). Women who stutter: Personality and speech characteristics. *Journal of Speech and Hearing Research, 22,* 553–564.

Silverman, F. (1974). Disfluency behavior of elementary-school stutterers and nonstutterers. *Language, Speech and Hearing Services in Schools, 5,* 32–37.

Silverman, F. (1988). The monster study. *Journal of Fluency Disorders, 13,* 225–231.

Silverman, F. (2004). *Stuttering and other fluency disorders* (3rd ed.). Long Grove, IL: Waveland Press.

Silverman, F., & Silverman, E. (1971). Stuttering-like behavior in manual communication of the deaf. *Perceptual and Motor Skills, 33,* 45–46.

Silverman, F., & Williams, D. (1967). Loci of disfluencies in the speech of stutterers. *Perceptual and Motor Skills, 24,* 1085–1086.

Silverman, F., & Williams, D. (1971). The adaptation effect for six types of speech disfluency. *Journal. of Speech and Hearing Research., 14,* 525–530.

Skinner, B. (1953). *Science and human behavior.* New York, NY: Macmillan.

Smith, A. & Zelaznik, H. (2004). The development of functional synergies for speech motor coordination in childhood and adolescence. *Developmental Psychobiology, 45,* 22–33.

Smith, A. (1989). Neural drive to muscles in stuttering. *Journal of Speech and Hearing Research, 32,* 252–264.

Smith, A. (1990). Toward a comprehensive theory of stuttering: A commentary. *Journal of Speech and Hearing Disorders, 55,* 398–401.

Smith, A. (1999). Stuttering: A unified approach to a multifactorial, dynamic disorder. In N. B. Ratner and E. C. Healey (Eds.), *Stuttering research and practice: Bridging the gap.* Mahwah, NJ: Erlbaum.

Smith, A., & Kelly, E. (1997). Stuttering: A dynamic, multifactorial model. In R. Curlee & G. Siegel (Eds.), *Nature and treatment of stuttering: New directions* (2nd ed.). Boston, MA: Allyn & Bacon.

Smith, A., Denny, M., Shaffer, L., Kelly, E., & Hirano, M. (1996). Activity of intrinsic laryngeal muscles in fluent and disfluent speech. *Journal of Speech and Hearing Research, 39,* 329–348.

Smith, A., Sadagopan, N., Walsh, B., and Weber-Fox, C. (2010). Phonological complexity affects speech motor dynamics in adults who stutter. *Journal of Fluency Disorders, 35,* 1–18.

Smith, M. (1975). *When I say no, I feel guilty.* New York, NY: Dial Press.

Smits-Bandstra, S., & De Nil, L. (2009). Speech skill learning of persons who stutter and fluent speakers under single and dual task conditions. *Clinical Linguistics & Phonetics, 23,* 38–57.

Smits-Bandstra, S., De Nil, L. &, Rochon, E. (2006). The transition to increased automaticity during finger sequence learning in adult males who stutter. *Journal of Fluency Disorders, 31,* 22–42.

Smits-Bandstra, S., De Nil, L. F., & Saint-Cyr, J. (2006). Speech and nonspeech sequence skill learning in adults who stutter. *Journal of Fluency Disorders, 31,* 116–131.

Snidecor, J. (1947). Why the Indian does not stutter. *Quarterly Journal of Speech, 33,* 493–495.

Snow, D. (1994). Phrase-final syllable lengthening and intonation in early child speech. *Journal of Speech and Hearing Research, 37,* 831–840.

Soderberg, G. (1967). Linguistic factors in stuttering. *Journal of Speech and Hearing Research, 10,* 801–810.

Sommer, M., Koch, M., Paulus, W., Weiller, C., & Buchel, C. (2002). Disconnection of speech-relevant brain areas in persistent developmental stuttering. *Lancet, 360,* 380–383.

Song, L., Peng, D., Jin, Z., Yao, L., Ning, N., Guo, X., & Zhang, T. (2007). Gray matter abnormalities in developmental stuttering determined with voxel-based morphometry. *National Medical Journal of China, 87,* 2884–2888.

Sparks, G., Grant, D., Millay, K., Walker-Batson, D., & Hynan, L. (2002). The effect of fast speech rate on stuttering frequency during delayed auditory feedback. *Journal of Fluency Disorders, 27,* 187–201.

Spielberger, C., Gorsuch, R., Luschene, R., Vagg, P., & Jacobs, G. (1983). *Manual for the state-trait anxiety inventory.* Palo Alto, CA: Consulting Psychologists Press.

Ssikorski, J. (1891). *Uber das stottern* (About Stuttering). Berlin, Germany: Hirschwald.

St. Louis, K. (1986). *The atypical stutterer.* San Diego, CA: Academic Press.

St. Louis, K. (2007). A group therapy model for adults who stutter. Tenth International Stuttering Awareness Day On-Line Conference. http://www.mnsu.edu/comdis/isad10/ papers/therapy10/stlouis10.htm

St. Louis, K., Myers, F., Cassidy, L., Michael, A., Penrod, S., Litton, B., Olivera, J., & Brodsky, E. (1996). Efficacy of delayed auditory feedback for treating cluttering: Two case studies. *Journal of Fluency Disorders, 21,* 305–314.

St. Louis, K., & Schulte, K. (2011). Defining cluttering: The lowest common denominator. In D. Ward, & K. Scaler Scott (Eds.), *Cluttering: A handbook of research, intervention and education* (pp. 233–253). Hove, East Sussex, UK: Psychology Press.

St. Louis, K., Myers, F., Bakker, K., & Raphael, L. (2007). Understanding and treating cluttering. In E. Conture & R. Curlee (Eds.), *Stuttering and related disorders of fluency* (3rd ed., pp. 297–325. New York: Thieme.

St. Louis, K., Myers, F., Faragasso, K., Townsend, P., & Gallagher, A. (2004). Perceptual aspects of cluttered speech. *Journal of Fluency Disorders, 29,* 213–235.

St. Onge, K., & Calvert, J. (1964). Stuttering research. *Quarterly Journal of Speech, 50,* 159–165.

Stager, S., Calis, K., Grothe, D., Block, M., Berensen, N., Smith, P., et al. (2005). Treatment with medications affecting dopaminergic and serotonergic mechanisms: Effects on fluency and anxiety in persons who stutter. *Journal of Fluency Disorders, 30,* 319–335.

Stager, S., Jeffries, K., & Braun, A. (2003). Common features of fluency-evoking conditions studied in stuttering subjects and controls: An H(2)15O PET study. *Journal of Fluency Disorders, 28,* 319–335.

Starkweather, C. W. (1987). *Fluency and stuttering.* Englewood Cliffs, NJ: Prentice-Hall.

Starkweather, C. W., & Givens-Ackerman, J. (1997). *Stuttering.* Austin, TX: Pro-Ed.

Starkweather, C. W., & Gottwald, S. (1984, November). *Children's stuttering and parents' speech rate.* Paper presented at the convention of the American Speech-Language-Hearing Association, San Francisco, CA.

Starkweather, C. W., & Gottwald, S. (1990). The demands and capacities model: II. Clinical implications. *Journal of Fluency Disorders, 15,* 143–157.

Starkweather, C. W., Gottwald, S., & Halfond, M. (1990). *Stuttering prevention: A clinical method.* Englewood Cliffs, NJ: Prentice-Hall.

Starkweather, W. (1995). A simple theory of stuttering. *Journal of Fluency Disorders, 20,* 91–116.

Stephanson-Opsal, D., & Bernstein Ratner, N. (1988). Maternal speech rate modification and childhood stuttering. *Journal of Fluency Disorders, 13,* 49–56.

Stern, E. (1948). A preliminary study of bilingualism and stuttering in four Johannesburg schools. *Journal of Logopaedics, 1,* 15–25.

Stevens, T. (2005). Assertion training. Retrieved from http://www.csulb.edu/~tstevens/asser tion_training.htm

Still, A., & Griggs, S. (1979). Changes in the probability of stuttering following a stutter: A test of some recent models. *Journal of Speech and Hearing Research, 22,* 565–571.

Stocker, B., & Goldfarb, R. (1995). *The Stocker probe for fluency and language* (3rd ed.). Vero Beach, FL: Speech Bin.

Stromsta, C. (1965). A spectrographic study of disfluencies labeled as stuttering by parents. *De Therapia Vocis et Loquelae, 1,* 317–318.

Stuart, A., Kalinowski, J., Rastatter, M., Saltuklaroglu, T., & Dayalu, V. (2004). Investigations of the impact of altered auditory feedback in-the-ear devices on the speech of people who stutter: Initial fitting and 4-month follow-up. *International Journal of Language and Communication Disorders, 39,* 93–119.

Stuart, G., Treat, T., & Wade, W. (2000). Effectiveness of an empirically based treatment for panic disorder delivered in a service clinic setting. *Journal of Consulting and Clinical Psychology, 68*(3), 506–512.

Sturm, J., & Seery, C. (2007). Speech and articulatory rates of school-age children in conversation and narrative contexts. *Language, Speech, and Hearing Services in Schools, 38,* 47–59.

Subramanian, A., & Yairi, E. (2006). Identification of traits transmitted in association with stuttering. *Journal of Communication Disorders, 39,* 200–216.

Subramanian, A., Yairi, E., & Amir, O. (2003). Second formant transitions in fluent speech of persistent and recovered preschool children who stutter. *Journal of Communication Disorders, 36,* 59–75.

Suresh, R., Ambrose, N., Roe, C., Pluzhnikov, A., Wittke-Thompson, J., C-Y Ng, M., et al. (2006). New complexities in the genetics of stuttering: Significant sex-specific linkage signals. *American Journal of Human Genetics, 78,* 554–563.

Sutton, S., & Chase, R. (1961). White noise and stuttering. *Journal of Speech and Hearing Research, 4,* 72.

Tani, T., & Sakai, Y. (2011). Analysis of five cases with neurogenic stuttering following brain injury in the basal ganglia. *Journal of Fluency Disorders, 36,* 1–16.

Taylor, G. (1937). *An observational study of the nature of stuttering at its onset* (Unpublished master's thesis). State University of Iowa, Iowa City.

Taylor, I., & Taylor, M. (1967). Test of predictions from the conflict hypothesis of stuttering. *Journal of Abnormal Psychology, 72,* 431–433.

Temple, L. (2000). Second language learner speech production. *Studia Linguistica, 54,* 288–297.

Theys, C., Van Wieringen, A., & De Nil, L. (2008). A clinician survey of speech and non-speech characteristics of neurogenic stuttering. *Journal of Fluency Disorders, 33,* 1–23.

Thomas, C., & Howell, P. (2001). Assessing efficacy in stuttering treatment. *Journal of Fluency Disorder, 26,* 311–333.

Thordardottir, E., & Weismer, E. (2002). Content mazes and filled pauses in the spontaneous speech of school-aged children with specific language impairment. *Brain and Cognition, 48,* 587–592.

Throneburg, R. (1997). *Temporal characteristics of disfluencies as predictors of persistency and recovery in early childhood stuttering* (Unpublished doctoral dissertation). University of Illinois.

Throneburg, R., & Yairi, E. (1994). Temporal dynamics of repetitions during the early stage of childhood stuttering: An acoustic study. *Journal of Speech and Hearing Research, 37,* 1067–1075.

Throneburg, R., & Yairi, E. (2001). Durational, proportionate, and absolute frequency characteristics of disfluencies: A longitudinal study regarding persistence and recovery. *Journal of Speech, Language, and Hearing Research, 44,* 38–51.

Throneburg, R., Yairi, E., & Paden, E. (1994). The relation between phonologic difficulty and the occurrence of disfluencies in the early stage of stuttering. *Journal of Speech and Hearing Research, 37,* 504–509.

Till, J., Goldsmith, H., & Reich, A. (1981). Laryngeal and manual reaction times of stuttering and nonstuttering adults. *Journal of Speech and Hearing Research, 24,* 192–196.

Tomaiuoli, D., Del Gado, F., Falcone, P., Marchese, C., Pasqua, E., & Grazia Spinetti, M. (2007). The use of drama-therapy in the rehabilitation of stuttering patients. Retrieved from http://www.mnsu.edu/comdis/ isad10/papers/tomaiuoli10.html

Tomblin, B., Morris, H., & Spriestersbach, D. (2000). *Diagnosis in speech-language pathology* (2nd ed.). San Diego, CA: Singular.

Toomey, G., & Sidman, M. (1970). An experimental analogue of the anxiety-stuttering relationship. *Journal of Speech and Hearing Research, 13,* 122–129.

Tourville, J., Cai, S., & Guenther, F. (2013). Exploring auditory-motor interactions in normal and disordered speech. Proceedings of the 21st International Congress on Acoustics (ICA), Montréal, Canada. *POMA, 19,* 060180). doi:10.1121/1.4800684

Toyoda, B. (1959). A statistical report. *Clinical Paediatrica, 12,* 788.

Travis, L. (1931). *Speech Pathology.* New York, NY: Appleton-Century-Crofts.

Travis, L. (1934). Dissociation of the homologous muscle function in stuttering. *Archives of Neurological Psychiatry, 31,* 127–133.

Travis, L. (1957). The unspeakable feelings of people, with special reference to stuttering. In L. Travis (Ed.), *Handbook of speech pathology*(Chapter 29). New York, NY: Appleton-Century-Crofts.

Travis, L. (1978a). Neurophysiological dominance. *Journal of Speech and Hearing Disorders, 43,* 275–277.

Travis, L. (1978b). The cerebral dominance theory of stuttering, 1931–1978. *Journal of Speech and Hearing Disorders, 43,* 278–281.

Travis, L., & Knott, J. (1936). Brain potential from normal speakers and stutterers. *Journal of Psychology, 2,* 137–150.

Travis, L., & Malamud, W. (1937). Brain potential from normal subjects, stutterers, and schizophrenic patients. *American Journal of Psychiatry, 93,* 929–936.

Travis, L., Johnson, W., & Shover, J. (1937). The relation of bilingualism to stuttering. *Journal of Speech Disorders, 2,* 185–189.

Trotter, W. (1955). The severity of stuttering during successive readings of the same material. *Journal of Speech and Hearing Disorders, 20,* 17–25.

Trotter, W., & Lesch, M. (1967). Personal experience with a stutter-aid. *Journal of Speech and Hearing Disorders, 32,* 270–272.

Tsao, Y.-C., & Weismer, G. (1997). Inter-speaker variation in habitual speaking rate: Evidence of a neuromuscular component. *Journal of Speech, Language, and Hearing Research, 40,* 858–866.

Tucker, G. (1998). A global perspective on multilingualism and multilingual education. In J. Cenos & F. Genese (Eds.), *Beyond bilingualism: Multilingualism and multilingualism education* (pp. 3–15). Clevendon, UK: Multilingual Matters.

Tudor, M. (1939). An experimental study of the effect of evaluative labeling on speech fluency (Unpublished master's thesis). University of Iowa, Iowa City.

Tuthill, C. (1946). A quantitative study of extensional meaning with special refernce to stuttering. *Speech Monograph, 13,* 81–98.

Tyre, T., Maisto, S., & Companik, P. (1973). The use of systematic desensitization in the treatment of chronic stuttering behavior. *Journal of Speech and Hearing Disorders, 38,* 514–519.

Ujihira, A. (2011). Stuttering in Japanese. In P. Howell & J. Van Borsel (Eds.), *Multilingual Aspects of Fluency Disorders,* Bristol, UK: Multilingual Matters.

van Beijsterveldt, CEM, Felsenfeld, S., Boomsma, DI. (2010). Bivariate genetic analysis of stuttering and nonfluency in a large sample of 5-year-old-twins. *Journal of Speech, Language, and Hearing Research, 53,* 609–619.

Van Borsel, J., & Britto Pereira, M. (2005). Assessment of stuttering in a familiar versus an unfamiliar language. *Journal of Fluency Disorders, 30,* 109–124.

Van Borsel, J., & Taillieu, C. (2001). Neurogenic stuttering versus developmental stuttering: An observer judgment study. *Journal of Communication Disorders, 34,* 385–395.

Van Borsel, J., Beck, C., & Delanghe, J. (2003). *Stuttering and medication: A look at the symptoms.* Poster session presented at the Fourth World Congress on Fluency Disorders, Montreal, Quebec, Canada.

Van Borsel, J., Goethals, L., & Vanryckeghem, M. (2004). Disfluency in Tourette Syndrome: Observational study in three cases. *Folia Phoniatrica et Logopaedica, 56,* 358–366.

Van Borsel, J., Leahy, M., & Britto Pereira, M. (2008). Judging stuttering in an unfamiliar language: Importance of the closeness to the mother tongue. *Clinical Linguistics and Phonetics, 22,* 59–67.

Van Borsel, J., Maes, E., & Foulon, K. (2001). Stuttering and bilingualism: A review. *Journal of Fluency Disorders, 26,* 179–205.

Van Borsel, J., Moeyaert, E., Rosseel, M., Van Loo, E., & Van Renterghem, L. (2006). Prevalence of stuttering in regular and special school population in Belgium based on teacher perception. *Folia Phoniatrica et Logopaedica, 58,* 289–302.

Van Borsel, J., Van Lierde, K., Van Cauweberge, P., Guldemont, I., & Van Orshoven, M. (1998). Severe acquired stuttering following injury of the left supplementary motor region: A case report. *Journal of Fluency Disorders, 23,* 49–58.

van Lieshout, P., Peters, H., Starkweather, C. W., & Hulstijn, W. (1993). Physiological differences between stutterers and nonstutterers in perceptually fluent speech: EMG amplitude and duration. *Journal of Speech and Hearing Research, 36*(1), 55–63.

Van Riper, C. (1954). *Speech correction: Principles and methods* (3rd ed.). New York, NY: Prentice-Hall.

Van Riper, C. (1971). *The nature of stuttering.* Englewood Cliffs, NJ: Prentice-Hall.

Van Riper, C. (1973). *The treatment of stuttering.* Englewood Cliffs, NJ: Prentice-Hall.

Van Riper, C. (1975). The stutterer's clinician. In J. Eisenson (Ed.), *Stuttering, a second symposium* (pp. 453–492). New York, NY: Harper & Row.

Van Riper, C. (1982). *The nature of stuttering* (2nd ed.). Englewood Cliffs, NJ: Prentice-Hall.

Van Riper, C. (1992). Stuttering? *Journal of Fluency Disorders, 17,* 81–84.

Vanryckeghem, M., & Brutten, G. (1993). The Communication Attitude Test: A test–retest reliability investigation. *Journal of Fluency Disorders, 17,* 177–190.

Vanryckeghem, M., & Brutten, G. (1997). The speech associated attitude of children who do and do not stutter and the differential effect of age. *American Journal of Speech-Language Pathology, 6,* 67–73.

Vasic, N., & Wijnen, F. (2005). Stuttering as a monitoring deficit. In R. J.Hartsuiker, Y. Bastiaanse, A. Postma, and F. Wijnen (Eds.), *Phonological encoding and monitoring in normal and pathological speech.* (pp. 226–247). Hove, UK: Psychology Press.

Venkatagiri, H. (2009). What do people who stutter want: Fluency or freedom? *Journal of Speech, Language, and Hearing Research, 52,* 500–515.

Virginia Department of Education. (2003). English standards of learning. Retrieved from http://www.doe.virginia.gov/VDOE/Superintendent/Sols/home.shtml

Viswanath, N., Lee, H., & Chakraborty, R. (2004). Evidence for a major gene influence on persistent developmental stuttering. *Human Biology, 76,* 401–412.

Vlasova, N. (1962). Prevention and treatment of children's stuttering in U.S.S.R. *Ceskoslovenska Otolaryngologie, 11,* 30–32.

von Sarbo, A. (1901). Statistik der an Sprachstorungen Leidenden Schulkinder Ungarns, *Medizinisch-padagogische Monatsschrift fur die gesamte Sprachheilkundo* (Statistics from Hungarian school children afflicted by speech disorders), 65–89.

Wakaba, Y. (1983). Group play therapy for Japanese children who stutter. *Journal of Fluency Disorders, 8,* 93–118.

Wakaba, Y. (1999). *Research on remedial process of stuttering with early onset* (Unpublished doctoral dissertation). Nagoya University, Nagoya, Japan.

Walden, T., Frankel, C., Buhr, A., Johnson, K., Conture, E., & Karrass, J. (2012). Dual diathesis-stressor model of emotional and linguistic contributions to developmental stuttering. *Journal of Abnormal Child Psychology, 40,* 633–644.

Walker, V. (1988). Durational characteristics of young adults during speaking and reading tasks. *Folia Phoniatrica, 40,* 13–20.

Wallach, G., & Butler, K. (1994). *Language learning disabilities in school-age children and adolescents.* New York, NY: MacMillan.

Wallin, J. (1916). A census of speech defects. *School Sociology, 3,* 213.

Walnut, F. (1954). A personality inventory item analysis of individuals who stutter and individuals who have other handicaps. *Journal of Speech and Hearing Disorders, 19,* 220–227.

Walsh, B. & Smith, A. (2002). Articulatory movements in adolescents: Evidence for protracted development of speech motor control processes. *Journal of Speech, Language, and Hearing Research, 45,* 1119–1133.

Walsh, B. & Smith, A. (2013). Oral electromyography activation patterns for speech are similar in preschoolers who do and do not stutter. *Journal Speech Language and Hearing Research, 56,*1441–1454.

Waltzman, S., & Cohen, N. (2000). *Cochlear implants.* New York, NY: Thieme.

Ward, D. (2006). *Stuttering and cluttering: Frameworks for understanding and treatment.* New York, NY: Psychology Press.

Watkins, K. (2011). Developmental disorders of speech and language: From genes to brain structure and function. In O. Braddick, J. Atkinson, & G. M. Innocenti (Eds.), *Progress in brain research* (Vol. 189, pp. 225–238). Burlington, VT: Academic Press.

Watkins, K., Smith, S., Davis, S., & Howell, P. (2008). Structural and functional abnormalities of the motor system in developmental stuttering. *Brain, 131,* 50–59.

Watkins, R. (2005). Language abilities of young children who stutter. In E. Yairi & N. Ambrose (Eds.), *Early childhood stuttering* (pp. 235–253). Austin, TX: Pro-Ed.

Watkins, R., Yairi, E., & Ambrose, N. (1999). Early childhood stuttering: III. Initial status of expressive language abilities. *Journal of Speech, Language, and Hearing Research, 42,* 1125–1135.

Watkins, R., Yairi, E., Ambrose, N., Evans, K., DeThorne, L., & Mullen, C. (2000, November). *Grammatical influences on stuttering in young children.* Paper presented at the convention of the American Speech-Language-Hearing Association, Washington, DC.

Watkins, R., & Johnson, B. (2004). Language abilities in children who stutter: Toward improved research and clinical applications. *Language, Speech, and Hearing Services in Schools, 35,* 82–89.

Watkins, R., & Yairi, E. (1997). Language production abilities of children whose stuttering persisted or recovered. *Journal of Speech, Language, and Hearing Research, 40,* 385–399.

Watson, B., & Alfonso, P. (1987). Physiological bases of acoustic LRT in nonstutterers, mild stutterers, and severe stutterers. *Journal of Speech and Hearing Research, 30,* 434–447.

Watson, B., & Freeman, F. (1997). Brain imaging contributions. In R. Curlee & G. Siegel (Eds.), *Nature and treatment of stuttering: New directions* (2nd ed.). Boston, MA: Allyn & Bacon.

Watson, B., Byrd, C., & Carlo, E. (2011). Effects of length, complexity, and grammatical correctness of stuttering in Spanish-speaking preschool children. *American Journal of Speech-Language Pathology, 20,* 209–220.

Watson, B., Freeman, F., Devous, M., Chapman, S., Finitzo, T., & Pool, K. (1994). Linguistic performance and regional cerebral blood flow in persons who stutter. *Journal of Speech and Hearing Research, 37,* 1221–1228.

Watson, B., Pool, K., Devous, M., Freeman, F., & Finitzo, T. (1992). Brain blood flow related to acoustic laryngeal reaction time in adult developmental stutterers. *Journal of Speech and Hearing Research, 35,* 555–561.

Watson, J., & Anderson, R. (2001). Disfluencies of 2- and 3-year-old Spanish-speaking children from Puerto Rico. *Contemporary Issues in Communication Science and Disorders, 28,* 140–150.

Watson, J., Byrd, C., & Moore, B. (2011). Ethics in stuttering treatment in the schools: Issues and intersections. *Seminars in Speech and Language, 32*(4), 319–329.

Watzl, J. (1925). Statistische Erhebungen uber das Vorkommen von Sprachstorungen in den Weiner Schulen (Statistical investigation over the results from speech disorders in the Vienna Schools). In *Proceedings of the First International Congress of Logopedics and Phoniatrics,* Vienna, Austria.

Weber, C., & Smith, A. (1990). Autonomic correlates of stuttering and speech assessed in a range of experimental tasks. *Journal of Speech and Hearing Research, 33,* 690–706.

Weber-Fox, C., & Hampton, A. (2008). Stuttering and natural speech processing semantic and syntactic constraints on verbs. *Journal of Speech, Language, and Hearing Research, 51,* 1058–1071.

Webster, L. (1977). A clinical note on psychotherapy for stuttering. *Journal of Fluency Disorders, 2,* 253–255.

Webster, R. (1979). Empirical considerations regarding *stuttering* therapy. In H. Gregory (Ed.), *Controversies about stuttering therapy* (pp. 209–240). Baltimore, MD: University Park.

Webster, R. (1980a). *The precision fluency shaping program: Speech reconstruction for stutterers (Clinician's program guide).* Roanoke, VA: Communication Development.

Webster, R. (1980b). Evolution of target-based behavioral therapy for stuttering. *Journal of Fluency Disorders, 5,* 303–320.

Wendahl, R., & Cole, J. (1961). Identification of stuttering during relatively fluent speech. *Journal of Speech and Hearing Research, 4,* 281–186.

West, R. (1958). An agnostic's speculations about stuttering. In J. Eisenson (Ed.), *Stuttering: A symposium* (pp. 167–222). New York, NY: Harper & Row.

West, R., & Nusbaum, E. (1929). A motor test for dysphemia. *Quarterly Journal of Speech, 25,* 469–479.

West, R., Nelson, S., & Berry, M. (1939). The heredity of stuttering. *Quarterly Journal of Speech, 25,* 23–30.

West, T., & Bauer, P. J. (1999). Assumptions of infantile amnesia: Are there differences between early and later memories? *Memory, 7,* 257–278.

White House Conference Committee Report on Child Health and Protection. (1931). Section III, *Special Education: The Handicapped and the Gifted.* New York, NY: Appleton Century.

White, A., Kraus, C., Flom, J., Kestenbaum, L., Mitchell, J., Shah, K., et al. (2005). College students lack knowledge of standard drink volumes: Implications for definitions of risky drinking based on survey data. *Alcoholism, Clinical and Experimental Research, 29,* 631–638.

White, E. (2002). Normal disfluency in young adults across three speech tasks (Unpublished master's thesis). University of Wisconsin-Milwaukee.

Wikipedia (2007). Psychotherapy. Retrieved from http://en.wikipedia.org/wiki/Psychotherapy.

Williams, D. (1955). Masseter muscle action potentials in stuttered and nonstuttered speech. *Journal of Speech and Hearing Disorders, 20,* 242–261.

Williams, D. (1957). A point of view about stuttering. *Journal of Speech and Hearing Disorders, 22,* 390–397.

Williams, D. (1968). Stuttering therapy: An overview. In H. Gregory (Ed.), *Learning theory and stuttering therapy.* Evanston, IL: Northwestern University Press.

Williams, D. (1971). Stuttering therapy for children. In E. Travis (Ed.), *Handbook of speech pathology and audiology* (pp. 1073–1096). New York, NY: Appleton-Century-Crofts.

Williams, D., & Brutten, G. (1994). Physiologic and aerodynamic events prior to the speech of stutterers and nonstutterers. *Journal of Fluency Disorders, 19,* 83–111.

Williams, D., & Kent, R. (1958). Listener evaluations of speech interruptions. *Journal of Speech and Hearing Research, 1,* 124–131.

Williams, D., Melrose B., & Woods, L. (1969). The relationship between stuttering and academic achievement in children. *Journal of Communication Disorders, 2,* 87–98.

Williams, D., Silverman, F., & Kools, J. (1968). Disfluency behavior of elementary school stutterers and nonstutterers: The adaptation effect. *Journal of Speech and Hearing Research, 11,* 622–630.

Wingate, M. (1972). Deferring the adaptation effect. *Journal of Speech and Hearing Research, 15,* 547–550.

Wingate, M. (1964). A standard definition of stuttering. *Journal of Speech and Hearing Disorders, 29,* 484–489.

Wingate, M. (1975). Expectancy as basically a short-term process. *Journal of Speech and Hearing Research, 18,* 31–42.

Wingate, M. (1976). *Stuttering: Theory and treatment.* New York, NY: Wiley.

Wingate, M. (1979). The loci of stuttering: Grammar or prosody. *Journal of Communication Disorders, 12,* 283–290.

Wingate, M. (1984). Stutter events and linguistic stress. *Journal of Fluency Disorders, 9,* 295–300.

Wingate, M. (1986). Adaptation, consistency and beyond: I. Limitations and contradictions. *Journal of Fluency Disorders, 11,* 1–36.

Wingate, M. (1988). *The structure of stuttering.* New York, NY: Springer-Verlag.

Wingate, M. (1997). *Stuttering: A short history of a curious disorder.* Westport, CT: Bergin & Garvey.

Wingate, M. (2002). *The foundations of stuttering.* San Diego, CA: California Academic Press.

Winkelman, N. (1954). Chlorpromazine in the treatment of neuropsychiatric disorders. *Journalof the American Medical Association, 155,* 18–21.

Wischner, G. (1950). Stuttering behavior and learning: A preliminary theoretical formulation. *Journal of Speech and Hearing Disorders, 15,* 324–335.

Wittke-Thompson, J., Ambrose, N., Yairi, E., Roe, C., Ober, C., & Cox, N. (2007). Linkage analyses of stuttering in a founder population. *Journal of Fluency Disorder, 32,* 33–50.

Wolk, L., Blomgren, M., & Smith, A. (2000). The frequency of simultaneous disfluency and phonological errors in children: A preliminary investigation. *Journal of Fluency Disorders, 25*(4), 269–281.

Wolk, L., Edwards, M., & Conture, E. (1993). Coexistence of stuttering and disordered phonology in young children. *Journal of Speech and Hearing Research, 36,* 906–917.

Wolpe, J. (1958). *Psychotherapy by reciprocal inhibition.* Stanford, CA: Stanford University Press.

Wolpe, J. (1990). *The practice of behavior therapy.* Tarrytown, NY: Pergamon Press.

World Health Organization. (1977). *Manual of the International Statistical Classification of Diseases, Injuries, and Causes of Death* (Vol. 1, p. 202). Geneva: Author.

Wu, J., Maguire, G., Riley, G., Lee, A., Keator, D., Tang, C., et al. (1997). Increased dopamine activity associated with stuttering. *Neuroreport, 8,* 767–770.

Wyatt, G., & Herzan, H. (1962). Therapy with stuttering children and their mothers. *American Journal of Orthopsychiatry, 23,* 645–659.

Yairi, E. (1976). Effects of binaural and monaural noise on stuttering. *Journal of Auditory Research, 16,* 114–119.

Yairi, E. (1981). Disfluencies of normally speaking two-year-old children. *Journal of Speech and Hearing Research, 24,* 490–495

Yairi, E. (1983). The onset of stuttering in two- and three-year-old children: A preliminary report. *Journal of Speech and Hearing Disorders, 48,* 171–177.

Yairi, E. (1993). Epidemiology and other considerations in treatment efficacy research with preschool-age children who stutter. *Journal of Fluency Disorders, 18,* 197–220.

Yairi, E. (1997). Disfluency characteristics of early childhood stuttering. In R. F. Curlee & G. M. Siegel (Eds.), *Nature and treatment of stuttering: New directions* (2nd ed., pp. 49–78). Boston, MA: Allyn & Bacon.

Yairi, E. (2006). The Tudor study and Wendell Johnson. In Goldfarb R. (Ed.), *Ethics: A case study from fluency.* San Diego, CA: Plural Publishing.

Yairi, E. (2007). Subtyping stuttering I: A review. *Journal of Fluency Disorders, 32,* 165–196.

Yairi, E. (2013). Defining stuttering for research purposes. *Journal of Disfluency Disorders, 38,* 294–298.

Yairi, E., & Ambrose, N. (1992a). A longitudinal study of stuttering in children: A preliminary report. *Journal of Speech and Hearing Research, 35,* 755–760.

Yairi, E., & Ambrose, N. (1992b). Onset of stuttering in preschool children: Selected factors. *Journal of Speech and Hearing Research, 35,* 782–788.

Yairi, E., & Ambrose, N. (2005). *Early childhood stuttering.* Austin, TX: Pro-Ed.

Yairi, E., & Ambrose, N. (2013). Epidemiology of stuttering: 21st century advancements. *Journal of Fluency Disorders. 38*, 66–87.

Yairi, E., & Ambrose, N. (1999). Early childhood stuttering: I. Persistency and recovery rates. *Journal of Speech, Language, and Hearing Research, 42*, 1097–1112.

Yairi, E., & Carrico, D. (1992). Early childhood: Pediatricians' attitudes and practices. *American Journals of Speech-Language Pathology, 1*, 54–62.

Yairi, E., & Clifton, N. (1972). The disfluent speech behavior of preschool children, high school seniors, and geriatric persons. *Journal of Speech and Hearing Research, 15*, 714–719.

Yairi, E., & Lewis, B. (1984). Disfluencies at the onset of stuttering. *Journal of Speech and Hearing Research, 27*, 154–159.

Yairi, E., & Seery, C. (2011). *Stuttering: Foundations and Clinical Applications*. Boston: Pearson.

Yairi, E., & Williams, D. (1970). Speech clinicians' stereotypes of elementary school boys who stutter. *Journal of Communication Disorders, 3*, 161–170.

Yairi, E., Ambrose, N., & Cox, N. (1996). Genetics of stuttering: A critical review. *Journal of Speech and Hearing Research, 39*, 771–784.

Yairi, E., Ambrose, N., & Niermann, R. (1993). The early months of stuttering: A developmental study. *Journal of Speech and Hearing Research, 36*, 521–528.

Yairi, E., Ambrose, N., Paden, E. P., & Throneburg, R. N. (1996). Predictive factors of persistence and recovery: Pathways of childhood stuttering. *Journal of Communication Disorders, 29*, 51–77.

Yairi, E., Gintautas, J., & Avent, J. (1981). Disfluent speech associated with brain damage. *Brain and Language, 14*, 49–56.

Yaruss, J. S. (1997a). Clinical implications of situational variability in preschool children who stutter. *Journal of Fluency Disorders, 22*, 187–203.

Yaruss, J. S. (1997b). Utterance timing and childhood stuttering. *Journal of Fluency Disorders, 22*, 263–286.

Yaruss, J. S. (2000). Converting between word and syllable counts in children's conversational speech samples. *Journal of Fluency Disorders, 25*, 305–316.

Yaruss, J. S., & Conture, E. (1993). F2 transitions during sound/syllable repetitions of children who stutter and predictions of stuttering chronicity. *Journal of Speech and Hearing Research, 36*, 883–896.

Yaruss, J. S., & Conture, E. (1996). Stuttering and phonological disorders in children: Examination of the Covert Repair Hypothesis. *Journal of Speech and Hearing Research, 39, ,* 349–364.

Yaruss, J. S., & Quesal, R. (2006). Overall Assessment of the Speaker's Experience of Stuttering (OASES): Documenting multiple outcomes in stuttering treatment. *Journal of Fluency Disorders, 31*, 90–115.

Yaruss, J. S., LaSalle, L., & Conture, E. (1998). Evaluating young children who stutter: Diagnostic data. *American Journal of Speech and Language Pathology, 7*(4), 62–76.

Yaruss, J. S., Quesal, R., Reeves, L., Molt, L., Kluetz, B., Caruso, A., et al. (2002). Speech treatment and support group experiences of people who participate in the National Stuttering Association. *Journal of Fluency Disorders, 2*, 115–134.

Young, E., & Hawk, S. (1955). *Moto-kinesthetic speech training*. Stanford, CA: Stanford University.

Young, M. (1961). Predicting ratings of severity of stuttering. *Journal of Speech and Hearing Disorders, Monograph Supplement, 7*, 31–54.

Young, M. (1984). Identification of stuttering and stutterers. In R. Curlee & W. Perkins (Eds.), *Nature and treatment of stuttering: New directions* (pp. 13–30). San Diego, CA: College-Hill.

Young, M. (1985). Increasing the frequency of stuttering. *Journal of Speech and Hearing Research, 28*, 282–293.

Weiss, D. (1967). Cluttering. *Folia Phoniatrica, 19*, 233–263.

Zebrowski, P. (1994). Duration of sound prolongation and sound/syllable repetition in children who stutter. *Journal of Speech and Hearing Research, 37*, 254–263.

Zebrowski, P., & Conture, E. (1989). Judgment of disfluency by mothers of stuttering and normally fluent children. *Journal of Speech and Hearing Research, 32*, 625–634.

Zebrowski, P., Weiss, A., Savelkoul, E., & Hammer, C. (1996). The effect of maternal rate reduction on the stuttering, speech rates and linguistic productions of children who stutter: Evidence from individual dyads. *Clinical Linguistics and Phonetics, 10*, 189–206.

Zimmerman, G., & Hanley, J. (1983). A cinefluorographic investigation of repeated fluent productions of stutterers in an adaptation procedure. *Journal of Speech and Hearing Research, 26*, 35–42.

Zimmerman, I., Steiner, V., & Pond, R. (1979). *Preschool Language Scale*. San Antonio, TX: Harcourt Brace Jovanovich.

Zimmermann, G. (1980a). Articulatory dynamics of fluent utterances of stutterers and nonstutterers. *Journal of Speech and Hearing Research, 23*, 95–107.

Zimmermann, G. (1980b). Articulatory behaviors associated with stuttering. *Journal of Speech and Hearing Research, 23*, 108–121.

Zimmermann, G. (1980c). Stuttering: A disorder of movement, *Journal of Speech and Hearing Research, 23*, 122–136.

Zimmermann, G., Liljebald, S., Frank, A., & Cleeland, C. (1983). The Indians have many terms for it: Stuttering among the Bannoch-Shoshoni. *Journal of Speech & Hearing Research, 26*, 315–318.

Index